Foreword

This report is the fourth National Survey of Morbidity in General Practice. It took place in 1991-92. It presents statistics on the reasons as perceived by the doctor or practice nurse for which people consult in general practice. These are linked with the socio-economic characteristics of each patient providing a comparison of the incidence and prevalence of disease among different groups in the community.

The study results from collaboration between the Office of Population Censuses and Surveys, the Royal College of General Practitioners and the Department of Health. It would not have been possible without the voluntary co-operation and painstaking work of many doctors and their practice staff throughout the country.

Thanks are also due to colleagues at the Department of Health for their advice and guidance. The staff of the Royal College of General Practitioners Research Unit in Birmingham gave continuous and unstinted support throughout the project. Many at the Office of Population Censuses and Surveys and elsewhere contributed their expertise to the collection, analysis and interpretation of the data and in the collation of this report. In particular we are indebited to Professor Shah Ebrahim and Professor Michael Pringle for their invaluable and constructive comments during the preparation of the text.

The study was funded by the Department of Health.

KAREN DUNNELL
Head of Health Statistics, OPCS

Contents

List of text tables

Chapter 3

Chapter 4

Chapter 5

Chapter 6

Acknowledgements

We are pleased to acknowledge the contribution made by participating practices, recognising that involvement in the study required considerable commitment from all members of the practice teams.

The practices are identified by the principal general practitioners listed below.

R J Abbatt	Denton
A S Abdul Karim	Peterborough
R K Aggarwal	Pontefract
P Anand	Thamesmead
J E Anderson	Burnhope
H Arshi	Plymouth
M W Ashmore	Leamington Spa
M G Askew	Gosport
M Aylett	Wooler
S P Babbington	St Neots
K N Badiani	Loughborough
J Bailey	Eynsham
D R Bainbridge	East Grinstead
V K Bajpal	Thamesmead
D J Barford	Birmingham
R Baxter	Corby
D Beckitt	Warlingham
A Benn	Birmingham
R J Bennett	South Shields
S Benstead	Bishop Auckland
N C Beriwal	Ashton-under-Lyne
W D Bevington	Guildford
K S Bhogal	Birmingham
J P D Blacker	Bromsgrove
P A Booth	Crewe
N Booth	Prudhoe
P Bowron	Bishop Auckland
P Bradley	Chester
C Bradshaw	South Shields
I H Bridges	Ware
D Brown	Corby
R N Bryant	Newton Abbott
S Burcombe	Thamesmead
M Burke	Wirral
K Bush	Wirral
D A Cadman	Cardiff
R J Calderhead	Crewe
F S Campbell	Leamington Spa
A M E T Carlyon	Guildford
K Carroll	Beckenham
A Carswell	Bristol
G A Carter	Whalley
A C Chadha	Aldershot
R Chandler	Bristol
H J M Charles	Cardiff
B Christopher	East Grinstead
J H Clarke	East Grinstead
F D Clayton	Wirral
C E H Coate	Derby
P P Coffey	Eynsham
T D Coleman	Walsall
R J Collis	Bristol
A R Colman	Bristol
D Cooke	Derby
J Cooper	Crewe
H L Courtenay	South Shields
A V Cowan	Bromsgrove
M S Cranney	Liverpool
S Craven	Swansea
D L Crombie	Birmingham
N E Curt	Dunstable
D Darvill	Bristol
B C Dawe	Bingley
A G Doherty	Crewe
M Duffy	Liverpool
A R Dunn	Newton Abbott
D Dwyer	Plymouth
P A Dykes	Bromsgrove
A H Eaton	Hartlepool
M G Edward	Birmingham
P H Edwards	Cardiff
S Edwards	Stockport
K B Edwards	Wirral
D J Egan	Stowmarket
J Eggleston	South Shields
A E Eldred	Prudhoe
P Ellis	Kirkby
J M English	Hayes
H W Evans	Eynsham
C M V Evans	Guildford
K J Evans	Loughborough
D A Evans	Gosport
D P Feeney	Stocksfield
S P Felton	Birmingham
J D S Fielder	Stowmarket
S M Findlay	Bishop Auckland
D M Fleming	Birmingham
V Foulger	East Grinstead
P A Fox	Pontefract
P Freeman	Leamington Spa
R A Freeman	Whalley
S H Garside	Oldham
A M Gibbons	Oldham
S H Gibson	Ware
I Gilchrist	Bishop's Stortford
R W Graham	Stocksfield
M J Green	Leamington Spa
R E Grundy	Stowmarket
M G Hackman	Huntingdon
T D Hall	Loughborough
E A Hall	Loughborough
E Hamnett	Birmingham

M Haque	Ashton-under-Lyne
S C Harris	Ware
M Harrison	Beckenham
C R Harry	Swansea
S Hart	Plymouth
G H Haslam	Bingley
J G Heath	Kirkby
T Heller	Sheffield
M C N Henchy	Peterborough
D B V Hewitt	Derby
J H W Hill	Weedon
K E Hill	Weedon
A R Holmes	Hartlepool
A P Hoodbhoy	Manningtree
D Howton	Corby
P G Hulse	Dunstable
E Hunt	Peterborough
B J Hyde	Eynsham
C Hyland	Warrington
M J Jameson	St Albans
A P K John	Loughborough
M A Johnson	Oldham
N K Jones	South Shields
G O Jones	Swansea
C F M Jones	Aberystwyth
R R Jones	Swansea
D Kinch	Birmingham
S P Kumaraswamy	Warrington
R C Lambert	Bingley
A T Law	Derby
M Lee	Newton Abbott
N E Leech	Minehead
V Letchumanan	Warrington
H Levycky	Wirral
H Lindsey	Cardiff
I G Lloyd	Bishop Auckland
S de Lusignan	Guildford
S MacDonald	Chester
M D MacLeod	Aldershot
J P Maddock	Dunstable
P Main	Bristol
J Main	Bristol
N Masters	Thamesmead
W Maxwell	Stockport
S R Mayhew	St Neots
A McCullagh	Thamesmead
P F McGowan	Hartlepool
G S McGregor	Bishop Auckland
D C McNutt	Gosport
M K Mehta	Aldershot
J Mellor	Corby
N Merwaha	Ware
P A Milstein	Thamesmead
M J Moor	St Neots
G F Morgan	Cardiff
A J Muchall	South Shields
V Murthy	Peterborough
S Navamani	Peterborough
M R Newby	St Neots
O B O'Toole	Dunstable
P Orton	Bishops Stortford
K Orton	Bishops Stortford
P Owens	Chester
G R Parry	Liverpool
R Paterson	Aldershot
V Patton	Birmingham
C A Pearson	Aldershot
K S Penry	Aberystwyth
J Perks	Plymouth
D J M Peterson	Eynsham
A J C Pickering	Denton
B R Pike	Bishop Auckland
D J Poll	Derby
B J Porter	Warrington
G M Powell	East Grinstead
P M Prasad	Swansea
R Pratt	Sheffield
J Pratt	Sheffield
A Priest	Pontefract
S J Quilliam	Prudhoe
Z R T Qureshi	Ashton-under-Lyne
A L Raeburn	Crewe
G R D Ralston	Birmingham
L Ratnam	Birmingham
R M Reid	Gosport
B A Roberts	Aberystwyth
W J Roberts	Aberystwyth
T C Ross	Minehead
A M Ross	Birmingham
N Sahatheva-Rajan	Pontefract
K Santos	Cardiff
S Sathiyeseelan	Warrington
K Scott	Beckenham
P J Searle	St Neots
C M E Shire	Stocksfield
M Simpson	Birmingham
J R Simpson	Eynsham
T Sinclair	Oldham
G P Singh	Leeds
G Singh	Loughborough
P J B Slade	Minehead
R N Smith	Birmingham
B Smith	Whalley
G D Smith	Warrington
R Smith	Sheffield
C J Southgate	Manningtree
D Stanley	Bristol
P B O Stephenson	Eynsham
P Stubbs	Bristol
P F Stuckey	Birmingham
D Swithinbank	Bristol
B M Thomas	Hayes
H G Thomas	Minehead
T H R Thompson	Cardiff
V A Todd	Thamesmead
C Trounce	Plymouth
V S Tudor	Birmingham
W Van Marle	Birmingham
S C Vaughan Jones	Guildford
J J Vevers	East Grinstead
J C Vickers	Crewe
S Wadsworth	Corby
P Walker	Hitchin
P A Wells	Ashton-under-Lyne

R Wells	Beckenham	J F Wilmot	Leamington Spa
R Welton	Oldham	I S Wilson	Warrington
R N Whittaker	Corby	R Winterburn	Kirkby
I D Whyte	Whalley	K C Wishart	Huntingdon
P J Wilczynski	Corby	K K Wlodarczyk	Whalley
J E A Williams	Crewe	J M Wright	Oldham
I Williams	Huntingdon	R Wynne	Bromsgrove
P H Williams	St Neots	J Youens	Peterborough
S Williams	Wirral	J M S Young	Ware

Notes to tables

Rates have been rounded and may not sum to totals.

'0' denotes less than 0.5

'-' denotes none.

Italic type in standardised ratio tables denotes a ratio based on twenty or fewer events.

Summary and conclusions

Introduction

This report covers the fourth study of morbidity in England and Wales. It was commissioned by the Department of Health (DH) and carried out between September 1991 and August 1992 under the guidance of a Project Board representing DH, the Royal College of General Practitioners (RCGP) and the Office of Population Censuses and Surveys (OPCS).

It was recognised in the 1950s that the reasons why people consult their GPs could provide useful indicators of the general health of the nation. Prevalence trends in sickness, including the increasing or decreasing incidence of particular conditions, could help to inform health service practitioners and planners. The first study (NMS1) took place in 1955-6, and further studies took place in 1970-6 (NMS2) and 1981-2 (MSGP3) (see chapter 1). As the result of increased computerisation in general practice and the collection of socio-economic data within the practices, the results from this study are available earlier than previous studies.

Objectives of this study

The objectives of this study included:

- to examine the pattern of disease seen by GPs, by the age, sex and socio-economic status of the patient and to give an indication of the care provided;

- to provide information to those planning health care resources;

- to compare the results of this study with those of the earlier studies.

Scope of the study

The study covered a one per cent sample of the population of England and Wales (502,493 patients, 468,042 person years at risk). These people were on the NHS lists of 60 practices which volunteered to take part. All the health regions were represented and the practices varied in size between 1,900 and 16,500 patients (for further details, see chapter 1).

The sample was compared with the 1991 Census. It was representative of the population of England and Wales in terms of age, sex, marital status, tenure of housing, economic position, occupation and whether living in an urban or rural area. There were small differences by social class (as defined by occupation) and some under-representation of minority ethnic groups and those living alone. The proportion who smoked was similar to that recorded by the General Household Survey.

An evaluation exercise carried out at the end of the study compared the study records with lists of patients who either attended a surgery, were visited at home or were referred to outpatients. This suggested that 96 per cent of contacts with a doctor in the surgery and 95 per cent in patients' homes were reported. However, only an estimated 61 per cent of referrals to outpatient departments were reported; this varied between 50 per cent by practices using software from one company to 88 per cent by those supplied by another. Comparison with copies of manual notes for a sample of patients suggested that 93 per cent of diagnoses were correctly reported (see chapter 1).

Methods used

The first three morbidity surveys were based on GPs keeping manual records of patients' details and diagnoses which were sent to OPCS for processing. For the 1991-2 study the process was streamlined. Using specially designed software, data were entered on computers in the practices and transferred to OPCS on disks. Socio-economic information was collected by interviewers for about 83 per cent of patients on practice lists, and transferred in the same format (chapter 1 explains the methods used in more detail).

Characteristics of the practices taking part

The practices which took part were different in some ways from the average of all practices in England and Wales. The ones in the study had a larger average number of patients on their lists, 7,700 compared with 5,200, and they employed more assistants and trainee doctors. Principal doctors in the study practices were, on average, younger than those in all practices with 80 per cent being aged under 50 compared with 72 per cent overall. The nurse/patient ratio was similar in each group.

Main results from the study

Chapter 2 describes the main results from the study. During the year 78 per cent of patients consulted at least once, an increase from 71 per cent in the 1981-2 study. Based on the chapters in the International Classification of Diseases (ICD), the proportion who consulted increased for every ICD disease chapter except mental disorders and symptoms, signs and ill-defined conditions. The highest proportion consulted for respiratory diseases (31 per cent), followed by diseases of the nervous system and sense organs (17 per cent), musculoskeletal disorders and diseases of the skin (15 per cent each) (see Fig 2.2).

Between the ages of 10 and 70 years the overall proportion of females who consulted exceeded that of males (Fig 2.1). This difference was most evident in the ICD chapters covering genitourinary conditions and diseases of the blood and blood-forming organs and, to a smaller degree, mental disorders, respiratory diseases, symptoms, signs and ill-defined conditions, and for reasons in the Supplementary Classification. A higher proportion of women between 15 and 64 consulted than men in this age-group for reasons classified as minor or intermediate (Figs 2.5 and 2.6). However, in all age-groups the rates for illnesses classified as serious were similar for men and women (Fig 2.4).

Males aged between 16 and 64 and living in the North or in the Midlands & Wales were more likely to consult than those living in the South of England. This difference did not apply to women in those regions. In particular, a higher proportion of men in the North than in the South consulted with serious illness.

Consulting rates were highest for children aged under five years, many of whom were born during the year of the study (Fig 2.1). They were more likely to consult than people in any other age-group for respiratory conditions, diseases of the nervous system and sense organs, largely accounted for by infections of the ear, infectious and parasitic diseases and diseases of the skin.

Among the elderly, a higher proportion consulted the doctor or practice nurse for circulatory disorders and respiratory diseases than for any other groups of illnesses, although many consulted for reasons coded in the Supplementary Classification, particularly for immunisation against influenza and tetanus and for general medical examinations. The proportion of people who consulted for neoplasms and circulatory, digestive and musculoskeletal disorders increased with age.

There were over 1.3m contacts recorded with study doctors during the year: an average of 3.8 contacts by each patient who consulted, equivalent to 2.9 by each person on the practice registers. Each diagnosis recorded during a contact was called a consultation. There were over 1.6m consultations: an average of 1.2 consultations during each contact. Eighty-nine per cent of contacts with a doctor took place in the surgery, 10 per cent in the patient's home and the remainder elsewhere. The average number of consultations per person increased by 2 per cent compared with the 1981-2 study.

A synopsis of the findings and some comparisons with the findings of MSGP3 follows under the ICD chapter headings.

Infectious and parasitic diseases

Of the 14 per cent of people diagnosed with diseases in this group, a high proportion consulted for thrush, viral warts, intestinal infections and ringworm. Chickenpox was the most common childhood infection included in this chapter. Compared with the 1981-2 study the proportion of people who consulted for herpes simplex, ringworm, thrush, viral warts and scabies increased.

Malignant neoplasms

The highest proportion who consulted for cancer among women was of the breast and of the prostate among men.

Relatively high rates were also shown for cancer of the trachea, bronchus and lung, and of the skin other than melanomas. These rates include people who consulted for the whole duration of illness from diagnosis through treatment to appropriate aftercare. The proportion of people with malignant neoplasms increased in the decade since the last study as, to a greater extent, did that for benign neoplasms. The proportion who consulted for cancer of the lung declined over this period, except among people aged 75 and over, while the prevalence of cancer of the female breast increased although, except among the very old, the incidence of new cases declined.

Endocrine, nutritional and metabolic diseases

Diabetes was the most common condition in this chapter. One per cent of the sample consulted for this. Although the rate of newly-diagnosed cases of diabetes declined since 1981-2, the proportion of people with diabetes increased over this period. A high proportion consulted for obesity, acquired hypothyroidism and gout. Since 1981-2 the consulting rate for thyrotoxicosis declined while that for acquired hypothyroidism increased. A higher proportion consulted for gout in 1991-2 than in 1981-2.

Diseases of the blood and blood-forming organs

Less than one per cent consulted for a disease in this chapter with a high proportion of those, mainly women, having iron and other deficiency anaemias. There was a small increase in the proportion of people consulting for diseases in this group: from 78 per 10,000 in 1981-2 to 97 in 1991-2.

Mental disorders

Over 7 per cent consulted with a condition in this chapter: the highest rates being for neurotic and depressive disorders and for affective psychotic conditions. This is the only ICD chapter of specific diseases which showed an overall decline since 1981-2. Rates were higher among women than men. While there was an increase for serious mental problems, mainly the affective psychoses, there was a decrease for conditions categorised as intermediate or trivial, mainly depressive disorders and anxiety states.

Diseases of the nervous system and sense organs

Seventeen per cent of patients were diagnosed with diseases in this chapter. A high proportion consulted for otitis media and external ear problems, conjunctivitis and migraine. Between 1981-2 and 1991-2 the rates for migraine, vertiginous syndromes, conjunctivitis, glaucoma and cataract all increased.

Diseases of the circulatory system

Nine per cent of the population consulted for a circulatory problem: this was an increase of nearly 10 per cent over the 1981-2 findings. Consulting rates were highest for essential hypertension and angina pectoris which, together with cerebrovascular disease, showed an increase over the 1981-2 rates. Consulting rates for haemorrhoids and varicose veins were also relatively high. The rate for acute myocardial infarction decreased since 1981-2.

Respiratory diseases

More than 30 per cent of the sample consulted for a respiratory illness. The majority were for upper respiratory tract infections, but there was also a high proportion for acute bronchitis and bronchiolitis, asthma, allergic rhinitis and influenza. In comparison with the 1981-2 study there was an increase of 14 per cent in the proportion of those who consulted for a respiratory disease. In particular, a higher proportion consulted for asthma although the number of new asthmatics did not change. There was also an increase in acute bronchitis, but a decline in chronic bronchitis.

Diseases of the digestive system

Nine per cent of the sample population consulted for diseases in this chapter with a high proportion having dyspepsia, oesophagitis, diaphragmatic hernias, gastritis and duodenitis. A smaller proportion consulted for constipation and irritable bowel syndrome. Compared with 1981-2 there were higher patient consulting rates for oesophagitis, gastritis, duodenitis and dyspepsia, while rates for diagnosed peptic ulcers were unchanged.

Diseases of the genito-urinary system

Eleven per cent of patients consulted at least once for diseases in this chapter, a 31 per cent increase in the proportion consulting in 1981-2. The increase was largely due to urinary tract infections which, with cystitis, were the most frequent reasons for patients to consult for diseases of the genitourinary system. The majority who consulted were women. Also among women a relatively high proportion consulted for inflammatory diseases of the cervix, vagina and vulva, for non-malignant diseases of the breast and for problems with menstruation and menopausal and postmenopausal disorders, all of which showed an increase over 1981-2.

Diseases of the skin

Fifteen per cent consulted for a disease of the skin, mainly for eczema, acne, psoriasis, impetigo and other infections. An increase of 24 per cent in the proportion of patients consulting for diseases in this chapter since 1981-2 is largely due to the fact that the rate for eczema more than doubled, while that for acne also increased.

Diseases of the musculoskeletal system

Fifteen per cent consulted for a disease in this chapter. The highest proportion related to disorders of the back, in particular unspecified backache, followed by osteoarthritis and unspecified pains in the joints, and specified problems with joints. Since 1981-2 the proportion who consulted for osteoarthritis and osteoporosis increased, while rates for rheumatoid arthritis declined.

Injury and poisoning

Fourteen per cent of the sample consulted for these reasons, an increase from 11 per cent in 1981-2. Rates were higher for men than women among young adults, but higher for women among older people. The majority had sprains and superficial injuries.

Socio-economic and geographic variations

Chapter 4 considers variations in the proportions of people who consulted according to single socio-economic and geographic characteristics. The main findings are that for all diseases and conditions men aged 16-64 living in the North of England are more likely to consult than those in the Midlands & Wales or the South. Other groups more likely to consult are those in council housing or other rented accommodation, widowed or divorced people, particularly if they are not cohabiting, those with children under five years of age, men living alone, men in Social Classes IV and V, the unemployed and long term sick, men looking after the home/family and people aged 16-64 years who smoke. These findings do not, however, take account of the effect individual socio-economic characteristics may have on each other. For example, council house tenants may be more likely to be in Social Classes 1V and V and to smoke, and it may be that their morbidity is affected more by those two factors than the fact that they are council house tenants.

Chapter 5 describes a technique, multi-variate analysis, which is designed to estimate the effect of one of the characteristics of those consulting independent of the patient's other characteristics. The likelihood of a patient consulting, for example by tenure of housing, was compared with the likelihood of a patient in a selected reference group (in this case those living in owner-occupied premises), after all other socio-economic factors have been accounted for.

The results show that people in Social Classes IV and V are more likely to consult than those in classes I and II, although the difference is diminished if all other socio-economic factors are taken into account. Similarly, people living in council housing or other rented accommodation are more likely to consult for serious illnesses and for mental and respiratory disorders than owner occupiers. Permanently sick and unemployed people are more likely to consult than those in work. A higher proportion of people in the Indian subcontinent ethnic groups consult than white people, particularly for serious conditions. Widowed, separated and divorced people are more likely to consult then those who are single or married. Female smokers aged 16-44 are more likely to consult than non-smokers, but smokers in older age-groups are less likely. People living in rural areas are less likely to consult than those in towns.

Morbidity levels for small areas

Information about morbidity is usually only available at national level but there is a need for information for small areas, for example, for FHSAs, DHAs and fundholding GPs. Local figures can be estimated from national ones using age/sex specific data, but this procedure does not take into account the effect of more than one socio-economic factor on the likelihood of a person consulting. Chapter 6 describes how the results obtained from the analysis in chapter 5 were applied to a 2 per cent sample of individual census records from the 1991 Census to estimate the numbers, by age and sex, consulting for small areas. The analysis covered the percentage consulting in the 16-44 age-group for serious illness - to illustrate a method of estimating consultation rates at local level. MSGP4 provides a wide variety of information which could be used to compile further estimates. OPCS is producing a range of synthetic estimates for other categories described in chapter 5 and these will be made available on floppy disk.

Conclusion

This study presents the best data currently available on the level and detail of morbidity seen in general practice. Combination with socio-economic information about all patients, irrespective of whether they consulted, helps to identify those most at risk and provides a basis for estimat-ing expected local morbidity levels. Vulnerable groups in the population can be targeted with health education and health care facilities. The results can be used for health care planning and compared with any local studies to identify unexpected differences. Trends for individual conditions may reflect changes in the incidence or prevalence of disease, or changes in the number of cases seen in general practice as a result of developments in the way health care is delivered.

Further tables and datasets available are listed in appendices E and F. We hope they will be widely used.

1 Background and methods

1.1 Background

The need for information about the illnesses for which patients attend their general practitioners was recognised by Logan in the 1950s. With Cushion and with the collaboration of the newly-founded College of General Practitioners he set up the first national study of morbidity in general practice in 1955-56.[1] In all, 171 principal doctors in 106 practices took part, covering a population of 380,000 people. Details of each consultation by a patient with his doctor were recorded on a patient-orientated card which included the patient's name, date of birth or age, sex, and, for 280,000 patients, occupation. These cards were sent to the General Register Office (now the Office of Population Censuses and Surveys) at the end of the study for processing and analysis.

The second and third studies in 1970-76[2-3-4] and 1981-82[5-6] were based on morbidity-orientated records in what was called the 'E-book', or episode book. This contained a page for each diagnosis and space for recording each attendance for each patient consulting for that condition. At the end of the studies the E-books were sent to the Office of Population Censuses and Surveys (OPCS) for processing. Information from the E-books was linked at OPCS with the age/sex register from each practice and with each person's 1971 or 1981 census form. These linkages created records for the total population included in the study, complete with socio-economic data for each patient. Fifty-three practices took part in the 1970-71 study, covering a population of 292,247 people. This study was extended by 43 of the practices for a further year (1971-72) and 24 practices representing 123,000 patients continued collecting morbidity data for a further four years (1972-76). Linkage with census data was achieved for 78 per cent of patients in the 1971-72 study. In the 1981-82 study, 48 practices participated, covering a population of 332,270 people. Of these, an attempt to link each patient with his census form to obtain socio-economic data was made for patients on the register of 25 practices. Linkage was achieved for 140,049 (80 per cent) of these patients, equivalent to 133,350 person years at risk after accounting for births, deaths and migration during the study year.

Linking morbidity data with the age/sex register and census forms in the second and third studies proved to be time-consuming because of the difficulty in correctly identifying census records for each individual patient. Incompatible addresses on practice records and on census forms and people who had moved by the date of the census meant that socio-economic information on 34,267 patients registered with the 25 practices in the third study could not be found.

For these reasons, a different method of obtaining socio-economic data was used for the 1991-92 study (MSGP4).

This was based on direct interviews and proved to be quicker and more successful. The direct interview approach was successfully tested for feasibility and acceptability by both doctors and patients for two weeks in each of four practices, two weeks in 1986 when socio-economic data alone were collected by two practices, and two weeks in 1987 when both morbidity and socio-economic data were recorded by the other two practices.

1.2 Introduction

Data collection for the fourth study (MSGP4) took place between 1 September 1991 and 31 August 1992. All doctors and practice-employed nurses in 60 practices in England and Wales recorded each face-to-face contact with patients on the NHS age/sex register (ASR). Telephone contacts and private or temporary patients were excluded. The ASRs provided the basis for calculating the denominator which, to allow for people who were only present for part of the study year, was converted to person years at risk. There were 502,493 patients on the ASRs at some time during the study year, representing 468,042 person years at risk.

Doctors and nurses recorded diagnoses, where the patient was seen and whether and to which agency the patient was referred. A specially trained interviewer in each practice collected socio-economic data about each patient on the ASR at any time during the study year. Collection of socio-economic data was successfully achieved for 83 per cent of the 502,493 patients. Comparison of the socio-economic characteristics of this population with the population of England and Wales enumerated by the 1991 census suggests that the population covered by the study was generally representative of the national population (see section 1.5).

This study differed from previous studies carried out by the Royal College of General Practitioners (RCGP) and OPCS in four ways. First, all morbidity data were entered on computers in the practices and sent to OPCS on disks instead of manual records. Second, socio-economic data were collected and entered on computers by interviewers in the practices, instead of being obtained from census forms. Third, diagnostic Read codes were used (see page 13). Fourth, except where a specific Read code was entered in the computer, the appropriate code for the diagnostic term entered was automatically assigned by the software in the practices.

The study was planned, guided and monitored by a Project Board. The Department of Health, the RCGP and OPCS were represented on the Board. The study was commissioned by the Department of Health. Ethical approval was obtained from the British Medical Association Ethical Committee.

1

Objectives of the study

The objectives of the study were as follows:

1. To examine the pattern of disease in the community as presented to general practice, including diagnoses and an indication of the severity and persistence of disease by age and sex;

2. To compare the results from the present study with the three earlier studies;

3. To provide an indication of the care given to patients in general practice, through statistics on contacts in the surgery and at home, and on referrals to other agencies;

4. To compare the demographic and socio-economic structure of the sampled population with that of the 1991 census in England and Wales on a national and regional basis;

5. To relate the pattern of disease observed to the socio-economic characteristics of the population;

6. To provide health authorities with information designed to assist in planning health care resources;

7. To provide participating practices with statistics relating to their own practices.

1.3 Methods

Recruitment of practices

Practices taking part in the study were volunteers. They received a small sum for setting up the extra computer requirements and a payment based on the number of patients on their ASR to cover the costs of capturing morbidity data from every consultation and for socio-economic data collection. Practices were recruited by the RCGP Research Unit in Birmingham. All practices contributing to the RCGP Weekly Return Service and others known to be interested in data collection were invited to recruitment meetings. At these the proposed study was described and discussed and an information booklet about the study was distributed.

Only three software companies supplying general practice systems agreed to enhance their product to meet the requirements of the study. Participation in the study had to be restricted to practices using this software. Many keen practices which were experienced in computing and in morbidity data collection had to be excluded. The limited number of doctors able to contribute to the study meant that no attempt could be made to achieve a random sample of practices. Initially all practices expressing a firm interest were accepted. In an attempt to obtain some degree of geographical representation across England and Wales, additional efforts were made to recruit practices in health regions where none had previously shown an interest. No practice withdrew from the study during the course of data collection. It was a condition of participation that *all* doctors within a practice would be committed to contributing to the study.

Training of practices

The RCGP and OPCS jointly held a total of six two-day training sessions for practice staff, three on morbidity data recording for doctors and three on socio-economic data collection for interviewers. Administrators and other practice staff also attended. The sessions were held in three centres, Harrogate, Birmingham and Reading. The morbidity sessions were held about four months before the start of the study to allow practices sufficient time to train other practice staff and to review their organisational procedures. The courses for socio-economic data collection were held four to six weeks before the start of the study. Advice was given about appropriate registration by practices under the Data Protection Act for the purposes of the study. Detailed manuals for both morbidity and socio-economic data collection were discussed during the training sessions and distributed to each practice. A video was sent to each practice to reinforce the instruction given and for use by members of the practice who had not attended the training sessions.

Practices collected morbidity data for two to four weeks during July and August 1991, before the start of the study. The data were sent on disk to OPCS where they were scrutinised and any irregularities reported back to the practices. Throughout the data collection year, morbidity and socio-economic data were sent from the practices regularly to OPCS for scrutiny and feedback. When a widespread problem was identified a circular was sent to all practices to clarify procedures and correct ambiguities. In addition, 31 practices were visited at least once by OPCS staff during the study year to help sort out problems. Visits were initiated by practices or OPCS.

Selection of general practice software

A number of options were considered for providing participating practices with appropriate software for recording during the study year. Many practices already had software installed and would have been unwilling to change. It was therefore decided that the Department of Health should commission purpose-built software from companies already supplying general practices.

In July 1989 fifteen companies were invited to a meeting at which the proposed study was described and tenders for the work invited. Seven companies expressed a firm interest and were asked to submit specifications based on requirements issued by OPCS. Six of these signed contracts to provide suitable software. Eventually only three companies met the requirements specified. They provided study practices with a special version of their existing software, enhanced to allow recording of morbidity for the study. The companies also provided practices with software for entering socio-economic data. This was produced independently from the morbidity software as it was firstly a temporary requirement and secondly the most economic programming option. The morbidity and socio-economic data were linked at OPCS using the unique practice and patient identification numbers generated by the system.

Transfer of data to OPCS

Data were transferred from the practices on disks supplied by OPCS. OPCS despatched the disks immediately each practice notified them that it was ready to download the data. The disks were checked for quality using Norton Disk Utilities and for viruses using Dr Solomon's Anti-virus Toolkit before despatch from OPCS and for viruses on receipt from the practices. Disks were transported between the practices and OPCS by TNT carrier.

Editing the data

All socio-economic and morbidity queries found during the edit process were listed and sent to the appropriate practice for completion or amendment and the lists returned to OPCS for correction of the file on the mainframe.

The data were transmitted from each practice in two files. The patient file contained information from the practice age/sex register (ASR) such as date of birth, sex, the number of days in the study, and the socio-economic information gathered by the interviewers. The consultation file contained the records of each face-to-face contact between the doctor or practice nurse and the patient.

Editing was carried out in three stages. First, an initial scrutiny was made on data from each practice on a PC. They were then examined to ensure that the appropriate practice number was present for each record, that patient study identification numbers were within prescribed ranges, that the data had been correctly downloaded by the practice software, and that there were no obvious signs of corruption. Backup copies were produced and stored on a different site.

Data from the age/sex register (ASR)

Practice number

Study identification number

Date of birth

Sex

Number of days in study

Second, the files were loaded on to a database on the mainframe. They were then examined separately and comparisons made between the two. The patient files were checked for duplicate patients and, where these were found, the most complete record was retained and duplicate(s) deleted. The consultation files were also checked for duplications where the date of consultation, doctor seen, place where seen, referral code and Read diagnostic code were each identical and, if found, one entry was deleted.

Socio-economic data collected

Marital status

Cohabiting status

Tenure of housing

Ethnic group

Sole adult in household

Children in household

Smoking

Economic position

Occupation

Employment status

Children living with sole adult

Finally, the patient and consultation files from each practice were combined and the main editing process begun. This included range checks, cross field checks and checks against external control files.

Data from the patient file from each practice were checked automatically for completeness of data entry to ensure that a code was present in each field. Codes included 'not applicable' and 'not known'. Each item of socio-economic information was checked to ensure that the code was within the defined range. The occupation code was matched against a 1991 Occupation Component Control File list compiled by OPCS, to ensure that acceptable codes for occupation and employment status had been recorded and were compatible combinations. Postcodes were compared with the Postcode Directory to ensure that each was valid.

As a result of these checks on the patient file, practices were sent a printout of all queries raised by OPCS and asked to amend the paper record as appropriate. Further information was requested for a total of 63,000 items of information on patient files. Over 46 per cent of these were for clarification of employment status, and a further three per cent for more precise information on occupation, both required for coding social class. A quarter of all socio-economic queries was for further information about the postcode.

Data from the consultation files were automatically checked to ensure that the day and month of each consultation had been recorded, and whether the place of contact, the doctor consulted, the consultation type and the referral type had been recorded and were within prescribed code limits. The

3

Key definitions

Patient   a person who was on a study practice age/sex register for part or all of the year (*see page 7*)

Contact   a face-to-face meeting between a GP or practice nurse and a patient (*see page 27*)

Consultation   each diagnosis or reason for contact recorded during a contact (*see page 15*)

Consultation type   *First*   first consultation ever by a patient with a GP or practice nurse for that
(*see page 16*)   illness or reason.

                          New   first consultation for a new occurrence of an illness or reason for which
                                        the patient has previously consulted a GP or practice nurse.

                          Ongoing   any consultation for continuing illness following a first or new consultation.

Episode   a single or sequence of consultations covering the duration of a continuing illness or reason for consulting.

Episode type   *First*   first ever episode for an illness or reason for consulting a GP or practice nurse.
(*see page 17*)
                          New   new episode of illness for which the patient has previously consulted a GP or practice nurse.

                          Ongoing   an episode for which the patient had consulted a GP or practice nurse before the start of the study year.

Person years at risk   the sum of the number of days each patient in a particular category was registered with a study practice during the year, divided by the number of days (366) in the year (*see page 7*)

Rates   rates for persons are per 10,000 person years at risk. This applies to each sex, age and socio-economic group, eg: patient consulting rates for males aged 0-4 years in social class IIIN per 10,000 males aged 0-4 years in social class IIIN expressed as person years at risk.

Patient consulting   rates of patients who consulted at least once during the year at a defined level of
rates   diagnostic detail (eg for any illness, or for a respiratory illness, or for acute bronchitis) (*see page 16*).

Prevalence rates   patient consulting rates (*see pages 16 and 24*)

Incidence rates   first and new episode rates (*see page 24*)

Category of severity   serious, intermediate or minor, assigned by OPCS to each diagnostic code (*see page 15*)

Referrals   referral by a GP to a medically or dentally qualified practitioner (*see page 18*)

Age standardised ratio   the ratio between the observed and expected numbers of occurrences in a subgroup of the population, where the expected number is the number which would be expected if those in that subgroup were to experience the same morbidity in each (five-year) age group as the study population as a whole.

Read diagnostic codes were matched against a Diagnostic Control file. If no code had been entered for a contact, the practice was asked to supply one. The diagnostic control file was used to convert four-digit Read codes to five-digit Read codes. The control file was also the means of converting five-digit Read codes to four-digit ICD9 codes and aggregating these to three-digit ICD9 codes, to ICD9 diagnostic related groups (ICD subheadings) and to ICD9 chapters. Each code on the diagnostic control file was allocated by OPCS to a category of severity, allowing analyses of morbidity by whether each illness is usually serious (S), intermediate (I) or minor (M) in nature (see page 15). The diagnostic control file was used to identify diagnoses which were invalid, for example because they were incompatible with the patient's sex or age such as prostatic hyperplasia in a female, or senile dementia in a newborn. It also identified diagnoses which were unlikely and for scrutiny, either on the grounds of sex, such as carcinoma of the breast in a male, or age, or of rarity, such as tetanus or cholera. When these were identified, the practice was asked to review the codes used and send an amendment if appropriate. A total of nearly 13,000 queries on morbidity records were referred back to practices.

All diagnoses finally given by the practice were not altered by OPCS which explains why a few unexpected occurrences appear in the tables and datasets.

Once the data from each practice were complete and acceptable, certain items were automatically derived from the data. Age as at 1 March 1992, the mid-study date, was derived from the date of birth. The age of children born during the study year was derived in months from the date of birth and date of first contact. Social class was derived from occupation and employment status. The urban/rural indicator was obtained from the postcode. Episodes were derived from the consultation type.

1.4 Characteristics of the study practices

Of the 60 practices which took part in the study, the number in each health region varied between one and eight, 16 were in metropolitan districts. Figure 1.1 shows the locality of the practices.

Practice size varied from those with a single-handed doctor to those with eight principal doctors. The populations covered by each practice varied between 1,900 and 16,500.

Representativeness of the study practices

Study practices differed from all practices in England and Wales in a number of ways. The doctors taking part were self-selected and had an interest in collecting morbidity data. Most had previous experience of recording morbidity on computers. At the time of the study, only 34 per cent of all practices in England and Wales recorded at least some item of clinical information on computer for every contact with a patient on their list and the reason why they consulted. Many study practices already contributed to the RCGP Weekly Return Service, reporting the number of new episodes of illness seen each week.

The characteristics of the study practices are compared in table 1A with data on all practices in England and Wales supplied by the Department of Health.

Derived data from ASR data	Derived morbidity data
Age	4 digit ICD code
Person years at risk	3 digit ICD code
	ICD disease related group (ICD subheadings)
	ICD chapter
	All illnesses (ICD chapters I-XVII)
Derived socio-economic data	All diseases and conditions (ICD chapters I-XVIII)
Social class of men	Category of severity
Partner's social class of women	Episode type
Own social class of women	Patients consulting rates
Parent's/guardian's social class of children	Consultation rates
Urban/rural indicator	Referral rates

Figure 1A Location of the practices participating in the study

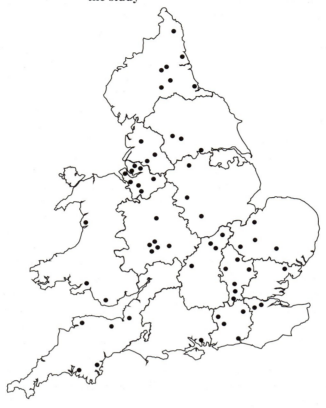

Table 1A Characteristics of practices in study, compared with England and Wales at 1 October 1991

Characteristic	Study practices				All practices			
	England and Wales	North	Midlands and Wales	South	England and Wales	North	Midlands and Wales	South
Average size of practice	7,733	7,092	9,190	7,305	5,239	5,239	5,456	5,105
Average number of patients per principal	1,917	1,960	1,910	1,888	1,571	1,937	1,907	1,811
Principals per practice	4.03	3.62	4.81	3.87	2.80	2.70	2.86	2.82
Assistants per practice	0.22	0.24	0.19	0.22	0.05	0.03	0.03	0.07
Trainees per practice	0.73	0.71	0.81	0.70	0.18	0.18	0.19	0.17
Practice nurses per practice (WTE)	1.44	1.28	1.61	1.48	0.95	0.82	0.99	1.00
Other ancillary staff per practice (WTE)	7.11	5.95	8.19	7.42	4.27	4.07	4.41	4.29
Assistants per 10,000 patients	0.3	0.3	0.2	0.3	0.1	0.0	0.1	0.1
Trainees per 10,000 patients	0.9	1.0	0.9	1.0	0.3	0.3	0.3	0.3
Practice nurses per 10,000 patients (WTE)	1.9	1.8	1.8	2.0	1.8	1.6	1.8	2.0
Other ancillary staff per 10,000 patients (WTE)	9.2	8.4	8.9	10.2	8.1	7.8	8.1	8.4
Percentage of principals aged:								
under 40 years	48	57	39	47	39	42	40	37
40 to 49 years	32	22	44	30	33	31	33	33
50 to 59 years	15	14	16	16	21	20	21	21
60 years and over	5	7	1	7	7	7	6	8
Percentage of principals:								
Male	74	74	73	76	75	76	78	73
Female	26	26	27	24	25	24	22	27
Percentage of principals working full time	92	95	86	96	93	94	93	92
Percentage of practices authorised to conduct minor surgery	72	86	50	74	56	49	51	40

Notes: 1. North   Northern, Yorkshire, North Western and Mersey RHAs.
        Midlands and Wales   West Midlands, Trent, East Anglian RHAs and Wales.
        South   South Western, Wessex, SW Thames, SE Thames, NE Thames, NW Thames and Oxford RHAs.
     2. This table includes restricted and unrestricted principals.

The average number of patients on the study practice lists was larger than for other practices, particularly in the Midlands and Wales. Although there were also more principal doctors in the study practices, these practices had a lower principal/patient ratio than other practices. This was possible because study practices employed both more assistants and more trainee doctors than other practices.

While study practices employed more practice nurses than the average practice in England and Wales, the nurse/patient ratio was similar. Study practices employed more ancillary staff for every 10,000 patients than other practices, although this may partly have been to carry out extra tasks associated with routine data collection and computer recording before the start of the study.

The average age of principal doctors within the study practices was lower than that of those working in other practices. Forty-eight per cent of study principal doctors were aged under 40 years and 80 per cent under 50 years, compared with 39 per cent and 72 per cent respectively in all practices in England and Wales. There was little difference in the proportion of principal doctors who were women or who worked full-time between the study practices and others.

The clinical activities undertaken by study practices may have differed from those of other practices. For example, 72 per cent of study practices were authorised to undertake minor surgery compared with 46 per cent of all practices in England and Wales.

1.5 The study population

The NHS age/sex register (ASR) in each practice was the basis for identifying the population covered by the study. Temporary and private patients were excluded. As a consequence of births, deaths and migration, some patients were on the ASRs of practices for only part of the study year. Each person's contribution to the study denominator was combined to produce the total person years at risk. This true denominator was derived by totalling the number of days that every person was present in the study and dividing this by 366 (1992 was a leap year). A similar calculation provided the denominator for each sex, age and socio-economic group.

Calculation of person years at risk

Total person years at risk $= \dfrac{\Sigma x_j}{366}$

where j = each patient

x = number of days patient j was in the study

Before the start of the study, each practice checked and updated their ASR with that held by the Family Health Services Authority (FHSA). The date of entry of each patient to the practice and the date of withdrawal during the study year was recorded by each practice on the practice ASR. The date of entry for those already on the register at the start of the study was recorded as 1 September 1991. For any person joining the practice during the study year, the date of entry was defined as the date the person expressed a wish to register with the practice or a newborn baby was brought for consultation. This was because many patients do not register with a new practice until they need to consult a doctor and it may take some time before they are placed on the practice register held by the FHSA. Those patients on the practice register at the end of the study were given a date of withdrawal of 31 August 1992. For any patient dying or leaving the practice during the study year, the date of withdrawal was defined as the date they were removed from the FHSA register. Although this was a compromise solution, it was considered that delay by some patients in registering with the practice, having moved into the area and therefore technically being at risk, would roughly equal the delay in being removed from the FHSA register. If a patient re-entered the practice or withdrew more than once during the study year, the same procedure was followed, but on re-entry his previous medical record was reinstated and he was allocated his original study patient identification number. The total number of days each patient was in the study was calculated by the practice software immediately before the file was transferred to OPCS at the end of the study.

Data held on the practice ASRs included a unique study patient identification number, the patient's date of birth and sex. Practices were asked to record the postcode of the patient's place of residence which they could obtain from the local Post Office postcode directory. If the postcode of a patient's place of residence could not be provided, the postcode of the practice was assigned to that patient. This was necessary for one per cent of patients. The place of residence was assigned to urban or rural categories by linking the postcode to the census enumeration district, and by linking the enumeration district to an urban/rural indicator supplied by the Department of the Environment. The practice ASR also served as a list of patients to be interviewed about their socio-economic circumstances.

No data sent to OPCS from practices included the patient's name or address. The only link held by OPCS and the practice by which an individual could be identified was the patient's study identification number, ensuring complete confidentiality. The patient's record could be identified in the practice by practice staff to answer any queries raised by OPCS.

Representativeness of the sample population

The study population for whom socio-economic data are available has been compared with the population enumerated in the 1991 census wherever comparable figures were available. Smoking data has been compared with the General Household Survey.

In general, the study sample was representative of the population enumerated in the census by age, sex, marital status, tenure of housing, economic position, occupation and whether they lived in an urban or rural area. The proportion who smoked was similar to that recorded by the General Household Survey. There were small differences in the proportions of people by social class. Ethnic minority groups were under-represented in the study sample. The proportion of people living alone in the study sample was lower than that identified in the census. The South of England was under-represented compared with the North and Midlands & Wales. People living in metropolitan districts were slightly under-represented in the study.

Age and sex

The age distribution of the study population was similar to that in the census. There was a slightly higher proportion of people of both sexes aged 25-44 years in the study population and a slightly lower proportion of people aged 65-84 years (table 1B). In the study population, 49 per cent were male compared with 48 per cent in the census.

Table 1B   Age and sex: population (percentages)

	All ages Persons	0-4	5-15	16-24	25-44	45-64	65-74	75-84	85 and over
Study	100	7	14	13	31	21	8	5	1
North	100	7	14	12	29	22	9	5	1
Midlands & Wales	100	7	14	13	31	20	8	5	1
South	100	7	13	13	32	21	8	5	1
1991 Census	100	7	13	13	29	22	9	6	2
North	100	7	14	13	29	22	9	5	1
Midlands & Wales	100	7	14	13	28	22	9	5	1
South	100	7	13	13	30	21	9	6	2

	All ages		0-4		5-15		16-24		25-44		45-64		65-74		75-84		85 and over	
	M	F	M	F	M	F	M	F	M	F	M	F	M	F	M	F	M	F
Study	100	100	7	7	15	13	13	13	31	30	22	21	7	9	4	6	1	2
North	100	100	7	6	15	13	12	11	30	29	23	22	8	10	4	6	1	2
Midlands & Wales	100	100	7	6	15	14	14	13	31	30	21	20	7	9	4	6	1	2
South	100	100	8	7	14	13	13	13	33	31	21	20	7	8	4	6	1	2
1991 Census	100	100	7	6	14	13	13	12	30	29	22	21	8	10	4	7	1	2
North	100	100	7	6	15	13	13	12	29	28	23	22	8	10	4	7	1	2
Midlands & Wales	100	100	7	6	14	13	13	12	29	28	23	22	9	10	4	7	1	2
South	100	100	7	6	14	12	13	12	31	29	22	21	8	9	4	7	1	2

Table 1C   Marital status: population (percentages)

	16-24 Persons	25-44	45-64	65-74	75-84	85 and over
Study	100	100	100	100	100	100
Single	90	23	6	6	7	11
Married	9	70	81	67	42	16
Widowed/Divorced	0	7	12	27	50	73
1991 Census	100	100	100	100	100	100
Single	89	24	7	7	8	11
Married	11	67	79	64	42	18
Widowed/Divorced	1	9	14	28	50	71

	16-24		25-44		45-64		65-74		75-84		85 and over	
	M	F	M	F	M	F	M	F	M	F	M	F
Study	100	100	100	100	100	100	100	100	100	100	100	100
Single	94	86	28	18	8	5	6	6	6	9	6	12
Married	6	13	67	72	84	78	80	55	67	27	43	7
Widowed/Divorced	0	1	5	9	8	17	14	39	28	64	51	81
1991 Census	100	100	100	100	100	100	100	100	100	100	100	100
Single	93	85	28	19	9	5	8	7	6	10	6	13
Married	7	14	64	70	81	76	78	54	66	28	43	10
Widowed/Divorced	0	1	7	11	10	18	15	39	27	63	50	78

Marital status

The study sample was very similar to that of the total population regarding marital status, with only small variations within each age group (table 1C).

Geographical distribution

The South of England was under-represented in the study sample whereas the North and Midlands & Wales were over-represented. This held for every age group and both sexes (table 1D).

Urban/rural place of residence

In the total study sample the proportions living in urban and rural areas was the same as those found in the census (table 1E). There was very little variation between the two populations by age group.

The 16 practices in metropolitan districts represented 27% of the total study sample. In comparison, 35% of the census population of England and Wales lived in metropolitan districts.

Table 1D Broad geographical region: population (percentages)

	All ages Persons	0-4	5-15	16-24	25-44	45-64	65-74	75-84	85 and over
Study	100	100	100	100	100	100	100	100	100
North	31	30	31	29	30	33	34	33	32
Midlands and Wales	32	32	33	34	32	31	31	33	33
South	36	39	35	37	38	36	34	35	35
1991 Census	100	100	100	100	100	100	100	100	100
North	26	26	27	26	25	26	26	25	24
Midlands and Wales	29	29	30	29	28	30	30	29	28
South	45	44	44	45	46	44	44	46	48

	0-4		5-15		16-24		25-44		45-64		65-74		75-84		85 and over	
	M	F	M	F	M	F	M	F	M	F	M	F	M	F	M	F
Study	100	100	100	100	100	100	100	100	100	100	100	100	100	100	100	100
North	30	30	31	32	30	28	30	30	33	34	34	35	33	33	29	33
Midlands and Wales	32	32	33	34	34	34	32	33	31	31	31	32	32	33	34	33
South	39	39	36	35	37	37	38	37	36	36	35	34	35	34	37	34
1991 Census	100	100	100	100	100	100	100	100	100	100	100	100	100	100	100	100
North	26	26	27	27	26	26	25	25	26	26	26	26	24	26	23	25
Midlands and Wales	29	29	30	30	30	29	29	28	30	30	31	30	29	29	28	27
South	44	44	44	44	45	45	46	46	44	44	43	44	47	46	49	48

Table 1E Urban/rural place of residence: population (percentages)

	All ages Persons	0-4	5-15	16-24	25-44	45-64	65-74	75-84	85 and over
Study	100	100	100	100	100	100	100	100	100
Urban	88	89	88	87	88	86	88	89	88
Rural	12	11	12	13	12	14	12	11	12
1991 Census	100	100	100	100	100	100	100	100	100
Urban	88	89	88	89	88	86	87	87	87
Rural	12	11	12	11	12	14	13	13	13

	0-4		5-15		16-24		25-44		45-64		65-74		75-84		85 and over	
	M	F	M	F	M	F	M	F	M	F	M	F	M	F	M	F
Study	100	100	100	100	100	100	100	100	100	100	100	100	100	100	100	100
Urban	89	89	88	88	87	88	88	88	86	86	87	89	88	89	86	89
Rural	11	11	12	12	13	12	12	12	14	14	13	11	12	11	14	11
1991 Census	100	100	100	100	100	100	100	100	100	100	100	100	100	100	100	100
Urban	89	89	87	88	88	89	88	88	86	86	86	87	86	88	86	88
Rural	11	11	13	12	12	11	12	12	14	14	14	13	14	12	14	12

Table 1F   Tenure of housing: population (percentages)

	All ages Persons	0-4	5-15	16-44	45-64	65-74	75-84	85 and over
Study	100	100	100	100	100	100	100	100
Owner-occupied	70	66	70	71	79	65	56	44
Council house	18	24	21	16	14	26	27	21
Other rented	9	10	7	12	6	8	11	9
Communal	2	0	1	2	0	1	7	25
1991 Census	100	100	100	100	100	100	100	100
Owner-occupied	70	64	71	71	77	65	56	44
Council house	18	25	21	15	15	25	25	21
Other rented	10	11	8	12	7	9	13	12
Communal	2	0	0	1	1	1	6	24

	0-4		5-15		16-44		45-64		65-74		75-84		85 and over	
	M	F	M	F	M	F	M	F	M	F	M	F	M	F
Study	100	100	100	100	100	100	100	100	100	100	100	100	100	100
Owner-occupied	66	65	70	71	71	70	79	78	68	63	61	53	53	42
Council house	24	24	21	21	15	17	14	15	24	27	25	28	22	21
Other rented	10	11	7	7	11	12	7	6	7	8	10	11	10	9
Communal	0	0	1	1	2	2	0	0	1	2	4	8	15	28
1991 Census	100	100	100	100	100	100	100	100	100	100	100	100	100	100
Owner-occupied	64	64	71	70	72	71	77	77	67	63	60	53	53	41
Council house	25	25	21	21	14	17	14	16	23	26	23	26	20	21
Other rented	11	11	8	8	12	12	8	7	9	10	12	14	12	12
Communal	0	0	0	0	2	1	1	1	1	1	4	7	15	26

Tenure of housing

A similar proportion of the total study sample lived in owner-occupied premises, council housing, other rented accommodation and communal establishments as in the census (table 1F). Among the elderly, a slightly lower proportion of the study sample lived in other rented premises than found in the census.

Table 1G   Household composition: population (percentages)

	16 and over Persons	16-64	65 and over
Study	100	100	100
Living alone	9	5	26
Not living alone	91	95	74
1991 Census*	100	100	100
Living alone	13	8	32
Not living alone	87	92	68

	16 and over		16-64		65 and over	
	M	F	M	F	M	F
Study	100	100	100	100	100	100
Living alone	6	12	5	6	15	34
Not living alone	93	88	95	94	85	66
1991 Census*	100	100	100	100	100	100
Living alone	11	16	9	6	20	38
Not living alone	89	84	91	94	80	62

* Census: females 16-59 and 65 and over.

Household composition

The proportion of people living alone was lower in the study sample than in the census (table 1G). This was consistent for adult men and the elderly of both sexes. The disparity may be due to a difference in the census and study definitions of a household.

Comparable census data on whether there were children in the household are only available for people aged 25-34 and 35-54 years (table 1H). In the study sample a lower proportion had no children in the household, particularly those aged 25-34 years, than in the census. A higher proportion in the study in both age groups had children aged under five years, but a similar proportion had children aged 5-15 years only.

Table 1H   Children in households of adults: population (percentages)

	25-54 Persons	25-34	35-54
Study	100	100	100
None	50	44	54
Under 5 years	22	41	12
5-15 years only	27	15	34
1991 Census	100	100	100
None	53	48	56
Under 5 years	21	37	11
5-15 years only	27	15	34

Economic position in the previous week

The proportion of people working full-time and of those who were economically inactive (which includes housewives, students and retired people) together made up 81 per cent of the total aged 16 years and over (table 1I). The proportion in each of these two groups were the same in the study sample as found in the census. A slightly higher proportion of people in the study were working part-time and a slightly lower proportion were unemployed.

Social class

The study and census data on social class (as defined by occupation) are not strictly comparable, for several reasons. First, social class in the study was considered to be that of the partner for married or cohabiting women and that of the parent or guardian for children. In the census, married or cohabiting women and children were allocated the social class of the head of the household, this being the person who filled in the census form. Second, the study data were aggregated to 16-64 years, whereas the census data relate to people of working age (16-64 years for men, 16-59 years for women). Third, the census question requested information on the type of occupation held only during the previous ten years. In the study no time limit was referred to. With these limitations, the data from the study and the census are given in table 1J.

Table 1J Social class (as defined by occupation): population (percentages)

	All ages Persons	0-15	16-64*	65 and over†
Study	100	100	100	100
I & II	30	34	31	24
IIIN	13	11	13	15
IIIM	29	31	29	26
IV & V	20	20	19	24
Other	8	4	8	11

	All ages	0-15	16-64*	65 and over†
1991 Census	100	100	100	100
I & II	37	37	38	35
IIIN	12	11	12	15
IIIM	28	29	28	22
IV & V	18	18	18	24
Other	4	5	4	3

* Including males 16-64 and females 16-59.
† Including males 65+ and females 60+.

Table 1I Economic position last week: population (percentages)

	16 and over Persons	16-24	25-44	45-64	65-74	75 and over
Study	100	100	100	100	100	100
Working full-time	46	55	61	49	2	0
Working part-time	11	4	16	15	3	1
Unemployed	5	10	6	4	0	0
Long-term sick	3	1	2	6	1	1
Other economically inactive	35	30	15	25	94	98
1991 Census	100	100	100	100	100	100
Working full-time	46	53	63	50	4	1
Working part-time	10	7	13	13	4	1
Unemployed	6	11	7	5	0	0
Long-term sick	4	1	2	8	3	3
Other economically inactive	35	28	15	24	89	95

	16 and over		16-24		25-44		45-64		65-74		75 and over	
	M	F	M	F	M	F	M	F	M	F	M	F
Study	100	100	100	100	100	100	100	100	100	100	100	100
Working full-time	64	30	60	50	86	40	71	28	3	1	1	0
Working part-time	2	19	2	6	1	28	2	27	4	3	1	1
Unemployed	8	3	14	7	9	3	7	2	0	0	0	0
Long-term sick	4	2	1	1	3	2	9	4	1	1	1	1
Other economically inactive	23	47	23	36	2	28	11	38	92	95	97	98
1991 Census	100	100	100	100	100	100	100	100	100	100	100	100
Working full-time	63	30	59	48	85	41	71	28	6	2	2	1
Working part-time	2	17	4	9	1	25	2	24	4	3	1	0
Unemployed	8	3	14	8	9	4	8	3	0	0	0	0
Long-term sick	5	3	1	1	3	2	11	6	4	2	2	3
Other economically inactive	22	47	23	34	2	28	8	39	85	93	94	96

Table 1K Occupation: population (percentages)

	Study 16-64 Persons	16-44	45-64	1991 Census 16-64 Persons	16-44	45-64
	100	100	100	100	100	100
1a Corporate managers/administrators	7	7	8	10	9	11
1b Managers/proprietors in agriculture	5	5	6	6	6	7
2a Science and engineering professionals	2	2	3	2	2	2
2b Health professionals	1	1	1	1	1	1
2c Teaching professionals	4	3	5	4	3	4
2d Other professional occupations	2	2	2	2	2	2
3a Science associated professionals	2	2	1	2	3	2
3b Health associated professionals	3	3	2	3	3	2
3c Other associated professionals	3	4	3	4	4	4
4a Clerical occupations	12	13	10	12	13	9
4b Secretarial occupations	5	5	5	5	5	4
5a Skilled construction trades	3	3	3	3	3	3
5b Skilled engineering trades	4	4	4	4	5	5
5c Other skilled trades	8	8	8	8	8	7
6a Protective service occupations	2	2	1	2	2	2
6b Personal service occupations	8	9	7	7	7	7
7a Buyers, brokers, sales reps	2	2	1	2	2	2
7b Other sales occupations	6	6	5	5	6	4
8a Industrial plant operators, assemblers	7	7	7	6	6	7
8b Drivers and machinery operators	4	3	4	4	3	5
9a Other occupations in agriculture etc.	1	1	1	1	1	1
9b Other elementary occupations	9	8	11	8	7	9

	Study 16-64		16-44		45-64		1991 Census 16-64		16-44		45-64	
	M	F	M	F	M	F	M	F	M	F	M	F
	100	100	100	100	100	100	100	100	100	100	100	100
1a Corporate managers/administrators	10	4	8	5	12	4	12	7	12	7	15	6
1b Managers/proprietors in agriculture	6	5	5	4	6	5	7	5	6	5	9	6
2a Science and engineering professionals	4	1	4	1	5	0	4	1	4	1	4	0
2b Health professionals	1	1	1	1	1	0	1	0	1	1	1	0
2c Teaching professionals	3	5	2	5	4	7	2	5	2	5	3	6
2d Other professional occupations	3	2	3	2	3	2	3	2	3	2	3	1
3a Science associated professionals	3	1	3	1	2	1	3	1	4	1	2	1
3b Health associated professionals	1	5	1	5	1	4	1	5	1	6	0	5
3c Other associated professionals	4	3	4	3	4	2	4	4	4	4	4	3
4a Clerical occupations	7	17	8	19	6	15	7	18	7	20	5	15
4b Secretarial occupations	0	10	0	10	0	11	0	10	0	10	0	10
5a Skilled construction trades	6	0	6	0	5	0	5	0	5	0	5	0
5b Skilled engineering trades	9	0	9	0	9	0	8	0	8	0	8	0
5c Other skilled trades	12	4	13	4	10	5	11	3	12	3	9	3
6a Protective service occupations	3	0	3	1	2	0	3	1	4	1	2	0
6b Personal service occupations	3	13	3	14	2	11	3	13	3	12	2	13
7a Buyers, brokers, sales reps	2	1	2	1	2	1	3	1	2	1	3	1
7b Other sales occupations	2	10	3	10	1	10	2	9	3	10	1	9
8a Industrial plant operators, assemblers	8	6	8	5	9	6	8	5	8	5	8	5
8b Drivers and machinery operators	7	0	6	0	8	0	7	0	6	0	8	0
9a Other occupations in agriculture etc.	1	1	1	1	1	1	1	0	1	0	1	0
9b Other elementary occupations	8	10	8	8	7	15	7	9	6	7	7	14

Among adults and the elderly, the study under-represented people in Social Classes I & II, and over-represented people in the 'other' group, which includes students, the armed forces and those whose occupations were inadequately described. Among children the same differences occurred, but to a smaller extent.

Among married and cohabiting women, social class based on their own occupation instead of that of their partner shows that Social Classes I & II and IIIN were under-represented in the study sample compared with the census, while those in the 'other' group were over-represented.

Occupation

The study population was representative of the population in the census (table 1K). With the exception of corporate managers, managers in agriculture and those in the personal services occupations, the proportion in each of the twenty-two major subgroups did not differ by more than one per cent between the study population and the census. In the study, 7 per cent of the population aged 16-64 years were corporate managers compared with 10 per cent in the census, and 5 per cent were managers in agriculture compared with just over 6 per cent in the census. These differences were greater for men than for women. The study slightly over-represented people in personal services occupations: 8 per cent, compared with 7 per cent in the census.

Ethnic group

A higher proportion of the study population were white than in the census population (table 1L): 98 per cent, compared with 94 per cent. The proportions of Black Afro-Caribbean, Indian and Pakistani/Bangladeshi groups in the study sample were a third of that identified by the census.

Smoking

No question on smoking was asked in the 1991 census. Estimates are available from the General Household Survey (GHS).[7] Among the study population aged 16 years and over, 29 per cent said they had smoked some type of tobacco product during the previous week. Of people aged 16 years and over in the 1992 GHS, 29 per cent said that they smoked cigarettes.

1.6 Recording morbidity data

The type of contacts reported are shown in figure 1.2 (page 17). The items of information recorded for each face-to-face contact between a patient and a doctor or practice nurse were the date, diagnosis or diagnoses, consultation type, where the patient was seen and the referral type if the patient was referred (see fig 1.3 page 18).

Recording diagnosis

In March 1990 the Department of Health acquired the copyright to the Read Clinical Classification System.[8] This

Table 1L Ethnic group: population (percentages)

	All ages Persons	0-4	5-15	16-24	25-44	45-64	65-74	75-84	85 and over
Study	100	100	100	100	100	100	100	100	100
White	98	97	97	97	97	98	99	100	100
Black Afro-Caribbean	1	1	1	1	1	0	0	0	0
Indian	1	1	1	1	1	1	0	0	0
Pakistani & Bangladeshi	0	1	1	1	0	0	0	0	0
Other	1	1	1	1	1	0	0	0	0
1991 Census	100	100	100	100	100	100	100	100	100
White	94	90	90	93	93	96	98	99	99
Black Afro-Caribbean	2	3	2	2	2	1	1	0	0
Indian	2	2	3	2	2	1	1	0	0
Pakistani & Bangladeshi	1	3	3	2	1	1	0	0	0
Other	1	2	2	2	2	1	0	0	0

	0-4		5-15		16-24		25-44		45-64		65-74		75-84		85 and over	
	M	F	M	F	M	F	M	F	M	F	M	F	M	F	M	F
Study	100	100	100	100	100	100	200	100	100	100	100	100	100	100	100	100
White	97	96	97	96	97	97	97	97	98	99	99	99	100	100	100	100
Black Afro-Caribbean	1	1	1	1	1	1	1	1	0	0	0	0	0	0	0	0
Indian	1	1	1	1	1	1	1	1	1	0	0	0	0	0	0	0
Pakistani & Bangladeshi	1	1	1	1	1	0	0	0	0	0	0	0	0	0	0	0
Other	1	1	1	1	1	1	1	1	0	0	0	0	0	0	0	0
1991 Census	100	100	100	100	100	100	100	100	100	100	100	100	100	100	100	100
White	90	90	90	90	93	92	94	93	96	96	98	99	99	99	99	100
Black Afro-Caribbean	3	3	2	2	2	2	2	2	1	1	1	0	0	0	0	0
Indian	2	2	3	3	2	2	2	2	1	1	1	0	0	0	0	0
Pakistani & Bangladeshi	3	3	3	3	2	2	1	1	1	1	0	0	0	0	0	0
Other	2	2	2	2	2	2	2	2	1	1	0	0	0	0	0	0

classification is a structural hierarchy of medical terms designed for use by clinicians in day-to-day patient care. They exist as a medical dictionary in computer files. The dictionary is more extensive than the ICD9 list of terms. The codes can be converted into ICD9 codes as shown below. The codes are structured as a 5 level hierarchy, with up to 58 separate codes at each level. Successive levels provide greater clinical detail.

Level code	Read term	Read code	ICD9
1	Circulatory system disease	G....	4599
2	Ischaemic heart disease	G3...	4149
3	Acute myocardial infarction	G30..	410-
4	Other acute myocardial infarct	G30y.	410-
5	Acute papillary muscle infarct	G30y1	410-

The diagnostic section of this system was used for recording morbidity data in the study. At the time, two versions were in use. The four-character codes (Read 4) were already installed in software distributed by one company to 37 of the study practices. Practices supplied by the other two companies were required to change from another diagnostic coding system to Read and were supplied through their software companies with the five-character version (Read 5).

The software allowed the practices to enter either the Read or a similar term which was stored as the appropriate Read code, or the Read code itself. They could also enter a high level Read code or term and choose options at each more detailed level.

Because the purpose of the study was to collect data on the illnesses for which patients consulted, practices were guided towards using 'acceptable' morbidity codes rather than, for example, social reasons for consulting.

An acceptable diagnostic code was a Read code prefixed by an upper case alpha character, equivalent to the International Classification of Diseases Revision 9 (ICD9) Chapters I-XVII, or a Read code prefixed by a numeric character, many equivalent to the ICD9 supplementary classification which had been selected by OPCS to describe a consultation for which no alpha prefixed code was appropriate. The practice software used a (V) prefix to distinguish numeric codes which were acceptable from those which were not acceptable.

Doctors were able to record, in addition, any 'unacceptable' codes for their own purposes; these were either not selected by the practice software for transfer to OPCS or were later removed from the file during the edit process at OPCS after the end of the study, depending upon the practice software.

Doctors were encouraged to record morbidity in as much detail as possible, avoiding codes for such general terms as 'respiratory illness' (so that data could later be aggregated in different ways for different analyses). Alpha character codes which were unacceptably vague were indicated on the practice software with an (X). The options for choice of diagnostic code for a consultation were given in an order of priority (see box on page opposite). Those prefixed by an alpha code equivalent to ICD9 Chapters I-XVII excluding Chapter XVI (Signs, symptoms and ill-defined conditions) were preferred. These were followed in order of preference by Read codes equivalent to ICD9 Chapter XVI, and Read codes prefixed by a numeric character. Finally, doctors were asked, if no other code listed above was appropriate, to record a 'dustbin' Read code equivalent to the ICD9 'Disease not otherwise specified' code. When recording an 'injury and poisoning' Read code (e.g. Colles fracture), equivalent to ICD9 Chapter XVII, doctors were asked to record, in addition, a Read code equivalent to an ICD9 external cause code (e.g. fell down stairs).

If a patient on the practice ASR consulted the doctor or nurse about some other person, irrespective of whether that person was also on the register, an appropriate code such as that for medical counselling or psychosexual counselling was recorded.

When a definite diagnosis which had been recorded for a consultation was subsequently found to have been incorrect,

Chapter headings of the Read clinical classification

Read 4	Description	Read 5
1	History/symptoms	1
2	Examination/signs	2
3	Diagnostic procedures	3
4	Laboratory procedures	4
5	Radiology/physics in medicine	5
6	Preventive procedures	6
7	Surgical procedures	7
8	Other therapeutic procedures	8
9	Administration	9
@	Health status assessment	@
A	Infectious/parasitic diseases	A
B	Neoplasms	B
C	Endocrine/nutrition/metabolic diseases	C
D	Blood diseases	D
E	Mental disorders	E
F	Nervous system/sense organ diseases	F
G	Circulatory system diseases	G
H	Respiratory system diseases	H
I	Digestive system diseases	J
J	Genitourinary system diseases	K
K	Pregnancy/childbirth/puerperium	L
L	Skin/subcutaneous tissue diseases	M
M	Musculoskeletal/connective tissues	N
N	Congenital anomalies	P
O	Perinatal conditions	Q
R	Symptoms/signs/ill-defined conditions	R
P	Injury and poisoning	S
Q	Causes of injury and poisoning	T
Z	Disease NOS	-

recorded reason for consultation was coded as ZV (no operation, condition resolved), this was changed to R2z.. (ICD 7999: other unknown and unspecified cause). There were 167 of these.

While practices were asked to assign an appropriate 'external injury' code (a five-digit Read code starting with T), such as that for 'fell down stairs', when recording an 'injury and poisoning' code (a five-digit Read code starting with S), such as 'Colles fracture' and vice versa, this was not always done. In this case, OPCS generated an S code (SN5z. = ICD 9958) to accompany the recorded T code, or a T code (TN8z. = ICD E9889) to accompany the recorded S code if it was a first or new consultation. Because both these codes reflected a single consultation, the occurrence of the T code was omitted from routine analysis to prevent double-counting.

Practices recorded every face-to-face contact between a doctor or a practice nurse with any patient on the practice ASR between 1 September 1991 and 31 August 1992. For each contact, the doctor or nurse recorded at least one diagnostic code. If the patient had more than one condition, each was recorded. Each diagnostic code recorded during a contact was regarded as a consultation, so that more than one consultation may have taken place during a single contact.

A doctor visiting a patient at home who had died was considered to have been providing clinical care and the contact was recorded with an appropriate diagnostic code if the cause of death was known, or the 'other ill-defined and unknown causes of morbidity and mortality' code if no cause of death could be identified.

The procedure adopted for morbidity data entry varied between practices. In some the doctors or nurses entered all the data themselves, either during the contact or later. In others, the doctor recorded the diagnostic details in longhand on the patient's notes and this information was later transferred to the computer by another member of the practice staff. In many practices a combination of these two methods was used.

After receipt of the morbidity data by OPCS at the end of the study, the Read 4 codes were converted to Read 5 codes. These were retained on the file, but were also converted to equivalent ICD9 codes for analysis.

Category of severity

Each ICD9 code was assigned by OPCS to a degree of severity category: serious, intermediate or minor. This was therefore independent of the the doctor's opinion of the degree of severity of an individual patient's condition. The definition of each was as follows:

Serious
Invariably or frequently serious or possibly life threatening, *or*
Invariably or frequently requiring major surgery or intensive care, *or*
With a high probability of serious complications or significant disability.

for example if a patient had been referred to hospital with a diagnosis of cholecystitis and appendicitis was diagnosed at operation, the doctor was asked to substitute the original diagnosis recorded with the updated one and, for legal reasons, to record for his own purposes the original diagnosis in textual form. If the original diagnosis recorded was subsequently improved (for example, if a cough or acute bronchitis was later diagnosed as carcinoma of the lung), the doctor was not asked to alter the original diagnosis because it was not factually incorrect, but to record the improved diagnosis at the next contact. An original unamended diagnosis for which an improved diagnosis was later recorded would result in that episode being analysed as two different episodes. However, the original diagnosis will usually have been non-specific, resulting only in inflation in the number of episodes in the symptoms, signs and ill-defined conditions ICD chapter.

Certain unacceptable Read codes were identified at this stage during the editing procedure at OPCS. Where cancer morphology codes (those starting with BB) instead of and without a code identifying the site had been recorded these were changed to code BAOz. (ICD 2399: neoplasm unspecified nature). This accounted for 1,855 alterations. Where the only

Typical patient's morbidity record

Date of contact	Diagnosis	ICD 3-digit code	ICD sub-heading code	ICD chapter	Category of severity	All diseases and conditions		
							Serious	
							Intermediate	
							Minor	
						ICD Chapter III		
6/11	Diabetes	250	028	III	S		Serious	
	Hyperlipidaemia	272	030	III	I		Intermediate	
	Infective otitis externa	380	041	VI	M	ICD Chapter IV		
	Angina pectoris	413	045	VII	S		Intermediate	
						ICD Chapter VI		
7/11	Diabetes	250	028	III	S		Minor	
						ICD Chapter VII		
18/11	Iron deficiency anaemia	280	031	IV	I		Serious	
	Menorrhagia	626	069	X	I	ICD Chapter X		
							Intermediate	
30/1	Diabetes	250	028	III	S	ICD subheading	028	
						ICD subheading	030	
30/4	Peripheral vascular disease	443	049	VII	S	ICD subheading	031	
	Diabetes	250	028	III	S	ICD subheading	041	
						ICD subheading	045	
						ICD subheading	049	
						ICD subheading	069	

This patient consulted at least once for conditions listed in right hand column

ICD 3-digit code	250
ICD 3-digit code	272
ICD 3-digit code	280
ICD 3-digit code	380
ICD 3-digit code	413
ICD 3-digit code	443
ICD 3-digit code	626

Intermediate
Other than serious or minor.

Minor
Illnesses commonly treated without recourse to medical advice, *or*
Minor self-limiting illnesses which require no specific treatment, *or*
Reasons for contact in the ICD9 supplementary classification.

Prevalence

The definition of prevalence for the purpose of this study is the number of patients who consulted at least once during the year for a condition or group of conditions. This is expressed as a patient consulting rate per 10,000 person years at risk.

The first occurrence of a patient making a contact for a five-digit Read code, a four-digit ICD9 code, a diagnostic related group code (ICD subheading), an ICD9 chapter or for any diagnosis (Chapters I-XVIII) or illness (Chapters I-XVII) was flagged independently, so that the number of patients consulting for conditions in each of these groups could be derived. The same was done for patients consulting by category of severity for consultations for all diseases and conditions, and within each ICD9 chapter. A patient may therefore be counted once, for example, under the heading for all diseases and conditions but would be counted once under each of the severe, intermediate and minor headings if he had consulted for conditions in each of these categories. An example is given in the box above.

Recording consultation type

For each consultation, that is to say, each diagnosis recorded during a contact, the doctor recorded whether that was the first time the patient had ever seen a general practitioner in his life for that illness (an F, or 'first ever' consultation), or whether he had seen a general practitioner for the same illness previously but had not suffered from that illness in the meantime (an N, or 'new' consultation), or whether the current consultation was for a continuing illness (an O, or 'ongoing', consultation).

During processing at OPCS, consultations by each patient for the same diagnosis were grouped to form an episode of illness. This was done both at the five-digit Read code level and independently at the three-digit ICD9 level.

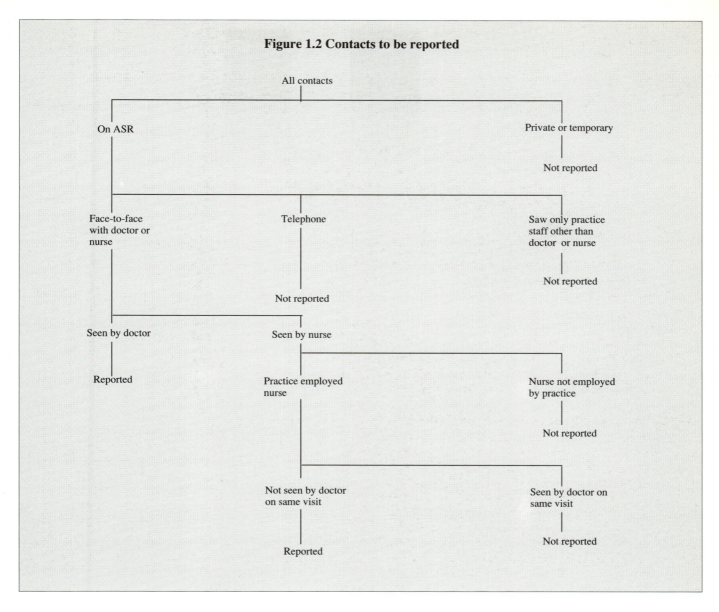

Figure 1.2 Contacts to be reported

Episode typing

An episode was defined as a *first* (F) consultation or a *new* (N) consultation together with any *ongoing* (O) consultations for the same diagnosis which occurred subsequently. Data from practices sometimes showed inconsistencies in the assignation of consultation types, entering, for example, an F for a diagnosis for which the patient had consulted previously. This occurred most frequently when the same patient was seen for the same illness by different doctors. To remedy this, the edit process at OPCS examined the consultations by each patient for the same diagnosis in date of consultation order. If a consultation assigned F followed another F or an N or an O consultation for the same five-digit Read diagnosis, the later F consultation was changed to an O consultation if it occurred within 28 days of the first F consultation, and to N if it occurred more than 28 days after the first consultation. Similarly, if an N consultation followed an F or an N or an O consultation, the later N was changed to an O if it occurred within 28 days of the F or the first N consultation. The same principle was applied to the derivation of episodes at the three-digit ICD9 level. All consultations assigned to a Read code equivalent to one in ICD Chapter XVI (Signs, symptoms and ill-defined conditions) were given consultation type O because if a more definite diagnosis was subsequently made and assigned, correctly, to consultation type F or N, the number of first or new episodes would otherwise have been inflated. As a result, all F and N episode rates indicate incidence of a condition or group of conditions.

All consultations with the same date, place of contact and doctor or practice nurse seen were grouped together to form a single contact.

The detailed diagnostic coding available within the Read system makes it possible for consultations for the same illness to be recorded using different codes. OPCS therefore carried out most analyses after the Read codes had been converted to the less detailed ICD9 codes. This prevented some duplication of episodes derived from the consultation type codes.

Doctor or nurse consulted

Practices allocated codes to each of the doctors and practice nurses working in the practice. These codes had different prefixes for principal doctors, assistant doctors, locums, trainees and practice nurses. Practice nurses were included

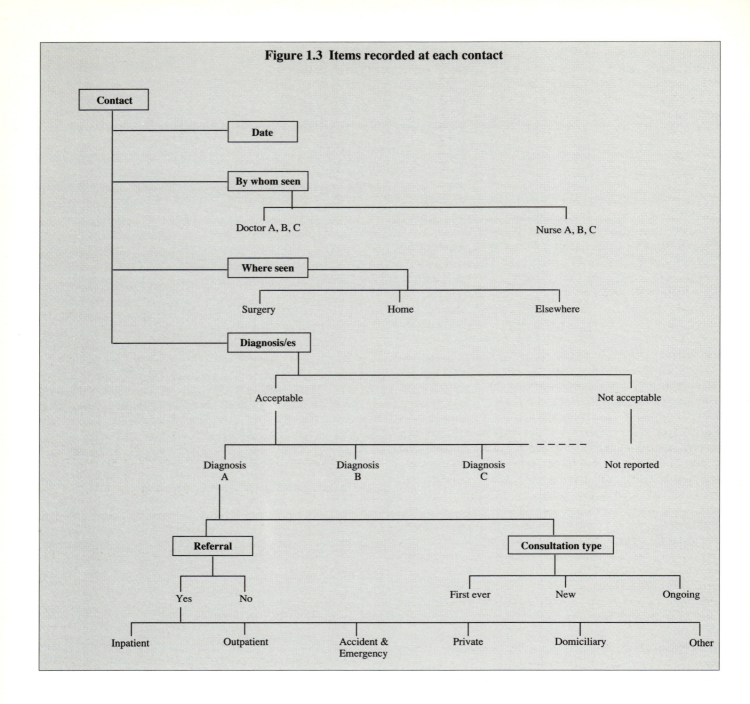

Figure 1.3 Items recorded at each contact

Contact
- Date
- By whom seen
  - Doctor A, B, C
  - Nurse A, B, C
- Where seen
  - Surgery
  - Home
  - Elsewhere
- Diagnosis/es
  - Acceptable
    - Diagnosis A
    - Diagnosis B
    - Diagnosis C
  - Not acceptable
    - Not reported

Diagnosis A
- Referral
  - Yes
    - Inpatient
    - Outpatient
    - Accident & Emergency
  - No
- Consultation type
  - First ever
  - New
  - Ongoing
  - Private
  - Domiciliary
  - Other

because some of the work previously carried out by doctors has now been delegated to practice nurses. Nurses not employed by the practices were not included because they do not come under the direct control of general practitioners and usually perform a different range of tasks.

A doctor/nurse code was assigned to each patient contact. If a patient was seen by another doctor or a nurse immediately after having been seen by a doctor and without leaving the premises, the first contact only was recorded. If a doctor saw a patient immediately after having been seen by a nurse, only the contact with the doctor was recorded.

Place of contact

Practices recorded whether the contact took place in the surgery (S), at home (V) or elsewhere (E). If a doctor held a routine general practice-type clinic in an institution such as a boarding school or old people's home, these were recorded as surgery consultations. If on the other hand he was called to see a patient in an institution as an emergency it was recorded as a home visit. When a doctor, while carrying out sessions in a local accident and emergency department, saw a patient on his ASR in the course of his accident and emergency duties the contact was not recorded. Attendance on one of a doctor's patients in a factory or in the road, for example, was recorded as having taken place elsewhere. Any consultations for which no place of contact was recorded were assumed to have taken place in the surgery because this was the most frequent location. For 8 per cent of contacts attributed to the surgery the place of contact was not stated.

Referral type

For each consultation, the doctor recorded whether the patient was referred to a medically or dentally qualified practitioner, and if so to which of the following agencies: inpatients, outpatients, an accident and emergency department, a private consultation, a domiciliary consultation or some other. If a patient was referred to outpatients or an accident and emergency department in the expectation that he would be admitted, the referral was an inpatient one.

The completeness of reporting morbidity data

At the end of the study year, each practice was asked to provide information from their manual practice records so that OPCS could compare these with the data on the computer files. Data was requested for four Tuesdays during the study: 8 October 1991, 14 January, 14 April and 14 July 1992. These included lists of people who attended the surgery, those who were visited at home, and those who were referred to outpatients. The study depended upon practices providing OPCS with accurate lists of persons seen in the surgery and those visited at home. They had not been warned beforehand that they would be required to produce these lists. It is possible that some practices sent lists which, particularly for surgery visits, had not been revised if people did not attend or were seen without appointment.

The comparison between over 28,000 manual and computer records studied suggests that 96 per cent of contacts with the doctor in the surgery and 64 per cent with the nurse were reported to OPCS. Of home visits made by a doctor, an estimated 95 per cent were reported. The proportion of referrals reported to OPCS was estimated to be 61 per cent. Staff in practices using software from one software company found it difficult to record referrals. These practices recorded only 50 per cent, compared with 78 and 88 per cent respectively for the practices using software from the other two companies. Although some practices were unable to send part of the data requested, 51 of the 60 practices sent all or most of the records required.

We asked practices to select a number of patients seen on each of the four dates mentioned above from the appointments book. The selection was random, the study person identification number being noted for the seventh person and every subsequent fifth person on the list until the required number, depending upon the size of the practice, was reached. They were asked to photocopy the medical notes for each of these patients and to include the date on which they were seen. The manual medical notes were compared with a computer list generated by OPCS to check whether the correct diagnosis had been transferred from the manual record to the computer record in the practice and whether there were any diagnoses on the manual record which had not been entered on the computer.

Diagnoses were considered correct if the Read code entered was compatible though not exactly what might be expected, and would fall within the same ICD disease related group. Diagnoses were considered wrong if they were outside this definition and the manual notes made no mention of a drug likely to be prescribed for the diagnosis recorded on the computer file. The number of unreported diagnoses was those on the medical records but missing from the computer record.

Morbidity data

Strengths

Practices scattered over England and Wales

Practices varied in terms of characteristics

Most practices were experienced recorders

Large population sample (1% of England and Wales)

Denominators consistent with numerators (person years at risk)

Full year's data

Every event recorded, not selective items

  - 96% of contacts in surgery reported

  - 95% of home visits reported

  - 93% of diagnoses correctly reported

Prevalence and incidence at each level of diagnostic detail

Data recorded by doctors and nurses at grass roots

Service utilisation reported

Combined with socio-economic data for 83% of patients

Weaknesses

Practices covered clusters of population

Not a random sample of practices

Too small sample for rare diseases

Based only on patients presenting for GP care

Referrals and nurse contacts poorly reported by some practices

---

A total of 999 records were examined from 49 practices.

Number of correct diagnoses reported	931
Number of wrong diagnoses reported	41
Number of unreported diagnoses	27
Proportion of correct diagnoses	93%

1.7 Recording socio-economic data

The aim of this part of the study was to obtain information about individuals comparable with that collected in the 1991 census.

Interviewers were appointed by each practice and employed specifically for this purpose. Many were permanent members of the practice staff, seconded for the study and replaced by temporary staff to cover their normal duties. Interviewers received intensive training which involved working through exercises to provide experience and to generate confidence. Patients were handed a standard letter in the surgery before the interview took place, describing the study and assuring them that all information would be treated in confidence and no information identifying individuals would leave the practice. Interviewers were issued with an official authorisation card.

The vast majority of patients were interviewed in the surgery while waiting to see the doctor, either in the waiting room or in a private room. No children were interviewed, the information about them being provided by an adult member of their family. Those interviewed were also asked to give information by proxy about other members of the family who were also on the practice ASR. Patients for whom socio-economic information had not been collected towards the end of the study year were sent a standard letter from the doctors in their practice describing the study and asking them to visit the surgery or to receive a visit at home by the interviewer. If the interviewer was unsuccessful in seeing the patient in his home, a telephone interview was carried out.

Socio-economic information was obtained for 83 per cent of patients, 36 per cent by direct interview and 47 per cent by proxy. Just over one per cent refused to be interviewed. Of the remainder, four per cent were not at the address on the practice ASR having moved or gone away, and eight per cent were not at the stated address and could not be contacted. Three per cent were not interviewed for other reasons. The variation between practices in response rates ranged from 50 per cent in a practice with a population of 11,000 to 98 per cent in each of two practices with populations of 2,000 and 3,000 respectively.

Once the interview was completed, no alterations to the record were made. Missing data were added to records if they became available. For patients who died before interview, a member of the family was asked to supply information applicable to the day before death. Socio-economic interview record forms were used for manual recording of data (see appendix A). These were in similar format to the data entry computer screen used in the practice. Most items on the form were pre-coded. The exceptions were country of birth and occupation which were written in full on the record form and coded later.

Interviewers used prescribed wording when introducing themselves and the study to patients and when asking the questions. Items included in the 1991 census were asked in the same wording as on the census form. However, for the census, the head of the household was deemed to be the person named in the first column of the census form. For this study, the socio-economic details for children related to the child's parent or guardian who may not have been the person who filled in the census form. Where appropriate, a card was shown to the patient listing the alternatives for reply, in the order set out on the census form. This had the added advantage that the patient could point to the answer to minimise possible embarrassment about sensitive issues. For each item the letter R could be ringed if the patient refused to answer that question.

The combinations of codes used for analytical purposes are shown below:

(i) Marital status and cohabiting status
One question was used to provide legal marital status for comparison with the census, and also the cohabiting status of the patient as this was felt to be more relevant for analysis purposes.

The patient was shown a card and asked 'Which describes your marital status?'

Precoded answers	*Legal marital status*
1. Single	Single (1,2)
2. Single living together as a couple	Married (3,4,5)
3. Married	Widowed and divorced (6,7,8,9)
4. Separated	
5. Separated living together as a couple	*Cohabiting status*
6. Divorced	Single (1)
7. Divorced living together as a couple	Married/cohabiting (2,3,5,7,9)
8. Widowed	Separated, widowed and divorced not cohabiting (4,6,8)
9. Widowed living together as a couple	

(ii) Tenure of housing
The patient was shown a card and asked 'Which best describes how you occupy your accommodation?'

Precoded answers	*Tenure*
Owner occupier	Owner occupied (1,2)
1. Buying through mortgage or loan	Council house (4,5)
2. Owns outright (no loan)	Other rented (3,6,7,8)
	Communal establishment (9)
Renting, rent free or by lease	
3. With a job, farm, shop or other business	
4. From a local authority (council)	
5. From a new town development corporation (or commission) or from a housing action trust	
6. From a housing association or charitable trust	
7. From a private landlord - furnished	
8. From a private landlord - unfurnished	
9. Living in a communal establishment	

(iii) Ethnic group

The patient was shown a card and asked 'To which group do you consider you belong?'

Precoded answers	*Ethnic group*
1. White	White (1)
2. Black-Caribbean	Afro-Caribbean (2,3)
3. Black-African	Indian (4)
4. Indian	Pakistani/Bangladeshi (5,6)
5. Pakistani	Other (7,8,9)
6. Bangladeshi	
7. Chinese	
8. Sri Lankan	
9. Other	

The option of 'Black — other' which appeared on the census form list was excluded because the number in the survey was estimated to be small.

(iv) Sole adult in household — yes or no

Patients aged 16 years and over were asked 'Are there any other adults in your household, even if they are not registered with this practice?'

(v) Children under five in household — yes or no

Patients aged 16 years and over were asked 'Are there any children under five years of age living in your household?'

(vi) Children aged five to fifteen in household — yes or no

Patients aged 16 years and over were asked 'Are there any children aged 5 to 15 years in your household?'

(vii) Smoked in the last week — yes or no

Patients aged 16 years and over were asked 'Did you smoke at all in the last seven days?' This applied to the smoking of any tobacco product.

(viii) Economic position last week

Patients aged 16 and over were shown a card and asked 'What were you doing last week?' A similar card was used to ask 'What were you doing one year ago?'

Precoded answers	*Economic position*
1. Working full-time (more than 30 hours a week)	Working full-time (1,3)
2. Working part-time (one hour or more up to and including 30 hours a week)	Working part-time (2)
3. On a government employment or training scheme	Unemployed (4,5)
4. Waiting to start a job which had already been accepted	Permanently sick (7)
5. Unemployed and looking for a job	Home/family (9)
6. At school or other full-time education	Other (6,8)

7. Unable to work because of long-term sickness or disability
8. Retired from paid work
9. Looking after the home or family

(ix) Occupation

Patients aged 16 and over were asked to state their main occupation. This referred to their current job. If they had more than one job, they were asked to state the most remunerative. If they had retired from their main job they were asked to state their main job before retirement. Interviewers were trained to ask for sufficient information about industry and the type of work done to assign an occupation code from a coding list supplied by OPCS. If they had any doubt about coding an occupation, they were asked to telephone the Occupation Information Unit at OPCS for advice.

For analysis in the tables in this volume, codes have been aggregated to the Standard Occupational Classification (SOC)[9] minor group codes (see appendix C).

(x) Employment status

Patients aged 16 and over were shown a card and asked 'Which of these apply to your job?'

Precoded answers
1. Employee
2. Self-employed, employing others
3. Self-employed, no employees
4. Foreman
5. Manager
6. Non-working, i.e. housewife, student, no occupation, etc.

Each patient's social class (for married or cohabiting women their own and their partner's social class, for children their parent or guardian's social class) was derived from the relevant occupation and employment status.

Social class		*Social class groups*
1. I	Professional etc occupations	I & II (1 and 2)
2. II	Intermediate occupations	
3. IIIN	Skilled occupations — non-manual	IIIN (3)
4. IIIM	Skilled occupations — manual	IIIM (4)
5. IV	Partly skilled occupations	IV & V (5 and 6)
6. V	Unskilled occupations	Other (7, 8 and 9)
7. Armed forces		
8. Inadequately described		
9. Unoccupied — includes students, housewives, persons of independent means, permanently sick or disabled, persons who have never worked and occupation not stated		

(xi) Living with sole adult — yes or no

For patients aged under 16 years, the interviewee was asked whether there was only one adult living in the child's household.

Socio-economic data

Strengths

Reliable collection by interview

Response rate was 83%

Questions generally consistent with census

Sample representative for age, sex, marital status, tenure of housing, economic position, occupation, urban or rural place of residence and smoking

Postcode information reported

Weaknesses

No data for 17% of the sample

Social class data not entirely comparable with 1991 census

Ethnic minority groups, people living alone and those in metropolitan areas were under-represented in the sample

---

Questions about the economic position, occupation and employment status of the parents or guardians of children aged under 16 years, and of the partners of married or cohabiting women, were asked in the same way as that described above. A child's parent or guardian was taken to be his father or, if the father did not live in the same household, his stepfather or his mother's cohabitee, or his mother if she was the sole adult in the household, or the head of the household if none of the above was applicable.

Questions about whether there was only one adult in the household and about the parent's economic position, occupation and employment status were not asked of children living in communal establishments. Because age was calculated from the date of birth to be that on 1 March 1992, there were a few children whose sixteenth birthday fell between the date of interview and 1 March 1992 and who were asked questions appropriate to those aged 16 years or over. This will have inflated the number apparently aged 16 or over who were still in full-time education. Conversely, those whose 16th birthday fell between 1 March 1992 and the end of the study year were not asked questions applicable to those aged 16 years and over, being under 16 for the purposes of the study.

No attempt was made to validate the socio-economic data collected.

1.8 Interpretation of the data

An understanding of how the data have been collected and processed is needed for correct interpretation. A few of the points to be considered are listed here.

- The results indicate the levels of illness seen in general practice, which may be different from those in the population as a whole.

- The pattern of care is constantly changing. Devolution from hospitals to general practice, and from doctors to nurses, has increased over recent years. The number of practice-employed nurses has increased. Targets and related payments for health promotion have induced greater activity in this area of work. As a result, comparisons with previous studies require care.

- The terms used in this volume should be understood. In particular, the terms for patients consulting, consultations and contacts should not be confused. (See appendix B)

- Some of the data were not reported by practices. For 17 per cent of patients no socio-economic data were collected. The place of contact was not recorded for 8 per cent of contacts, and these were assumed to have taken place in the surgery. Referrals were under-reported, and the referral data based on the full study population are therefore unreliable. Researchers using the datasets are advised to use referral data about the patients whose records have been flagged appropriately. These patients attended 28 practices which are each estimated to have reported at least 60 per cent of referrals to outpatient departments. The practices cared for 236,000 patients and, overall, reported 77 per cent of referrals. Contacts between patients and practice nurses were also under-reported. As a result, patient consulting rates for conditions for which only the nurse may be seen are unreliable.

- There is some variation between the diagnosis assigned by different doctors, or by the same doctor on different occasions. A patient may therefore be counted as a patient consulting for the same illness more than once at a detailed level of coding. These rates cannot be summed to estimate a rate at a less detailed diagnostic level because some patients may be counted more than once.

- About half the practices used the four-character version of the Read classification. These codes were mapped to the more detailed five-character version at OPCS. The numbers in individual five-character codes are therefore biased towards those which corresponded to a four-character code.

- Some diagnostic codes, notably those corresponding to ICD 239.9 (neoplasm of unspecified nature, site unspecified), ICD 995.8 (other specified adverse effects not elsewhere classified), ICD E988.9 (injury by other and unspecified means) and ICD 799.9 (other unknown and unspecified cause) were used as default codes. As a result the numbers and rates for these conditions are unreliable.

- The Read code corresponding to the external cause (E) ICD9 code was recorded whenever a Read code corresponding to an ICD9 code in the injury and poisoning chapter was recorded and the consultation was a first ever (F) or new (N) one. The E codes should therefore not be included in the calculation of rates for all causes or all illnesses because patients with these codes would be counted twice.

- The assignment of the severity of an illness to each diagnostic code was done at OPCS. This was therefore independent of whether the reporting doctor considered an individual patient's illness to be serious, intermediate or minor.

- The prevalence of an illness is expressed in this volume as the rate of persons consulting at least once during the year for that illness. This rate is increased if the duration of the illness, or the survival time between diagnosis and death, lengthens, although the incidence or 'new cases' rate may not have altered.

1.9 Some uses of the data from this survey

This survey, like its predecessors, was a surveillance survey. It was designed to collect data which are routinely available in general practice. It was not intended to answer specific hypotheses, but to form a basis from which hypotheses could be generated. The results provide much useful information about who consults the primary care services, where they are seen and for which conditions. Combined with the socio-economic data collected about individuals, they give an estimate of the services which need to be planned for the care of particular population groups.

The data themselves give an estimate of the incidence and prevalence of disease in the community as a whole, and of the changes over time. The commentary in this volume covers a brief and necessarily superficial analysis of some aspects of the expressed need for general practitioner services. It is hoped that others will use the data both to help them solve their own problems and to delve more deeply into some of the questions which the data generate.

The results from this survey can be used for health care planning. In particular, they provide an estimate of the prevalence of disease over a large population which can be compared with local studies of the same nature. Any differences found will raise questions. Is this an artefact due to different definitions or methods of data collection or analysis? Are all cases being diagnosed? Are there really differences in prevalence and, if so, why? By the use of synthetic estimation, the results of this study can be applied to different, perhaps local, populations, taking account of any differences in the socio-economic structure of the population. The expected incidence, prevalence or consultation rates in that population can be estimated. This can be used for health care planning, or for health education, targeting the groups most at risk. The relationship between incidence and prevalence rates will give an estimate of duration of the disease or the survival time from diagnosis, and the difference over time may indicate both the effect of treatment and changes in the kind of care which will be needed.

Researchers with particular interests can use the data for many purposes. For example, the relationship between one condition and another can be studied, as can the association between a disease and people in a particular socio-economic group. The prevalence of a disease found in this survey can be of help in estimating the sample size required for other studies on a particular subject. Individuals with specific problems can, with the necessary ethical approval and the collaboration of the appropriate participating practices, be co-opted into more detailed and longer-term studies. These data can be compared with those from other sources such as mortality statistics. The incidence to mortality ratio among people in different socio-economic groups of the population or those in different regions of the country can then be identified.

Anonymised data from this survey are available on disk and can be obtained from OPCS (see appendix F). It is hoped that they will be widely used to their full potential.

2 Results

2.1 Introduction

The results of this study give the most comprehensive information available about the people who consult their general practitioners and the doctor's perception of what is wrong with them. The sample covered is large: 500,000 people, one per cent of the population of England and Wales. The level of reporting contacts was high and the diagnoses recorded on computer corresponded well with those on manual notes kept in the practices.

The main aim of the study was to collect data on illness seen in general practice. It is accepted that this does not reflect all morbidity in the community although it is likely that patients with the more serious conditions will consult their general practitioner at some time during their illness. In deciding whether to consult a general practitioner a patient may be influenced by the severity of the problem, the expectation that he may be helped, the accessibility of the surgery premises, the need for sickness certification and the availability of alternative sources of care such as accident and emergency departments and family planning clinics.

As a result, morbidity presenting to general practitioners measures a need expressed by individuals to one source of health care. Over the last few years, the pattern of much work done in general practice has changed. For example, health promotion has become more a feature of primary care than it was in the past. The routine care of many with chronic conditions such as diabetes has fallen on general practice rather than hospital clinics. Such changes are reflected in the results of studies of morbidity seen in primary care, but do not necessarily indicate any change in the incidence or prevalence of disease.

Prevalence of ill-health can also be estimated by population interview surveys such as the General Household Survey.[7] This provides data on self reported long-standing illness and includes those for which the patient did not contact his general practitioner. The new Health Survey for England[10] concentrates on cardiovascular disease and estimates the prevalence of symptoms, conditions and risk factors. Some of the latter are derived by taking standard measurements in the interviewee's home.

The population covered by a national survey such as MSGP4 comprises groups of people clustered around the sites of participating practices. Such a sample is adequate for estimating the incidence and prevalence of common diseases which tend to be randomly distributed within broad areas of the country. However, some diseases, such as many communicable diseases, frequently occur in clusters and a clustered sample may not produce such reliable estimates for the country as a whole.

Doctors, both individually and collectively, may be inconsistent in assigning particular diagnostic codes to the same conditions. For example, one doctor may record depression as the reason for a consultation, while another may record a marital problem as being the cause of the depression. This diversity in diagnostic recording has been discussed by Crombie.[11] He concluded from studies of the data collected during the second National Morbidity Study that individual doctors are consistent from year to year in assignment of codes within ICD chapters and that if the population at risk is sufficiently large, variations between ICD chapters cancel out.

The data provide estimates of the incidence and prevalence of disease seen in general practice. In this report, the *incidence*, or number of new episodes of a condition or group of conditions diagnosed during the year, is the sum of first ever (F) and new (N) episodes reported. This holds good both for acute self-limiting disease, such as acute infections, where a subject returns to the denominator after recovery. However, for most chronic degenerative diseases such as strokes, heart attacks or chronic obstructive airways conditions, a subsequent episode represents a recurrence. Examples of these from the study are shown in the box below.

Episodes per 10,000 person years at risk

ICD		First	First & New
410	Acute myocardial infarction	15	23
413	Angina pectoris	21	52
436	Acute but ill-defined cerebrovascular disease	11	18
493	Asthma	81	297
496	Chronic airways obstruction NEC	4	24

Prevalence is the term used for annual period prevalence. This is the level of presence of a disease during the year and is defined as being the number of persons who consulted at least once for a condition or a group of conditions during the year. Incidence and prevalence are shown in the main tables as rates per 10,000 person years at risk, or, in the case of tables by sex, as rates per 10,000 years at risk for that sex. It is possible for an individual to contribute once to the *prevalence* of a disease, but several times to the *incidence* of that disease if he has experienced more than one distinct episode of that disease during the year.

These data provide an insight into the demand made on the health service at the main point of entry. They apply to activity during 1991-92 and there are many reasons, such as the new general practice contract and implementation of NHS reforms, why the occurrence of disease seen in general practice in that year may differ from that seen in previous or in subsequent years.

2.2 Use of services

Patient consulting rates

During the year, 78 per cent of patients consulted at least once. Rates were highest among small children (fig 2.1). Many consultations were for children born during the year. While most of these will have consulted, they were only in the study for part of the year, contributing relatively few days to the person years at risk, thus diminishing the size of the denominator. As an example, if each of four children were registered with a practice for only three months they would together contribute one person year at risk. If each consulted they would be counted as four persons consulting: a rate of 40,000 per 10,000 person years at risk. This explains the 102 per cent patient consulting rate among children aged under five years. It is surprising that only 92 per cent of people aged 85 years and over apparently consulted during the year. This may be due to an inflated denominator caused by delay in the removal of patients from the ASR after death or transfer to an institution from which they may not have had to call upon the general practitioner's services.

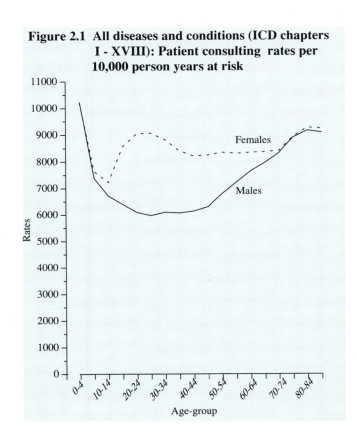

Figure 2.1 All diseases and conditions (ICD chapters I - XVIII): Patient consulting rates per 10,000 person years at risk

A higher proportion of people consulted for respiratory conditions at least once during the year (31 per cent) than for diseases in any other single ICD chapter, apart from reasons for consulting in the supplementary classification (fig 2.2). The rate was highest among small children (fig .25). Next in order of magnitude was the proportion of people who consulted for diseases of the nervous system and sense organs. Seventeen per cent of people of all ages consulted for these conditions, the highest rate being again among small children (fig 2.20), largely accounted for by infections of the ear. Diseases of the musculoskeletal system caused 15 per cent of people to consult, the rate increasing with age (fig 2.30). For diseases of the skin 15 per cent consulted; these were fairly evenly distributed across all ages, although the rate was once again highest among children under five years of age (fig 2.29). Overall, 14 per cent consulted for infectious or parasitic diseases. The highest rate was among small children and decreased with advancing age except among the elderly (fig 2.12). While 14 per cent of people of all ages consulted for injury or poisoning, rates were higher for males than for females under 30 years of age and lower among older age groups (fig 2.32).

Overall, 20 per cent of people consulted at least once for a condition assigned to the serious category. The rate increased with age (fig 2.3). For diseases in the intermediate category of severity, 54 per cent consulted at least once. The highest rate was among the young (fig 2.4). Within the intermediate category, a large proportion of children aged under five years consulted for infectious and parasitic diseases (33 per cent) and for diseases of the nervous system and sense organs (30 per cent), the respiratory system (25 per cent) and the skin (23 per cent). For the minor group of conditions, 62 per cent consulted (fig 2.5). Again, the rate was highest among young children. A large proportion of the total population consulted for minor diseases of the respiratory system (52 per cent), and for reasons in the supplementary classification (53 per cent). (The supplementary classification of the ICD consists of codes prefixed by 'V'. These cover circumstances other than disease or injury not found elsewhere in the ICD. They include encounters for prophylactic immunisation or to discuss a problem which is not in itself a disease or injury, such as contraception. In the tables the supplementary classification is sometimes referred to as ICD Chapter XVIII.) Patient consulting rates for all illnesses, which excludes the supplementary classification, are shown in figure 2.6.

The main reasons for which children consulted included procedures in the supplementary classification, notably immunisations and health supervision, respiratory illnesses and otitis media.

Between the ages of 15 and 64 years the consulting rate for women exceeded that for men (fig 2.1). The chapters for which this difference was most evident include genitourinary disease, mental disorders, diseases of the blood and blood-forming organs, symptoms, signs and ill-defined conditions, and for reasons in the supplementary classification.

Among the elderly, a higher proportion consulted for circulatory disorders and respiratory diseases than for any other group of illnesses, although many consulted for reasons coded in the supplementary classification, particularly immunisation against influenza and tetanus, and general medical examinations.

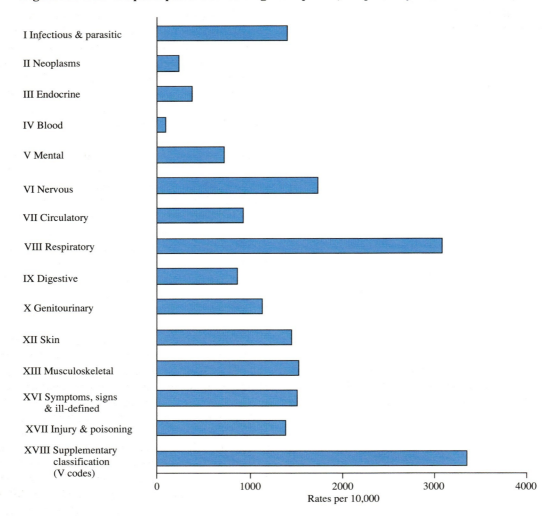

Figure 2.2 ICD chapters patient consulting rates per 10,000 person years at risk

I Infectious & parasitic

II Neoplasms

III Endocrine

IV Blood

V Mental

VI Nervous

VII Circulatory

VIII Respiratory

IX Digestive

X Genitourinary

XII Skin

XIII Musculoskeletal

XVI Symptoms, signs & ill-defined

XVII Injury & poisoning

XVIII Supplementary classification (V codes)

Rates per 10,000

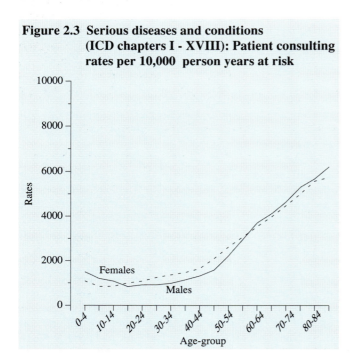

Figure 2.3 Serious diseases and conditions (ICD chapters I - XVIII): Patient consulting rates per 10,000 person years at risk

Rates

Females

Males

Age-group

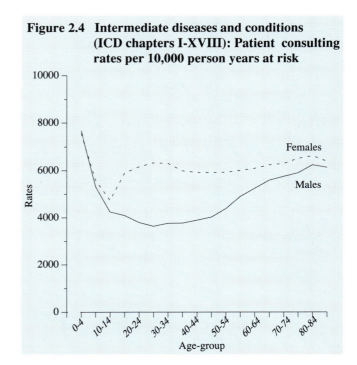

Figure 2.4 Intermediate diseases and conditions (ICD chapters I-XVIII): Patient consulting rates per 10,000 person years at risk

Rates

Females

Males

Age-group

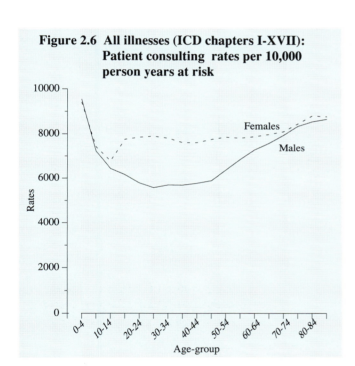

Figure 2.5 Minor diseases and conditions (ICD chapters I-XVIII): Patient consulting rates per 10,000 person years at risk

Females

Males

Rates

Age-group

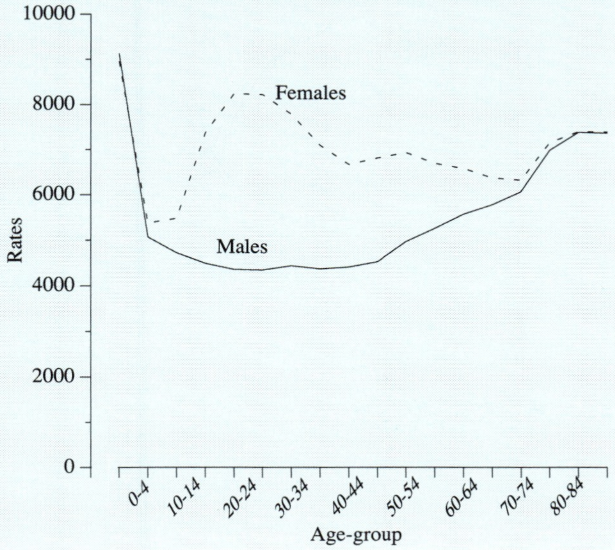

Figure 2.6 All illnesses (ICD chapters I-XVII): Patient consulting rates per 10,000 person years at risk

Females

Males

Rates

Age-group

The number and locations of contacts with a doctor

Each face-to-face meeting between a patient and a doctor and/or a practice nurse was considered to be a *contact*. There were a total of 1,374,014 contacts made with a doctor during the year, representing 29,358 per 10,000 person years at risk. On average, each person saw a doctor 2.9 times during the year. However, because only 78 per cent of patients consulted at least once during the year, those who did consult saw the doctor on average 3.8 times.

The number of contacts reported in the study can be validated against the General Household Survey (GHS). This is a continuous national survey carrying out approximately 19,000 interviews in private households each year. Respondents are asked whether they have spoken to a doctor for any reason during the previous two weeks, either on behalf of themselves or another person, and if so, how many times. In 1991 eight per cent of these contacts were by telephone and have been excluded for the purposes of this comparison. Annual estimates of contacts with a general practitioner are reached by multiplying the contact rate by twenty-six.

Comparison of GHS and MSGP4 rates for reported contacts shows that GHS rates are consistently higher than the MSGP4 rates, except among elderly women (table 2A and fig 2.7). However, it is estimated that 96 per cent of contacts were recorded on the MSGP4 survey (see page 19). The discrepancy may have resulted for a number of reasons. The GHS relies upon correct recall by the patient, and a reported contact may have been outside the two week period. The patient may not have been clear whether they saw the doctor himself or only the practice nurse. In both these circumstances the GHS rate would be inflated. The MSGP4 rate for all contacts with the doctor or practice nurse approximate more closely than that with the doctor alone to the GHS figure.

MSGP4 contact rates were half as high again for females than for males. This difference occurred among women of all age groups except the young and very old, and was mainly confined to visits to the surgery (fig 2.8). It was greatest among women aged 15-44 years. Contact rates were highest for people aged 85 years and over, who saw a doctor on average 4.7 times; nearly two-thirds of these contacts were in the patient's home (table 2B). Among 75-84 year olds, 4.4

Table 2A Average contact rates per 10,000 person years at risk, recorded by the General Household Survey and the Morbidity Survey

	0-4	5-15	16-44	45-64	65-74	75 and over
Males						
GHS	6.8	2.8	2.4	3.5	4.8	6.9
MSGP4						
- doctor contacts	5.1	2.3	2.1	3.0	4.2	5.6
- all contacts	5.5	2.4	2.2	3.3	4.8	6.4
Females						
GHS	6.5	2.9	4.8	4.9	5.4	5.4
MSGP4						
- doctor contacts	4.8	2.6	4.2	4.0	4.6	6.3
- all contacts	5.3	2.7	4.6	4.5	5.3	7.1

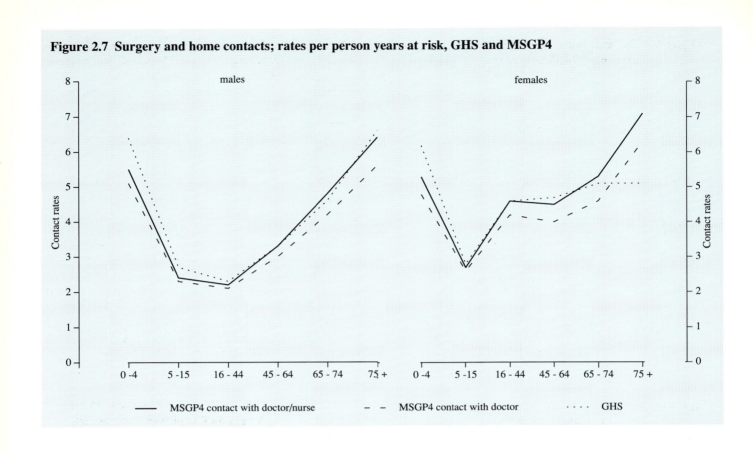

Figure 2.7 Surgery and home contacts; rates per person years at risk, GHS and MSGP4

males

females

Contact rates

Contact rates

| 0 -4 | 5 -15 | 16 - 44 | 45 - 64 | 65 - 74 | 75 + |

MSGP4 contact with doctor/nurse — — — MSGP4 contact with doctor · · · · GHS

Table 2B Patient contacts with practice, by age, sex, place of consultation, and whom consulted
Rates per 10,000 persons years at risk

	Total	0-4	5-15	16-24	25-44	45-64	65-74	75-84	85 and over
All doctors									
Surgery	26,216	39,976	18,192	24,458	24,875	28,179	31,460	28,322	16,257
Home	2,953	4,716	1,252	997	1,111	1,655	5,583	15,027	29,828
Elsewhere	189	244	176	176	135	196	182	379	570
Principals									
Surgery	23,174	34,205	15,525	20,624	21,760	25,616	29,251	26,516	15,142
Home	2,446	3,252	902	771	885	1,390	4,801	13,235	26,396
Elsewhere	176	210	163	161	123	190	171	361	568
Assistants									
Surgery	478	863	382	495	502	427	420	425	185
Home	56	161	38	23	29	29	80	223	281
Elsewhere	1	5	1	1	2	0	1	1	4
Trainees									
Surgery	2,195	4,322	2,017	2,712	2,237	1,821	1,542	1,216	881
Home	293	583	157	106	106	151	542	1,360	2,837
Elsewhere	3	4	2	5	3	2	4	7	18
Locums									
Surgery	395	647	320	643	392	329	267	210	136
Home	181	751	167	121	102	98	178	340	505
Elsewhere	11	32	12	14	9	6	10	14	9
Practice nurses									
Surgery	3,114	4,129	1,298	1,976	2,492	3,981	5,711	5,656	2,840
Home	50	37	8	6	7	11	44	549	718
Elsewhere	3	5	2	2	2	2	5	9	12

Figure 2.8 Contacts with a doctor in the surgery, rates per 10,000 person years at risk

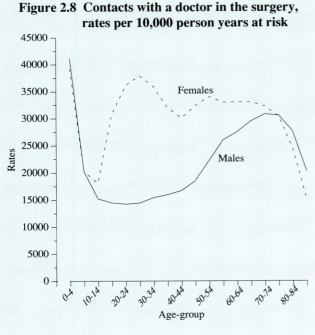

Figure 2.10 Contacts with a practice nurse in the surgery, rates per 10,000 person years at risk

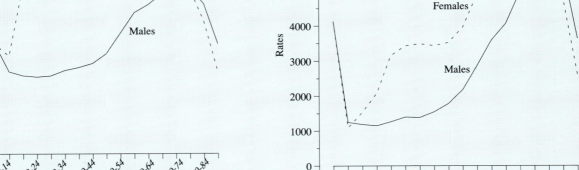

Figure 2.9 Contacts with a doctor at home, rates per 10,000 person years at risk

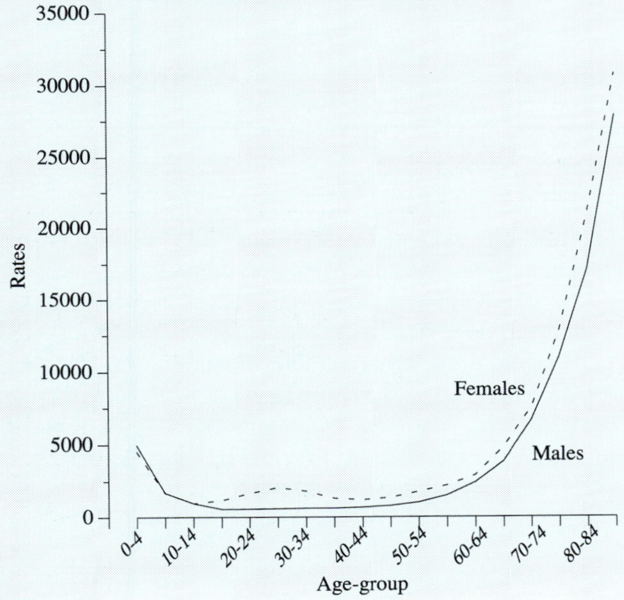

Figure 2.11 Contacts with a practice nurse at home, rates per 10,000 person years at risk

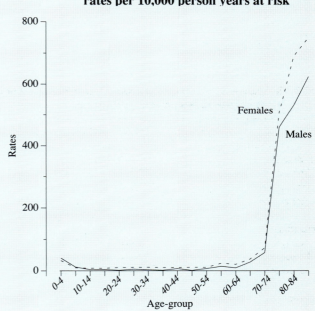

contacts were made on average by each patient, about one third being in the patient's home. Children under five years of age saw the doctor on average 4.5 times, although this figure may be a high estimate because of the diminution in the size of the denominator as described earlier (page 25).

Of all contacts with a doctor, 89 per cent took place in the surgery, 10 per cent in the patient's home and the remaining one per cent elsewhere (table 2D). Home visiting rates by doctors were low among adults but increased steadily with advancing age among the elderly and were slightly higher for all ages among females than males (fig 2.9). Of all home visits made by a doctor, 25 per cent were to people aged 75-84 years and 15 per cent to people aged 85 years and over; 11 per cent were to children aged under one year (table 2E).

Of the 1,374,014 contacts with a doctor, 88 per cent were with a principal doctor, 8 per cent with a trainee, 2 per cent with a locum and 2 per cent with an assistant (table 2C). Between 88 and 90 per cent of contacts with principal, assistant or trainee doctors were in the surgery, compared with 67 per cent with a locum doctor. Between 9 and 12 per cent of contacts with principal, assistant or trainee doctors were made in the patient's home, 31 per cent of contacts by a locum were home visits (table 2D).

Of all home visits carried out by a doctor, 82 per cent were made by a principal doctor, 10 per cent by a trainee, 6 per cent by a locum and 2 per cent by an assistant (table 2C).

Table 2C   Per cent of all doctor contacts, by type of doctor, place of contact and age group of patient

	Total	0-4	5-15	16-24	25-44	45-64	65-74	75-84	85 and over
All doctors									
Surgery	100	100	100	100	100	100	100	100	100
Home	100	100	100	100	100	100	100	100	100
Elsewhere	100	100	100	100	100	100	100	100	100
Total	100	100	100	100	100	100	100	100	100
Principals									
Surgery	88	85	85	84	87	91	93	93	93
Home	82	69	71	76	79	83	86	87	88
Elsewhere	92	84	91	89	90	96	92	94	95
Total	88	84	84	84	87	90	92	91	90
Assistants									
Surgery	2	2	2	2	2	2	1	1	1
Home	2	3	3	2	3	2	1	1	1
Elsewhere	1	2	1	1	1	0	0	0	1
Total	2	2	2	2	2	2	1	1	1
Trainees									
Surgery	8	11	11	11	9	6	5	4	5
Home	10	12	12	10	9	9	10	9	9
Elsewhere	2	1	1	3	2	1	2	2	3
Total	8	11	11	11	9	7	6	6	8
Locums									
Surgery	2	2	2	3	2	1	1	1	1
Home	6	16	13	12	9	6	3	2	2
Elsewhere	6	13	7	8	6	3	5	4	1
Total	2	3	3	3	2	1	1	1	1

Table 2D   Per cent of contacts by place of contact for different types of doctor

	All contacts	Surgery	Home	Elsewhere
All doctors	100	89	10	1
Principals	100	90	9	1
Assistants	100	89	10	0
Trainees	100	88	12	0
Locums	100	67	31	2

The number and place of contacts with a practice nurse

Practice nurses were reported to have made 148,299 contacts with patients who had not been seen immediately before by a doctor during the year. From the evaluation study it is clear that many of these practice nurse contacts were not reported, so this figure is clearly an underestimate For these reasons, the data do not reflect the entire range of work carried out by practice nurses. However, the distribution by age of patient and place of contact may give an indication of practice nurses' activity (table 2E).

Table 2E   Per cent of all contacts by doctors/practice nurses by place of contact and age of patient

	All contacts	0-4	5-15	16-24	25-44	45-64	65-74	75-84	85 and over
Doctors									
Surgery	100	10	10	12	29	23	10	5	1
Home	100	11	6	4	12	12	15	25	15
Elsewhere	100	9	13	12	22	22	8	10	4
All sites	100	11	9	11	27	22	10	7	2
Practice nurses									
Surgery	100	9	6	8	25	27	15	9	1
Home	100	5	2	1	4	5	7	55	21
Elsewhere	100	12	10	8	20	17	14	15	6
All sites	100	9	6	8	24	27	15	10	2

Table 2F Number of contacts and consultations, and consultation/contact ratio, by age of patient

	All ages	0-15	16-64	65-74	75 and over
Number of contacts	1,374,014	271,956	826,086	142,332	133,640
Number of consultations	1,628,042	299,546	992,110	174,092	162,294
Consultation/contact ratio	1.2	1.1	1.2	1.2	1.2

The highest contact rate by a practice nurse was with patients aged 75-84 years, with a slightly lower rate with those aged 65-74 years. In the surgery, contact rates were high among children and among women aged 15-45 years. Above that age, rates increased steadily for both sexes until 75 years of age (fig 2.10). Contact rates by nurses in the patient's home were low until 70 years of age and then increased to a relatively high rate among the elderly: nine per cent for patients aged 75-84 and 20 per cent for those aged 85 years over, compared with less than two per cent for patients of all ages (fig 2.11).

Of all home visits made by a practice nurse, 76 per cent were to those aged 75 years and over (table 2E).

Consultations

Each diagnosis reported during each contact was considered to be a consultation.

There were 1,628,042 consultations with a doctor during the year, a rate of 34,785 per 10,000 person years at risk. This was an average of 1.2 consultations during each contact. The ratio did not vary between different age groups (table 2F).

Referrals

Practices were asked to report all referrals to a qualified medical or dental practitioner. The evaluation exercise carried out after the end of the study suggested that only 61 per cent of referrals to outpatient departments were reported. This was partly due to problems with recording referrals on the practice software. In particular, the software from one company was so designed that referrals to outpatient departments were frequently coded as 'other' referrals. The data presented should therefore be interpreted with caution and most of the 'other' referrals assumed to be to outpatient departments. However, assuming that there is no other bias in the referrals that were reported, the distribution by age and sex is of interest and is shown in table 2G.

Over the age of four years, the referral rate increased steadily with age. In each age group, some patients were referred more than once. Between 16 and 64 years, the rates were higher for women than for men. This was reversed among those aged 65 and over. Under the age of five years, the ratio of boys to girls for all referrals was 1.4.

The highest referral rates among all age groups and both sexes were to outpatient departments, irrespective of whether these included referrals of the 'other' type. A relatively high proportion of children aged under five years were referred to accident and emergency departments, the rate for them only being exceeded by that for people aged 75 years and over.

Referral rates to inpatient beds were also relatively high among children aged under five years and did not reach the same level among adults until 65-74 years. Inpatient referral rates were higher for women than for men in the 16-44 age group, but this pattern was reversed among older adults. Referral rates for private consultations were highest for both males and females aged 45-64 years. Rates for domiciliary referrals were low for people aged under 75 years and highest among the very elderly.

Table 2G Persons referred and referrals, by age, sex, and type of referral
Rates per 10,000 person years at risk

	Age-group and sex															
	0-4		5-15		16-24		25-44		45-64		65-74		75-84		85 and over	
	M	F	M	F	M	F	M	F	M	F	M	F	M	F	M	F
Persons referred	1,158	834	701	641	719	1,183	822	1,452	1,191	1,429	1,664	1,610	2,304	2,042	2,555	2,138
Referrals, by type																
All referrals	1,321	925	766	700	781	1,352	915	1,688	1,376	1,661	2,013	1,919	2,900	2,548	3,304	2,733
In-patient	149	101	37	37	34	97	32	85	81	73	199	166	455	343	666	561
Out-patient	577	390	360	337	357	712	458	955	685	880	1,008	1,000	1,112	997	1,052	798
Accident and emergency	258	180	101	73	71	123	59	109	115	95	225	159	427	343	707	506
Private consultation	35	26	25	30	21	41	66	83	100	117	75	70	82	72	48	45
Domiciliary	4	-	1	1	1	2	4	6	5	7	20	14	71	63	113	118
Other	300	228	242	223	297	377	296	450	390	490	486	510	753	730	719	703

2.3 ICD Chapters

Infectious and parasitic diseases

In all, 14 per cent of people consulted at least once for a disease in this group. Prevalence was highest among small children and diminished with age (fig 2.12).

The highest prevalence rate among the disease related groups (ICD subheadings) was for the mycoses (fungi), particularly for candidiases (thrush) among small children of both sexes and among young adult and middle-aged women. Candidiasis accounted for 699 consultations per 10,000 children under five years of age, the majority being infections of the mouth, and nearly 1,200 consultations per 10,000 among women aged 16-44 years, mostly for vulvovaginitis. On average, nearly half the women infected consulted more than once for this infection (table 2H).

More children with chickenpox saw their doctor than with any other childhood infection. The rate for people consulting for herpes zoster was highest among the elderly (table 2H). Herpes simplex was prevalent among young adult women, genital herpes occurring three times as often among women aged 16-44 years as among men of the same age (table 2H). There was a high number of older children of both sexes who consulted for 'other diseases due to viruses and Chlamydiae', compared with a smaller number among women in early adulthood. These were nearly all viral warts, prevalence being highest among children aged 5-15 years, and higher among females than males in all age groups up to 45-64 years (table 2H). Infectious mononucleosis (glandular fever) showed peak prevalence among young adults aged 16-24 years (table 2H).

There was also a high prevalence of intestinal infections, nearly all of ill-defined nature and predominantly among young children, although occurring among people of all ages (table 2H).

Among the ICD group termed 'other intestinal helminth infections', 40 persons per 10,000 consulted for threadworms, the rate being highest among children. Headlice was the reason for 27 per 10,000 to consult, being more prevalent

Figure 2.12 Infectious and parasitic diseases (ICD chapter I): Patient consulting rates per 10,000 person years at risk

among children aged under 5 years (81 per 10,000) and 5-15 years (112 per 10,000). Scabies occurred among people in all age groups, with a high rate among the very elderly (table 2H), and a slight predominance among females.

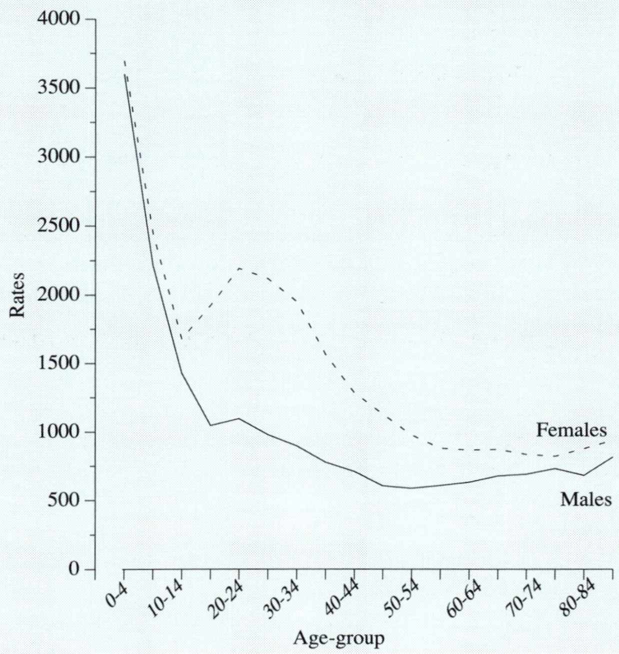

A few reported cases of infections which are rare in this country may reflect incorrect coding; the infection itself may have been recorded instead of immunisation against it. A number of these were identified during editing at OPCS and the codes were rectified by the practices, but when these were not amended by the practices they were left unchanged on the files held by OPCS. For example, one in 10,000 people were reported to have had tetanus, when only a single case would have been expected in a sample of this size. For the same reason, the prevalence of measles, mumps, rubella, diphtheria, whooping cough and poliomyelitis may be inflated.

Table 2H Summary for selected infectious and parasitic diseases

	0-4	5-15	16-24	25-44	45-64	65-74	75-84	85+
Candidasis (ICD 112.0, 112.1 + 112.2): *prevalence rates per 10,000 person years at risk, by sex*								
Mouth								
Males	305	13	10	13	23	57	82	77
Females	343	18	19	29	48	84	78	81
M/F ratio	0.9	0.7	0.5	0.4	0.5	0.7	1.1	1.0
Urogenital								
Males	109	12	58	53	30	24	23	6
Females	234	93	837	813	239	84	52	47
M/F ratio	0.5	0.1	0.1	0.1	0.1	0.3	0.4	0.1

Table 2H - *continued*

	0-4	5-15	16-24	25-44	45-64	65-74	75-84	85+
Candidiasis (ICD 112): *rates per 10,000 female years at risk*								
Incidence	674	127	1,041	998	319	188	158	146
Prevalence	644	123	887	870	302	181	150	146
Consultations	832	149	1,195	1,164	385	240	200	171
Herpes zoster (ICD 053): *rates per 10,000 person years at risk*								
Incidence	10	27	24	28	61	108	118	130
Prevalence	10	27	24	29	63	119	138	146
Consultations	13	32	31	42	102	240	259	308
Herpes simplex (ICD 054.1, 054.2): *Prevalence rates per 10,000 person years at risk, by sex*								
Genital								
Males	18	21	30	27	18	20	9	-
Females	24	38	89	85	48	35	19	14
M/F ratio	0.7	0.6	0.3	0.3	0.4	0.6	0.5	-
Oral								
Males	29	11	6	6	3	8	7	-
Females	27	16	16	22	12	8	8	2
M/F ratio	1.1	0.7	0.4	0.3	0.2	1.0	0.9	-
Viral warts (ICD 078.1): *prevalence rates per 10,000 person years at risk, by sex*								
Males	126	551	231	117	71	59	35	42
Females	131	627	301	150	76	50	42	14
M/F ratio	1.0	0.9	0.8	0.8	0.9	1.2	0.8	3.0
Infectious mononucleosis (ICD 075): *rates per 10,000 person years at risk*								
Incidence	2	14	38	5	1	1	-	-
Prevalence	3	16	46	7	1	1	-	-
Consultations	4	23	77	10	1	2	-	-
Ill-defined intestinal infections (ICD 009): *rates per 10,000 person years at risk*								
Incidence	2,011	387	366	284	198	233	311	445
Prevalence	1,827	379	362	281	201	234	313	435
Consultations	2,541	428	428	337	242	296	415	580
Scabies (ICD 133.0): *prevalence rates per 10,000 person years at risk, by sex*								
Males	50	51	45	24	13	8	15	30
Females	47	66	69	35	21	8	18	49
M/F ratio	1.1	0.8	0.7	0.7	0.6	1.0	0.8	0.6

Neoplasms

The ICD chapter of neoplasms includes both malignant and benign growths. While 239 patients per 10,000 person years at risk consulted for a neoplastic disorder (fig 2.13), less than half of these consulted for malignant disease (fig 2.14). The prevalence of malignant disease in both sexes increased with advancing age, while that of benign disease was greatest among adults, mainly women, and declined among the elderly (fig 2.15).

Where it is usual for patients to continue in a programme of follow-up checks, the relationship between incidence and prevalence gives some idea of the length of time between diagnosis and death, the greater the difference indicating a longer average survival time. For example, among those aged 45-64 years, the ratio of prevalence to incidence for cancer of the breast is 5.5, reflecting survival time of approximately five years, compared with a ratio of two for cancer of the lung, for which the average survival time is much shorter, often less than a year.

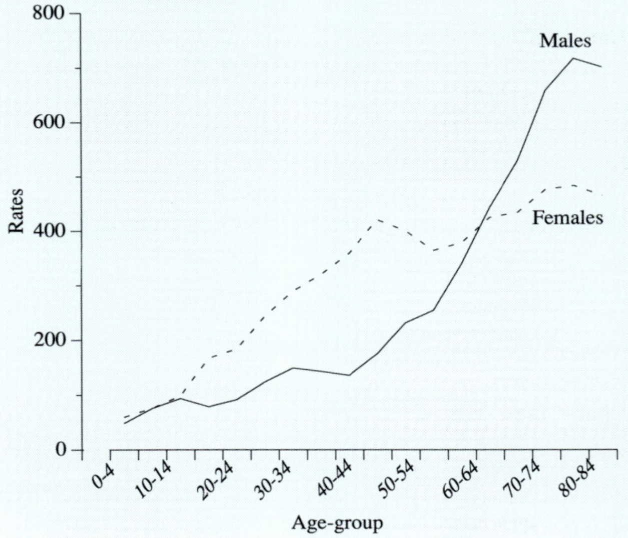

The average number of consultations made by each person who consulted for a condition gives an indication of the amount of care required for people with that disease. This may be biased because a relatively small difference between the number of patients consulting and the number of consultations may reflect the success of treatment, with a high proportion of people consulting rarely for a checkup, while a large difference may reflect those in the early or terminal stages of a more rapidly developing disease who would be expected to consult more frequently.

The incidence rates for individual cancers found in this study are compared with the rates of new cases reported to cancer registries in England and Wales, which are published by OPCS.[12] Registrations are made by clinicians and pathologists to regional cancer registries. The method of reporting varies between regions. There are several reasons why the incidence of cancers reported in MSGP4 may differ from

cancer registrations. The incidence of some cancers varies geographically and areas with high incidence may not have been represented in the study sample. While registrations of most cancers, particularly cancer of the lung, are thought to be complete, it is known that reporting of melanomas is incomplete, which explains the higher incidence rate found in the study. It is also possible that patients with a cancer of short duration may be diagnosed in hospital and never return to the practice.

Figure 2.13 Neoplasms (ICD chapter II): Patient consulting rates per 10,000 person years at risk

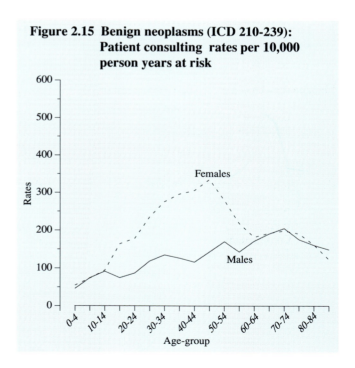

Figure 2.14 Malignant neoplasms (ICD 140-208): Patient consulting rates per 10,000 person years at risk

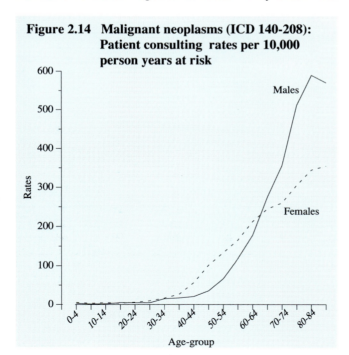

Figure 2.15 Benign neoplasms (ICD 210-239): Patient consulting rates per 10,000 person years at risk

Tables 2I Summary for selected neoplasms

	0-4	5-15	16-24	25-44	45-64	65-74	75-84	85 and over
Cancer of the breast (ICD 174): *rates per 10,000 female years at risk*								
Incidence	-	-	-	4	22	27	29	37
Prevalence	-	-	-	10	61	81	88	87
Consultations	-	-	-	25	176	186	231	193
Cancer of the prostate (ICD 185): *rates per 10,000 male years at risk*								
Incidence	-	-	-	-	4	19	46	36
Prevalence	-	-	-	-	7	45	137	155
Consultations	-	-	-	-	34	176	465	671
Cancer of the bladder (ICD 188): *rates per 10,000 person years at risk, by sex*								
Males								
Incidence	-	-	-	-	2	7	17	18
Prevalence	-	-	-	0	5	27	50	71
Consultations	-	-	-	0	21	82	149	256
Females								
Incidence	-	-	-	-	0	1	10	6
Prevalence	-	-	-	-	1	3	12	18
Consultations	-	-	-	-	4	10	29	57
M/F prevalence ratio	-	-	-	-	5.0	9.0	4.2	3.9
Cancer of the trachea, bronchus and lung (ICD 162): *rates per 10,000 person years at risk, by sex*								
Males								
Incidence	-	-	-	0	7	19	31	53
Prevalence	-	-	0	0	14	45	61	71
Consultations	-	-	1	3	56	191	247	267
Females								
Incidence	-	-	-	-	4	8	14	10
Prevalence	-	-	-	0	9	15	17	16
Consultations	-	-	-	0	38	85	75	51
M/F prevalence ratio	-	-	-	-	1.6	3.0	3.6	4.4
Malignant melanoma of the skin (ICD 172): *rates per 10,000 person years at risk*								
Incidence	-	0	1	2	2	3	2	4
Prevalence	-	0	1	2	4	4	4	6
Consultations	-	0	2	3	10	6	8	18
Other malignant neoplasm of skin (ICD 173): *rates per 10,000 person years at risk*								
Incidence	-	-	0	1	6	20	39	41
Prevalence	-	-	0	1	9	25	49	50
Consultations	-	-	0	1	12	36	69	68

	0-4	5-15	16-24	25-44	45-64	65-74	75-84	85 and over
Benign neoplasms of the skin (ICD 216): *rates per 10,000 person years at risk, by sex*								
Males								
Incidence	18	46	42	53	64	65	37	12
Prevalence	21	50	47	58	70	75	40	18
Consultations	24	62	59	72	87	99	46	18
Females								
Incidence	18	53	102	125	94	64	43	20
Prevalence	21	57	111	135	104	71	47	24
Consultations	22	71	127	163	129	89	51	43
M/F prevalence ratio	1.0	0.9	0.4	0.4	0.7	1.1	0.9	0.7

Of the malignant neoplasms, prevalence was highest for cancers of the bone, connective tissue and breast ICD sub-heading (table 2J). However, the consultation rate for this group, indicating the care provided by general practice, was exceeded by that for cancers of the genitourinary organs, most of which were for cancer of the prostate and of the bladder among elderly men.

Of individual cancers, the commonest was cancer of the breast, with a prevalence rate of 30 per 10,000 female years at risk, and an incidence rate of 11. Incidence increased steadily with age to a rate of 37 among women aged 85 and over (table 2I) compared with the National Cancer Registry rate of 36 for this age group. The incidence rate for women of all ages was similar to that of registrations.

The second most prevalent cancer reported was that of the prostate, with an overall rate of 11 per 10,000 male years at risk. The incidence rate of 4 per 10,000 was slightly lower than that of registered cases. Prevalence increased with age, 155 men per 10,000 aged 85 years and over consulting for this condition. They consulted on average over four times during the year, and the high prevalence to incidence ratio indicates a long survival time between diagnosis and death (table 2I). Four people per 10,000 consulted for neoplasm of the bladder, which was nearly five times more prevalent among men than among women and increased with age; nearly all patients were aged 65 years or over (table 2I). The incidence rate of one per 10,000 was half that of registrations, with a similar sex distribution. As for cancer of the prostate, the indications were that the survival time was long and consultations were frequent.

The rate consulting for cancer of the body of the uterus was 2 per 10,000 women, for cancer of the cervix, 3 per 10,000, for cancer of the uterus of an unspecified site, one per 10,000. The incidence rate of cancer of the cervix was less than half that of registrations. Four per 10,000 females consulted for cancer of the ovary, with an incidence rate of two, similar to that of registrations. This condition was prevalent among females in all age groups, with two per 10,000 among those aged under five years, three per 10,000 aged 5-15, and peaking at 11 per 10,000 among those aged 45-64 years. The age distribution of incidence rates differed from that of registrations, which showed a steady increase with increasing age.

For cancer of the trachea, bronchus and lung, 7 per 10,000 consulted. The incidence rate of 4 per 10,000 was half that of registrations. The youngest patient who consulted was aged between 16 and 24 years, and prevalence increased with age. The incidence rate of cancer of the lung was nearly twice as high among men than among women (table 2I), a slightly lower ratio than that of registrations. Each person who consulted did so on average four times during the year. The prevalence to incidence ratio suggests a relatively short survival time compared with cancer of the breast, prostate or bladder, particularly among the elderly.

The prevalence of cancer of the colon was 5 per 10,000, with an incidence rate of two per 10,000, compared with a registration rate of 3.5. The incidence of cancer of the rectum and anus was one per 10,000 compared with a registration rate of two, and a prevalence rate of three. Prevalence rates for both these conditions increased with age and were higher among men than women.

Malignant melanoma is relatively uncommon but serious, with an overall five year mortality of about 50%. The incidence of melanoma of the skin was two per 10,000 person years at risk, compared with less than one for registrations. Cases occurred among all age groups except the very young, and with only a small increase with age (table 2I). This differed from registration rates, which increased more steadily with age. There was little difference between the sexes except among people aged 85 years and over, for whom all the cases reported were female. Registrations, however, showed a general predominance among females. Compared with melanoma, there was a relatively high prevalence rate of other malignant neoplasms of the skin, which are less serious in terms of mortality but very common. Seven per 10,000 person years at risk consulted with an incidence rate of 6, similar to that of registrations. The prevalence rate increased with age and was highest among those aged 75 years and over (table 2I). There was no difference in incidence between men and women, although registrations show a higher incidence among men. The face was the most common site, suggesting that many may have been rodent ulcers for which there is no specific ICD code.

The proportion of all malignant neoplasms by disease related group by age is shown in table 2J.

No other individual cancer showed an incidence rate of one or more per 10,000 person years at risk, or a prevalence rate of more than two. However, a number were reported of ill-defined or secondary sites, which may either represent an under-estimate of cancers of a specific site or double-counting of those reported under a specific site at an earlier stage of the disease.

Among benign neoplasms, growths of the skin were the most prevalent, occurring in 75 per 10,000 persons. The age distribution peaked among people aged 25-44 years and they occurred predominantly among women (table 2I).

The second most commonly found benign neoplasms were lipomas, with a prevalence rate of 21 per 10,000. These occurred in all age groups, but prevalence was highest among people aged 25-74 years. There was no difference between the sexes, except for a small predominance among elderly women.

Table 2J   Patients consulting as a proportion for all malignant neoplasms, by age

	All ages	0-4	5-15	16-24	25-44	45-64	65-74	75-84	85 and over
All cancers	100	100	100	100	100	100	100	100	100
Lip, oral cavity and pharynx (ICD 140-149)	1	-	-	-	-	2	1	1	1
Digestive organs and peritoneum (ICD 150-159)	15	-	-	-	5	12	16	19	20
Respiratory and intrathoracic organs (ICD 160-165)	9	-	-	-	-	10	11	8	7
Bones connective tissues skin and breast (ICD 170-175)	30	-	33	40	43	35	25	25	28
Genitourinary organs (ICD 179-189)	20	25	33	20	24	17	18	23	20
Other and unspecified sites (ICD 190-199)	20	25	-	-	19	19	21	19	21
Lymphatic and haematopoietic tissue (ICD 200-208)	6	50	33	40	10	6	6	5	3

Endocrine, nutritional and metabolic diseases and immunity disorders

Four per cent of patients consulted for disorders in this ICD chapter. Above five years of age, the proportion consulting increased until 65-74 years and decreased thereafter. In all age groups between 16-24 and 75-84 a higher proportion of women consulted than of men (fig 2.16).

More people consulted for diabetes mellitus than for any other single condition in this chapter. Prevalence was highest among people aged 75-84 years and more common among males than females in every age group (table 2K, Fig 2.17). The high ratio of consultations with a doctor to the rate of persons consulting indicates the level of care provided for people with this disease, particularly as many with asymptomatic disease may see only the practice nurse for routine checks. Of all consultations with a doctor for diabetes by those aged over 75 years, 25 per cent were made in the patient's home.

The next highest prevalence rate in this group of disorders was for obesity. A rate of 82 per 10,000 persons was recorded, with a peak at 45-64 years of age. This disorder was predominately a problem among females (table 2K). Comparison with the Health Survey for England 1991 and 1992,[10] suggests considerable under-consultation for, or recognition of, obesity, particularly among men. In the Health Survey, 64 per cent of men and 45 per cent of women were found by clinical assessment to be overweight or obese, with highest rates among both men and women aged 55-64 years. Based on this information, the MSGP4 study suggests that women who are overweight are more likely to be concerned about this than men and more likely to consult their doctor for advice. However, the higher rate among women may have been the result of diagnosis of obesity during a contact for other reasons such as contraception. In addition, in our survey, 61 per 10,000 people consulted for disorders of lipoid metabolism, nearly all between 45 and 74 years of age. Although some of these people may have also consulted for obesity and been counted twice, most people found to have high serum lipid levels are identified as a result of a family history of heart disease or because of the presence of hypertension.

The prevalence of acquired hypothyroidism was found to be 50 per 10,000 persons. This increased with age from 27 among 25-44 year olds to 167 among people aged 85 years and over, and was considerably more common among women than among men (table 2K). The large difference between incidence and prevalence illustrates the chronic nature of this illness. Thyrotoxicosis on the other hand was far less common, affecting 9 persons in 10,000. Like hypothyroidism, it was more prevalent among women than men, but the peak age was younger.

Forty people per 10,000 consulted for gout which was more than twice as common among men than among women, with a slightly different age distribution (table 2K). Highest prevalence rates for men were for those aged 65-74 years, while for women there was an increase with advancing age with the highest rate among those aged 85 years and over.

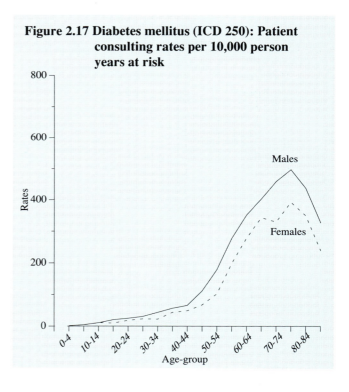

Figure 2.16 Endocrine, nutritional and metabolic diseases and immunity disorders (ICD chapter III): Patient consulting rates per 10,000 person years at risk

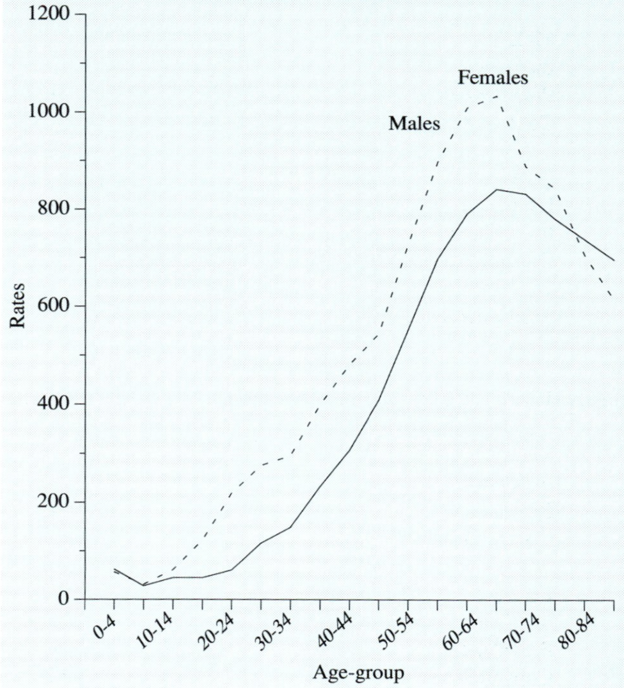

Figure 2.17 Diabetes mellitus (ICD 250): Patient consulting rates per 10,000 person years at risk

The prevalence rate for disorders of fluid, electrolyte and acid-base balance was 16 per 10,000 increasing with age and among adults much more common among women than among men, although this difference diminished with advancing age. These people were recorded as having 'fluid overload' which may have been used to describe peripheral oedema or fluid retention, mainly among women, with peak prevalence among those aged 45-64 years.

Table 2K   Summary for selected endocrine, nutritional and metabolic diseases and immunity disorders

	0-4	5-15	16-24	25-44	45-64	65-74	75-84	85 and over
Diabetes mellitus (ICD 250): *rates per 10,000 person years at risk, by sex*								
Males								
Incidence	-	2	7	15	58	109	120	65
Prevalence	1	8	24	49	217	428	475	327
Consultations	1	12	55	113	544	1053	1164	778
Females								
Incidence	1	3	4	8	43	95	103	71
Prevalence	1	7	15	34	154	337	374	238
Consultations	3	10	35	86	394	858	932	496
M/F prevalence ratio	1.0	1.1	1.6	1.4	1.4	1.4	1.3	1.4
Obesity (ICD 278): *rates per 10,000 person years at risk, by sex*								
Males								
Incidence	3	9	11	22	32	23	9	-
Prevalence	4	14	15	41	72	62	21	-
Consultations	5	13	15	47	89	80	19	-
Females								
Incidence	3	15	72	95	100	57	23	4
Prevalence	4	22	107	163	213	135	51	12
Consultations	4	28	128	213	289	169	53	10
M/F prevalence ratio	1.0	0.6	0.1	0.3	0.3	0.5	0.4	-
Acquired hypothyroidism (ICD 244): *rates per 10,000 person years at risk, by sex*								
Males								
Incidence	-	-	0	2	6	13	17	12
Prevalence	-	-	1	6	19	42	48	89
Consultations	-	-	2	9	33	76	92	178
Females								
Incidence	-	1	3	14	45	51	51	33
Prevalence	1	4	11	48	156	245	204	193
Consultations	2	7	22	93	320	429	378	351
M/F prevalence ratio	-	-	0.1	0.1	0.1	0.2	0.2	0.5
Gout (ICD 274): *rates per 10,000 person years at risk, by sex*								
Males								
Incidence	-	1	1	36	91	150	143	172
Prevalence	-	1	1	43	125	197	180	178
Consultations	-	1	0	73	221	340	289	273
Females								
Incidence	-	-	2	4	17	45	62	69
Prevalence	-	-	2	4	21	53	68	73
Consultations	-	-	2	5	39	105	117	120
M/F prevalence ratio	-	-	0.5	10.7	6.0	3.7	2.6	2.4

Diseases of the blood and blood-forming organs

Only one per cent of people consulted for a disease of the blood during the year. The rate increased with age and in every age group was higher among women than among men (fig 2.18).

The vast majority consulted for iron deficiency anaemia, with a smaller number reported to have suffered from other deficiency anaemias, which includes pernicious anaemia. Iron deficiency anaemia was much more common among women than among men, particularly among those aged 16-64 years and, to a lesser extent, among the elderly (table 2L). Among women of childbearing years, iron deficiency anaemia often results from menstruation and pregnancy.

Fourteen per 10,000 consulted for other and unspecified anaemia. These were reported predominately among women, and may have been additional cases of undiagnosed iron deficiency anaemia (table 2L). Prevalence of 'other deficiency anaemias' increased with age and were nearly all reported as pernicious anaemia, prevalence of which was higher among women than among men, except among the very elderly (table 2L).

The high prevalence rates among children were mostly attributed to non-specific mesenteric adenitis.

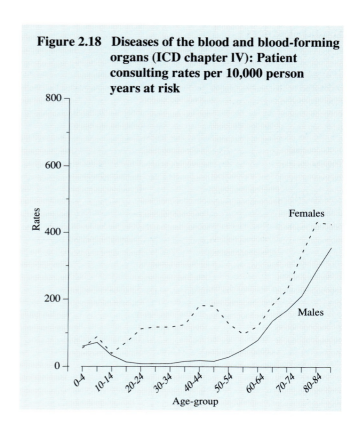

Figure 2.18 Diseases of the blood and blood-forming organs (ICD chapter IV): Patient consulting rates per 10,000 person years at risk

Table 2L Summary for diseases of the blood and blood forming organs

	0-4	5-15	16-24	25-44	45-64	65-74	75-84	85 and over
Iron deficiency anaemia (ICD 280): *rates per 10,000 person years at risk, by sex*								
Males								
Incidence	15	8	2	4	14	50	77	101
Prevalence	22	9	2	4	17	70	121	184
Consultations	30	17	4	6	33	131	194	428
Females								
Incidence	16	9	55	80	64	59	135	171
Prevalence	18	11	68	101	86	101	212	266
Consultations	31	15	92	134	138	162	390	433
M/F prevalence ratio	1.2	0.8	0.0	0.0	0.2	0.7	0.6	0.7
Other and unspecified anaemia (ICD 285.9): *prevalence rates per 10,000 person years at risk, by sex*								
Males	9	2	1	1	4	22	21	24
Females	5	5	19	20	21	34	59	67
M/F ratio	1.8	0.4	0.1	0.1	0.2	0.6	0.4	0.4
Pernicious anaemia (ICD 281.0): *prevalence rates per 10,000 person years at risk, by sex*								
Males	-	-	-	2	9	41	65	89
Females	-	0	1	4	22	53	91	63
M/F ratio	-	-	-	0.5	0.4	0.8	0.7	1.4

Mental disorders

Over seven per cent of people consulted for a mental illness. Prevalence was lowest among older children and increased with age. Among every age group in adults and the elderly, the rate was higher for women than for men (fig 2.19).

Of those who consulted, 85 per cent did so for neurotic, personality or other non-psychotic mental disorders. The number of consultations for this disease related group was exceeded only by that for acute respiratory infections. Within this group, it is often difficult to be precise when assigning a diagnosis. For example, an acute reaction to stress or an adjustment reaction may be recorded by another doctor as a neurotic disorder or depression. While the rate of people consulting for a condition in this disease group as a whole was 649 per 10,000 people, 729 per 10,000 consulted for an individual disease within the group, suggesting that about 12 per cent were assigned different diagnoses during the survey year. The prevalence estimates for individual disorders within this group is therefore unreliable, although it is clear that collectively these disorders present a problem of considerable size in general practice.

Among mental illnesses, prevalence was highest for neurotic disorders, the rate being 344 per 10,000 people. It was highest for both men and women aged 45-64 years and over twice as high among women than among men between 16 and 68 years. The specific conditions reported under the neuroses were anxiety states, neurotic depression and neurasthenia (table 2M).

Figure 2.19 Mental disorders (ICD chapter V): Patient consulting rates per 10,000 person years at risk

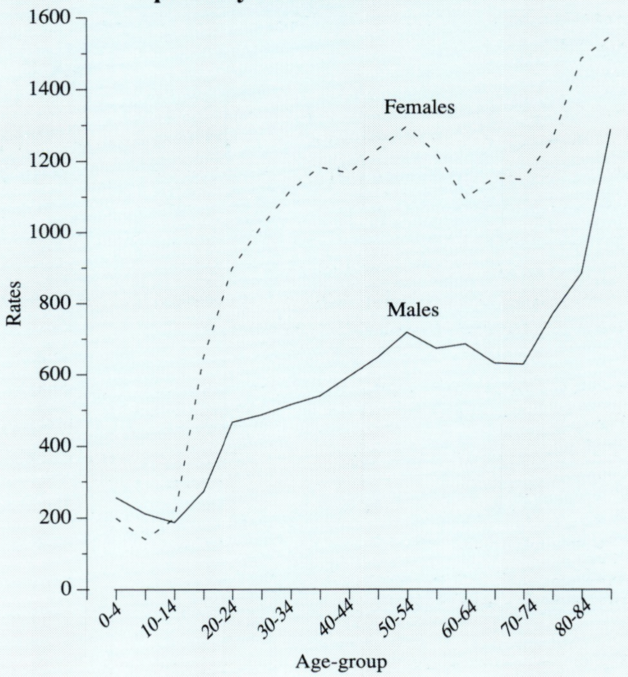

Table 2M Summary for selected mental disorders

	0-4	5-15	16-24	25-44	45-64	65-74	75-84	85 and over
Neurotic disorders (ICD 300): *rates per 10,000 person years at risk, by sex*								
Males								
Incidence	13	33	152	188	213	185	187	184
Prevalence	16	37	181	243	298	257	244	226
Consultations	18	48	325	524	656	577	499	440
Females								
Incidence	13	56	410	520	492	416	384	292
Prevalence	15	66	462	627	656	582	508	398
Consultations	18	81	761	1,313	1,431	1,178	1,023	804
M/F prevalence ratio	1.1	0.6	0.4	0.4	0.5	0.4	0.5	0.6
Unspecified anxiety states (ICD 300.0): *prevalence rates per 10,000 person years at risk, by sex*								
Males	9	13	106	173	204	176	151	125
Females	4	25	234	373	426	371	319	258
M/F ratio	2.2	0.5	0.5	0.5	0.5	0.5	0.5	0.5
Neurotic depression (ICD 300.4): *prevalence rates per 10,000 person years at risk, by sex*								
Males	1	2	30	34	50	47	55	59
Females	-	4	94	134	114	112	95	77
M/F ratio	-	0.5	0.3	0.3	0.4	0.4	0.6	0.8

	0-4	5-15	16-24	25-44	45-64	65-74	75-84	85 and over

Neurasthenia (ICD 300.5): *prevalence rates per 10,000 person years at risk, by sex*

	0-4	5-15	16-24	25-44	45-64	65-74	75-84	85 and over
Males	5	18	45	37	49	41	40	36
Females	10	28	139	132	121	103	103	69
M/F ratio	0.5	0.6	0.3	0.3	0.4	0.4	0.4	0.5

Depressive disorder not elsewhere classified (ICD 311): *rates per 10,000 person years at risk, by sex*

	0-4	5-15	16-24	25-44	45-64	65-74	75-84	85 and over
Males								
Incidence	1	3	32	45	62	62	65	113
Prevalence	1	3	37	67	99	94	112	190
Consultations	1	7	84	170	300	240	239	315
Females								
Incidence	-	7	103	156	140	101	135	126
Prevalence	-	8	119	215	221	174	207	175
Consultations	-	12	283	536	595	451	462	329
M/F prevalence ratio	-	0.4	0.3	0.3	0.4	0.5	0.5	1.1

Drug dependence (ICD 304): *rates per 10,000 person years at risk, by sex*

	0-4	5-15	16-24	25-44	45-64	65-74	75-84	85 and over
Males								
Incidence	-	1	23	10	5	1	5	6
Prevalence	-	1	34	30	16	10	11	12
Consultations	-	1	146	241	58	23	24	18
Females								
Incidence	-	1	6	6	9	12	6	8
Prevalence	-	2	8	20	32	43	23	16
Consultations	-	2	70	142	80	96	30	28
M/F prevalence ratio	-	0.5	4.2	1.5	0.5	0.2	0.5	0.7

Affective psychoses (ICD9 296): *rates per 10,000 person years at risk, by sex*

	0-4	5-15	16-24	25-44	45-64	65-74	75-84	85 and over
Males								
Incidence	-	1	18	24	33	23	39	59
Prevalence	-	2	25	35	62	48	80	107
Consultations	-	3	57	95	187	148	239	273
Females								
Incidence	-	1	36	62	78	75	79	99
Prevalence	-	1	44	90	126	128	127	136
Consultations	-	3	100	272	379	359	342	278
M/F prevalence ratio	-	2.0	0.6	0.4	0.5	0.4	0.6	0.8

Table 2M - *continued*

		0-4	5-15	16-24	25-44	45-64	65-74	75-84	85 and over
Selected problems affecting the elderly: prevalence rates per 10,000 person years at risk, by sex									
Senile dementia:	M						10	97	309
(ICD 290.0)	F						18	139	307
Acute confusional state:	M						17	65	155
(ICD 293.0)	F						18	66	154
Manic depressive psychosis:	M						46	78	107
(ICD 296.0, 296.1)	F						120	125	140
Anxiety states unspecified:	M						176	151	125
(ICD 300.0)	F						371	319	258

Depression not elsewhere classified had a prevalence rate of 110 per 10,000 people, and special syndromes or syndromes not elsewhere classified a rate of 97 per 10,000. These were mainly disorders of sleep, and pains of mental origin (psychalgia). In addition, 26 per 10,000 people consulted for acute reaction to stress, and 36 for adjustment reaction.

Of other conditions in this group, 15 per 10,000 people consulted for personality disorders. This rate increased with age among women, but showed little association with age among adult and elderly men. Sexual deviations and disorders accounted for 15 per 10,000 persons consulting, but occurred more commonly among men than women, and was highest among those men aged 45-74 years. Alcohol dependence was also more prevalent among men than women, particularly among those aged 25 to 64 years. For drug dependence 19 per 10,000 people consulted. This was higher among men aged 16-44 years than among women, but higher among women in all older age groups (table 2M). The incidence rate among men was highest among those aged 16-24 years. The high ratio between consultation and prevalence rates indicates the frequency with which people with drug dependence consult their general practitioner. Non-dependent drug abuse showed peak prevalence rate among those

aged 16-64 years, with a small predominance among men.

For non-organic psychoses, 77 per 10,000 people consulted. Among these, 58 per 10,000 consulted for affective psychoses. Prevalence increased with age and was higher among women than among men (table 2M). For schizophrenia, 11 per 10,000 consulted, with higher rates among males up to 45-64 years of age and no consistent difference between the sexes in older age groups. Each person who consulted for either of these conditions saw a doctor for this reason on average three times during the year.

Among children, 11 per 10,000 aged under five years consulted for the hyperkinetic syndrome and 51 for specific delays in mental development. Both were more common among boys than girls.

The prevalence of selected mental conditions for which the elderly consulted are shown in the last part of table 2M. These data should be interpreted bearing in mind that 15 per cent of men aged 65 years and over in the study lived alone, compared with 34 per cent of women. The prevalence of dementia was lower than in other community studies in England and Wales.[13] This is probably due to the broader definition used for these studies.

Diseases of the nervous system and sense organs

Of the sample in the study, 17 per cent consulted for a disease in this ICD chapter. The highest rate was among children aged under five years. There was a steady increase with advancing age among adults and the elderly. Between the ages of 10 and 65 years, prevalence was higher among females than among males (fig 2.20).

Highest prevalence among the disease related groups was for diseases of the ear and mastoid process. This was largely accounted for by the high rate among small children and older children, most commonly for infections of the middle ear. For disorders of the eye and adnexa, 20 per cent of children aged under five years consulted.

Otitis media was the most prevalent condition in this chapter for which people consulted. The incidence rate was highest among children aged under five years and fell to a third of this rate among those aged 5-15 years (table 2N). There was very little difference between the sexes. On the other hand, disorders of the external ear were more common among older adults and the elderly, largely due to excess wax. Prevalence was higher among men than women (table 2N).

The next most common reason for people to consult was for disorders of the conjunctiva, occurring mainly among small children, 18 per cent of whom consulted at least once. These were nearly all for acute conjunctivitis. A relatively large number of people consulted for vertiginous syndromes causing dizziness, which increased with age, and deafness, which affected children and to a greater extent the elderly.

Among diseases of the eye, 21 per 10,000 people consulted for glaucoma and 34 for cataract. Both conditions were rare before 45-64 years of age and prevalence increased with age.

Figure 2.20 Diseases of the nervous system and sense organs (ICD chapter VI): Patient consulting rates per 10,000 person years at risk

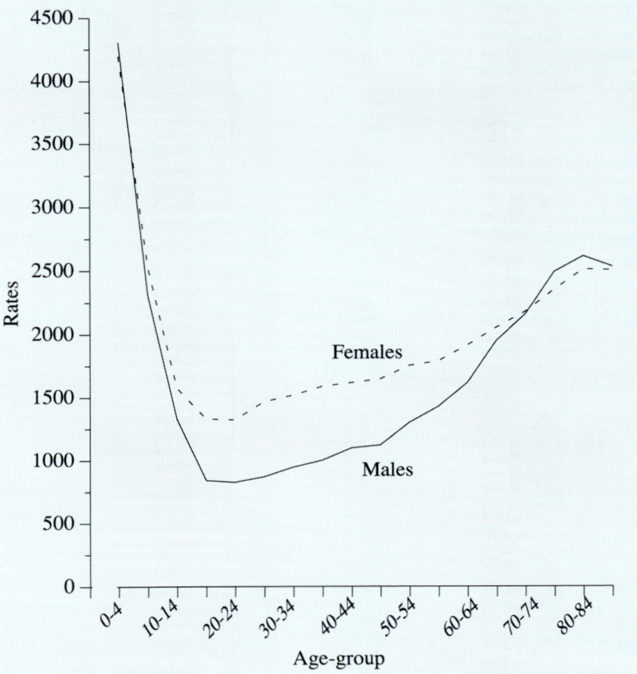

There was no sex difference for glaucoma, but cataract was slightly more common among women than among men.

For diseases of the nervous system other than the sense organs, over one per cent consulted for migraine. This was most common among people aged 16-44 years and prevalence was considerably higher among women than among

Table 2N   Summary for selected diseases of the nervous system and sense organs

	0-4	5-15	16-24	25-44	45-64	65-74	75-84	85 and over
Non-suppurative otitis media and Eustachian tube disorders (ICD 381): *rates per 10,000 person years at risk*								
Incidence	2,426	853	179	167	114	84	51	36
Prevalence	1,899	757	181	168	119	88	53	36
Consultations	3,155	1,076	218	218	152	115	71	55
Suppurative and unspecified otitis media (ICD 382): *rates per 10,000 person years at risk*								
Incidence	1,269	395	69	64	45	39	27	18
Prevalence	1,033	355	68	64	47	44	30	21
Consultations	1,680	523	88	94	74	68	45	28
Disorders of the external ear (ICD 380): *rates per 10,000 person years at risk, by sex*								
Males								
Incidence	230	197	249	385	555	883	1,024	981
Prevalence	230	198	242	368	541	851	1,005	927
Consultations	303	243	286	432	563	901	890	891
Females								
Incidence	212	280	295	399	487	568	685	751
Prevalence	205	273	285	375	471	546	681	727
Consultations	270	334	343	478	542	613	686	782
M/F prevalence ratio	1.1	0.7	0.8	1.0	1.1	1.6	1.5	1.3

Table 2N - *continued*

	0-4	5-15	16-24	25-44	45-64	65-74	75-84	85 and over
Migraine (ICD 346): *rates per 10,000 person years at risk, by sex*								
Males								
Incidence	3	77	56	53	41	29	18	6
Prevalence	4	89	67	65	56	36	24	6
Consultations	4	118	88	100	89	64	41	6
Females								
Incidence	3	99	200	208	146	55	34	14
Prevalence	3	109	233	251	197	75	42	16
Consultations	3	148	329	382	324	107	51	18
M/F prevalence ratio	1.3	0.8	0.3	0.3	0.3	0.5	0.6	0.4
Epilepsy (ICD 345): *rates per 10,000 person years at risk, by sex*								
Males								
Incidence	10	13	19	9	10	16	18	12
Prevalence	15	25	45	36	40	38	46	30
Consultations	29	47	95	89	99	84	85	107
Females								
Incidence	15	12	15	11	8	16	16	14
Prevalence	18	24	45	38	36	43	40	35
Consultations	33	48	103	99	78	92	83	65
M/F prevalence ratio	0.8	1.0	1.0	0.9	1.1	0.9	1.2	0.9
Multiple sclerosis (ICD 340): *rates per 10,000 person years at risk, by sex*								
Males								
Incidence	-	-	1	2	2	1	-	-
Prevalence	-	-	1	6	11	6	5	-
Consultations	-	-	1	20	46	10	11	-
Females								
Incidence	-	-	2	5	5	1	-	-
Prevalence	-	-	2	14	20	11	1	-
Consultations	-	-	3	50	56	35	2	-
M/F prevalence ratio	-	-	0.5	0.4	0.6	0.5	5.0	-
Parkinson's disease (ICD 332): *rates per 10,000 person years at risk, by sex*								
Males								
Incidence	-	-	0	1	4	19	61	83
Prevalence	-	-	0	1	14	64	149	155
Consultations	-	-	0	1	45	181	421	362
Females								
Incidence	-	-	-	0	2	21	36	43
Prevalence	-	-	-	1	9	51	91	128
Consultations	-	-	-	1	29	165	220	278
M/F prevalence ratio	-	-	-	1.0	1.6	1.3	1.6	1.2

men (table 2N). A smaller number, 36 per 10,000 people, consulted for epilepsy, the distribution of which was similar for each sex (table 2N). The relationships between the incidence, prevalence and consultation rates emphasise the long duration of this condition, and the frequency of the need to consult the doctor. Seven people per 10,000 consulted for multiple sclerosis, nearly all between 25 and 74 years of age.

The prevalence to incidence ratio was high, reflecting the long duration of the disease. This affected women twice as often as men (table 2N). The prevalence of Parkinson's disease was low among people aged under 65. It was more prevalent among men than women in each age group among the elderly. Like multiple sclerosis, the prevalence to incidence ratio was high (table 2N).

Diseases of the circulatory system

Of the total study sample, 9 per cent consulted for a circulatory problem. This proportion was small for those under 45 years of age and increased in each successive age group (fig 2.21). There was little overall difference in prevalence between the sexes. Approximately 36 per cent were in the serious category.

The most common reason was for essential hypertension. This was most prevalent among people aged 65-84 years, affecting 16 per cent aged 65-74 and 14 per cent aged 75-84 (fig. 2.22). In every age group of 45-64 years and over, prevalence was higher among women than among men. The male to female ratio was 0.9 for those aged 45-74 and 0.7 for those aged 75 and over (table 2O). This difference in prevalence between the sexes is similar to that found by the Health Survey for England in 1991 and 1992,[10] for which a systolic pressure over 159 mmHg was interpreted as being hypertensive.

The ratio of prevalence to incidence rates for essential hypertension, which increased gradually with age from three times among 25-44 year olds to seven times among the very elderly, indicates the long-term nature of this health problem (table 2O).

For ischaemic heart disease, two per cent of all people consulted. Prevalence was highest among those aged 75-84 years, 8 per cent of whom consulted. In contrast to hypertension, ischaemic heart disease was more prevalent among men in every age group than among women (fig. 2.23), the male to female ratio being highest (2.6) among people aged 25-44 years and decreasing with age (table 2O). One per cent of the population were reported to have consulted for angina pectoris. Prevalence increased with age up to 75-84 years and was higher among men than women (table 2O). A

Figure 2.21 Diseases of the circulatory system (ICD chapter VII): Patient consulting rates per 10,000 person years at risk

similar age and sex distribution occurred for acute myocardial infarction as for angina (table 2O), for which 29 people per 10,000 consulted at least once.

For cerebrovascular disease, 66 per 10,000 people consulted at least once. Prevalence increased with age (fig. 2.24); it was uncommon among those aged under 45-64 years, but affected 7 per cent of people aged over 85. As for ischaemic heart disease, and in contrast to hypertension, the male to female ratio shows a predominance among men, and the ratio was highest among the younger age groups, then decreased with age (table 2O).

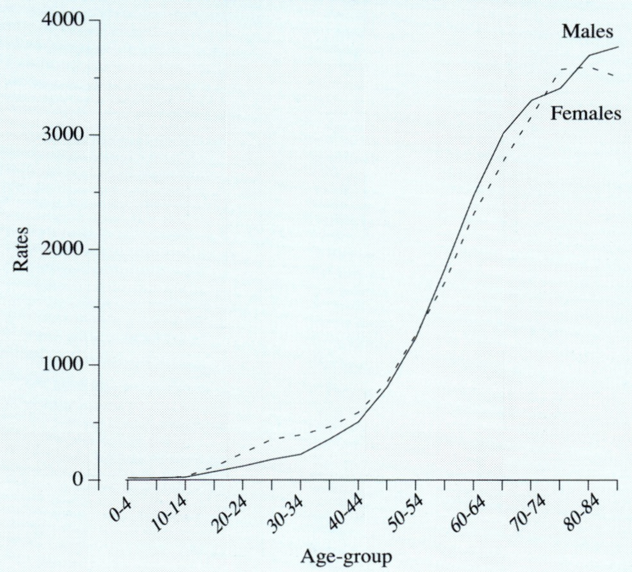

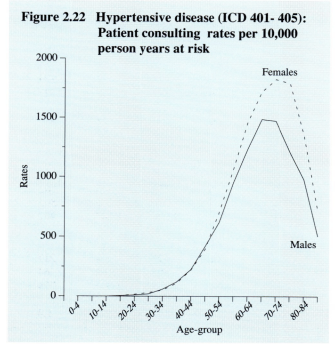

Figure 2.22 Hypertensive disease (ICD 401- 405): Patient consulting rates per 10,000 person years at risk

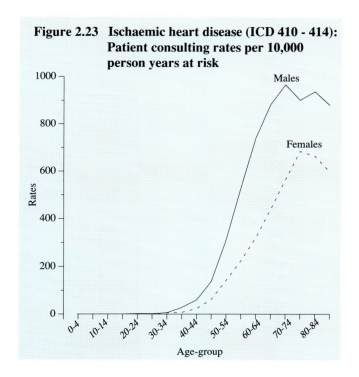

Figure 2.23 Ischaemic heart disease (ICD 410 - 414): Patient consulting rates per 10,000 person years at risk

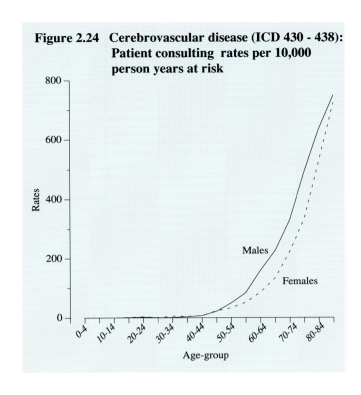

Figure 2.24 Cerebrovascular disease (ICD 430 - 438): Patient consulting rates per 10,000 person years at risk

Nearly all patients who consulted for cerebrovascular disease did so for transient cerebral ischaemia or for acute but ill-defined cerebrovascular disease. Some patients may have been recorded as consulting for both of these diagnoses. The prevalence of each increased with age and was higher among men than women.

Heart failure was rare among people under 65-74 years of age and increased steeply to 14 per cent among those aged 85 and over. There was a small predominance among men in each age group.

Of the remaining circulatory diseases, 89 per 10,000 consulted for varicose veins of the lower extremities and 103 for haemorrhoids. Rates were higher among females for varicose veins and among males, except for young adults, for haemorrhoids (table 2O).

Table 2O   Summary for selected diseases of the circulatory system

	0-4	5-15	16-24	25-44	45-64	65-74	75-84	85 and over
Hypertension (ICD 401-405), **ischaemic heart disease** (ICD 410-414) **and cerebrovascular disease** (ICD 430-438): *prevalence rates per 10,000 person years at risk, by sex*								
Hypertensive disease								
Males	1	2	9	103	762	1,482	1,124	505
Females	1	1	13	99	861	1,773	1,606	715
M/F ratio	1.0	2.0	0.7	1.0	0.9	0.8	0.7	0.7
Ischaemic heart disease								
Males	-	0	1	23	397	920	915	879
Females	1	-	0	9	176	498	675	597
M/F ratio	-	-	-	2.6	2.3	1.8	1.4	1.5
Cerebrovascular disease								
Males	-	0	2	3	72	272	546	749
Females	-	-	3	4	46	177	417	723
M/F ratio	-	-	0.7	0.7	1.6	1.5	1.3	1.0
Angina pectoris (ICD 413): *rates per 10,000 person years at risk, by sex*								
Males								
Incidence	-	-	-	9	108	225	273	202
Prevalence	-	-	0	14	257	580	586	505
Consultations	-	-	0	31	670	1,281	1,247	927
Females								
Incidence	1	-	-	4	66	176	224	217
Prevalence	1	-	0	7	133	364	466	364
Consultations	1	-	0	19	337	809	1,006	774
M/F prevalence ratio	-	-	-	2.0	1.9	1.6	1.3	1.4

Table 20 - *continued*

	0-4	5-15	16-24	25-44	45-64	65-74	75-84	85 and over
Essential hypertension (ICD 401): *rates per 10,000 person years at risk, by sex*								
Males								
Incidence	1	1	2	33	187	293	227	71
Prevalence	1	1	9	99	743	1,458	1,108	493
Consultations	1	1	11	238	1,927	3,479	2,548	981
Females								
Incidence	-	-	5	32	198	372	327	102
Prevalence	1	1	10	95	849	1,757	1,584	703
Consultations	1	1	21	238	2,138	4,333	3,717	1,487
M/F prevalence ratio	1.0	1.0	0.9	1.0	0.9	0.8	0.7	0.7
Acute myocardial infarction (ICD 410): *rates per 10,000 person years at risk, by sex*								
Males								
Incidence	-	-	0	3	53	126	153	143
Prevalence	-	-	0	6	73	158	188	166
Consultations	-	-	0	14	163	278	309	273
Females								
Incidence	-	-	-	1	15	58	94	104
Prevalence	-	-	-	1	20	71	117	112
Consultations	-	-	-	2	35	124	176	183
M/F prevalence ratio	-	-	-	6.0	3.7	2.2	1.6	1.5
Varicose veins (ICD 454) **and haemorrhoids** (ICD 455): *prevalence rates per 10,000 person years at risk, by sex*								
Varicose veins								
Males	1	1	10	31	97	197	232	232
Females	1	1	33	96	186	263	307	244
M/F ratio	1.0	1.0	0.3	0.3	0.5	0.7	0.8	1.0
Haemorrhoids								
Males	5	3	51	116	134	159	143	125
Females	3	6	94	173	137	140	118	91
M/F ratio	1.7	0.5	0.5	0.7	1.0	1.1	1.2	1.4

Diseases of the respiratory system

More people consulted for respiratory illnesses than for any other single ICD chapter of illnesses. More than 30 per cent consulted at least once during the year. Nearly 20 per cent consulted for a minor respiratory condition, 13 per cent for intermediate illnesses and 6 per cent for serious ones. Some consulted for an illness in more than one category of severity. Prevalence for all respiratory diseases was highest among children aged under five years, the rate being roughly twice as high as any other age group. Only among children aged under 16 years and people aged 65-74 and over was the prevalence rate higher among males than females (fig 2.25).

For the disease related groups, prevalence was over four times higher for acute respiratory infections than for any other group of diagnoses in this chapter. It was highest among small children, lowest among those aged 45-64 years and then increased with age. Prevalence was similar between the sexes among the very young and the very old. Between 16 and 64 years women were almost twice as likely as men to consult for an acute respiratory infection (table 2P), possibly because these conditions were mentioned in passing during a contact for preventive health such as contraception. The acute infections group includes the common cold and more specific diagnoses such as acute sinusitis, pharyngitis and tonsillitis which often occur simultaneously and are therefore difficult to analyse individually. Acute bronchitis and bronchiolitis are also included in the acute infections group. Acute bronchitis was prevalent among small children, of whom 14 per cent consulted, and among the elderly, of whom 17 per cent of those aged 85 years and over consulted. Among those aged under 15 years and over 65 years, acute bronchitis was more prevalent among males, but between these ages it was more prevalent among females (table 2P). In addition, three per cent of children were reported to have consulted at least once during the year for acute bronchiolitis (table 2P).

The group of diseases under the heading 'chronic obstructive pulmonary disease' includes chronic and unspecified bronchitis, emphysema, asthma and chronic airways obstruction not elsewhere classified. Prevalence rates for this group are shown in table 2P. Although there is potential for overlap in the assignment of diagnostic codes, only seven per cent of patients who consulted for a condition in this diagnostic group (ICD 490-496) were assigned more than one diagnosis during the year.

A total of 45 per 10,000 person years at risk consulted for chronic bronchitis. This increased with age and was more prevalent in each age group of 45-64 years and over among men (table 2P). Forty-six per 10,000 people were also reported to have consulted for bronchitis which was not specified as acute or chronic (table 2P), but some of these may have also been reported to have had acute or chronic bronchitis at a different consultation.

Four per cent of the total sample consulted for asthma (fig 2.26). This was most prevalent among children, some of whom experienced more than one episode. Prevalence was higher among boys than girls. This ratio was reversed among people aged 16 to 74 years (table 2P). On average, each

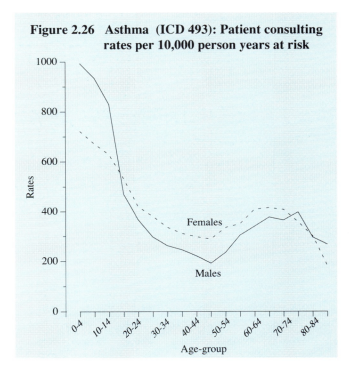

Figure 2.25 Diseases of the respiratory system (ICD chapter VIII): Patient consulting rates per 10,000 person years at risk

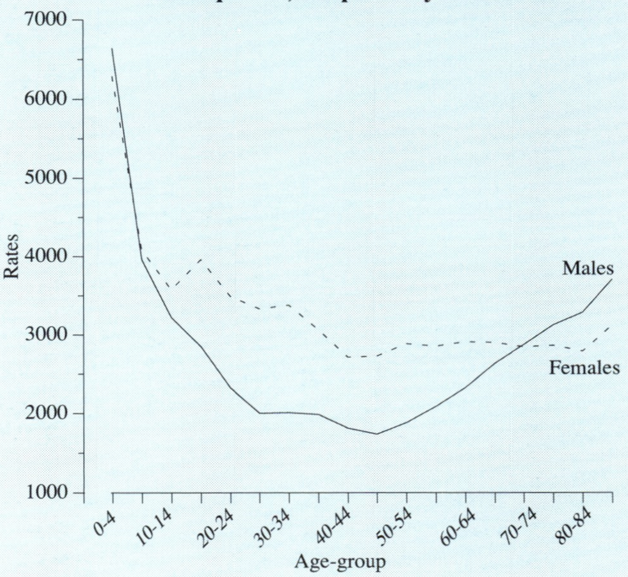

Figure 2.26 Asthma (ICD 493): Patient consulting rates per 10,000 person years at risk

person consulting a doctor for asthma did so more than twice during the year. Chronic airways obstruction, not elsewhere classified, was reported among the elderly. It was most prevalent among those aged 75-84 years and the rate among men was roughly twice that among women. Interpretation of these data is difficult because at individual diagnosis level the same patient may be recorded as having different illnesses during the same episode.

Allergic rhinitis includes hay fever. Three per cent consulted for this illness which was most prevalent among those aged 5-44 years. There was no consistent sex difference.

Table 2P   Summary for selected diseases of the respiratory system

	0-4	5-15	16-24	25-44	45-64	65-74	75-84	85 and over
Acute respiratory infections (ICD 460-466): *prevalence rates per 10,000 person years at risk, by sex*								
Males	6,191	2,620	1,784	1,389	1,413	1,936	2,268	2,716
Females	5,966	3,115	2,954	2,511	2,253	2,201	2,170	2,480
M/F ratio	1.0	0.8	0.6	0.6	0.6	0.9	1.0	1.1
Acute bronchitis (ICD 466.0) **and acute bronchiolitis** (ICD 466.1): *prevalence rates per 10,000 person years at risk, by sex*								
Acute bronchitis								
Males	1,447	433	356	372	630	1,144	1,516	1,913
Females	1,295	397	501	613	892	1,134	1,237	1,586
M/F ratio	1.1	1.1	0.7	0.6	0.7	1.0	1.2	1.2
Acute bronchiolitis								
Males	316	8	1	2	4	5	10	6
Females	251	6	1	4	3	3	8	6
M/F ratio	1.3	1.3	1.0	0.5	1.3	1.7	1.3	1.0
Chronic obstructive pulmonary disease and allied conditions (ICD 490-496): *prevalence rates per 10,000 person years at risk, by sex*								
Males	1,075	876	417	285	417	886	1,032	1,105
Females	794	661	480	374	479	691	676	534
M/F ratio	1.4	1.3	0.9	0.8	0.9	1.3	1.5	2.1
Chronic bronchitis (ICD 491): *prevalence rates per 10,000 person years at risk, by sex*								
Males	5	2	5	6	73	270	319	279
Females	4	4	6	9	57	130	135	73
M/F ratio	1.3	0.5	0.8	0.7	1.3	2.1	2.4	3.8
Bronchitis not specified as acute or chronic (ICD 490): *prevalence rates per 10,000 person years at risk, by sex*								
Males	103	20	18	19	39	92	124	232
Females	87	16	17	32	57	89	127	197
M/F ratio	1.2	1.3	1.1	0.6	0.7	1.0	1.0	1.2
Asthma (ICD 493): *rates per 10,000 person years at risk, by sex*								
Males								
Incidence	1,017	626	249	157	150	197	158	125
Prevalence	994	860	396	258	260	372	360	267
Consultations	2,347	1,719	651	465	613	953	875	541
Females								
Incidence	742	460	301	224	215	244	194	104
Prevalence	722	645	459	334	342	412	334	181
Consultations	1,727	1,242	841	710	858	1,129	826	437
M/F prevalence ratio	1.4	1.3	0.9	0.8	0.8	0.9	1.1	1.5
Chronic airways obstruction NEC (ICD 496): *prevalence rates per 10,000 person years at risk, by sex*								
Males	1	0	-	3	80	299	363	374
Females	-	1	-	4	58	137	170	136
M/F ratio	0.0	0.0	-	0.7	1.4	2.2	2.1	2.7

Diseases of the digestive system

Nine per cent of the sample population consulted for a disease of the digestive system. Among children under five years of age, 8 per cent consulted, mainly for teething problems and others of the soft tissues of the mouth. Over the age of 15, prevalence increased steadily with age, reaching 18 per cent among people aged 85 and over (fig 2.27). Although prevalence was relatively low among those aged 16 to 44 years, it was higher among women of these ages than among men.

Between the disease related groups, prevalence was highest for diseases of the oesophagus, stomach and duodenum, for which 4 per cent of people consulted. This increased with age among those between 5 and 84 years, with no consistent difference between the sexes. In this disease group, the most common reason for people to consult was for disorders of function of the stomach for which 153 per 10,000 consulted, these were mostly for dyspepsia. Also reported were 211 people per 10,000 who consulted for functional disorders of the digestive system not classified elsewhere. These were mainly for constipation and irritable colon. Prevalence of constipation was common in young children and the elderly, while irritable colon was most common among those aged 25-44 years. Both these conditions occurred more often among females than males (table 2Q). Diseases of the oesophagus accounted for 103 persons per 10,000 consulting, mostly for oesophagitis, which was most prevalent among those aged 65-74 years, and commoner among females than males.

The prevalence of peptic ulceration is reflected in the separate consulting rates for gastric ulcer, duodenal ulcer and peptic ulcer in unspecified site (table 2Q). The rate for gastric ulcer increased with age, with no consistent difference between the sexes. Duodenal ulcers were most prevalent among those aged 45 to 74 years, the rate for men being twice as high as that for women (table 2Q). The ratio between incidence, prevalence and consultation rates shows how this illness is of fairly long duration and initiates a considerable number of consultations (table 2Q). Twelve per 10,000 people were also reported to have consulted for a gastrointestinal haemorrhage, of which 7 were for haematemesis, 3 for melaena and two unspecified, higher rates occurring among men than

Figure 2.27 Diseases of the digestive system (ICD chapter IX): Patient consulting rates per 10,000 person years at risk

women in each age group. In addition, 24 per 10,000 consulted for haemorrhage of the rectum or anus, which were included under the code for 'other disorders of the intestine'. Some of these may also have been reported as consulting for a peptic ulcer, haemorrhoids or some other condition.

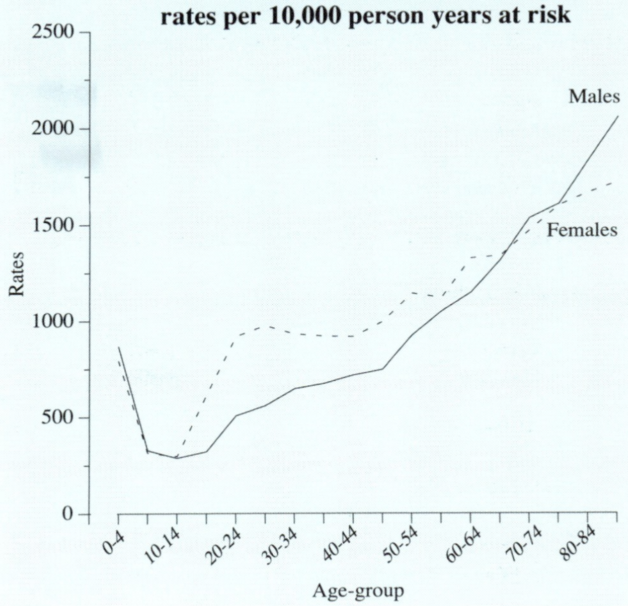

Inguinal hernia was more prevalent among men than women, the ratio varying between five to one among 5-15 year olds and sixteen to one among those aged 75-84 years (table 2Q). In contrast, the prevalence of abdominal hernia, which were nearly all diaphragmatic, was highest among those aged 45-64 years and over, with a predominance, though to a smaller extent, among women (table 2Q). Femoral hernias were rarely reported, but occurred in both men and women.

Gallstones (cholelithiasis) were most prevalent among women aged 45-64 years. The male to female ratio for this age group was 0.4 to one. This predominance among women occurred in every age group (table 2Q).

Table 2Q Summary for selected diseases of the digestive system

	0-4	5-15	16-24	25-44	45-64	65-74	75-84	85+
Constipation (ICD 564.0): *prevalence rates per 10,000 person years at risk, by sex*								
Males	182	47	20	20	44	169	396	683
Females	200	69	105	85	79	181	337	554
M/F ratio	0.9	0.7	0.2	0.2	0.6	0.9	1.2	1.2
Irritable colon (ICD 564.1): *prevalence rates per 10,000 person years at risk, by sex*								
Males	1	8	35	54	54	61	34	12
Females	1	17	187	206	180	130	86	49
M/F ratio	1.0	0.5	0.2	0.3	0.3	0.5	0.4	0.2

	0-4	5-15	16-24	25-44	45-64	65-74	75-84	85+

Peptic ulcers (ICD 531, 532, 533): *prevalence rates per 10,000 person years at risk*

	0-4	5-15	16-24	25-44	45-64	65-74	75-84	85+
Gastric ulcers	-	-	1	4	10	16	26	33
Duodenal ulcers	-	0	9	34	64	66	50	36
Peptic ulcers, site unspecified	-	0	6	13	22	20	27	19

Duodenal ulcer (ICD 532): *prevalence rates per 10,000 person years at risk, by sex*

	0-4	5-15	16-24	25-44	45-64	65-74	75-84	85+
Males	-	0	14	49	85	96	69	42
Females	-	-	4	18	42	42	38	33
M/F ratio	-	-	3.5	2.7	2.0	2.3	1.8	1.3

Duodenal ulcer (ICD 532): *rates for males per 10,000 person years at risk*

	0-4	5-15	16-24	25-44	45-64	65-74	75-84	85+
Incidence	-	-	12	34	47	45	37	30
Prevalence	-	0	14	49	85	96	69	42
Consultations	-	0	30	88	144	169	120	113

Inginal hernia (ICD 550): *prevalence rates per 10,000 person years at risk, by sex*

	0-4	5-15	16-24	25-44	45-64	65-74	75-84	85+
Males	52	10	14	25	83	156	262	267
Females	7	2	2	3	7	10	18	35
M/F ratio	7.4	5.0	7.0	8.3	11.9	15.6	14.6	7.6

Diaphragmatic hernia (ICD 553.3): *prevalence rates per 10,000 person years at risk, by sex*

	0-4	5-15	16-24	25-44	45-64	65-74	75-84	85+
Males	1	0	3	10	35	78	61	30
Females	2	1	1	11	50	105	119	85
M/F ratio	0.5	-	3.0	0.9	0.7	0.7	0.5	0.4

Cholelithiasis (ICD 574): *prevalence rates per 10,000 person years at risk, by sex*

	0-4	5-15	16-24	25-44	45-64	65-74	75-84	85+
Males	-	0	0	2	10	18	18	12
Females	-	-	7	16	32	28	23	16
M/F ratio	-	-	-	0.1	0.3	0.6	0.8	0.8

Diseases of the genitourinary system

For genitourinary complaints, 11 per cent consulted at least once during the year. With the exception of children under five years of age, the rate was higher among females than among males, particularly among those aged 16-64 years, for whom the ratio of men to women consulting was one to twelve. This sex difference gradually diminished with increasing age (fig 2.28). This predominance among women was due to high prevalence rates for cystitis and for conditions affecting the female genital organs.

One per cent of all people consulted for cystitis. This was 44 times more prevalent among females than males aged 16-24 and the difference between the sexes became less marked among those in older age groups. The relationship between prevalence and incidence shows that some women in every age group had more than one episode of cystitis during the year (table 2R). Under the diagnostic term 'other disorders of the urethra and urinary tract', 280 per 10,000 persons were reported to have consulted. Nearly all of these were for urinary tract infections of unspecified site. Prevalence of these infections was higher in every age group among females than among males (table 2R).

Among diseases of the male genital organs, 28 per 10,000 males consulted for hyperplasia of the prostate, prevalence

Figure 2.28 Diseases of the genitourinary system (ICD chapter X): Patient consulting rates per 10,000 person years at risk

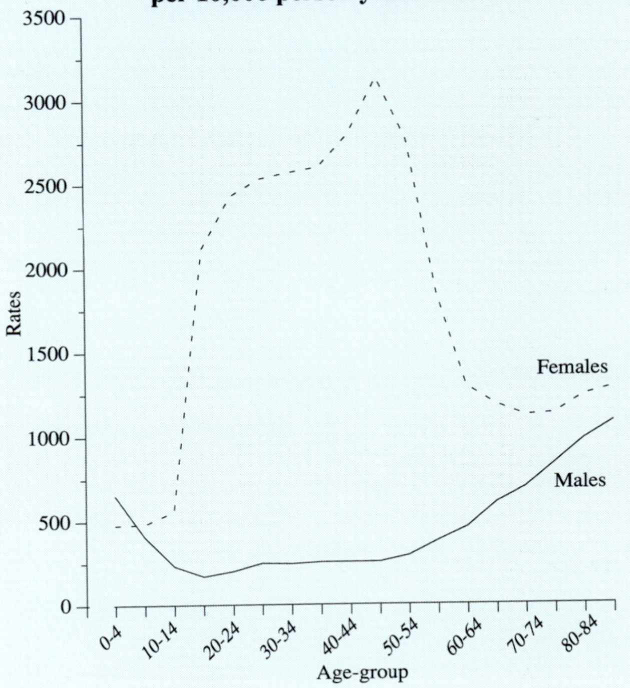

Table 2R Summary for selected diseases of the genitourinary system

	0-4	5-15	16-24	25-44	45-64	65-74	75-84	85+
Cystitis (ICD 595): *prevalence rates per 10,000 person years at risk, by sex*								
Males	5	6	6	10	20	36	42	71
Females	43	56	262	240	225	249	246	197
M/F ratio	0.1	0.1	0.0	0.0	0.1	0.1	0.2	0.4
Cystitis (ICD 595): *rates for females per 10,000 person years at risk*								
Incidence	41	59	290	262	246	274	272	227
Prevalence	43	56	262	240	225	249	246	197
Consultations	54	65	336	304	305	357	373	284
Urinary tract infection (ICD 599.0): *prevalence rates per 10,000 person years at risk, by sex*								
Males	127	60	39	57	108	265	440	636
Females	302	220	499	433	361	464	600	831
M/F ratio	0.4	0.3	0.1	0.1	0.3	0.6	0.7	0.8
Menopausal and postmenopausal disorders (ICD 627): *rates for females per 10,000 person years at risk*								
Incidence	-	-	1	115	678	134	75	87
Prevalence	-	-	1	170	1,219	197	106	106
Consultations	-	-	1	293	2,219	302	144	181
Pelvic inflammatory disease (ICD 614, 615, 616): *prevalence rates for females per 10,000 person years at risk*								
Ovary, etc	1	1	159	129	14	0	1	-
Uterus	-	-	16	18	2	-	1	-
Cervix, vagina and vulva	103	65	204	217	113	77	74	73

being highest among those aged 75-84 years. Thirty per 10,000 males consulted for orchitis or epididymitis, prevalence of which was highest among those aged 25-44 years.

For disorders of menstruation and other abnormal bleeding from the genital tract, 449 per 10,000 females consulted. The largest number of these were for excessive or frequent menstruation, with many also for amenorrhoea, metrorrhagia and unspecified disorders of menstruation. Among women aged 16-24 and 25-44, 476 and 553 per 10,000 women respectively consulted for pain and other symptoms associ-ated with the female genital organs. These were mostly for dysmenorrhoea and premenstrual tension. Among women aged 45-64 years, 12 per cent of women consulted for menopausal and postmenopausal disorders (table 2R). Among other diseases of females, inflammatory disease of the vagina and vulva showed a prevalence of 142 per 10,000 females, of the uterus 8, and of the ovary, fallopian tube, pelvic cellular tissue and peritoneum 62. Prevalence was highest for each of these conditions among women aged 16 to 44 years.

Diseases of the skin and subcutaneous tissue

Fifteen per cent of the study population consulted for a condition in this chapter. The highest rate was among children aged under five years, with little variation in prevalence in older age groups. In every age group, the rate for females was higher than that for males (fig 2.29).

The most prevalent conditions affecting the skin were atopic dermatitis, which includes eczema and nappy rash, and contact dermatitis, which includes dermatitis of unspecified cause. Three per cent of people consulted for the former and two per cent for the latter, although some may have been assigned to both diagnoses on different visits. Each was more prevalent among small children, some of whom had more than one episode (table 2S). Up to the age of 64 years, atopic dermatitis was slightly more prevalent among females, while this was so among all ages for contact dermatitis. For psoriasis, one per cent of people consulted, with a consultation rate of 113 per 10,000. Prevalence increased with age up to 16-24 years, showed little variation between the ages of 25 and 74, and decreased thereafter.

Two per cent of people consulted for diseases of the sebaceous glands, which includes acne. Acne was most prevalent among people aged 16-24 years. The rate for females was slightly higher than for males. The majority of people aged 5-15 and 16-24 years with diseases of the sebaceous glands consulted more than once (table 2S).

Among infections of the skin, 60 per 10,000 people consulted for carbuncles and furuncles, 61 for cellulitis or abscesses of the fingers and toes, and 105 for other cellulitis and abscesses. Prevalence of the last of these increased steadily with age, reaching 348 per 10,000 among those aged 85 years

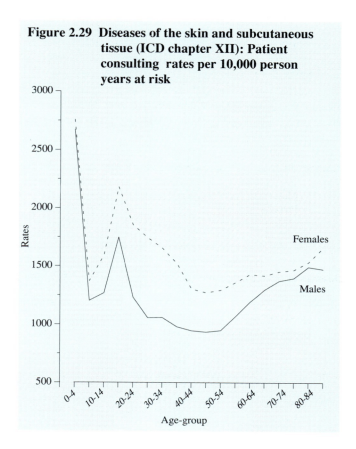

Figure 2.29 Diseases of the skin and subcutaneous tissue (ICD chapter XII): Patient consulting rates per 10,000 person years at risk

and over, for whom the rate was twice as high among women as among men. The highest rate for impetigo was among children aged under five years, three per cent of whom consulted for this infection (table 2S).

Table 2S   Summary for selected diseases of the skin and subcutaneous tissue

	0-4	5-15	16-24	25-44	45-64	65-74	75-84	85 and over
Atopic dermatitis (eczema) (ICD 691.8): *prevalence rates per 10,000 person years at risk, by sex*								
Males	977	253	149	133	144	218	200	166
Females	924	342	355	240	189	183	157	165
M/F ratio	1.1	0.7	0.4	0.6	0.8	1.2	1.3	1.0

54

Table 2S - *continued*

	0-4	5-15	16-24	25-44	45-64	65-74	75-84	85 and over
Dermatitis, unspecified cause (ICD 692.9): *prevalence rates per 10,000 person years at risk, by sex*								
Males	349	129	114	98	104	155	149	131
Females	334	176	258	199	156	167	148	148
M/F ratio	1.0	0.7	0.4	0.5	0.7	0.9	1.0	0.9
Atopic dermatitis (ICD 691) **and contact dermatitis and other eczema** (ICD 692): *rates per 10,000 person years at risk*								
Atopic dermatitis								
Incidence	1,624	240	201	149	135	154	127	135
Prevalence	1,602	297	252	186	166	199	175	169
Consultations	2,458	384	346	245	222	291	262	237
Contact dermatitis								
Incidence	333	155	225	166	141	155	146	118
Prevalence	371	178	247	193	166	195	173	161
Consultations	542	221	321	238	218	268	248	228
Psoriasis (ICD 696): *prevalence rates per 10,000 person years at risk, by sex*								
Males	24	47	62	77	79	80	56	53
Females	15	70	110	93	76	80	55	26
M/F ratio	1.6	0.7	0.6	0.8	1.0	1.0	1.0	2.0
Diseases of sebaceous glands (ICD 706): *rates per 10,000 person years at risk*								
Incidence	33	184	411	173	93	70	59	43
Prevalence	36	217	549	219	106	83	69	49
Consultations	41	346	873	306	144	116	102	58
Acne (ICD 706.1): *prevalence rates per 10,000 person years at risk, by sex*								
Males	4	162	467	73	13	10	10	6
Females	3	221	497	183	15	5	4	2
M/F ratio	1.3	0.7	0.9	0.4	0.9	2.0	2.5	3.0
Impetigo (ICD 684): *prevalence rates per 10,000 person years at risk, by sex*								
Males	294	173	55	25	16	20	24	36
Females	275	156	73	31	18	19	18	14
M/F ratio	1.1	1.1	0.8	0.8	0.9	1.1	1.3	2.6

Diseases of the musculoskeletal system

Fifteen per cent of the population consulted for a problem in this ICD chapter. The patient consulting rate was low among those aged under 25-44 years and then increased steadily with age (fig 2.30). Five per cent consulted for a serious disease, nine per cent for an intermediate one and three per cent for those in the minor category. Some consulted for a problem in more than one category of severity. In every age group from 5-15 years upwards, prevalence rates were higher among females than among males.

Among the four disease related groups in this chapter, an equal number of people consulted for an arthropathy (disease of the joints), and a dorsopathy (disease of the back), and a slightly smaller number for the group titled rheumatism, which includes joints, muscle and other soft tissue problems. While the prevalence of each group of conditions increased with age, this was most marked for the arthropathies.

Apart from unspecified backache, osteoarthritis was the most common reason in this chapter for patients to consult. Prevalence increased with age. The incidence to prevalence ratio, which decreased with increasing age, confirmed that osteoarthritis is a long term problem (table 2T). Among those aged 45 and over, each patient on average consulted twice during the year for this condition. In every age group from 25-44 years upwards, prevalence among women was half as high again as among men (table 2T).

Prevalence of rheumatoid arthritis was only one-eighth that of osteoarthritis. Each patient with this condition consulted on average nearly three times during the year (table 2T). The prevalence rate in every age group among adults and the elderly was at least twice as high among women as among men (table 2T).

Other and unspecified disorders of the joint include stiffness, swelling, effusion and pain in the joints. For one or more of these conditions, 241 per 10,000 people consulted. These were nearly all for joint pains. Joint pains were increasingly prevalent among the older age groups, among whom more women than men consulted (table 2T).

It is difficult to estimate the total number of people who consulted for back problems because they may have been assigned to a number of different codes, both in this ICD chapter and as sprains and strains in the injury and poisoning chapter. Spondylosis and allied disorders were the most prevalent among specific conditions affecting the back. The rate was highest among people aged 65-74 years, and in every age group was more prevalent among women than men. Most were for cervical spondylosis, with a smaller number for that of the lumbosacral region. Other and unspecified disorders of the back includes back pain. Four per cent of people consulted for these conditions, the rate increasing with age, and being higher among women than men, although this is certainly an underestimate for all people consulting for 'back pain'. The highest number consulted for unspecified backache, with smaller numbers of people diagnosed as having sciatica and lumbago (table 2T), although some were included in more than one category.

Figure 2.30 Diseases of the musculoskeletal system and connective tissue (ICD chapter XIII): Patient consulting rates per 10,000 person years at risk

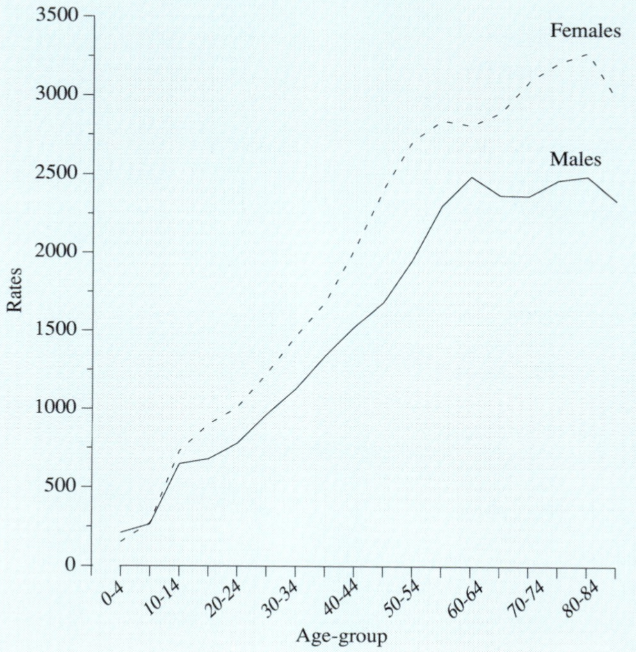

Two per cent of the total population consulted for at least one of the enthesopathies or tendonitis, bursitis and synovitis, the highest rate being among those aged 45-64 years. There was no consistent difference between the sexes. The elbow was the most frequent site, and the shoulder the second most common.

Complications of pregnancy, childbirth and the puerperium, congenital anomalies, and certain conditions originating in the perinatal period

The most prevalent complications of pregnancy were those leading to haemorrhage in early pregnancy (table 2U). Some women may have been assigned more than one diagnosis at different consultations. Of other reasons why women consulted, infections of the breast and nipple were the most common. Forty-nine per 10,000 women aged 16-24 years and 33 per 10,000 aged 25-44 years consulted for excessive vomiting in pregnancy. Urinary tract infections occurred during pregnancy in 41 and 26 per 10,000 women aged 16-24 and 25-44 years respectively.

Among children aged under five years, two per cent consulted for a congenital anomaly. Over half of these were in the serious category. The conditions for which children most frequently consulted at least once are shown in the table. The highest prevalence rate was for anomalies of the genital organs. These were mainly cryptorchidism and hypospadias. 'Other specified anomalies of the skin' includes birthmarks; this group of conditions was twice as common among girls as

Table 2T Summary for selected diseases of the musculoskeletal system

	0-4	5-15	16-24	25-44	45-64	65-74	75-84	85 and over
Rheumatoid arthritis and other inflammatory polyarthropathies (ICD 714): *rates per 10,000 person years at risk*								
Incidence	0	1	3	11	24	29	23	25
Prevalence	1	3	6	21	71	111	101	71
Consultations	1	3	10	57	225	313	268	107
Osteoarthritis (ICD 715): *rates per 10,000 person years at risk*								
Incidence	0	1	6	49	325	560	676	645
Prevalence	1	1	10	69	559	1038	1370	1444
Consultations	1	1	15	103	1056	1893	2637	2699
Rheumatoid arthritis (ICD 714.0) **and osteoarthritis** (ICD 715): *prevalence rates per 10,000 person years at risk, by sex*								
Rheumatoid arthritis								
Males	-	-	1	9	44	69	52	18
Females	-	2	5	22	85	133	122	85
M/F ratio	-	-	0.2	0.4	0.5	0.5	0.4	0.2
Osteoarthritis								
Males	1	1	11	55	466	818	1017	1022
Females	-	1	9	82	654	1217	1581	1584
M/F ratio	-	1.0	1.2	0.7	0.7	0.7	0.6	0.6
Pain in joint (ICD 719.4): *prevalence rates per 10,000 person years at risk, by sex*								
Males	36	104	141	176	227	245	246	273
Females	22	121	165	242	365	344	371	319
M/F ratio	1.6	0.9	0.9	0.7	0.6	0.7	0.7	0.9
Other and unspecified disorders of the back (ICD 724): *rates per 10,000 person years at risk*								
Incidence	6	53	233	392	463	410	425	374
Prevalence	9	59	257	452	556	495	517	481
Consultations	10	67	390	804	1025	772	831	756
Lumbago (ICD 724.2), **sciatica** (ICD 724.3) **and backache unspecified** (ICD 724.5): *prevalence rates per 10,000 person years at risk, by sex*								
Lumbago								
Males	-	5	41	91	98	89	94	71
Females	-	5	54	101	117	93	89	67
M/F ratio	-	1.0	0.8	0.9	0.8	1.0	1.1	1.1
Sciatica								
Males	1	-	18	85	149	141	128	107
Females	1	3	28	108	174	179	159	83
M/F ratio	1.0	-	0.6	0.8	0.9	0.8	0.8	1.3
Backache unspecified								
Males	5	26	115	214	237	193	204	303
Females	1	43	205	261	293	236	271	292
M/F ratio	5.0	0.6	0.6	0.8	0.8	0.8	0.8	1.0

Table 2U Summary for selected complications of pregnancy, childbirth and the puerperium, congenital anomalies, and certain conditions originating in the perinatal period

	5-15	16-24	25-44	45-64
Conditions causing haemorrhage in early pregnancy: *prevalence rates per 10,000 female years at risk*				
Missed abortion (ICD 632)	1	11	11	-
Ectopic pregnancy (ICD 633)	0	13	14	-
Spontaneous abortion (ICD 634)	0	71	65	1
Legally induced abortion (ICD 635)	2	36	16	0
Unspecified abortion (ICD 637)	-	2	1	-
Haemorrhage in early pregnancy (ICD 640)	2	105	93	1

	0-4		5-15	
	M	F	M	F
Congenital anomalies: *prevalence rates per 10,000 person years at risk, by sex*				
Eyelids, lacrymal system, & orbit (ICD 743.6)	15	17	-	1
Ventricular septal defect (ICD 745.4)	11	13	2	2
Ostium secundum atrial septal defect (ICD 745.5)	2	5	1	0
Patent ductus arteriosus (ICD 747.0)	1	3	-	-
Tongue tie (ICD 750.0)	15	7	2	0
Congenital hypertrophic pyloric stenosis (ICD 750.5)	10	4	-	-
Cryptorchidism (ICD 752.5)	82	-	32	-
Hypospadias (ICD 752.6)	10	-	2	-
Congenital dislocation of hip (ICD 754.3)	9	11	-	1
Varus deformities of feet (ICD 754.5)	10	14	2	2
Vulgus deformities of feet (ICD 754.6)	7	6	2	3
Other specified skin anomalies (ICD 757.3)	19	35	3	6
Down's syndrome (ICD 758.0)	2	5	1	1

boys. The reverse applied to tongue tie. Pyloric stenosis occurred nearly twice as often among boys than girls. A total of 17 per 10,000 children consulted for bulbus cordis and cardiac septal closure anomalies, nearly all simple septal defects. Among chromosomal abnormalities, 4 per 10,000 children aged under five years consulted with Down's syndrome, which occurred more than twice as commonly among girls than boys.

The only conditions originating in the neonatal period for which more than a very few children were taken to the surgery were neonatal infections. These were mainly candida infections (thrush), for which 113 per 10,000 under five years consulted, and conjunctivitis, for which 5 per 10,000 under five years consulted.

Symptoms, signs and ill-defined conditions

The terms used in this chapter refer to patients for whom a specific diagnosis could not be made at the time of the consultation. Some patients may have been assigned a more definite diagnosis at a subsequent consultation.

Overall, 15 per cent of patients consulted at least once for a complaint in this chapter. The prevalence rate varied between 12 per cent among those aged 25-44, and 29 per cent among those aged 85 years and over. The rate was higher among females in all age groups except among the very young and the very old (fig 2.31). This was particularly so for people aged between 16 and 44 years, among whom the prevalence rate was twice as high among women as among men. Symptoms with a prevalence rate over 50 per 10,000 person years at risk are listed in table 2V.

Table 2V   Summary for selected symptoms, signs and ill-defined conditions

Symptoms: *prevalence rates per 10,000 person years at risk*

Dizziness & giddiness (ICD 780.4)	93
Rash & other non specific skin eruption (ICD 782.1)	122
Headache (ICD 784.0)	129
Dyspnoea & respiratory abnormalities (ICD 786.0)	54
Cough (ICD 786.2)	195
Chest pain (ICD 786.5)	107
Nausea & vomiting (ICD 787.0)	67
Abdominal pain (ICD 789.0)	255

Injury and poisoning

Fourteen per cent of all people consulted for a condition in this chapter. Prevalence was similar among all age groups except for those aged 75-84 and over, among whom it increased. Up to the age of 34 years, prevalence was higher among males than females, above that age it was higher among females (fig. 2.32). Of the categories of severity, one per cent consulted for a serious problem, four per cent for an intermediate one, while 11 per cent consulted for a minor one. A few consulted for a problem in more than one category.

Among the disease related groups in this chapter, prevalence was highest for sprains and strains of joints, for which 550 per 10,000 people consulted. Of these, 168 per 10,000 people consulted for sprains of the back, which was most prevalent among those aged 16-44 years and equally distributed between the sexes. Sprains of the ankle and foot occurred most commonly among those aged 5-24 years, and of the knee among those aged 16-24 years; both were more frequent among males than females. The other two groups for which many people consulted were superficial injuries and contusion with intact skin surfaces (bruising), with a prevalence rate of 154 and 124 per 10,000 people respectively. Superficial injuries were mainly to the lower limb, and to a lesser extent to the hands and face, with highest rates among children aged 5-15 years and the very old, particularly women. Contusions were most prevalent among the elderly, the commonest sites being the forehead and lower limb.

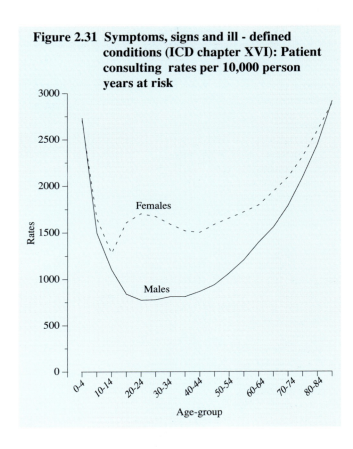

Figure 2.31 Symptoms, signs and ill - defined conditions (ICD chapter XVI): Patient consulting rates per 10,000 person years at risk

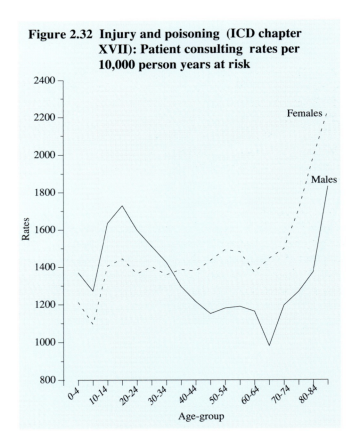

Figure 2.32 Injury and poisoning (ICD chapter XVII): Patient consulting rates per 10,000 person years at risk

Table 2W Summary for selected injuries and poisoning

	0-4	5-15	16-24	25-44	45-64	65-74	75-84	85 and over

Fractures of the neck of femur (ICD 820), **radius and ulna** (ICD 813), **and humerus** (ICD 812):
prevalence rates per 10,000 person years at risk, by sex

	0-4	5-15	16-24	25-44	45-64	65-74	75-84	85 and over
Femur								
Males	-	-	0	1	2	5	18	89
Females	-	-	-	0	3	23	63	193
M/F ratio	-	-	-	-	0.7	0.2	0.3	0.5
Humerus								
Males	2	6	4	2	2	3	5	12
Females	4	6	1	2	7	19	20	32
M/F ratio	0.5	1.0	4.0	1.0	0.3	0.2	0.2	0.4
Radius & ulna								
Males	12	35	23	14	10	7	9	24
Females	14	26	8	8	22	40	62	65
M/F ratio	0.9	1.3	2.9	1.8	0.5	0.2	0.1	0.4

Closed fracture of rib (ICD 807.0: *prevalence rates per 10,000 person years at risk, by sex*

	0-4	5-15	16-24	25-44	45-64	65-74	75-84	85 and over
Males	1	2	7	15	18	22	24	30
Females	1	1	3	5	14	18	25	41
M/F ratio	1.0	2.0	2.3	3.0	1.3	1.2	1.0	0.7

Among the open wound injuries, children under five years of age showed a high prevalence rate for open wounds of the head, 159 per 10,000 persons consulting, the most common site being the face. The rate among boys was nearly twice that of girls. Among the elderly, there was also a high prevalence rate for open wounds of the head compared with other age groups. Open wounds to the fingers were most common among men aged 16-24 years.

The prevalence of fractures of many sites increased with age, often with a considerable difference between males and females. For fractures of the neck of femur, humerus, and radius and ulna over the age of 45 years, the rate was higher among women than men (table 2W). Closed fractures of the ribs also showed increased prevalence with age, but were equally distributed between the sexes. Among younger ages, particularly those aged 16-24 years, fractures of the arm bones were more common among males than females.

Other complications of procedures, not elsewhere classified, for which 41 per 10,000 consulted, were nearly all post operative infections and other post operative complications. Very few patients were recorded as having poisoning.

Three per cent, spread fairly evenly over every age group, were reported to have suffered from certain adverse affects not elsewhere classified. This included ICD 995.8, which was the code used as a default for any consultation for which a cause of injury code, such as that for 'fell down stairs', had been recorded without an injury code such as 'fractured wrist'.

Supplementary classification of factors influencing health status and contact with health services

This classification comprises reasons for attending the practice other than for an illness. In the main tables it is referred to as ICD Chapter XVIII.

More patients consulted for reasons in this classification than for any single diagnostic chapter. The age distribution is shown in figure 2.33. Fourteen per cent of the total population attended for vaccination and other preventive procedures against communicable diseases. This proportion was highest among children aged under five years of age, of whom 45 per cent consulted at least once for this purpose, mainly for combined vaccines (table 2X). Above this age, the rate was low, but gradually increased with age to reach 28 per cent among those aged 75-84 years, who attended mainly for vaccination against influenza and, to a smaller extent, against tetanus (table 2X).

Of women aged 16-24 and 25-44 years, 47 per cent and 26 per cent respectively visited the practice for contraceptive management (table 2X). Among children aged under five years, 18 per cent were taken to the practice for health supervision which included routine child health checks.

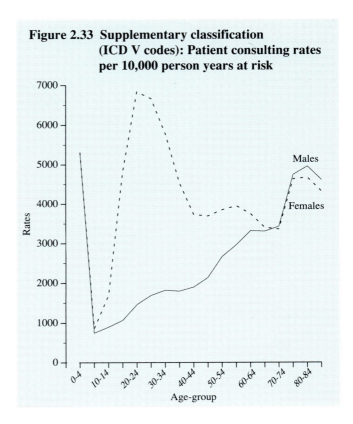

Figure 2.33 Supplementary classification (ICD V codes): Patient consulting rates per 10,000 person years at risk

Table 2X   Summary for selected reasons in the supplementary classification

	0-4	5-15	16-24	25-44	45-64	65-74	75-84	85+
Immunisation: *patient consulting rates per 10,000 person years at risk*								
Cholera (VO3.0)	7	10	23	28	26	13	5	-
Typhoid (VO3.1)	32	64	140	143	155	75	19	3
Tuberculosis (VO3.2)	6	77	3	0	0	-	0	-
Tetanus (VO3.7)	14	99	216	380	458	442	329	209
Poliomyelitis (VO4.0)	263	93	120	153	121	56	14	4
Rubella (VO4.3)	0	225	6	3	0	-	-	-
Influenza (VO4.8)	5	48	90	158	635	2,055	2,575	2,453
DPT (VO6.1)	182	1	-	0	0	-	0	-
DPT & poliomyelitis (VO6.3)	1,755	6	1	1	0	-	-	1
MMR (VO6.4)	1,615	46	2	0	0	-	-	-
Other combined (VO6.8)	1,310	206	59	54	37	18	7	-
Reproduction: *females consulting rates per 10,000 female years at risk*								
Normal pregnancy (V22)		9	683	666	3			
Postpartum care (V24)		3	427	471	1			
Contraceptive advice (V25)		138	4,707	2,559	147			
Screening for malignant neoplasms: *females consulting rates per 10,000 female years at risk*								
Breast (V76.1)	-	0	23	74	408	50	8	8
Cervix (V76.2)	-	6	1,045	1,331	918	167	12	2
Special screening: *patient consulting rates per 10,000 person years at risk*								
Thyroid disorders (V77.0)	1	1	4	9	20	28	34	28
Diabetes (V77.1)	1	1	5	16	36	43	45	25
Obesity (V77.8)	-	3	5	11	22	18	6	1
Hypertension (V81.1)	1	4	55	104	274	374	262	112
Other reasons: *patient consulting rates per 10,000 person years at risk*								
Medical certificate (V68.0)	8	10	438	577	822	146	43	62
Expert advice (V68.2)	7	5	46	108	126	60	80	50
Health examination (V70.5)	26	102	234	225	183	164	2073	1980

Five per cent of people visited the practice for administrative purposes such as the issue of medical certificates and medical examinations for expert advice, such as that required for insurance.

Among examinations for screening purposes during which no abnormality was found, four per cent attended for a general medical examination. These included 21 per cent of those aged 75-84 and 20 per cent of those aged 85 years and over. Nearly all who attended for screening for neoplasms were women. The majority of these were for cancer of the cervix (table 2X).

3 Trends in morbidity

3.1 Introduction

One of the purposes of these morbidity studies is to identify changes in morbidity seen in general practice. In this chapter, the results from the 1981-82 and 1991-92 studies are compared. Data from the 1971-72 survey are also included where these are compatible. The nature of general practice based surveys is such that the morbidity data to an extent reflect health care utilisation. The number of patients seen in general practice does not necessarily represent prevalence of disease in the total community. There are many factors which influence whether a patient takes a problem to his general practitioner. These may change over time, depending upon the patient himself and upon other circumstances.

3.2 Interpretation of results

The comparisons between the surveys presented here must be considered in relation to differences in the survey conditions and methods. Descriptions of the methods are given in this and previous publications,[3,5] but a few salient points are mentioned here.

In 1991-92, the morbidity data were usually entered using free-text terms which were automatically identified and stored in the computer as Read codes. This method was simpler than the manual diagnostic index used in the earlier studies, particularly when multiple problems were presented during a single contact. There was, however, increased scope for the use of different terms with similar meaning during the course of one episode of illness, particularly if the patient was seen by different doctors. This could produce inflated prevalence rates if the analysis were carried out on a detailed level of morbidity coding.

For some conditions, accurate comparisons cannot be made between the two studies because in 1981-82 the RCGP disease classification was used, which was not entirely compatible with the ICD9 classification used for analysis of the 1991-92 study. This commentary is restricted to conditions where a good comparison can be made.

The consultation type codes, first (F), new (N) and other or ongoing (O) used in the 1991-92 survey provided a simpler method of typing the consultation than the numeric coding used in the previous surveys. The terms serious, intermediate and trivial as an indication of severity were applied to ICD9 rubrics for the 1981-82 study, and have been applied in an identical way to data collected in the 1991-92 survey for the purpose of this comparison. The definition of each category is given in the box (page 63). This differs slightly from the revised designation of serious, intermediate and minor used elsewhere in this volume.

Between 1981-82 and 1991-92 the structure of general practice

altered. The number of nurses employed by practices and the scope of their activities increased substantially. This activity by nurses was not recorded in the 1981-82 survey. Practice responsibilities in delivering preventive health care increased in the ten years between the surveys. The selective reimbursement for health promotion clinics and the introduction of target payments influenced both practice performance and the quality of recording the appropriate data. Procedures for the certification of sickness were simplified between the two surveys, leading to a reduced requirement for general practitioners to issue certificates for short-term illness. The practice sample in the 1991-92 survey included only three fundholding practices, so the results of this comparison with data from the 1981-82 survey is not likely to be influenced by

---

Definition of category of severity used in the 1981/1991 comparison

Serious diseases include:

1. Those which at the time are invariably serious,

2. Those which invariably require surgical intervention,

3. Those which carry a high probability of serious complications or significant recurring disability.

Intermediate diseases include:

1. Those which though sometimes potentially serious are classified to a morbidity code which spans a wide range of severity, or embraced by a diagnostic term which is used with widely disparate meaning by general practitioners;

2. Those which though not often serious, are usually brought to the attention of the general practitioner.

Trivial diseases include:

1. Illnesses commonly treated without recourse to medical advice,

2. Minor self limiting illnesses which require no specific treatment,

3. Diseases which are not included above.

this innovation. Computerised information systems in general practice were uncommon during the 1981-82 survey, but used by all practices taking part in the 1991-92 survey. Computerisation has led both to greater accuracy of practice registers and to reduced errors in morbidity recording.

The interplay between the treatment of disease and patient expectation influences the proportion of people who consult. This may be one of the reasons why the rate of persons consulting for mental disorders has decreased. Complementary medicine has increased dramatically over the last decade and it may be that competition from alternative practitioners has contributed to the decline in people consulting for mental and other disorders. The reduction is particularly apparent for neurotic disorders. This was the group of conditions for which in the early 1980s, benzodiazepine tranquillisers were prescribed. There has subsequently been a considerable reduction in the use of these drugs. The possible explanation for the reduction in patients consulting for neurotic disorders is that their expectations of acceptable treatment such as tranquillisers have diminished. Likewise, obese patients are less likely to consult with this problem if they know they will not be prescribed appetite suppressants.

Any changes in consulting rates must be considered against a background of increased contact between patient and doctor. This is particularly so among the elderly, with the recent emphasis on preventive screening and community based care, and the discontinuation of hospital follow-up for less serious chronic conditions. These factors possibly account for the increased consulting rates for diabetes, hypothyroidism and serious mental disorders. The increased consulting rates for fungal infections may reflect greater expectations from medical care.

The reduced prevalence rates for respiratory cancers among men and for acute myocardial infarction are encouraging. They are supported by reduced rates of first diagnosis and may reflect the changing patterns of smoking in our society. A decline in the reported prevalence of chronic obstructive airways disease supports this interpretation.

The reduction in the consulting rate for thyrotoxicosis was substantial and there does not seem to be any explanation relating to changes in patterns of health care. The reduced prevalence of psoriasis appears to be real, particularly as increased contact between patients and their doctors might bring chronic diseases such as this to the attention of the doctor.

Among cardiovascular disorders, the increased consulting rates for angina contrast with the decrease for acute myocardial infarction. Ischaemic heart disease is managed more actively with regular medical review and medication than it was in 1981-82. In addition, if the incidence of myocardial infarction falls, and particularly if there are fewer deaths, more survive to consult for ischaemic heart disease. The prevalence of hypertension has changed little, except among the elderly for whom the importance of diagnosis and treatment has been recognised over recent years.

A variety of statistics indicate an increase in the prevalence of asthma, and the surveys since 1971-72 confirm this. The increase found in the 1991-92 study is greatest among the very young. Part of this may be an increased willingness by doctors to use the term, but the evidence is that acute bronchitis was not previously used as a substitute term for asthma because consulting rates for acute bronchitis have also increased.

Reduced consulting rates for rheumatoid arthritis are difficult to interpret because the term is now used more precisely by doctors than in 1981-82. Clinical management is more interventionist and for this reason an increased patient consulting rate might have been expected. The decrease in the rates for first diagnoses was greater than that for patient consulting rates, suggesting a real reduction in the incidence rate.

Increased consulting rates for osteoarthritic conditions is an example of disorders for which patients have come to expect greater intervention, either by medication or physiotherapy. As treatment improves, more people request care. It is only when treatment is curative that medical advances result in fewer people consulting.

There are many conditions for which there has been no change between the 1981-82 and 1991-92 studies in the proportion of people who consulted. Perhaps we should be asking ourselves why, as advances in medical care, prevention and improved socio-economic conditions might be expected to reduce burdens of illness.

Some conditions for which the proportion of people who consulted in 1981/82 and 1991/92 remained virtually unchanged are:

> Malignant disease of the oesophagus, stomach, colon, rectum and anus combined (ICD 150, 151, 153, 154)
> Parkinson's disease (ICD 332)
> Multiple sclerosis (ICD 340)
> Epilepsy (ICD 345)
> Varicose veins of lower extremities (ICD 454)
> Inguinal hernia (ICD 550)
> Diverticula of intestine (ICD 562)
> Necrosis, cirrhosis, abscess and other disorders of the liver (ICD 570-573)

3.3 Changes in morbidity

The comparison of morbidity between the 1981-82 and 1991-92 surveys which follows is chiefly concerned with changes in prevalence. Prevalence for this purpose is defined as the number of persons consulting at least once during the study year. This is expressed as a rate per 10,000 person years at risk. However, the prevalence rate may depend upon the survival time following initial diagnosis. This may be lengthened by earlier diagnosis or as the result of treatment. If the average survival time increased between the two surveys from, say, four to five years, the consulting rate will increase by one quarter. An example is cancer of the breast. The prevalence rate increased between 1981-82 and 1991-92, but the first incidence rate remained the same, suggesting that the chance of developing cancer of the breast is unchanged, but the average survival may have increased.

All diseases and conditions

Changes in the prevalence rates between 1981-82 and 1991-92 for all diseases and conditions, category of severity and each ICD chapter are shown in table 3A.

Between the 1981-82 and 1991-92 surveys there was an increase from 71 per cent to 78 per cent in the proportion of people who consulted at least once during the study year for any disease or condition. This increase was greatest among the elderly, but occurred among people in every age group and both sexes.

There was an increase in the proportion of people within each age group who consulted for serious, for intermediate and for trivial conditions. Patient consulting rates increased between 1981-82 and 1991-92 for conditions in every ICD chapter except mental disorders, and symptoms, signs and ill-defined conditions.

The number of consultations increased by 2.4 per cent, from 33,961 per 10,000 person years at risk in 1981-82 to 34,785 in 1991-92.

Infectious and parasitic diseases

There was a small increase from 12 per cent to 13 per cent between 1981-82 and 1991-92 in the proportion of people who consulted for conditions in this chapter. The increase, which occurred among people in every age group, was for trivial conditions.

Intestinal infections were the most frequently reported diseases within the chapter, and for these 4 per cent consulted, compared with 3 per cent in 1981-82. The relative increase was greatest among small children and the elderly, and probably reflects greater awareness of potentially serious enteric infections among these age groups.

Among the viral exanthemata, patient consulting rates were higher in 1991-92 for chickenpox, which doubled, and for herpes simplex, which almost trebled (table 3B). Increased rates for chickenpox occur every nine years, and were exceptionally low in 1981-82, which may account for the apparent increase. Numbers of cases of herpes simplex do not show marked annual fluctuations. The availability of treatment for herpes simplex over recent years may have encouraged patients to consult. The patient consulting rates for measles and rubella among children under 15 years of age decreased, although 1981-82 was not an epidemic year for either disease. Patient consulting rates for herpes zoster increased from 39 to 49 per 10,000 persons.

A larger proportion of patients in the 1991-92 survey consulted for tinea (ringworm) and fungal infections of the skin.

Consulting rates for candida (thrush), both of the mouth and to a greater extent of urogenital sites (table 3B) almost doubled between the two surveys. Increased awareness and concern may account for more people consulting the general practitioner for thrush. Consulting rates were also higher in 1991-92 for viral warts (table 3B), enterobiasis, which includes threadworms, and acariasis, which includes scabies (table 3B).

Neoplasms

Consulting rates for all neoplasms increased from 135 to 239 per 10,000 person years at risk between 1981-82 and 1991-92. For diseases in the serious category, most of which were malignant, the exception being some benign growths of the nervous system and endocrine glands, the rate increased from 68 to 86 per 10,000 persons (table 3C). For intermediate conditions, which were benign, the rate increased from 68 to 158 per 10,000 (table 3C). The patterns of increase in the serious and intermediate categories occurred among all age groups and both sexes.

The prevalence of cancer of the larynx, trachea, bronchus and lung is shown in table 3D. The prevalence of respiratory cancer has declined for men aged under 75 years, but for older men there has been a small increase between 1981-82 and 1991-92. This decline has not occurred among women, and the prevalence rate more than doubled between the two surveys for women aged 75 years and over. Among men aged 45-64 years, the first incidence rate in the 1991-92 survey was 75 per cent of that in the 1981-82 survey, for men aged 65-74 years, 55 per cent, and for men aged 75 years and over, 78 per cent (table 3D). The first incidence rate among younger women also declined, but was three times higher among those aged 75 years and over in 1991-92 compared with 1981-82. The changing patterns of smoking may explain these changes. Between 1972 and 1990, the proportion of men aged 16 years and over who smoked cigarettes declined from 52 to 31 per cent, and of women from 41 to 29 per cent.[7] The decline was greater among the elderly than young adults, and greater among those in Social Classes I & II than in Classes IV & V.

There was an increase in the prevalence rate for breast cancer between 1981-82 and 1991-92 (table 3D). This increase occurred in each age group. The rates of first incidence in the two surveys were similar, except for the very elderly, among whom the first incidence rate increased. This suggests that there has been no increase in the incidence of breast cancer except among those aged 75 years and over.

Between 1981-82 and 1991-92 there was no difference in the consulting rates for cancers of the gastrointestinal tract or for leukaemia.

The proportion of people of both sexes who consulted in 1991-92 for benign neoplasms of the skin increased compared with 1981-82 (table 3D). There was little change in the patient consulting rates for uterine fibroids between the two studies (table 3D).

Table 3A   All diseases and conditions, category of severity, ICD chapter: prevalence rates per 10,000 person years at risk

Chapter		Persons	All ages	0-4	5-14	15-24	25-44	45-64	65-74	75+
All diseases		1981–82	7,116	9,846	6,686	7,054	6,768	6,749	7,388	7,890
& conditions		1991–92	7,803	10,221	7,243	7,536	7,537	7,610	8,271	9,082
		Change	+10%	+4%	+8%	+7%	+9%	+13%	+12%	+15%
Serious		1981–82	1,439	649	538	653	865	1,959	3,411	4,439
		1991–92	1,829	1,200	995	940	1,088	2,352	4,015	5,114
		Change	+27%	+85%	+85%	+44%	+26%	+20%	+18%	+15%
Intermediate		1981–82	4,160	6,200	4,004	3,862	3,710	4,021	4,693	4,914
		1991–92	4,741	6,843	4,446	4,390	4,189	4,597	5,554	5,912
		Change	+14%	+10%	+11%	+14%	+13%	+14%	+18%	+20%
Trivial		1981–82	5,702	8,843	5,187	5,922	5,719	5,148	5,195	5,625
		1991–92	6,576	9,376	5,603	6,396	6,343	6,366	6,618	7,659
		Change	+15%	+6%	+8%	+8%	+11%	+24%	+27%	+36%
I	Infectious and parasitic	1981–82	1,172	3,472	1,759	1,297	1,022	595	530	580
		1991–92	1,339	3,648	1,946	1,573	1,298	789	776	819
		Change	+14%	+5%	+11%	+21%	+27%	+33%	+46%	+41%
II	Neoplasms	1981–82	135	28	29	52	111	193	315	361
		1991–92	239	54	86	131	218	317	452	548
		Change	+77%	+93%	+197%	+152%	+96%	+64%	+43%	+52%
III	Endocrine	1981–82	288	32	48	163	269	474	568	516
		1991–92	377	60	41	115	277	682	907	744
		Change	+31%	+88%	-15%	-29%	+3%	+44%	+60%	+44%
IV	Blood	1981–82	78	40	29	45	73	78	134	253
		1991–92	97	58	59	53	74	88	182	345
		Change	+24%	+45%	+103%	+18%	-	+13%	+36%	+36%
V	Mental	1981–82	854	317	172	637	1,053	1,159	1,111	1,292
		1991–92	728	228	185	584	824	946	919	1,228
		Change	-15%	-28%	+8%	-8%	-22%	-18%	-17%	-5%
VI	Nervous	1981–82	1,409	3,710	1,640	949	1,039	1,232	1,530	1,711
		1991–92	1,732	4,252	1,941	1,080	1,258	1,549	2,078	2,470
		Change	+23%	+15%	+18%	+14%	+21%	+26%	+36%	+44%
VII	Circulatory	1981–82	850	17	14	124	400	1,435	2,630	3,094
		1991–92	931	19	22	139	376	1,488	3,035	3,559
		Change	+10%	+12%	+57%	+12%	-6%	+4%	+15%	+15%
VIII	Respiratory	1981–82	2,696	6,188	3,414	2,594	2,307	2,024	2,258	2,241
		1991–92	3,070	6,471	3,715	3,134	2,546	2,405	2,817	3,038
		Change	+14%	+5%	+9%	+21%	+10%	+19%	+25%	+36%
IX	Digestive	1981–82	720	968	320	552	665	828	1,084	1,204
		1991–92	866	834	307	604	791	1,038	1,405	1,687
		Change	+20%	-14%	-4%	+9%	+19%	+25%	+30%	+40%
X	Genitourinary	1981–82	864	411	298	1,114	1,265	843	590	694
		1991–92	1,133	570	419	1,242	1,431	1,327	928	1111
		Change	+31%	+39%	+41%	+11%	+13%	+57%	+57%	+60%
XII	Skin	1981–82	1,178	2,085	1,141	1,468	1,064	948	1,041	1,089
		1991–92	1,455	2,715	1,354	1,732	1,288	1,177	1,387	1,504
		Change	+24%	+30%	+19%	+18%	+21%	+24%	+33%	+38%
XIII	Musculoskeletal	1981–82	1,328	170	413	820	1,345	2,004	2,215	2,395
		1991–92	1521	161	462	837	1,393	2,354	2,702	2,195
		Change	+15%	-5%	+12%	+2%	+4%	+17%	+22%	-8%

Table 3A - *continued*

Chapter		Persons	All ages	0-4	5-14	15-24	25-44	45-64	65-74	75+
XIV	Congenital	1981–82	26	174	46	18	10	7	8	10
		1991–92	53	217	60	34	34	42	46	46
		Change	+104%	+25%	+30%	+89%	+240%	+500%	+475%	+360%
XV	Perinatal	1981–82	3	40	1	0	-	-	-	-
		1991–92	13	173	0	2	2	0	-	2
		Change	+333%	+332%	-	-	-	-	-	-
XVI	Signs, symptoms & ill-defined	1981–82	1,595	2,961	1,497	1,343	1,338	1,406	1,805	2,535
		1991–92	1,510	2,721	1,386	1,234	1,195	1,403	1,855	2,480
		Change	-5%	-8%	-7%	-8%	-11%	-	+3%	-2%
XVII	Injury and poisoning	1981–82	1,135	1,131	1,176	1,358	1,074	1,031	1,011	1,290
		1991–92	1,390	1,293	1,351	1,528	1,375	1,306	1,293	1,745
		Change	+22%	+14%	+15%	+13%	+28%	+27%	+28%	+35%
XVIII	Supplementary classification	1981–82	2,003	3,604	727	2,926	2,515	1,440	1,282	1,682
		1991–92	3,348	5,313	1,040	3,620	3,525	3,254	3,380	4,652
		Change	+67%	+47%	+43%	+24%	+40%	+26%	+64%	+177%

Table 3B   Summary for selected infectious and parasitic diseases

		All ages	0-4	5-14	15-24	25-44	45-64	65-74	75+
Urogenital candida (ICD 112.1, 112.2): *prevalence rates per 10,000 person years at risk, by sex*									
Males	1981–82	23	70	5	31	28	14	10	16
	1991–92*†	43	109	12	58	53	30	24	20
	Change	+87%	+56%	+140%	+87%	+89%	+114%	+140%	+25%
Females	1981–82	219	122	28	438	434	82	26	22
	1991–92*†	445	234	93	837	813	239	84	51
	Change	+103%	+92%	+232%	+91%	+87%	+191%	+223%	+132%
Herpes simplex (ICD 054): *prevalence rates per 10,000 person years at risk, by sex*									
Males	1981–82	23	55	35	24	20	11	18	8
	1991–92	50	75	65	53	51	33	48	28
	Change	+117%	+36%	+86%	+121%	+155%	+200%	+167%	+250%
Females	1981–82	39	58	47	56	46	27	21	8
	1991–92	110	85	93	155	154	91	60	33
	Change	+182%	+47%	+98%	+177%	+235%	+237%	+186%	+312%
Dermatophytosis and dermatomycosis (ICD 110, 111): *prevalence rates per 10,000 person years at risk*									
Persons	1981–82	94	74	112	128	107	79	50	39
	1991–92	167	116	205	198	184	152	144	83
	Change	+78%	+57%	+83%	+55%	+72%	+92%	+188%	+113%
Viral warts (ICD 078.1): *prevalence rates per 10,000 person years at risk*									
Persons	1981–82	137	63	444	185	86	47	38	26
	1991–92	176	128	603	235	117	70	54	35
	Change	+28%	+103%	+36%	+27%	+36%	+49%	+42%	+35%
Scabies (ICD 133): *prevalence rates per 10,000 person years at risk*									
Persons	1981–82	22	29	36	48	18	8	5	5
	1991–92	34	49	59	57	30	17	8	23
	Change	+55%	+69%	+64%	+19%	+67%	+113%	+60%	+360%

* 1991–92 age groups are 5-15 and 16-24

† 1991–92 ICD 112 and 112.2 rates have been summed, possibly producing duplication

Table 3C Summary for neoplasms in the serious and intermediate categories

		All ages	0-4	5-14	15-24	25-44	45-64	65-74	75+
Neoplasms in the serious category: *prevalence rates per 10,000 person years at risk, by sex*									
Males	1981–82	64	3	3	4	11	91	276	426
	1991–92	77	3	2	5	15	95	327	572
	Change	+20%	-	-33%	+25%	+36%	+4%	+18%	+35%
Females	1981–82	71	-	1	4	29	113	212	255
	1991–92	95	5	4	6	30	156	266	355
	Change	+34%	-	+300%	+50%	+3%	+38%	+25%	+39%
Neoplasms in the intermediate category: *prevalence rates per 10,000 person years at risk, by sex*									
Males	1981–82	47	30	25	33	48	67	79	50
	1991–92	117	46	83	81	123	153	177	136
	Change	+149%	+53%	+240%	+145%	+156%	+128%	+124%	+172%
Females	1981–82	87	23	30	63	131	118	83	56
	1991–92	198	55	84	171	272	252	179	138
	Change	+128%	+139%	+180%	+171%	+108%	+114%	+116%	+146%

Table 3D Summary for selected neoplasms

		All ages	0-4	5-14	15-24	25-44	45-64	65-74	75+
Cancer of the larynx, trachea, bronchus & lung (ICD 161, 162): *prevalence rates per 10,000 person years at risk, by sex*									
Males	1971–72	14	1	-	-	2	28	68	60
	1981–82	14	-	-	-	2	24	66	66
	1991–92	10	-	-	0	1	16	51	67
	1981/91 change	-29%	-	-	-	-	-27%	-23%	+2%
Females	1971–72	3	-	-	-	1	6	13	4
	1981–82	4	-	-	-	0	10	18	7
	1991–92	5	-	-	-	0	10	17	17
	1981/91 change	+25%	-	-	-	-	-	-6%	+143%
Cancer of the larynx, trachea, bronchus & lung (ICD 161, 162): *first incidence rates per 10,000 person years at risk, by sex*									
Males	1981–82	6	-	-	-	1	8	33	41
	1991–92	4	-	-	-	0	6	18	32
	Change	-33%	-	-	-	-	-25%	-45%	-22%
Females	1981–82	2	-	-	-	0	6	8	3
	1991–92	2	-	-	-	0	3	6	9
	Change	-	-	-	-	-	-50%	-25%	+200%
Cancer of the breast (ICD 174): *prevalence rates per 10,000 female years at risk*									
	1971–72	19	-	-	1	8	35	51	67
	1981–82	23	-	-	-	8	44	72	69
	1991–92	30	-	-	-	10	61	81	88
	1981/91 change	+30%	-	-	-	+25%	+39%	+12%	+28%
Cancer of the breast (ICD 174): *first incidence rates per 10,000 female years at risk*									
	1981–82	8	-	-	-	4	15	26	18
	1991–92	8	-	-	-	4	15	20	25
	Change	-	-	-	-	-	-	-23%	+39%
Benign neoplasm of skin (ICD 216): *prevalence rates per 10,000 person years at risk, by sex*									
Males	1981–82	23	14	15	15	23	31	42	16
	1991–92	56	21	50	47	58	70	75	36
	Change	+143%	+50%	+133%	+213%	+152%	+126%	+79%	+125%
Females	1981–82	33	10	18	33	43	40	38	17
	1991–92	94	21	52	111	135	104	71	41
	Change	+185%	+110%	+189%	+136%	+214%	+160%	+87%	+141%
Uterine leiomyoma and other benign neoplasm of uterus (ICD 218, 219): *prevalence rates per 10,000 female years at risk*									
	1981–82	13	-	-	2	28	25	2	2
	1991–92	13	-	-	0	22	29	1	1
	Change	-	-	-	-	-21%	+16%	-100%	-100%

Endocrine, nutritional and metabolic diseases and immunity disorders

Consulting rates for diseases in this chapter increased from 288 to 377 per 10,000 person years at risk between 1981-82 and 1991-92. For serious disorders prevalence increased from 150 to 209 per 10,000 people. Prevalence rates increased from 25 to 104 for diseases in the intermediate category, but decreased from 125 to 82 for trivial conditions.

Consulting rates for thyrotoxicosis decreased from 14 per 10,000 people in 1981-82 to 9 in 1991-92. Decreases occurred across all age groups (table 3E). First incidence rates for thyrotoxicosis decreased from 4 to 2 per 10,000 between the two surveys. In contrast, prevalence rates for hypothyroidism increased from 33 to 51 per 10,000 persons (table 3E). First incidence rates were the same in the two surveys. This suggests that new incidence and prevalence of thyrotoxicosis have declined over the last ten years and that whilst the incidence of hypothyroidism has remained unchanged, its prevalence as measured by the proportion consulting for this disease has increased substantially.

Prevalence rates for diabetes increased from 74 to 111 per 10,000 person years between 1981-82 and 1991-92, although the first incidence rates declined. Prevalence and first incidence rates were higher among men than women in both surveys (table 3E).

The consulting rate for disorders of lipoid metabolism increased tenfold from 6 per 10,000 in 1981-82 to 61 in 1991-92, accounting for much of the increase in the intermediate category of severity in this chapter. Screening for cardiovascular risk factors including blood cholesterol is now commonplace in general practice, whereas it was performed infrequently in 1981-82. In contrast, the proportion of people recorded as having consulted for obesity decreased from 125 per 10,000 persons in 1981-82 to 85 in 1991-92 (table 3E). Obesity was categorised as a trivial disorder.

Consulting rates for gout increased from 27 per 10,000 to 40 between the surveys (table 3E). Increased prevalence was evident among people in all age groups.

Diseases of the blood and blood-forming organs

There was a small increase in the consulting rate for disorders included in this ICD chapter, from 78 per 10,000 persons in 1981-82 to 97 in 1991-92. Rates for serious conditions decreased from 17 to 8 per 10,000 persons. Prevalence of reported iron deficiency anaemia increased slightly (table 3F), as did the proportion of people who consulted for pernicious and other deficiency anaemias. Other and unspecified anaemias accounted for most of the overall increase in consulting rates for diseases of the blood.

Mental disorders

Reduced consulting rates between 1981-82 and 1991-92 were only found for two ICD chapters — mental disorders, and symptoms, signs and ill-defined conditions. This reduction in the patient consulting rate for mental disorders was greatest among women aged 25-74 years (table 3G). The decrease among mental conditions was mainly for those in the intermediate category of severity, but also to a lesser extent for trivial conditions. The decline in trivial conditions may have arisen from the increase in the availability of counsellors in primary care. Among intermediate illnesses, the reduction was mainly for depressive disorders. For trivial conditions, defined as 'minor self-limiting illnesses which require no specific treatment', the consulting rates for several, such as anxiety states (table 3G), hysteria, insomnia, and psychalgia (pains of mental origin) decreased, but for neurasthenia (a neurotic disorder characterised by fatigue, irritability, headache, insomnia, etc.) the rate increased seven-fold (table 3G), suggesting a change in diagnostic patterns. Consulting rates for serious mental disorders increased from 72 to 113 per 10,000 people, reflecting the move of patients with chronic psychiatric illness into the community. The increase was distributed evenly among all adult age groups of both sexes. This increase was mainly for the affective psychoses, from 21 per 10,000 in 1981-82 to 60 in 1991-92.

Disorders of the nervous system and sense organs

Consulting rates for nervous diseases increased from 1409 per 10,000 persons in 1981-82 to 1732 in 1991-92. Increases were evident among people in all age groups, but were greatest among the elderly. The relative increase was greater for intermediate disorders than for serious ones. There was a decrease in the proportion of people who consulted for trivial conditions.

There was little change between 1981-82 and 1991-92 in the proportion of people who consulted for Parkinson's disease, multiple sclerosis or epilepsy. Consulting rates for migraine increased between the two surveys from 82 per 10,000 in 1981-82 to 115 in 1991-92 (table 3H). For vertiginous syndromes, the rate increased from 49 to 73 per 10,000.

Increased consulting rates among the elderly were reported for glaucoma and cataracts (table 3H), perhaps partly reflecting the increase in the average age of the population within the 65-74 and 75 years and over age groups.

There was an increase in the proportion of patients who consulted for conjunctivitis from 284 per 10,000 in 1981-82 to 395 in 1991-92 (table 3H). The consulting rate for acute suppurative and unspecified otitis media decreased from 233 per 10,000 in 1981-82 to 164 in 1991-92, but this change was largely compensated for by an increase in the rate for non-suppurative otitis media, from 166 per 10,000 to more than 271.

Diseases of the circulatory system

The overall consulting rates for diseases in this chapter increased from 850 per 10,000 in 1981-82 to 931 in 1991-92. Increases occurred among people in all age groups except 25-44 years. Small increases were evident for each category of severity.

For this comparison, uncomplicated hypertension was categorised as an intermediate illness, and hypertension with organic damage as serious. Since people may have been assigned to one or more rubrics in each of these categories

Table 3E   Summary for selected endocrine, nutritional and metabolic diseases and immunity disorders

		All ages	0-4	5-14	15-24	25-44	45-64	65-74	75+
Thyrotoxicosis (ICD 242): *prevalence rates per 10,000 person years at risk, by sex*									
Males	1981–82	5	3	1	1	5	8	11	14
	1991–92	3	-	-	1	2	5	10	8
	Change	-40%	-	-	-	-60%	-38%	-9%	-43%
Females	1981–82	22	2	1	10	25	35	41	28
	1991–92	15	-	-	3	16	23	31	24
	Change	-32%	-	-	-70%	-36%	-8%	-24%	-14%
Hypothyroidism (ICD 243, 244): *prevalence rates per 10,000 person years at risk, by sex*									
Males	1971–72	5	1	1	1	4	8	13	15
	1981–82	8	1	1	2	4	18	23	17
	1991–92	12	1	1	2	6	19	42	55
	1981/91 change	+50%	-	-	-	+50%	+6%	+83%	+224%
Females	1971–72	32	2	1	3	14	58	106	74
	1981–82	56	-	2	7	25	110	154	138
	1991–92	87	1	4	11	49	157	245	201
	1981/91 change	+55%	-	+100%	+57%	+96%	+43%	+59%	+46%
Diabetes (ICD 250): *prevalence rates per 10,000 person years at risk, by sex*									
Males	1971–72	47	2	5	14	27	85	173	163
	1981–82	74	2	10	16	35	132	255	274
	1991–92	119	1	8	23	49	217	428	451
	1981/91 change	+61%	-50%	-20%	+44%	+40%	+64%	+68%	+65%
Females	1971–72	47	-	8	13	20	72	154	139
	1981–82	73	1	10	21	29	108	223	224
	1991–92	102	1	8	14	34	154	337	339
	1981/91 change	+40%	-	-20%	-33%	+17%	+43%	+51%	+51%
Diabetes (ICD 250): *first incidence rates per 10,000 person years at risk, by sex*									
Males	1981–82	19	2	5	3	9	33	57	74
	1991–92*	17	-	2	4	8	31	64	53
	Change	-11%	-	-60%	+33%	-11%	-6%	+12%	-28%
Females	1981–82	17	1	5	7	8	24	51	48
	1991–92*	15	1	3	1	5	22	55	44
	Change	-12%	-	-40%	-86%	-38%	-8%	+8%	-8%
Gout (ICD 274): *prevalence rates per 10,000 person years at risk, by sex*									
Males	1971–72	27	-	-	1	22	61	63	59
	1981–82	46	-	-	1	31	99	130	136
	1991–92	64	-	1	1	43	125	197	180
	1981/91 change	+39%	-	-	-	+39%	+26%	+52%	+32%
Females	1971–72	6	-	-	1	4	12	18	8
	1981–82	10	-	-	1	5	15	31	37
	1991–92	16	-	-	2	4	21	53	70
	1981/91 change	+60%	-	-	+50%	-20%	+40%	+71%	+89%
Obesity (ICD 278.0): *prevalence rates per 10,000 person years at risk, by sex*									
Males	1981–82	54	15	21	42	57	93	64	46
	1991–92	38	4	14	14	41	72	62	17
	Change	-24%	-73%	-33%	-67%	-28%	-23%	-3%	-63%
Females	1981–82	189	1	35	194	271	291	166	66
	1991–92	124	4	19	103	162	213	134	41
	Change	-34%	+300%	-46%	-47%	-40%	-27%	-19%	-38%

* 1991–92 age groups are 5-15 and 16-24

Table 3F   Summary for selected diseases of the blood and blood forming organs

		All ages	0-4	5-14	15-24	25-44	45-64	65-74	75+
Iron deficiency anaemia (ICD 280): *prevalence rates per 10,000 person years at risk, by sex*									
Males	1981–82	16	25	7	3	5	16	49	104
	1991–92	19	22	9	3	4	17	70	132
	Change	+19%	-12%	+29%	-	-20%	+6%	+43%	+27%
Females	1981–82	84	18	15	56	103	93	105	191
	1991–92	87	18	10	64	101	86	101	226
	Change	+4%	-	-33%	+14%	-2%	-8%	-4%	+18%

Table 3G   Summary for selected mental disorders

		All ages	0-4	5-14	15-24	25-44	45-64	65-74	75+
Mental disorders (ICD 290-319): *prevalence rates per 10,000 person years at risk, by sex*									
Males	1981–82	554	366	175	379	648	777	697	912
	1991–92	503	256	200	379	533	681	632	891
	Change	-9%	-30%	+14%	0	-18%	-12%	-9%	-2%
Females	1981–82	1,127	266	169	877	1,427	1,522	1,437	1,483
	1991–92	944	199	169	789	1,117	1,216	1,152	1,407
	Change	-16%	-25%	-	-10%	-22%	-20%	-20%	-5%
Anxiety states (ICD 300.0): *prevalence rates per 10,000 person years at risk, by sex*									
Males	1981–82	160	10	23	106	232	246	195	147
	1991–92	135	9	12	99	173	204	176	147
	Change	-16%	-10%	-48%	-7%	-25%	-17%	-10%	-
Females	1981–82	376	12	28	272	539	546	461	342
	1991–92	290	4	20	221	373	426	371	304
	Change	-23%	-67%	-21%	-19%	-31%	-22%	-20%	-11%
Neurotic depression and depressive disorder NEC (ICD 300.4, 311): *prevalence rates per 10,000 person years at risk, by sex*									
Males	1981–82	124	4	9	68	135	217	205	262
	1991–92	91	1	3	61	100	146	141	177
	Change	-27%	-75	-66%	-10%	-26%	-33%	-31%	-32%
Females	1981–82	383	2	13	295	508	559	510	441
	1991–92	246	-	7	197	342	329	283	285
	Change	-36%	-	-46%	-33%	-33%	-41%	-45%	-35%
Neurasthenia (ICD 300.5): *prevalence rates per 10,000 person years at risk, by sex*									
Males	1981–82	6	1	2	4	9	7	8	14
	1991–92*	35	5	18	45	37	49	41	39
	Change	+483%	+400%	+800%	+1,025%	+311%	+600%	+412%	+179%
Females	1981–82	14	5	1	16	18	17	15	21
	1991–92*	103	10	28	139	132	121	103	94
	Change	+636%	+100%	+2,200%	+769%	+633%	+612%	+587%	+348%

*   1991–92 age groups are 5-15 and 16-24

Table 3H Summary for selected diseases of the nervous system and sense organs

		All ages	0-4	5-14	15-24	25-44	45-64	65-74	75+
Migraine (ICD 346): *prevalence rates per 10,000 person years at risk, by sex*									
Males	1971–72	49	3	47	70	68	43	26	10
	1981–82	47	8	45	58	62	49	28	9
	1991–92	58	4	84	73	65	56	36	21
	1981/91 change	+23%	-50%	+87%	+26%	+5%	+14%	+29%	+133%
Females	1971–72	111	-	47	130	189	138	45	13
	1981–82	113	1	57	143	176	141	47	17
	1991–92	169	3	105	226	251	197	75	36
	1981/91 change	+50%	+200%	+84%	+58%	+43%	+40%	+60%	+112%
Glaucoma (ICD 365): *prevalence rates per 10,000 person years at risk*									
Persons	1971–72	8	-	-	-	1	9	41	39
	1981–82	12	-	0	0	2	18	46	67
	1991–92	21	-	-	0	3	29	77	120
	1981/91 change	+75%	-	-	-	+50%	+61%	+67%	+79%
Cataract (ICD 366): *prevalence rates per 10,000 person years at risk*									
Persons	1971–72	17	2	0	1	2	17	68	154
	1981–82	22	2	1	0	2	18	78	164
	1991–92	34	1	1	1	1	19	127	322
	1981/91 change	+55%	-50%	-	-	-50%	+6%	+63%	+96%
Conjunctivitis (ICD 372.0-372.3): *prevalence rates per 10,000 person years at risk*									
Persons	1981–82	284	1165	330	237	193	192	206	210
	1991–92	396	1828	394	224	246	272	371	401
	Change	+39%	+57%	+19%	-5%	+27%	+42%	+80%	+91%

during the year as their disease progressed, there is potential overlap in the prevalence data. Given the best comparison available, prevalence of uncomplicated hypertension was similar in the two surveys for people aged under 65 years. For people aged 65 years and over, there was a considerable increase in prevalence between 1981-82 and 1991-92 (table 3I).

The first incidence rate of acute myocardial infarction fell from 26 per 10,000 in 1981-82 to 15 in 1991-92. Among people aged 45-64 years, first incidence rates in 1991-92 were half those in 1981-82. While prevalence rates for myocardial infarction declined between the two surveys, those for angina increased for both sexes (table 3I), suggesting that treatment of early symptoms has an effect on the outcome.

Prevalence of cerebrovascular disease increased from 40 per 10,000 in 1981-82 to 66 in 1991-92 (table 3I). The prevalence rate for varicose veins was similar in the two surveys, but that for haemorrhoids increased from 82 to 103 per 10,000 people.

Diseases of the respiratory system

There was an increase of 14 per cent between 1981-82 and 1991-92 in the prevalence rate for respiratory disorders. This increase was evident in all age groups. Rates for serious conditions almost doubled between the two surveys, an

increase almost entirely attributable to the rise in the proportion of people who consulted for asthma (table 3J).

In children, patient consulting rates for asthma in 1991-92 were over three times those in 1981-82 and over six times those in 1971-72. First incidence rates for all ages for asthma in 1981-82 were similar to those in 1991-92, but among children aged under five years they increased from 192 per 10,000 in 1981-82 to 339 in 1991-92 (table 3J). Rates for new and first episodes combined, for all ages, increased from 214 per 10,000 people in 1981-82 to 297 in 1991-92. They increased among people in each age group up to 44 years, but the greatest increase, from 342 to 883 per 10,000, was among children under five years of age. These data suggest that an increased proportion of people are consulting for asthma, the rate of new cases of asthma is increasing among small children only, and asthmatics, particularly small children, consulted for more attacks in 1991-92 than in 1981-82. Possible changes in the balance of care between hospital and the community and increased concern, particularly among parents of small children, may have contributed to the increase in the number of consultations for this condition.

The prevalence rate for acute bronchitis and bronchiolitis among children changed only slightly between the two surveys (table 3J). This suggests that the increase in the prevalence rate for asthma is not due simply to a change in the assignation of a diagnosis from one condition to another.

Table 3I   Summary for selected diseases of the circulatory system

		All ages	0-4	5-14	15-24	25-44	45-64	65-74	75+

Uncomplicated hypertension (ICD 401.1, 401.9): *prevalence rates per 10,000 person years at risk, by sex*

		All ages	0-4	5-14	15-24	25-44	45-64	65-74	75+
Males	1981–82†	314	-	1	7	116	737	1,149	754
	1991–92	347	1	1	9	100	757	1,485	836
	Change*≠	+11%	-	-	+29%	-14%	+3%	+29%	+11%
Females	1981–82†	427	-	0	22	118	873	1,477	968
	1991–92*≠	459	1	0	10	96	867	1,789	1,127
	Change	+7%	-	-	-55%	-19%	-1%	+21%	+16%

Acute myocardial infarction (ICD 410): *prevalence rates per 10,000 person years at risk, by sex*

		All ages	0-4	5-14	15-24	25-44	45-64	65-74	75+
Males	1971–72	52	-	-	1	15	116	214	176
	1981–82**	55	-	-	0	16	117	199	224
	1991–92	38	-	-	0	6	73	158	186
	1981/91 change	-31%	-	-	-	-63%	-38%	-21%	-17%
Females	1971–72	21	-	-	1	4	32	72	104
	1981–82**	29	-	-	-	3	38	111	128
	1991–92	20	-	-	-	1	20	71	118
	1981/91 change	-31%	-	-	-	-67%	-47%	-34%	-8%

Angina pectoris (ICD 413): *prevalence rates per 10,000 person years at risk, by sex*

		All ages	0-4	5-14	15-24	25-44	45-64	65-74	75+
Males	1971–72≠	54	-	-	1	11	121	238	196
	1981–82≠	81	-	-	-	9	172	354	319
	1991–92	130	-	-	0	14	257	580	573
	1981/91 change	+60%	-	-	-	+56%	+49%	+64%	+80%
Females	1971–72≠	46	-	1	1	6	71	191	178
	1981–82≠	58	-	-	0	7	91	215	228
	1991–92	98	1	-	0	7	133	364	440
	1981/91 change	+69%	-	-	-	-	+46%	+69%	+93%

Cerebrovascular disease (ICD 430-438): *prevalence rates per 10,000 person years at risk, by sex*

		All ages	0-4	5-14	15-24	25-44	45-64	65-74	75+
Males	1971–72	46	2	0	1	3	6	247	444
	1981–82§	39	-	-	1	2	42	153	396
	1991–92	64	-	0	2	3	72	272	579
	1981/91 change	+64%	-	-	+100%	+50%	+71%	+78%	+46%
Females	1971–72	49	-	1	1	4	36	167	408
	1981–82§	43	-	-	1	1	26	125	332
	1991–92	67	-	-	2	4	46	177	496
	1981/91 change	+56%	-	-	+100%	+300%	+77%	+42%	+49%

*   1991–92 age groups are 5-15 and 16-24
≠   1991–92 ICD 401.1 and 401.9 rates have been summed, possibly producing duplication
†   1981–82 includes part of secondary hypertension (ICD 405)
** 1981–82 includes other acute and subacute forms of ischaemic heart disease (ICD 411)
≠   1971–72 and 1981–82 includes angina of effort only (ICD 413 part)
§   1981–82 excludes transient cerebral ischaemia (ICD 435) and hypertensive encephalopathy (ICD 437.2)

Table 3J   Summary for selected diseases of the respiratory system

		All ages	0-4	5-14	15-24	25-44	45-64	65-74	75+
Asthma (ICD 493): *prevalence rates per 10,000 person years at risk, by sex*									
Males	1971–72	106	148	193	88	79	82	104	28
	1981–82	200	333	375	186	121	139	215	162
	1991–92	429	994	883	414	258	260	372	345
	1981/91 change	+114%	+198%	+135%	+123%	+113%	+87%	+73%	+113%
Females	1971–72	86	72	89	74	84	101	91	59
	1981–82	159	183	205	147	121	181	187	129
	1991–92	422	722	650	470	334	342	412	295
	1981/91 change	+165%	+295%	+217%	+220%	+176%	+89%	+120%	+129%
Asthma (ICD 493): *rates per 10,000 person years at risk*									
First episodes	1981–82	82	192	146	80	53	58	70	53
	1991–92*	81	339	146	69	47	39	46	29
	Change	-1%	+77%	-	-14%	-11%	-33%	-34%	-45%
First and new episodes	1981–82	214	342	356	200	146	188	227	158
	1991–92*	297	883	545	275	190	182	223	134
	Change	+39%	+158%	+53%	+37%	+30%	-3%	-2%	-15%
Prevalence	1981–82	178	260	293	166	121	161	199	140
	1991–92*	425	861	755	428	296	300	394	312
	Change	+139%	+231%	+158%	+158%	+145%	+86%	+98%	+123%
Acute bronchitis, bronchiolitis and bronchitis not specified as acute or chronic (ICD 466, 490): *prevalence rates per 10,000 person years at risk, by sex*									
Males	1981–82	578	1,637	499	306	321	532	994	1,279
	1991–92	676	1,739	468	371	390	666	1,222	1,689
	1981/91 change	+17%	+6%	-6%	+21%	+21%	+25%	+23%	+32%
Females	1981–82	584	1,308	401	326	432	635	885	907
	1991–92	834	1,557	426	500	642	939	1,206	1,448
	1981/91 change	+43%	+19%	+6%	+53%	+49%	+48%	+36%	+60%
Chronic bronchitis (ICD 491): *prevalence rates per 10,000 person years at risk, by sex*									
Males	1981–82	81	2	1	0	13	123	379	475
	1991–92	54	5	2	5	6	73	270	313
	Change	-33%	+150%	+100%	-	-54%	-41%	-29%	-34%
Females	1981–82	40	-	0	1	14	67	136	123
	1991–92	37	4	3	6	9	57	130	119
	Change	-8%	-	-	+500%	-36%	-15%	-4%	-3%

* 1991–92 age groups are 5-15 and 16-24

There was a reduction in the proportion of both men and women who consulted for chronic bronchitis between 1981-82 and 1991-92 (table 3J). The prevalence of allergic rhinitis, which includes hay fever, increased from 197 per 10,000 in 1981-82 to 283 in 1991-92.

Diseases of the digestive system

Consulting rates for gastrointestinal disorders increased from 720 per 10,000 in 1981-82 to 866 in 1991-92. These increases were confined to adults and the elderly (table 3K). Rates for serious conditions, which include peptic ulcers, hernias and liver and gall bladder diseases, were similar in the two surveys, except for children among whom the rates were lower in 1991-92 compared with 1981-82.

The proportion of people who were diagnosed as having gastric, duodenal or peptic ulcers was unchanged between the surveys. However, the consulting rate for oesophagitis increased from 24 to 103 per 10,000 people, and the consulting rate for gastritis and duodenitis increased from 27 to 74 per 10,000 people between 1981-82 and 1991-92. There was also an increase in the proportion who consulted for disorders of the function of the stomach, which includes dyspepsia.

Consulting rates for gall bladder and liver diseases were similar in both surveys, as were those for diverticular disease and other disorders of the lower intestinal tract. The proportion of children and young adults who consulted for appendicitis decreased (table 3K). There was no change in the

Table 3K   Summary for selected diseases of the digestive system

		All ages	0-4	5-14	15-24	25-44	45-64	65-74	75+
Diseases of the digestive system (ICD 520-579): *prevalence rates per 10,000 person years at risk, by sex*									
Males	1981–82	678	1,015	319	441	615	813	1,090	1,304
	1991–92	742	870	308	423	645	943	1,410	1,752
	Change	+9%	-14%	-3%	-4%	+5%	+16%	+29%	+34%
Females	1981–82	758	917	322	656	711	843	1,079	1,154
	1991–92	1,009	796	305	785	938	1,134	1,400	1,652
	Change	+33%	-13%	-5%	+20%	+32%	+35%	+30%	+43%
Appendicitis (ICD 540-542): *prevalence rates per 10,000 person years at risk*									
Persons	1981–82	14	5	30	30	12	6	4	4
	1991–92	9	1	18	22	9	4	2	1
	Change	-36%	-80%	-40%	-27%	-25%	-33%	-50%	-75%

proportion consulting for inguinal hernias, but the rate increased for diaphragmatic hernias.

Diseases of the genitourinary system

There was an increase of 31 per cent in the proportion of people who consulted for conditions in this chapter, from 864 per 10,000 people in 1981-82 to 1133 in 1991-92. Increases were most evident in the rates for children aged under five years, from 411 per 10,000 in 1981-82 to 570 in 1991-92, and among adults aged 45 years and over. Rates for serious conditions declined from 34 to 23 per 10,000 people between the two surveys.

There was no change in the consulting rates for renal calculus, but for pyelonephritis there was a decrease from 23 to 14 per 10,000 people. In contrast, consulting rates for cystitis and urinary infections increased (table 3L). The now widespread use of the initials UTI for urinary tract infections as a generic term embracing all urinary infections limits direct comparison between the surveys, but it is estimated that there was an increase from 241 to approximately 315 per 10,000 persons.

The prevalence of orchitis and epididymitis increased from 19 to 30 per 10,000 males between the two surveys. Over the same period, the prevalence of prostatic hypertrophy decreased from 37 to 27 per 10,000 male years at risk (table 3L). For other male genitourinary problems, consulting rates remained unchanged.

The proportion of women consulting for benign mammary dysplasia declined from 50 to 36 per 10,000 female years at risk between 1981-82 and 1991-92. There was an increase in the consulting rate for a group of conditions termed 'other diseases of the breast', which includes lumps in the breast,

Table 3L   Summary for selected diseases of the genitourinary system

		All ages	0-4	5-14	15-24	25-44	45-64	65-74	75+
Cystitis and urinary tract infection site not specified (ICD 595, 599.0): *prevalence rates per 10,000 person years at risk, by sex*									
Males	1981–82	79	104	42	35	50	91	162	309
	1991–92	117	132	68	44	65	125	292	505
	Change	+48%	+27%	+62%	+26%	+30%	+37%	+80%	+63%
Females	1981–82	390	248	173	478	494	371	379	396
	1991–92	586	339	270	690	643	558	675	843
	Change	+50%	+37%	+56%	+44%	+30%	+50%	+78%	+113%
Hyperplasia of prostate (ICD 600): *prevalence rates per 10,000 male years at risk*									
	1981–82	37	-	-	1	1	49	173	284
	1991–92	27	-	-	-	1	41	136	177
	Change	-27%	-	-	-	-	-16%	-21%	-38%
Menopausal and postmenopausal disorders (ICD 627): *prevalence rates per 10,000 female years at risk*									
	1981–82	129	-	-	2	73	496	62	34
	1991–92	328	-	-	1	170	1,219	197	106
	Change	+154%	-	-	-50%	+133%	+146%	+218%	+212%

from 75 to 160 per 10,000 female years at risk. There was also an increase, from 47 to 70 per 10,000 females, in the consulting rate for pelvic inflammatory disease. Among problems associated with menstruation, an increased proportion of women consulted for premenstrual tension syndromes and dysmenorrhoea in 1991-92 than in 1981-82, and 328 per 10,000 women consulted for menopausal and postmenopausal symptoms compared with 129 in 1981-82 (table 3L).

Pregnancy, childbirth and the puerperium; congenital abnormalities; conditions arising in the perinatal period

These chapters are taken together because the increased emphasis on hospital confinements in 1991-92 compared with 1981-82 limits comparison.

The prevalence of women consulting for haemorrhage in early pregnancy increased from 69 to 98 per 10,000 females aged 15-24 years, and from 59 to 93 among those aged 25-44 years.

Among children aged under five years, there was an increase in the rate consulting for congenital abnormalities, from 209 to 265 per 10,000 boys and from 136 to 167 per 10,000 girls between 1981-82 and 1991-92. The proportion of boys aged under five years who consulted for undescended testicles increased from 62 to 82 per 10,000, but there was no difference above that age. Consulting rates by children aged under five years for conditions originating in the perinatal period increased from 40 to 173 per 10,000 persons. These were nearly all neonatal infections. Increased rates for conditions arising during the perinatal period reflect increased general practitioner involvement in neonatal care following early discharge after confinement in hospital.

Diseases of the skin and subcutaneous tissue

The proportion of people who consulted for skin diseases increased from 12 per cent in 1981-82 to 15 per cent in 1991-92. Increases were evident among people of all ages and both sexes, but were greatest among those aged 65 years and over.

The prevalence of psoriasis fell from 44 to 24 per 10,000 persons between 1981-82 and 1991-92, after having increased between 1971-72 and 1981-82. This decrease occurred among people of all ages (table 3M).

The proportion of people with eczema more than doubled, from 110 to 258 per 10,000 persons between the two surveys. This change affected people of all ages (table 3M). Prevalence rates for acne also increased between 1981-82 and 1991-92, from 90 to 132 per 10,000 persons, affecting mainly those aged 5-44 years (table 3M).

Diseases of the musculoskeletal system and connective tissue

The proportion of people who consulted for disorders in this chapter increased from 13 per cent in 1981-82 to 15 per cent in 1991-92. The greatest increase was for serious conditions, which include osteoarthritis and rheumatoid arthritis.

Patient consulting rates for osteoarthritis increased from 235 per 10,000 people in 1981-82 to 315 in 1991-92. This increase occurred for people in every age group and both sexes (table 3N). Osteoarthritis of the spine, which is coded separately, also increased, from 41 per 10,000 people in 1981-82 to 119 in 1991-92.

In contrast to osteoarthritis, the prevalence rate of rheumatoid arthritis decreased, from 56 per 10,000 people to between 38 and 42 in 1991-92. The uncertainty about the exact difference is because the 1981-82 data included ankylosing spondylitis (ICD 720.0) of which the consulting rate was 4 in 1991-92, compared with 38 for rheumatoid arthritis (ICD 714). The reduction in prevalence occurred in all age groups and both sexes (table 3N). There was also a decrease in the

---

Table 3M   Summary for selected diseases of the skin and subcutaneous tissue

		All ages	0-4	5-14	15-24	25-44	45-64	65-74	75+
Psoriasis (ICD 696.0, 696.1): *prevalence rates per 10,000 person years at risk*									
Persons	1971–72*	35	8	26	36	43	42	36	33
	1981–82	44	10	26	44	52	51	61	34
	1991–92	24	2	12	24	27	29	34	24
	1981/82 change	-45%	-80%	-54%	-45%	-46%	-43%	-43%	-29%
Atopic dermatitis and eczema (ICD 691.8): *prevalence rates per 10,000 person years at risk*									
Persons	1981–82	110	468	131	125	69	63	68	59
	1991–92†	258	951	296	252	186	166	199	171
	Change	+135%	+103%	+126%	+102%	+170%	+163%	+193%	+190%
Acne (ICD 706.0, 706.1): *prevalence rates per 10,000 person years at risk*									
Persons	1981–82	90	2	86	345	75	13	8	4
	1991–92	132	3	127	520	128	14	7	6
	Change	+47%	+50%	+48%	+51%	+71%	+8%	-13%	+50%

* 1971–72 includes all ICD 696 except 696.3
† 1991–92 age groups are 5-15 and 16-24

Table 3N   Summary for selected diseases of the musculoskeletal system

		All ages	0-4	5-14	15-24	25-44	45-64	65-74	75+
Osteoarthritis (ICD 715): *prevalence rates per 10,000 person years at risk, by sex*									
Males	1981–82	144	-	1	4	40	275	549	696
	1991–92	228	1	1	10	55	466	818	1,018
	Change	+58%	-	-	+150%	+37%	+69%	+49%	+46%
Females	1981–82	318	-	-	3	64	480	1,037	1,348
	1991–92	398	-	1	8	82	654	1,217	1,582
	Change	+25%	-	-	+167%	+28%	+36%	+17%	+17%
Rheumatoid arthritis (ICD 714, 720.0): *prevalence rates per 10,000 person years at risk, by sex*									
Males	1981–82	33	-	1	5	21	71	89	85
	1991–92	28	1	1	5	19	60	73	49
	Change	-15%	-	-	-	-10%	-15%	-18%	-44%
Females	1981–82	76	-	2	8	39	153	200	185
	1991–92	54	1	5	8	31	98	145	120
	Change	-29%	-	+150%	-	-21%	-36%	-28%	-35%
Rheumatoid arthritis (ICD 714, 720.0): *first incidence rates per 10,000 person years at risk, by sex*									
Males	1981–82	12	-	0	4	9	24	24	33
	1991–92*†	4	1	0	2	3	6	10	7
	Change	-66%	-	-	-50%	-67%	-75%	-58%	-79%
Females	1981–82	27	-	1	6	18	56	57	52
	1991–92*†	7	-	0	3	7	14	11	11
	Change	-74%	-	-	-50%	-61%	-75%	-81%	-79%
Back pain (ICD 720.1-720.9, 724.1, 724.2, 724.5-724.9): *prevalence rates per 10,000 person years at risk, by sex*									
Males	1981–82	276	4	44	228	397	397	303	319
	1991–92	259	12	41	180	335	374	317	356
	Change	-6%	+200%	-7%	-21%	-16%	-6%	+5%	+12%
Females	1981–82	304	5	52	272	401	423	337	346
	1991–92	339	4	62	285	422	476	391	406
	Change	+12%	-20%	+19%	+5%	+5%	+13%	+16%	+18%
Osteoporosis (ICD 733.0): *prevalence rates per 10,000 person years at risk, by sex*									
Males	1981–82	1	-	-	-	0	2	2	19
	1991–92	2	-	-	-	1	3	10	10
	Change	+100%	-	-	-	-	+50%	+50%	-47%
Females	1981–82	7	-	-	-	1	4	20	52
	1991–92	22	-	-	0	2	27	76	112
	Change	+214%	-	-	-	-100%	+575%	+180%	+115%

* 1991–92 age groups are 5-15 and 16-64
† 1991–92 excludes ankylosing spondylitis (ICD 720.0)

first incidence rates (table 3N), suggesting either that there is a real decline in prevalence of this condition in the community or that this diagnosis is used more restrictively.

The proportion of people who consulted at least once for any one or more of a number of conditions grouped together as back pain is shown in table 3N. Using these definitions of back pain, the rate declined among males and increased among females between 1981-82 and 1991-92.

The prevalence of osteoporosis increased between 1981-82 and 1991-92 among elderly women (table 3N).

Symptoms, signs and ill-defined conditions

The consulting rate for these problems decreased from 1595 per 10,000 people in 1981-82 to 1510 in 1991-92. The reduction occurred for both intermediate and trivial conditions. It is likely that more specific diagnoses have led to

Table 30   Summary for selected injuries and poisoning

		All ages	0-4	5-14	15-24	25-44	45-64	65-74	75+
Open wound (ICD 870-897): *prevalence rates per 10,000 person years at risk, by sex*									
Males	1981–82	172	298	237	252	135	114	108	91
	1991–92	167	289	252	226	128	108	120	164
	Change	-3%	-3%	+6%	-10%	-5%	-5%	+11%	+80%
Females	1981–82	109	195	142	96	72	84	124	194
	1991–92	116	189	134	83	77	95	137	257
	Change	+6%	-3%	-6%	-14%	+7%	+13%	+10%	+32%
Poisoning by drugs, medicaments and biological substances (ICD 960-979): *prevalence rates per 10,000 person years at risk, by sex*									
Males	1981–82	4	5	1	5	6	3	5	13
	1991–92	2	4	-	2	1	1	3	5
	Change	-50%	-20%	-	-60%	-83%	-67%	-40%	-62%
Females	1981–82	9	9	1	12	9	7	12	11
	1991–92	3	5	1	3	2	2	3	7
	Change	-67%	-44%	-	-75%	-78%	-71%	-75%	-34%

illnesses being assigned to other ICD chapters. Rates decreased for nearly every condition in this chapter. Examples are cough (from 250 to 195), nausea and/or vomiting (from 99 to 67), heartburn (from 25 to 10), abdominal pain (from 298 to 255), dysuria (from 41 to 25) and frequency of micturition (from 38 to 19).

Injury and poisoning

The proportion of people who consulted following an accident or injury increased from 11 per cent in 1981-82 to 14 per cent in 1991-92. In both surveys, consulting rates for males up to 25-44 years were higher than for females, but over this age the position was reversed.

Consulting rates for serious problems such as head injuries and the more serious fractures including those of the long bones of the leg increased among all adults but mainly the elderly. A smaller proportion of people consulted for intermediate conditions (mostly simple fractures) between 1981-82 and 1991-92. This decrease occurred among people of all ages and both sexes. The major increase in the consulting rates for conditions in this chapter was for trivial complaints not normally requiring specific treatment.

Consulting rates for fractures, burns and open wounds were similar in the two surveys, but there were increases for sprains, strains and contusions, particularly sprains and strains of the shoulder and arm, knee and neck. The proportion who

consulted for an open wound varied little overall between 1981-82 and 1991-92 but increased among the elderly (table 30). Prevalence of poisoning by drugs, medicaments, and biological substances fell by 50 per cent among males and 67 per cent among females (table 30).

Supplementary classification of factors influencing health status and contact with health services

This classification contains codes for reasons for consultation not directly associated with illness. It includes consultations for immunisation, health surveillance procedures and antenatal and contraceptive care. Consulting rates for reasons included in this chapter increased between 1981-82 and 1991-92 more than for any other ICD chapter except neoplasms, and congenital and perinatal conditions. In 1981-82, 20 per cent of people consulted at least once during the year, compared with 33 per cent in 1991-92. Increases were greatest among the elderly, for whom the consulting rate in 1991-92 was nearly three times that in 1981-82. All codes within this chapter were assigned to the trivial category of severity.

The changing role of general practice in health promotion is reflected in these comparative statistics. Influenza vaccination increased between the two surveys, from 71 to 533 per 10,000 people, tetanus toxoid alone from 59 to 311, and typhoid/ paratyphoid immunisation from 38 to 113, the last because of increased travel abroad. The rates for screening for cancer of the cervix increased from 362 to 750 per 10,000 female years at risk, and for hypertension from 25 to 143 per 10,000 people.

4 Variations in morbidity according to socio-economic characteristics and geographic region

4.1 Introduction

This chapter compares the proportion of people in different socio-economic groups who consulted at least once during the study year.

These data serve a different purpose from those presented in the following chapter. They allow comparison between one group, such as people living in council housing, with the whole sample population, in this case people living in any kind of accommodation. They also allow comparison between one group and another within that socio-economic characteristic, such as people living in council housing and those living in owner-occupied premises. This is a simple and easy method of comparison. The rates from this study can be applied to local communities to estimate local morbidity rates. However, it takes no account of other socio-economic characteristics which may influence the results. For example, people living in council housing may be more likely to be in Social Classes IV & V and to smoke, and these may be the characteristics of council housing tenants which influence their morbidity patterns, rather than the fact that they live in council housing. The regression analysis described in the next chapter looks at each socio-economic characteristic in turn, controlling for the effect of all other socio-economic characteristics. The method requires considerable resource to develop and to apply to local areas, but provides a more accurate comparison between people within a socio-economic characteristic. This chapter describes the results of analysis of single socio-economic characteristics without controlling for other characteristics.

Standardisation by five-year age groups minimises the effect that variations in the age distribution between those in different socio-economic groups may have on the proportion who consulted (see appendix B). This allows comparison between people in different groups for each socio-economic characteristic. These are presented here separately by sex, and, where appropriate, for children, adults and the elderly separately. The inclusion of 95 per cent confidence intervals indicates the significance of differences between socio-economic groups. Where these are large, the results should be treated with caution. No account has been taken of confounding factors, such as whether people living in council housing are more likely to belong to Social Classes IV & V. However, where appropriate, reference is made to the results of multivariate or regression analysis described in the following chapter.

The tables in the text show for each socio-economic group those ICD chapters for which the lower 95 per cent confidence limit of the standardised patient consulting ratio is above 100. Where this occurs, people within that socio-economic group were more likely to consult than the population as a whole within the same age/sex group. This is summarised in table 4A for all diseases and conditions and for category of severity. Each characteristic by ICD chapter is shown in the tables which follow.

The histograms illustrate the standardised patient consulting ratios for different groups within a socio-economic characteristic. Where the confidence limits do not overlap, the differences between the groups are significant at the 95 per cent level for that characteristic. These are discussed in the commentary.

4.2 Commentary

Summary of main findings

The main findings are summarised as follows (see also box). Men but not women living in the North or Midlands & Wales were more likely to consult than those living in the South of England. People living in urban areas were more likely to consult than those in rural areas. A higher proportion of council house tenants and those living in other rented accommodation, consulted than people living in owner occupied dwellings. By marital status, widowed and divorced people were more likely to consult than those who were single or married. Comparison between people who were cohabiting and not cohabiting showed that widowed, separated or divorced people who were not cohabiting were more likely to consult than people who were married or cohabiting, particularly for mental disorders. Adults with small children in the household were more likely to consult than those without children. By social class (as defined by occupation), a higher proportion of people in Classes IV & V consulted than those in Classes I & II, with a general gradient between these two extremes of class. This was reflected in the analysis by occupation, in which in general those in managerial and professional occupations were less likely to consult than those in construction, service and industrial occupations. People who were long term sick and, to a smaller extent, those who were unemployed were more likely to consult than those in full-time work. By ethnic group, a higher proportion of people who were not white consulted compared with those who were white, particularly for symptoms, signs and ill-defined conditions. Adults, but not the elderly, who smoked were more likely to consult than those who did not smoke.

Geographical region

The country was divided into three regions made up of regional health authorities: North (Northern, Yorkshire, Mersey and North Western), Midlands & Wales (Trent, East Anglian, West Midlands and Wales), and South (North West Thames, North East Thames, South East Thames, South West Thames, Wessex, Oxford and South Western). In the survey sample, 31 per cent of people lived in the North, 33 per cent in the Midlands & Wales, and 36 per cent in the South.

Table 4A People aged 16-64 years with socio-economic characteristics who were more likely to consult (lower SPCR confidence limit over 100)

		All diseases and conditions	Serious	Inter-mediate	Minor
Geographic region					
North	M	✓	✓		✓
Midlands & Wales	M			✓	✓
	F				✓
Tenure					
Council housing	M	✓	✓	✓	✓
	F	✓	✓	✓	✓
Other rented	M	✓	✓	✓	✓
	F	✓	✓	✓	✓
Communal	M		✓		
	F		✓		
Marital status					
Single	M		✓		
Widowed/divorced	M	✓	✓	✓	✓
	F	✓	✓	✓	✓
Cohabiting status					
Single	M		✓		
Separated/widowed/divorced not cohabiting	M	✓	✓	✓	✓
	F	✓	✓	✓	✓
Household composition					
Living alone	M	✓	✓	✓	✓
	F		✓	✓	✓
With children under 5 years only	M	✓		✓	✓
	F	✓		✓	✓
With children under 5 and 5-15 years	M			✓	✓
	F			✓	
Sole adult with children	F			✓	
Social class					
IIIM	M		✓	✓	
	F		✓	✓	
IV & V	M	✓	✓	✓	
	F		✓	✓	
Other	M		✓		
	F		✓		
Occupation					
5a	M		✓		
5c	M		✓	✓	
	F		✓		
6a	M				✓
6b	M	✓	✓	✓	✓
	F	✓	✓	✓	✓
8a	M		✓	✓	
	F		✓	✓	✓
8b	M	✓	✓	✓	✓
9b	M	✓	✓	✓	✓
	F		✓	✓	
Economic position					
Unemployed	M	✓	✓	✓	✓
	F	✓	✓	✓	✓
Long term sick	M	✓	✓	✓	✓
	F	✓	✓	✓	✓
Home/family	M	✓	✓	✓	
	F		✓	✓	
Ethnic group					
Indian	M				✓
	F		✓		
Pakistani/Bangladeshi	M		✓		✓
	F		✓		
Smokers	M	✓	✓	✓	
	F	✓	✓	✓	✓

Socio-economic characteristics associated with increased likelihood of consulting: people aged 16-64 years

Living in North or Midlands & Wales

In urban areas

Council property tenants

In other rented accommodation

Widowed and divorced

Living alone

Adults with young children

Social Classes IV & V

Construction, service and industrial occupations

Long-term sick

Unemployed

Ethnic minority group

Smokers

Men aged 16-64 years living in the North or in the Midlands & Wales were more likely to consult than those living in the South of England. This was most marked for circulatory, respiratory and musculoskeletal diseases, injury and poisoning, symptoms, signs and ill-defined conditions, and reasons in the supplementary classification. These differences were not on the whole apparent for women.

Comparison between those aged 16-64 years living in the North with those living in the Midlands & Wales shows no difference for all diseases and conditions. However, a higher proportion of men in the North consulted with serious illnesses and a higher proportion of women in the Midlands & Wales for minor ones. For conditions in each ICD chapter, the only difference for men was that those in the Midlands & Wales were more likely to consult than those in the North for symptoms, signs and ill-defined conditions. Women in the Midlands & Wales were more likely to consult than women in the North for infections, neoplasms, nervous, genitourinary and musculoskeletal illnesses, injury and poisoning, symptoms, signs and ill-defined conditions and for reasons in the supplementary classification.

Figure 4.1 Age standardised patient consulting ratios for people aged 16 - 64 by broad geographical region

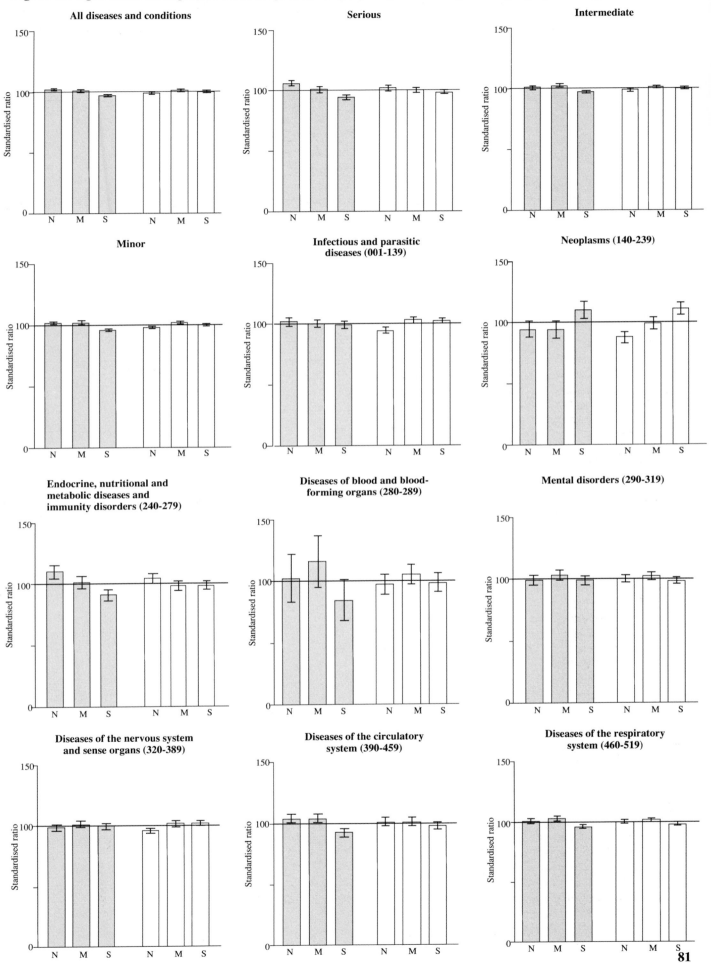

Figure 4.1 - Continued

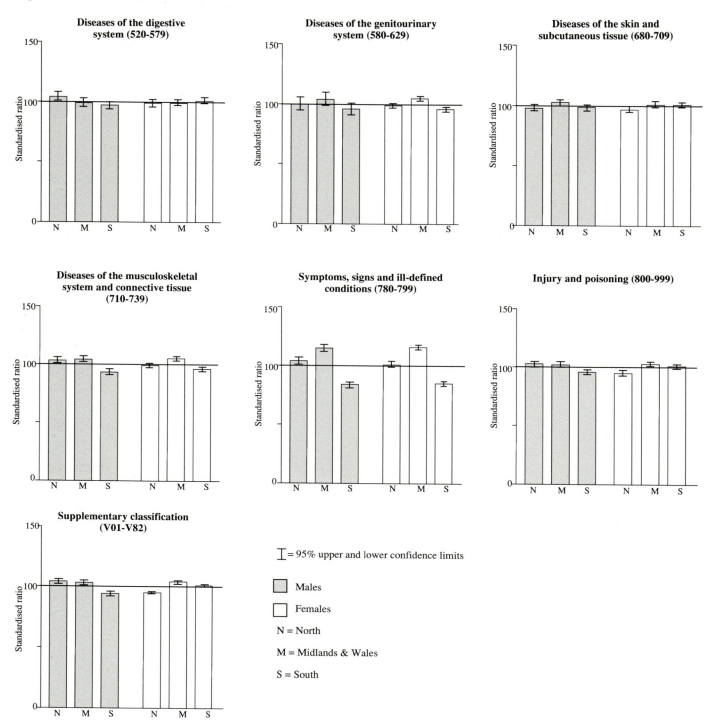

Compared with the South, a higher proportion of men in the North consulted for all diseases and conditions and for each category of severity, while the difference for women was insignificant. A higher proportion of people in the South consulted for neoplasms than people in the North, and women in the South also were more likely to consult for infections, nervous disorders, injury and poisoning, and for reasons in the supplementary classification. People living in the North were more likely than those in the South to consult for symptoms, signs and ill-defined conditions, and men in the North were also more likely to consult for circulatory, respiratory, digestive and musculoskeletal conditions and for reasons in the supplementary classification.

A higher proportion of men in the Midlands & Wales than in the South consulted for all diseases and conditions and for each category of severity. There was no difference among women who consulted for these groups of conditions. For diseases in individual ICD chapters for men and women, with the exception of neoplasms, either people in the Midlands & Wales were more likely to consult or the difference was not significant. A higher proportion of people in the Midlands & Wales consulted for musculoskeletal conditions and for symptoms, signs and ill-defined conditions. Men in the

Midlands & Wales were also more likely to consult for endocrine, circulatory and respiratory disorders, injury and poisoning and for reasons in the supplementary classification. Women in the Midlands & Wales were also more likely to consult for genitourinary illnesses than women in the South.

In contrast to adults, children living in the North were less likely to consult for all diseases and conditions and for each category of severity than those living in the Midlands & Wales, except for boys for serious conditions, for which there was no difference. Comparison shows few differences between children living in the North and South, except that children in the South were more likely to consult for intermediate illnesses. Between the Midlands & Wales and the South, the only difference in the proportion who consulted was that a higher proportion in the Midlands & Wales consulted for minor ailments.

Among the elderly, the only difference between those living in different parts of the country for all diseases and conditions and for each category of severity was for men in the Midlands & Wales who were more likely to consult for severe illnesses than those living in the South.

Urban and rural place of residence

The urban or rural place of residence was derived from the postcode. In the sample, 88 per cent of people lived in urban areas and 12 per cent in rural areas.

Among people aged 16-64 years, there was a consistent difference, with those living in urban areas more likely to consult than those living in a rural environment, for every category of severity. This was in marked contrast to children and the elderly, for whom there was no difference except for elderly women living in urban areas who were more likely to consult for severe conditions. Multivariate analysis suggests that when confounding factors have been removed, this difference is significant only for men aged 16-44 years, for all diseases and conditions and for illnesses in the serious category, and for men and women aged 45-64 years for serious conditions.

For diseases in individual chapters among adults, a higher proportion of urban dwellers of both sexes consulted for mental, circulatory, respiratory, digestive, skin and musculoskeletal diseases, injury and poisoning, symptoms signs and ill-defined conditions, and reasons in the supplementary classification. Women in urban areas were also

Table 4B ICD chapters for which people were more likely to consult (lower SPCR confidence limit over 100), by broad geographical region

Broad geographical region	I	II	III	IV	V	VI	VII	VIII	IX	X	XI	XII	XIII	XIV	XV	XVI	XVII	XVIII*
Males aged 0-15 years																		
North								✓	✓				✓			✓	✓	✓
Midlands & Wales		✓		✓		✓												✓
South																		✓
Females aged 0-15 years																		
North																		
Midlands & Wales								✓	✓				✓			✓	✓	✓
South																		✓
Males aged 16-64 years																		
North			✓				✓		✓				✓			✓		✓
Midlands & Wales							✓	✓					✓			✓		✓
South		✓																
Females aged 16-64 years																		
North																		
Midlands & Wales									✓				✓			✓	✓	✓
South		✓																
Males aged 65 & over																		
North							✓											
Midlands & Wales						✓								✓		✓		
South												✓						✓
Females aged 65 & over																		
North							✓											
Midlands & Wales			✓						✓					✓		✓		
South		✓				✓						✓						✓

* Supplementary classification (V codes).

Figure 4.2 Age standardised patient consulting ratios for people aged 16 - 64 by urban/rural place of residence

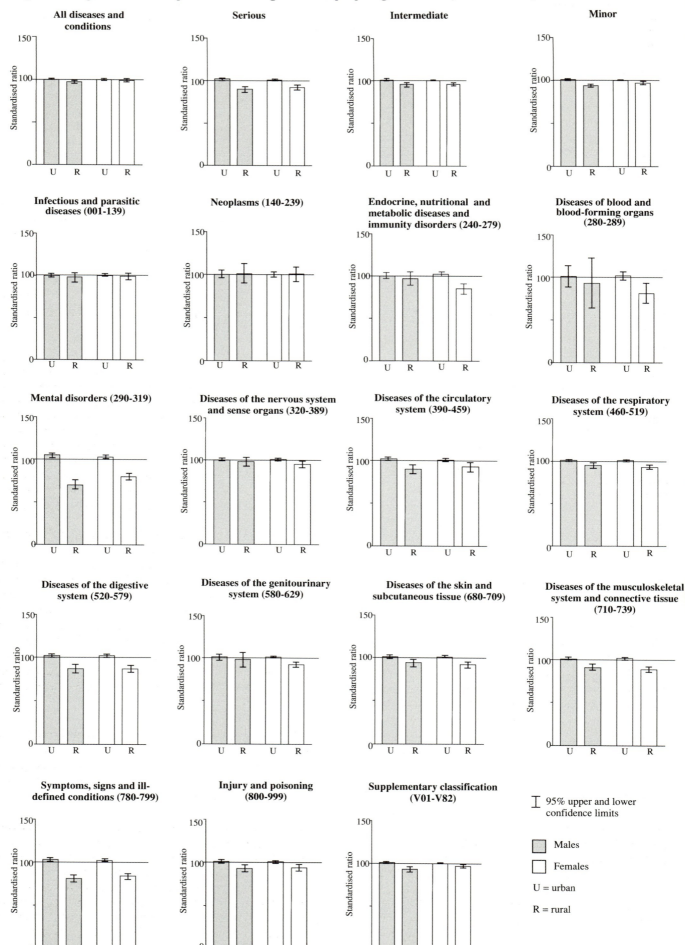

Table 4C ICD chapters for which people aged 16-64 years were more likely to consult (lower SPCR confidence limit over 100), by urban or rural place of residence

Urban/rural place of residence	I	II	III	IV	V	VI	VII	VIII	IX	X	XI	XII	XIII	XIV	XV	XVI	XVII	XVIII
Males																		
Urban					✓											✓		
Rural																		
Females																		
Urban					✓											✓		
Rural																		

more likely to consult for endocrine, blood and genitourinary disorders. There was no ICD chapter for which either men or women in rural areas consulted more than those in urban areas.

Children living in rural areas were in general as likely to consult as those living in urban areas. This was still true after the effect of other socio-economic factors had been taken into account. The only exceptions for which urban children were more likely to consult were for symptoms, signs and ill-defined conditions, among boys for respiratory diseases, and among girls for mental disorders.

Among the elderly there was very little difference between urban and rural dwellers. Women living in urban areas were more likely to consult for serious diseases, but the only ICD chapters for which they were more likely to consult than those in rural surroundings were respiratory and musculoskeletal diseases.

Housing tenure

In the study population, 70 per cent of people lived in owner occupied premises, 18 per cent in council housing, 9 per cent in other rented accommodation and 2 per cent in communal establishments.

The difference in the proportion of people aged 16-64 years who consulted by the kind of housing they occupied was marked. Adults who lived in council housing were very much more likely to consult than those in owner occupied premises. This was confirmed by regression analysis when confounding factors had been taken into consideration. Adults living in other rented accommodation were also more likely to consult than owner occupied dwellers. These differences were less marked among the elderly and children.

People aged 16-64 years who lived in council housing were more likely to consult for all diseases and conditions than people living in owner occupied dwellings. This discrepancy between owner occupiers and council house occupants was greatest for serious illnesses and confirmed by multivariate analysis, but also present for intermediate and to a smaller extent for minor conditions. A higher proportion of people of each sex in council housing consulted than those in owner occupied premises for diseases in every ICD chapter of illness except for neoplasms. The difference was greatest for mental disorders, but was also large for circulatory, digestive

and musculoskeletal diseases and among women for endocrine and nutritional disorders. The difference was relatively small for reasons in the supplementary classification.

For children, the differences between those in owner occupied housing and council accommodation were significant for girls in each category of severity, but for boys only for serious illnesses.

Among the elderly, these differences, in contrast to younger adults, were confined to the serious category for each sex, with no difference for all diseases and conditions and for other categories of severity. Both elderly men and elderly women in council housing were more likely to consult than those in owner occupied premises for mental, respiratory and digestive disorders. A higher proportion of women in council housing also consulted for endocrine and musculoskeletal diseases and injury and poisoning. Elderly men and women in council housing were less likely to consult for reasons in the supplementary classification than owner occupiers.

Comparison of the proportion of people aged 16-64 years living in other rented accommodation and those in owner occupied housing shows that for all diseases and conditions and for each category of severity those in other rented accommodation were more likely to consult. Without exception, within each ICD chapter those in other rented accommodation were more likely to consult than owner occupiers, or the difference was not significant. The ICD chapters for which the difference was significant were similar to those between owner occupiers and council house tenants. There was no difference between the proportion of each who consulted for neoplasms.

A higher proportion of children in other rented accommodation than in owner occupied premises consulted for all diseases and conditions. The only difference by category of severity was that girls in other rented accommodation were more likely to consult for minor ailments.

Among the elderly, there was no difference for all diseases and conditions or for intermediate or minor illnesses between those living in owner occupied housing and those in other rented premises, but the latter were more likely to consult for serious conditions. The only significant differences among the ICD chapters were that people in other rented accommodation were more likely to consult for symptoms, signs and ill-defined conditions, and while men also were more likely

Figure 4.3 Age standardised patient consulting ratios for people aged 16 - 64 by tenure

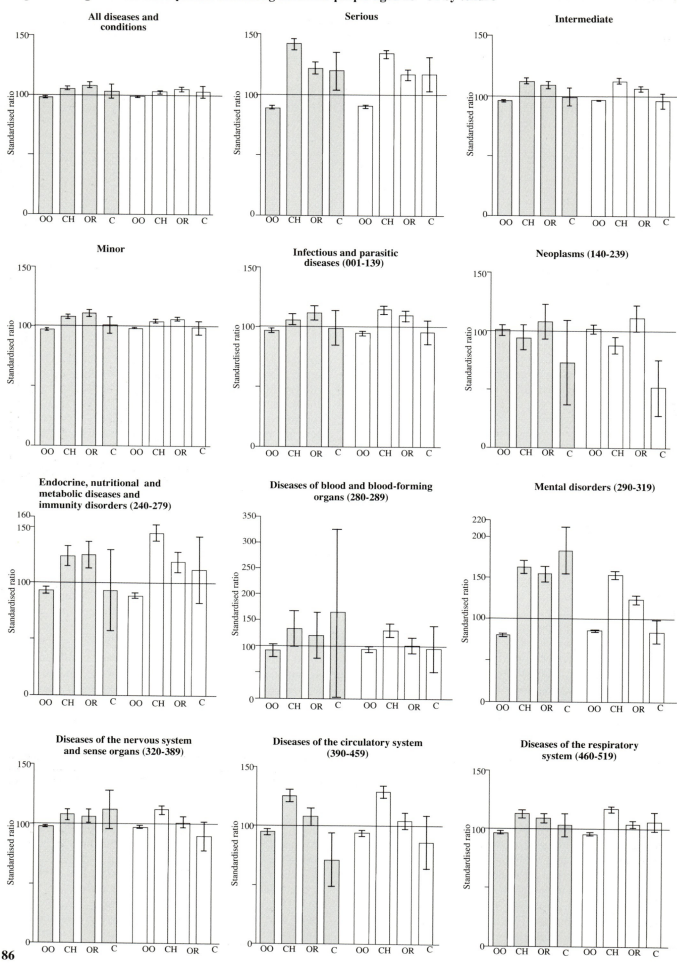

Figure 4.3 -Continued

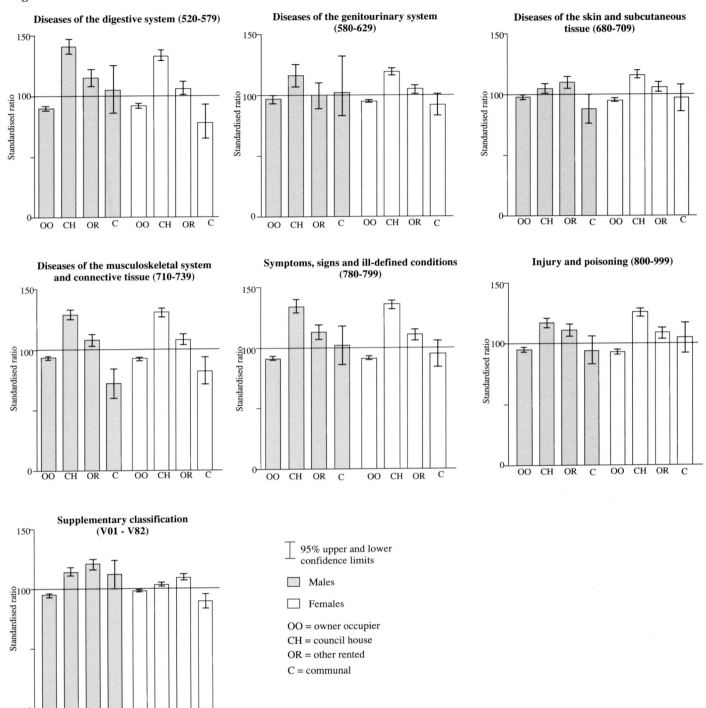

Table 4D ICD chapters for which people aged 16-64 years were more likely to consult (lower SPCR confidence limit over 100), by tenure of housing

Housing tenure	I	II	III	IV	V	VI	VII	VIII	IX	X	XI	XII	XIII	XIV	XV	XVI	XVII	XVIII
Males																		
Owner occupier																		
Council housing	✓		✓		✓	✓	✓	✓	✓	✓		✓	✓	✓		✓	✓	✓
Other rented	✓		✓		✓	✓		✓	✓			✓	✓			✓	✓	✓
Communal					✓													
Females																		
Owner occupier																		
Council housing	✓		✓	✓	✓	✓	✓	✓	✓	✓	✓	✓	✓	✓		✓	✓	✓
Other rented	✓		✓		✓		✓	✓	✓	✓	✓	✓	✓			✓	✓	✓
Communal																		

to consult for respiratory conditions, women were more likely to consult for nervous diseases.

Differences in the proportion of people aged 16-64 years living in council housing compared with those in other rented accommodation were smaller than between council house occupants and people living in their own homes. There was no significant difference for all diseases and conditions or for minor ailments. People in council housing were more likely to consult for serious disorders and women in council housing also for intermediate conditions. By ICD chapter, for men there were no significant differences except that a higher proportion of men in council housing consulted for circulatory, digestive and musculoskeletal conditions and symptoms, signs and ill-defined conditions. The situation was different among women of whom a higher proportion in council housing consulted for conditions in every ICD chapter except infectious diseases, neoplasms and reasons in the supplementary classification. Among children and the elderly there was no difference between those living in council housing and those living in other rented accommodation for all diseases and conditions or for any category of severity.

Marital status

In the sample population, of those aged over 15 years, 26 per cent were single, 60 per cent married and 14 per cent widowed or divorced.

In general there was little difference in the proportion of people aged 16-64 years who consulted between those who were single and those who were married. The exception was for mental disorders for which a higher proportion of single men, and to a smaller extent of single women, consulted than married men and women. There was, however, a marked difference between the proportion of widowed and divorced people who consulted, compared with single and with married people of each sex.

Among people aged 16-64 years, there was no difference between the proportion of single and married people who consulted for all diseases and conditions. Single men were more likely to consult for serious conditions, and married women were more likely to consult for intermediate illnesses. Apart from mental disorders, for which single people of both sexes were more likely to consult than those who were married, the only ICD chapter for which a single person was more likely to consult than a married one was men for endocrine disorders. A higher proportion of married than single men consulted for musculoskeletal disorders and of married than single women for blood, circulatory and genitourinary conditions and for reasons in the supplementary classification.

Comparison between married and widowed or divorced people aged 16-64 years shows that the latter of both sexes were more likely to consult for all diseases and conditions, confirmed by regression analysis, and for each category of severity. There was no single ICD chapter for which widowed or divorced men or women were less likely to consult than married men or women. Widowed or divorced men and women were more likely than married men and women to consult for infectious, mental, respiratory, digestive and musculoskeletal disorders, injury and poisoning, symptoms, signs and ill-defined conditions and reasons in the supplementary classification.

Among people aged 65 years and over, a higher proportion of single than married men consulted for mental disorders, but there was no difference for women. Single elderly people were less likely to consult than married people for respiratory and musculoskeletal conditions and for reasons in the supplementary classification. A higher proportion of married women also consulted than those who were single for circulatory and digestive conditions. Among the elderly, there was not the same disparity between widowed and divorced and other people as among younger adults. Where there was a difference, it was mostly among women. A higher proportion of widowed and divorced men and women consulted than married men and women for mental disorders and fewer for reasons in the supplementary classification. Widowed and divorced women were also more likely to consult than married women for circulatory illnesses, injury and poisoning and symptoms, signs and ill-defined conditions.

Table 4E ICD chapters for which people aged 16-64 years were more likely to consult (lower SPCR confidence limit over 100), by marital status

Marital status	I	II	III	IV	V	VI	VII	VIII	IX	X	XI	XII	XIII	XIV	XV	XVI	XVII	XVIII
Males																		
Single			✓		✓													
Married																		
Widowed/divorced	✓				✓		✓	✓	✓			✓	✓			✓	✓	✓
Females																		
Single																		
Married										✓								
Widowed/divorced	✓	✓	✓		✓	✓		✓	✓	✓		✓	✓			✓	✓	✓

Figure 4.4 Age standardised patient consulting ratios for people aged 16 - 64 by marital status

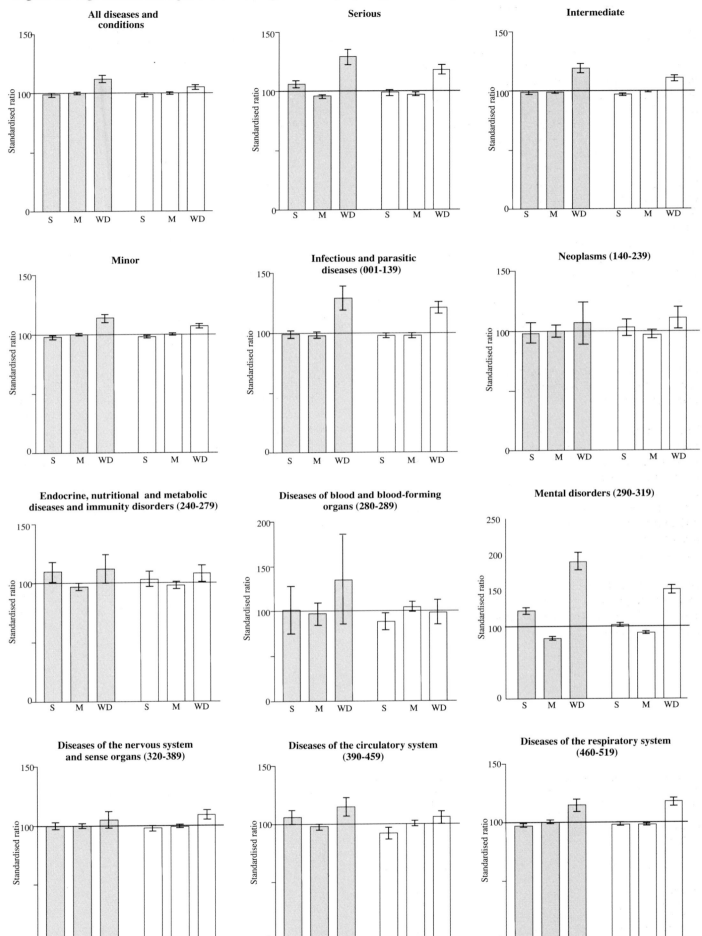

Figure 4.4 - continued

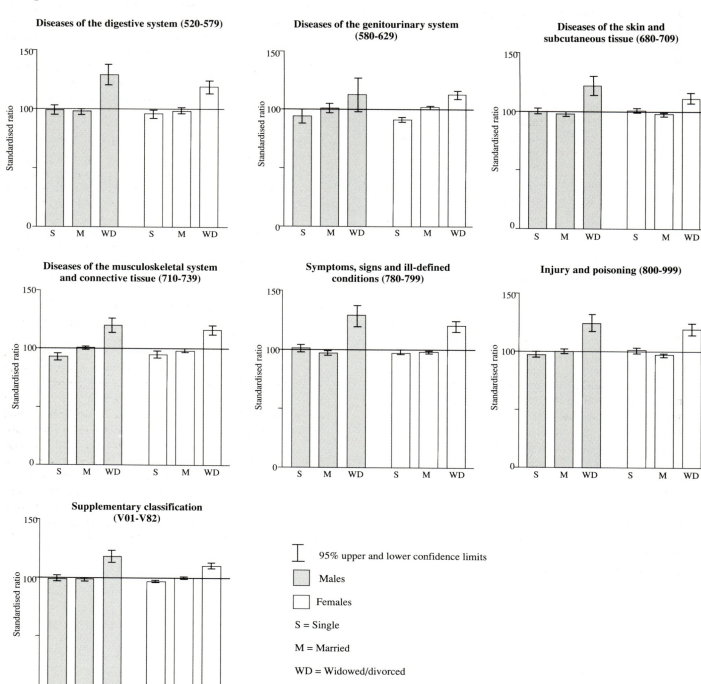

Diseases of the digestive system (520-579)

Diseases of the genitourinary system (580-629)

Diseases of the skin and subcutaneous tissue (680-709)

Diseases of the musculoskeletal system and connective tissue (710-739)

Symptoms, signs and ill-defined conditions (780-799)

Injury and poisoning (800-999)

Supplementary classification (V01-V82)

⊤ 95% upper and lower confidence limits

▨ Males

☐ Females

S = Single

M = Married

WD = Widowed/divorced

Cohabiting status

In the study sample, of those aged 16 years and over, 22 per cent were single and not cohabiting, 65 per cent were either married or cohabiting, and 14 per cent were widowed, separated or divorced and not cohabiting.

There was a fairly consistently higher proportion of people who were widowed, separated or divorced who were not cohabiting who consulted than those who were either single, or married or cohabiting. The difference was smaller among the elderly than among younger adults. The most marked difference was for mental disorders, for which single people and to a greater extent those who were widowed, separated or divorced were more likely to consult than those who were married or cohabiting.

Among people aged 16-64 years, people of both sexes who were single were less likely to consult for all diseases and conditions than those who were married or cohabiting. For the categories of severity the exception was among single men, who were more likely to consult for serious disorders. With the exception of mental disorders, and for men endocrine diseases, there was either no difference between the proportion of single and married or cohabiting people who consulted for conditions in single ICD chapters or a smaller proportion of single people consulted than those who were married or cohabiting. Married or cohabiting people of both sexes were more likely to consult than single people for genitourinary and musculoskeletal disorders. A higher proportion of married or cohabiting women also consulted for blood, circulatory and digestive conditions and for symptoms, signs and ill-defined conditions and reasons in the supplementary classification.

Comparison between married or cohabiting adults aged under 65 years and those who were widowed, separated or divorced who were not cohabiting shows that for all diseases and conditions and for each category of severity widowed, separated or divorced people were more likely to consult. For every ICD chapter, either the difference was not significant, or a higher proportion of widowed, separated or divorced than married or cohabiting people consulted. This difference was most marked for mental disorders, but also present for infectious, respiratory, digestive, skin and musculoskeletal conditions, injury and poisoning, symptoms, signs and ill-defined conditions and reasons in the supplementary classification.

Among the elderly, there was a less marked difference between people of different cohabiting states than among younger adults. There was no difference in the proportion who consulted between single and married or cohabiting, or between married or cohabiting and widowed, separated or divorced for all diseases and conditions. Single elderly men and women were more likely to consult for minor illnesses than married or cohabiting people. Elderly widowed, separated or divorced women were more likely to consult for serious conditions than married or cohabiting women.

There was no ICD chapter for which single elderly people were more likely to consult than those who were married or cohabiting and the difference for mental disorders was not significant. A higher proportion of both elderly men and women who were married or cohabiting consulted than single people for respiratory diseases and reasons in the supplementary classification and married or cohabiting women were also more likely to consult for digestive and genitourinary conditions. Among the elderly there was also little difference between the married or cohabiting and widowed, separated or divorced people in the number who consulted, the exception being mental disorders, for which widowed, separated or divorced people, particularly men, were more likely to consult than married or cohabiting people. A smaller proportion of men and women who were widowed, separated or divorced consulted for reasons in the supplementary classification than married or cohabiting men and women.

Table 4F ICD chapters for which people aged 16-64 years were more likely to consult (lower SPCR confidence limit over 100), by cohabiting status

Cohabiting status	I	II	III	IV	V	VI	VII	VIII	IX	X	XI	XII	XIII	XIV	XV	XVI	XVII	XVIII
Males																		
Single			✓		✓													
Married/cohabiting																		
Separated/widowed/ divorced not cohabiting	✓				✓		✓	✓	✓		✓	✓			✓	✓	✓	
Females																		
Single																		
Married/cohabiting								✓	✓									✓
Separated/widowed/ divorced not cohabiting	✓					✓	✓	✓	✓	✓	✓		✓	✓		✓	✓	✓

Figure 4.5   Age-standardised patient consulting ratios for people aged 16-64 by cohabiting status

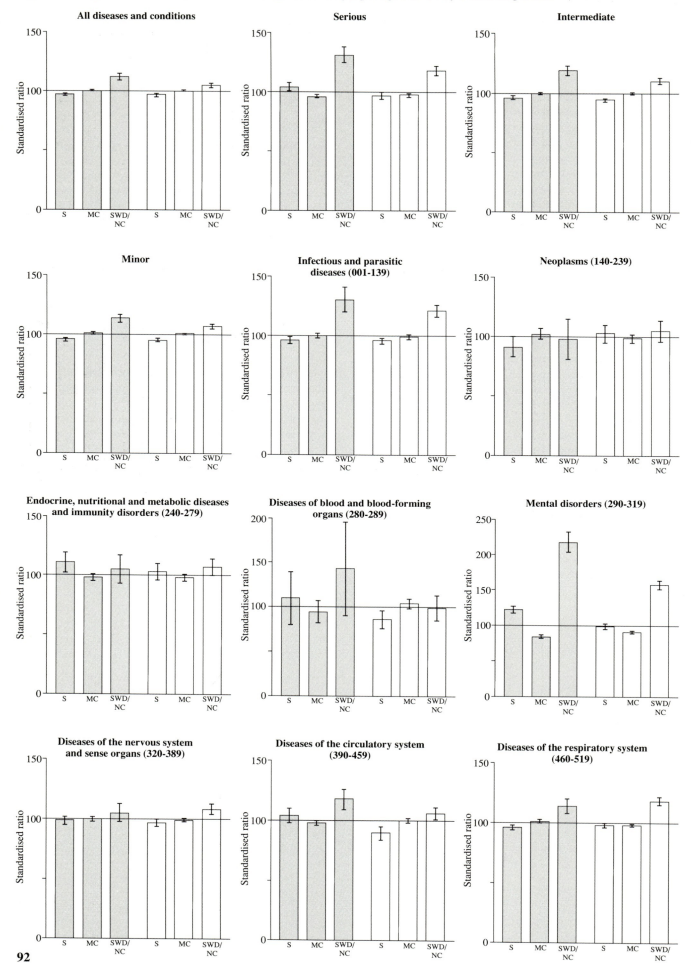

Figure 4.5 - Continued

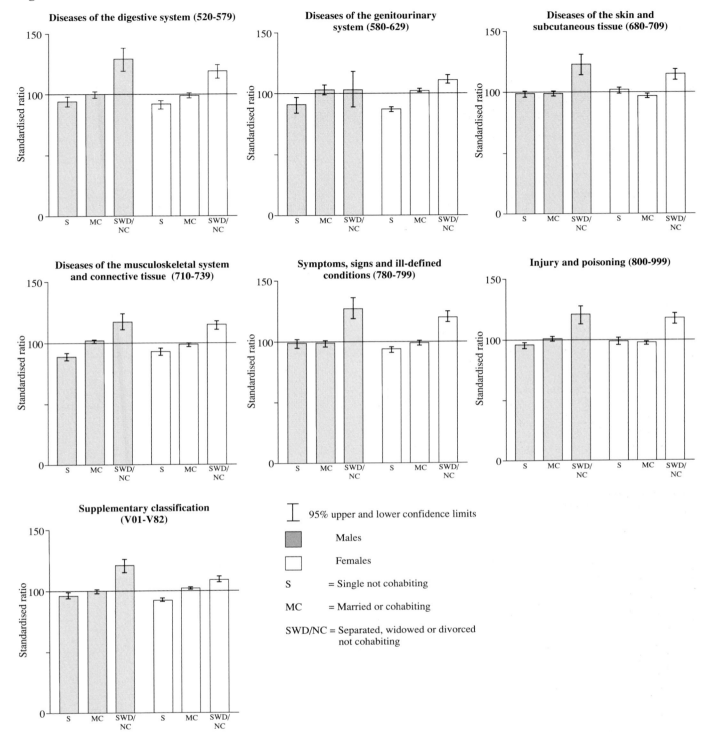

Figure 4.6 Age standardised patient consulting ratios for people aged 16-64 by whether living alone

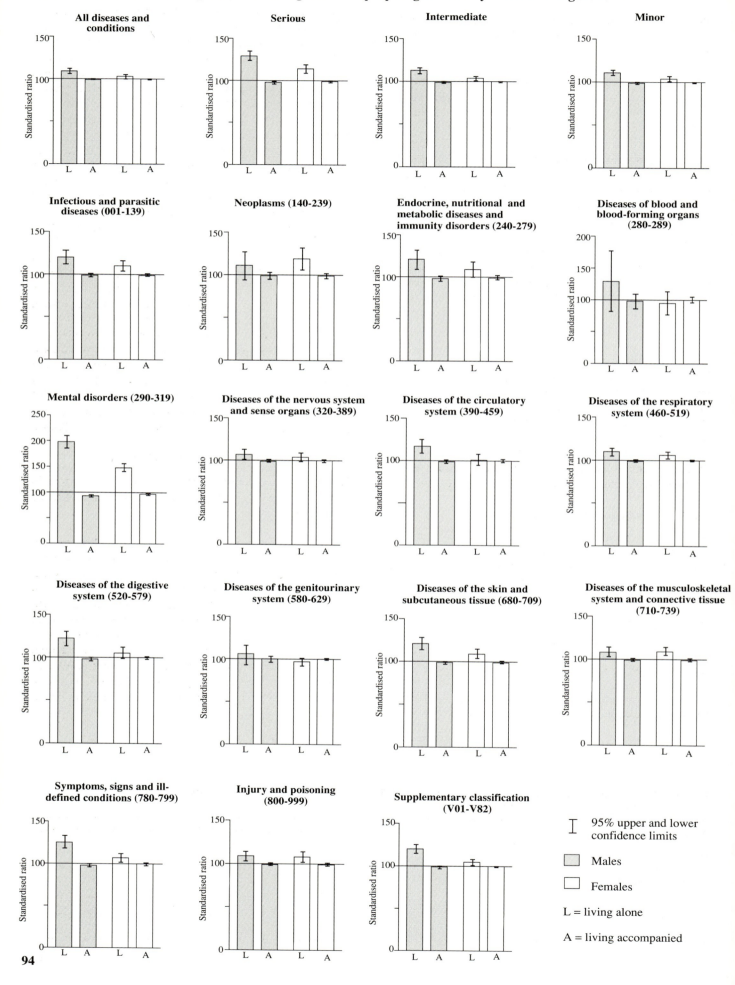

Adults living alone

In the sample population, 5 per cent of people aged 16-64 years and 26 per cent of those aged 65 years and over lived alone.

Among people aged 16-64 years, men living alone were more likely to consult for all diseases and conditions than those who did not. This was true for both men and women for serious, intermediate and minor conditions.

By ICD chapter the most marked difference was for mental disorders, people of both sexes who lived alone being much more likely to consult. Both men and women living alone were also more likely to consult for infectious diseases, respiratory, skin and musculoskeletal conditions, for injury and poisoning, symptoms, signs and ill-defined conditions, and for reasons in the supplementary classification. Men were more likely to consult also for endocrine and nutritional disorders, and circulatory and digestive diseases. Women living alone were also more likely to consult for neoplasms, but less likely to consult for complications of pregnancy, childbirth and the puerperium.

Among those aged 65 years and over there was no difference between those living alone and accompanied for all diseases and conditions, or for each category of severity. For individual ICD chapters, men not living alone were more likely to consult for diseases of the nervous system and sense organs and the genitourinary system. Elderly women living alone were more likely to consult for musculoskeletal diseases and injury and poisoning and less likely for genitourinary diseases and reasons in the supplementary classification.

Adults with children in the household

In the sample population aged 16 years and over, 73 per cent lived in a household with no children, 7 per cent with children under 5 years only, 15 per cent with children aged 5-15 years only and 5 per cent with children aged both under 5 and 5-15 years.

Adults with only small children were more likely to consult than those with no children. The difference was smaller where there were children aged both under 5 and 5-15 years and smaller still if there were children aged 5-15 only.

For all diseases and conditions, men and women aged 16-64 years were more likely to consult if there were only small children in the household than if there were no children, but there was no difference if there were both children aged under 5 and children aged 5-15, or if there were only children aged 5-15 years. The difference between those with no children and those with children under 5 years only was confined to intermediate and minor illnesses for both men and women. Men with children aged 5-15 only were less likely to consult for serious illnesses than men with no children.

For diseases in ICD chapters, men with children aged under 5 years only were more likely to consult than men with no children for nervous and respiratory diseases. Those with children aged both under 5 and 5-15 years were more likely to consult for respiratory diseases, injury and poisoning and symptoms, signs and ill-defined conditions. Among women, those with children under 5 years only were more likely than women with no children to consult for infectious, blood, mental, nervous, circulatory, respiratory and genitourinary conditions, and for symptoms, signs and ill-defined conditions and reasons in the supplementary classification. A higher proportion of women with children both under 5 and 5-15 years than women with no children consulted for infectious, nervous, respiratory, genitourinary and skin diseases, and for symptoms, signs and ill-defined conditions. Among adults with children aged 5-15 years only, men were not more likely to consult for diseases in any ICD chapter than those without children. Women with children aged 5-15 only were more likely to consult for blood and genitourinary diseases, and for symptoms, signs and ill-defined conditions.

Sole adults in the household with children

In the sample population, 39,550 adults were the sole adult in the household. Of these, 14 per cent lived with children in the household.

There was no difference between the proportion of sole adults in households who consulted, depending upon whether there were children in the household, for all diseases and conditions, or for serious or minor illnesses. Sole women with children were more likely than those without children to consult for intermediate conditions. A higher proportion of sole men and sole women with children consulted for infectious diseases. Sole women with children in the household were also more likely to consult than those without children for respiratory, digestive and genitourinary diseases, injury and poisoning, and symptoms, signs and ill-defined conditions.

Table 4G ICD chapters for which people aged 16-64 years were more likely to consult (lower SPCR confidence limit over 100), by whether they were living alone or accompanied

Whether living alone	I	II	III	IV	V	VI	VII	VIII	IX	X	XI	XII	XIII	XIV	XV	XVI	XVII	XVIII
Males																		
Living alone	✓		✓		✓	✓	✓	✓	✓			✓	✓			✓	✓	✓
Living accompanied																		
Females																		
Living alone	✓	✓			✓			✓				✓	✓	✓		✓	✓	✓
Living accompanied																		

Table 4H   ICD chapters for which people aged 16-64 years were more likely to consult (lower SPCR confidence limit over 100), by whether there were children in the household

Whether children in household	I	II	III	IV	V	VI	VII	VIII	IX	X	XI	XII	XIII	XIV	XV	XVI	XVII	XVIII
Males																		
None			✓		✓													✓
Under 5 yrs only	✓					✓		✓	✓									
5-15 yrs only																		
Under 5 and 5-15 yrs								✓								✓	✓	
Females																		
None																		
Under 5 yrs only	✓			✓	✓	✓	✓	✓		✓	✓					✓		✓
5-15 yrs only																		
Under 5 and 5-15 yrs	✓					✓		✓		✓		✓				✓		

Table 4I   ICD chapters for which people aged 16-64 years were more likely to consult (lower SPCR confidence limit over 100), by whether they were a sole adult in the house with or without children

Whether sole adult with children	I	II	III	IV	V	VI	VII	VIII	IX	X	XI	XII	XIII	XIV	XV	XVI	XVII	XVIII
Males																		
Sole adult with children	✓																	
Sole adult without children																		
Females																		
Sole adult with children	✓					✓		✓	✓	✓	✓		✓			✓	✓	
Sole adult without children																		

Children living with only one adult

Among those in the sample population aged under 16 years, 12 per cent lived in households with only one person aged 16 years or over, the remaining 88 per cent lived with more than one adult.

For all diseases and conditions there was no significant difference in the proportion who consulted between children living with one adult and those living with more than one adult. Regression analysis suggests that girls in single adult households were more likely to consult than those in households with more than one adult. For serious diseases there was, however, a slightly higher proportion of children living with one adult who consulted, although this is not apparent when the effect of other socio-economic characteristics is eliminated.

A higher proportion of children living with one adult consulted for infectious diseases. Boys in these circumstances were more likely to consult for mental disorders, and girls for respiratory, genitourinary and musculoskeletal illnesses and for signs, symptoms and ill-defined conditions. Among boys living with only one adult, a smaller proportion consulted for nervous disorders and for reasons in the supplementary classification. For every other ICD chapter there was no difference between those living with only one adult and those living with more than one.

Social class (as defined by occupation)

In the sample population, 30 per cent of people were in Social Classes I & II, 13 per cent in IIIN, 29 per cent in IIIM, and 20 per cent in IV & V. Eight per cent were in other categories.

Table 4J   ICD chapters for which children aged under 16 years were more likely to consult (lower SPCR confidence limit over 100), by whether they lived with a sole adult

Whether children living with a sole adult	I	II	III	IV	V	VI	VII	VIII	IX	X	XI	XII	XIII	XIV	XV	XVI	XVII	XVIII
Males																		
Living with sole adult	✓				✓											✓	✓	
Not living with sole adult																		
Females																		
Living with sole adult	✓						✓		✓							✓		
Not living with sole adult																		

In general, there was a gradient among people aged 16-64 years, with a smaller proportion of people in Social Classes I & II consulting than those in Social Classes IIIN, IIIM and IV & V. From regression analysis it would appear that this is not true for all diseases and conditions, although there was a slight gradient for serious illnesses. The gradient seen in univariate analysis was most marked for mental disorders. The single exception to this trend was for neoplasms, for which both men and women in Classes IV & V were less likely to consult than those in Classes I & II. These differences between people in different social classes were largely absent among the elderly.

For all diseases and conditions, this gradient among those of working age was true for men but there was no significant difference for women. However, the gradient was present for both men and women for serious conditions and confirmed by regression analysis, to a lower degree for intermediate illnesses, and only among men for minor ones.

The chapters for which the difference between those in Classes I & II and those in other classes, though not necessarily between each succeeding class, increased and were significant when compared with those in Classes IV & V for both men and women were mental, circulatory, digestive and musculoskeletal illnesses, injury and poisoning, and symptoms, signs and ill-defined conditions. Men in Classes I & II were also more likely to consult for reasons in the supplementary classification than those in other classes, but there was no difference for women. A higher proportion of women in Classes I & II also consulted for endocrine and skin disorders, but this did not apply to men. The single exception to this general gradient between those in Classes I & II and through to those in Classes IV & V was neoplastic conditions, for which women in Class IIIN and both men and women in Classes IV & V were less likely to consult than those in Classes I & II.

The gradients between Social Classes I & II and IV & V in the proportion of people of working age who consulted were almost completely absent among the elderly. A higher proportion of people aged 65 years and over in Classes IV & V consulted for serious illnesses and for musculoskeletal conditions than people in Classes I & II. There was no difference between people in Classes I & II and those in other classes for mental disorders, except for women in Classes IV & V who were more likely to consult. For reasons in the supplementary classification, elderly people in Classes I & II were more likely to consult than those in Classes IV & V.

Married or cohabiting women aged 16-64 years analysed by their own social class show almost identical differences as when analysed by the social class of their partner.

Occupation

The occupations of patients have been grouped by the Standard Occupational Classification (SOC) sub-major groups (see appendix C). The largest proportion, 12 per cent, worked in clerical occupations (group 4a), 9 per cent other elementary occupations (group 9b), 8 per cent protective service occupations (group 6a), 8 per cent other skilled trades (group 5c), 7 per cent corporate managers and administrators (group 1a) and 7 per cent industrial plant and machine operators (group 8a). Each of the remaining sub-major groups were represented to a smaller degree.

The most remarkable feature among men is the low consulting ratios for health professionals. They probably treat themselves and each other rather than seeking help from their general practitioners. In general, there was a gradual gradient with men in the managerial, administrative and professional occupations less likely to consult than those in the construction, service and industrial occupations. This was most marked for serious illnesses, but also to a lesser extent for intermediate and minor ones.

Conditions in each ICD chapter for which male workers in different occupations were significantly more likely than average to consult are shown below (see also Table 4L).

1b Managers/proprietors in agriculture and services: endocrine and nutritional disorders,

2a, 3a Science and engineering professionals and associate professionals: neoplasms,

2c Teaching professionals: infectious diseases, diseases of the nervous system and sense organs, respiratory diseases,

2d Other professional occupations: infectious diseases,

Table 4K ICD chapters for which people aged 16-64 years were more likely to consult (lower SPCR confidence limit over 100), by social class (married/cohabiting women by partner's social class)

Social class (as defined by occupation)	I	II	III	IV	V	VI	VII	VIII	IX	X	XI	XII	XIII	XIV	XV	XVI	XVII	XVIII
Males																		
I & II		✓																
IIIN																		
IIIM									✓				✓			✓	✓	✓
IV & V			✓		✓	✓	✓		✓				✓		✓	✓	✓	✓
Other					✓	✓						✓		✓				
Females																		
I & II		✓							✓									
IIIN																		
IIIM				✓	✓	✓	✓	✓	✓	✓	✓	✓		✓			✓	✓
IV & V	✓		✓	✓	✓	✓	✓	✓	✓	✓		✓				✓	✓	
Other					✓													

Figure 4.7 Age-standardised patient consulting ratios for people aged 16-64 by social class (as defined by occupation)

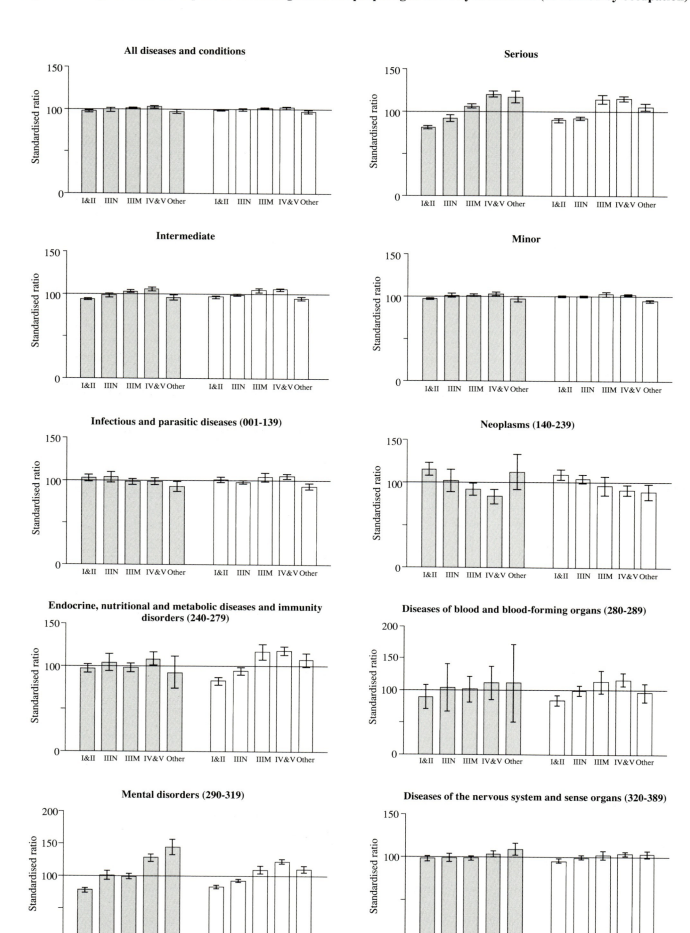

Figure 4.7 - Continued

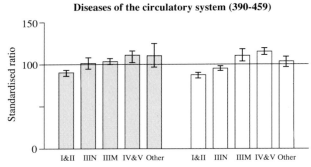

Diseases of the circulatory system (390-459)

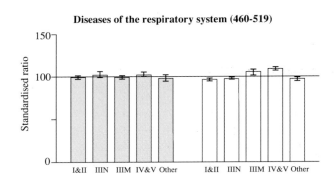

Diseases of the respiratory system (460-519)

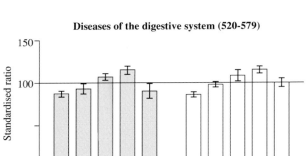

Diseases of the digestive system (520-579)

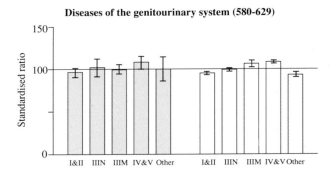

Diseases of the genitourinary system (580-629)

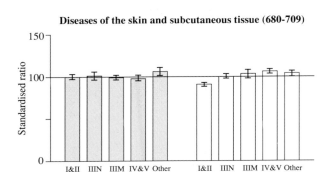

Diseases of the skin and subcutaneous tissue (680-709)

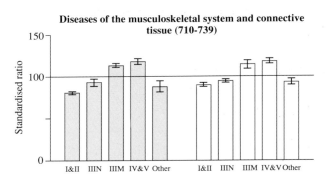

Diseases of the musculoskeletal system and connective tissue (710-739)

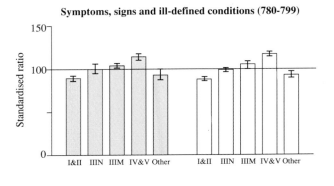

Symptoms, signs and ill-defined conditions (780-799)

Injury and poisoning (800-999)

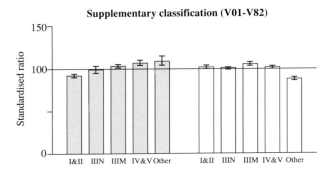

Supplementary classification (V01-V82)

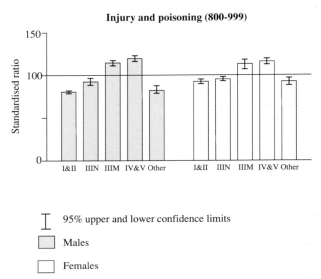

95% upper and lower confidence limits

Males

Females

3c Other associate professionals: diseases of the nervous system and sense organs, skin diseases,

4a Clerical workers: mental disorders,

5a, 5b, 5c Craft and related occupations: musculoskeletal diseases, injury and poisoning,

5c Other skilled trades: also symptoms, signs and ill-defined conditions,

6a, 6b Protective and personal service workers: musculoskeletal diseases, injury and poisoning, symptoms, signs and ill-defined conditions,

6a Protective service occupations: also reasons in the supplementary classification,

6b Personal service workers: also infectious diseases, endocrine and nutritional conditions, mental disorders, circulatory, respiratory and digestive diseases, symptoms, signs and ill-defined conditions,

7a Buyers, brokers and sales reps: infectious diseases,

8a, 8b Plant and machine operators: digestive and musculoskeletal diseases, injury and poisoning, symptoms, signs and ill-defined conditions,

8a Industrial plant and machine operators: also circulatory and genitourinary diseases,

8b Drivers and mobile machine operators: also endocrine and nutritional disorders, reasons in the supplementary classification,

Table 4L ICD chapters for which people aged 16-64 years were more likely to consult (lower SPCR confidence limit over 100), by occupation group

Occupation group	I	II	III	IV	V	VI	VII	VIII	IX	X	XI	XII	XIII	XIV	XV	XVI	XVII	XVIII
Males																		
1a																		
1b			✓															
2a		✓																
2b																		
2c	✓					✓		✓										
2d	✓																	
3a		✓																
3b																		
3c						✓						✓						
4a					✓													
4b																		
5a													✓			✓		
5b													✓			✓		
5c													✓		✓	✓		
6a													✓			✓	✓	
6b	✓		✓		✓		✓	✓	✓				✓			✓	✓	✓
7a	✓																	
7b																		
8a							✓		✓	✓			✓			✓	✓	
8b			✓						✓				✓			✓	✓	✓
9a			✓														✓	
9b					✓		✓	✓	✓				✓			✓	✓	✓
Females																		
1a		✓																✓
1b																		
2a																		
2b																		
2c	✓	✓									✓							
2d																		
3a																		✓
3b																		
3c																		
4a																		
4b			✓															
5a																		
5b							✓											
5c				✓		✓			✓	✓		✓				✓	✓	
6a																✓		
6b	✓			✓		✓	✓	✓	✓	✓			✓			✓	✓	✓
7a																		
7b							✓		✓			✓				✓		
8a		✓	✓	✓		✓	✓	✓	✓	✓	✓	✓				✓	✓	✓
8b		✓		✓												✓		
9a																		
9b			✓		✓		✓	✓	✓	✓		✓	✓			✓	✓	

For occupation codes see appendix C.

9a Other occupations in agriculture, forestry and fishing: endocrine and nutritional disorders, injury and poisoning,

9b Other elementary occupations: mental disorders, circulatory, respiratory, digestive and musculoskeletal diseases, injury and poisoning, symptoms, signs and ill-defined conditions, reasons in the supplementary classification.

For women there were less marked differences between the proportion in different occupations who consulted than for men. There was no significant difference for all diseases and conditions except for health professionals who were least likely to consult. In general, for serious illnesses corporate managers and administrators, teachers and those in secretarial occupations were less likely to consult than the average worker. Women in other skilled trades, personal service occupations, industrial plant and machine operators and other elementary occupations were most likely to consult. The differences for intermediate and minor illnesses were small.

Conditions in each ICD chapter for which female workers in different occupations were significantly more likely than average to consult are shown below (see also Table 4L).

1a Corporate managers and administrators: neoplasms, reasons in the supplementary classification,

2c Teaching professionals: infectious diseases, neoplasms, complications of pregnancy, childbirth and the puerperium,

3a Science and engineering professionals: reasons in the supplementary classification,

4b Secretarial occupations: neoplasms,

5b Skilled engineering trades: circulatory diseases,

5c Other skilled trades: endocrine and nutritional disorders, mental disorders, digestive and musculoskeletal conditions, complications of pregnancy, childbirth and the puerperium, injury and poisoning, reasons in the supplementary classification,

6a Protective service occupations: injury and poisoning,

6b Personal service occupations: infectious diseases, endocrine and nutritional disorders, mental disorders, nervous, circulatory, respiratory, digestive, genitourinary and musculoskeletal diseases, injury and poisoning, symptoms, signs and ill-defined conditions, reasons in the supplementary classification,

7b Other sales occupations: circulatory, genitourinary and musculoskeletal diseases, symptoms, signs and ill-defined conditions,

8a Industrial plant and machine operators: endocrine and nutritional disorders, diseases of the blood, mental disorders, circulatory, respiratory, digestive, genitourinary, skin and musculoskeletal diseases, complications of pregnancy, childbirth and the puerperium, injury and poisoning, symptoms, signs and ill-defined conditions, reasons in the supplementary classification,

8b Drivers and mobile machine operators: endocrine and nutritional disorders, mental disorders, injury and poisoning,

9b Other elementary occupations: endocrine and nutritional disorders, mental disorders, circulatory, respiratory, digestive, genitourinary, skin and musculoskeletal diseases, injury and poisoning, symptoms, signs and ill-defined conditions.

Economic position

In the sample population over 15 years of age, 46 per cent were employed full-time, 11 per cent worked part-time, 5 per cent were unemployed (waiting to start a job or seeking work), 3 per cent were long term sick and 11 per cent looked after the home. Twenty-four per cent had some other occupation which included students and retired people. The proportions for people aged 16-64 years by sex are shown in the box.

Compared with people aged 16-64 years working full-time, the most obvious difference was for the long term sick, who were more likely to consult for all diseases and conditions, each category of severity and diseases in every ICD chapter. People who were unemployed were more likely to consult than those who were employed full-time.

Between those working full-time and the unemployed, a higher proportion of people of both sexes who were unemployed consulted for all diseases and conditions and for each category of severity. This was still true when all confounding factors were removed by regression analysis for all diseases and conditions and for serious illnesses. People of both sexes who were unemployed were more likely to consult for endocrine, mental, nervous, circulatory, digestive, skin and musculoskeletal diseases, injury and poisoning and symptoms, signs and ill-defined conditions. More men who were unemployed also consulted for respiratory diseases and for reasons in the supplementary classification. Unemployed women were also more likely to consult for infectious and genitourinary disorders.

Economic position last week, percentages by sex, people aged 16-64 years		
	Men	Women
Working full time	76	38
Working part time	2	24
Unemployed	9	3
Long-term sick	5	2
Home/family	0	22
Other	8	11

Figure 4.8(a) Age standardised patient consulting ratios for males aged 16-64 years by occupation*

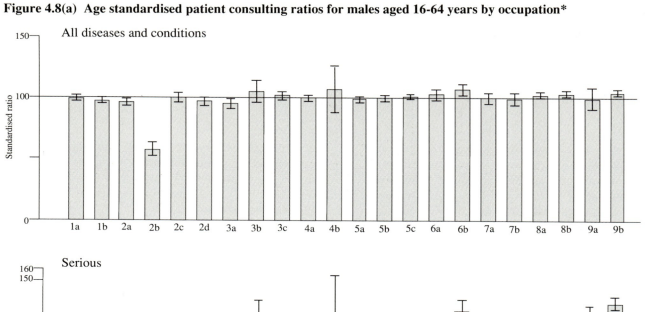

All diseases and conditions

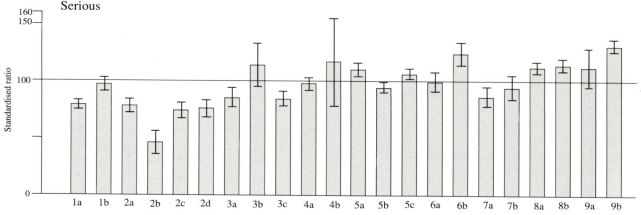

Serious

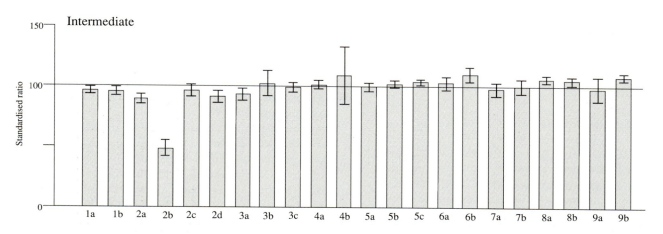

Intermediate

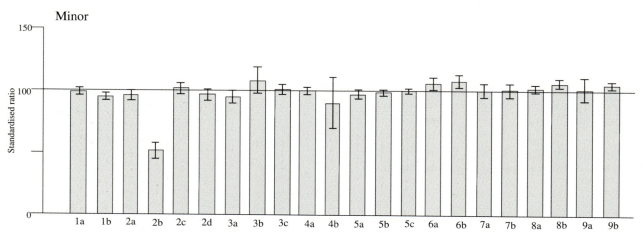

Minor

* For occupation codes see appendix C.

102

Figure 4.8(b) Age standardised patient consulting ratios for females aged 16-64 years by occupation

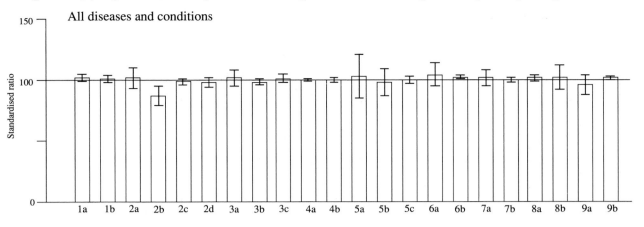

All diseases and conditions

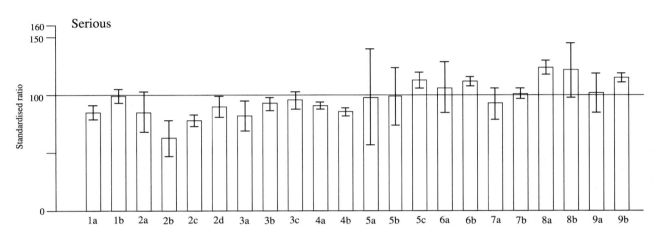

Serious

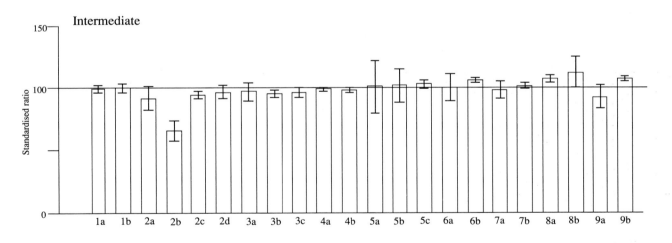

Intermediate

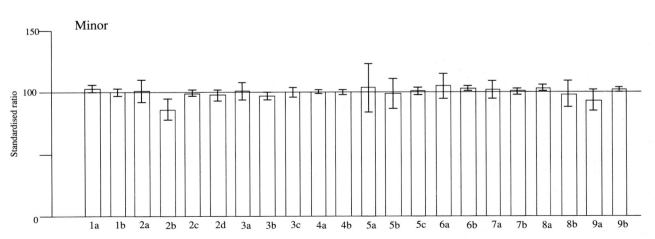

Minor

Comparison between full-time and part-time workers showed no significant difference for all diseases and conditions or each category of severity. However, men working part-time were more likely to consult for mental disorders and diseases of the skin, while part-time women were more likely to consult for diseases of the blood and genitourinary system.

A higher proportion people of both sexes looking after the home or family consulted for severe and intermediate diseases than full-time workers. Both men and women at home were more likely to consult for mental illnesses. Men were also more likely to consult for musculoskeletal disorders and reasons in the supplementary classification. Women were also more likely to consult for infectious, endocrine, blood, nervous, circulatory, digestive, genitourinary and skin diseases.

The economic position of a child's parent or guardian did not have such a marked effect on whether the child consulted. The parent or guardian was defined as being his father, stepfather, mother's cohabitee, mother or head of household in that order of preference. In the sample population aged under 16 years, the parent or guardian of 77 per cent of children were working full-time, 4 per cent part-time, 9 per cent were unemployed, 2 per cent were long term sick and 8 per cent were looking after the home.

The only difference among the categories of illness between children whose parent was a full-time worker and those in another economic position was for serious illness, for which children whose parent looked after the home were more likely to consult.

The economic position of the partners of married and cohabiting women did not influence the likelihood of women consulting to the same extent as their own economic position. For all diseases and conditions there was no significant difference between women whose partners were working full-time and those whose partners were in any other economic position. By category of severity and diseases in every ICD chapter, there was no difference between women whose partners worked full-time or those who worked part-time. Between women whose partners worked full-time and those whose partners were unemployed, women whose partners were unemployed were more likely to consult for serious and

intermediate illnesses, and for conditions in every ICD chapter except neoplasms, and blood and respiratory diseases. A higher proportion of women whose partners were long term sick consulted than those whose partners were fully employed for severe, intermediate and minor illnesses, and for diseases in every ICD chapter except neoplasms blood and genitourinary disorders, and reasons in the supplementary classification for which there was no difference. Women whose partners looked after the home were more likely than those whose partners worked full-time to consult for serious conditions, and for nervous and mental disorders.

Ethnic group

In the sample population, 98 per cent of people were white, one per cent Black Afro-Caribbean, one per cent Indian and less than 0.5 per cent Pakistani/Bangladeshi. One per cent belonged to other ethnic groups. Although the proportion of those in minority groups was small, they represented over 9,000 person years at risk.

The most remarkable difference between white people aged 16-64 years and those of all other ethnic groups was that a higher proportion of those in other ethnic groups of both sexes consulted for symptoms, signs and ill-defined conditions compared with white people. People of Indian subcontinent origin were also more likely to consult for serious illnesses than white people.

For all diseases and conditions there was no difference in the proportion who consulted between white people and those of any other ethnic group, although regression analysis suggests that men aged 16-44 years and women aged 45-64 years of Indian subcontinent origin were more likely to consult after other socio-economic factors had been accounted for. However, a higher proportion of Pakistani/Bangladeshi than white people and Indian women consulted for serious illnesses. This was confirmed by regression analysis. A higher proportion of Indian and Pakistani/Bangladeshi men than white men also consulted for minor ailments.

For diseases in individual ICD chapters, white men were more likely to consult than Afro-Caribbean men for neoplasms and white women were more likely to consult for neoplasms than women from the Indian subcontinent. A higher proportion of white than Indian people also consulted

Table 4M ICD chapters for which people aged 16-64 years were more likely to consult (lower SPCR confidence limit over 100), by economic position

Economic position	I	II	III	IV	V	VI	VII	VIII	IX	X	XI	XII	XIII	XIV	XV	XVI	XVII	XVIII
Males																		
Working full time																		
Working part time					✓							✓						
Unemployed					✓				✓				✓			✓	✓	
Long term sick	✓	✓	✓	✓	✓	✓	✓	✓	✓	✓		✓	✓	✓		✓	✓	✓
Home/family					✓												✓	✓
Females																		
Working full time																		
Working part time																		
Unemployed	✓		✓		✓				✓	✓		✓	✓			✓	✓	✓
Long term sick	✓	✓	✓	✓	✓	✓	✓	✓	✓	✓		✓	✓	✓		✓	✓	✓
Home/family	✓		✓	✓	✓				✓	✓	✓	✓				✓		✓

Figure 4.9 Age-standardised patient consulting ratios for people aged 16-64 by economic position

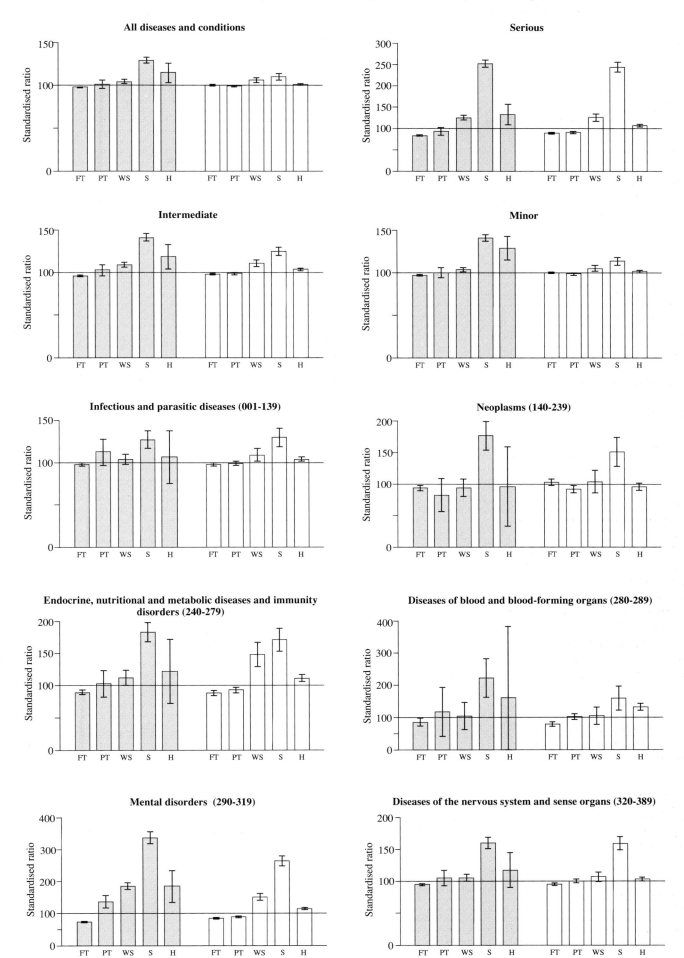

105

Figure 4.9 - Continued

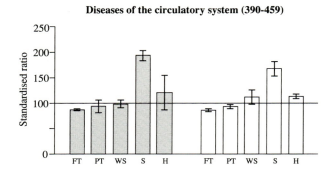

Diseases of the circulatory system (390-459)

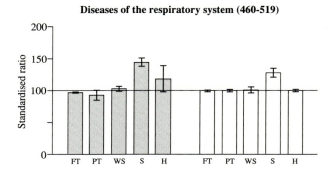

Diseases of the respiratory system (460-519)

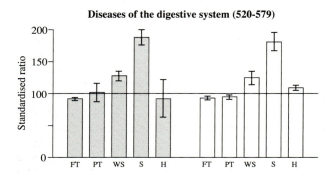

Diseases of the digestive system (520-579)

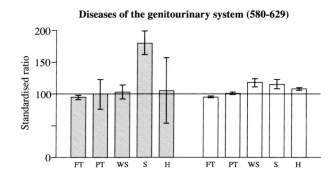

Diseases of the genitourinary system (580-629)

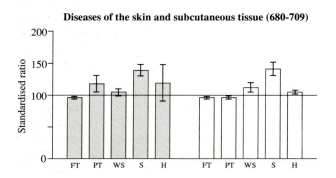

Diseases of the skin and subcutaneous tissue (680-709)

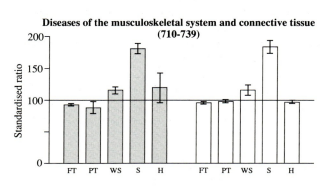

Diseases of the musculoskeletal system and connective tissue (710-739)

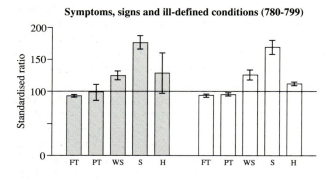

Symptoms, signs and ill-defined conditions (780-799)

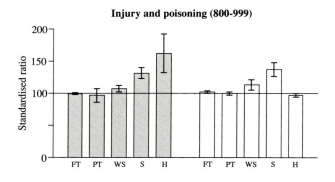

Injury and poisoning (800-999)

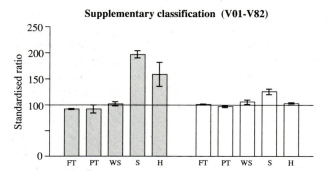

Supplementary classification (V01-V82)

I 95% upper and lower confidence limits

▨ Males

☐ Females

FT = Working full time
PT = Working part time
WS = Waiting/seeking work (unemployed)
S = Long term sick
H = Looking after home/family

106

Table 4N ICD chapters for which people aged 16-64 years were more likely to consult (lower SPCR confidence limit over 100), by ethnic group

Ethnic group	I	II	III	IV	V	VI	VII	VIII	IX	X	XI	XII	XIII	XIV	XV	XVI	XVII	XVIII
Males																		
White																		
Black Afro-Caribbean																✓		
Indian			✓				✓									✓		✓
Pakistani/Bangladeshi			✓				✓	✓			✓	✓				✓		✓
Other																		
Females																		
White																		
Black Afro-Caribbean			✓	✓			✓									✓		
Indian				✓									✓	✓		✓		
Pakistani/Bangladeshi			✓	✓		✓				✓			✓	✓		✓		
Other																✓		

for mental disorders. With the exception of neoplasms and mental disorders, people in the Black Afro-Caribbean, Indian and Pakistani/Bangladeshi ethnic groups were more likely to consult than white people for diseases in each ICD chapter where the difference was significant. In particular, all people in ethnic groups other than white were more likely to consult for symptoms, signs and ill-defined conditions than white people. Women in each of the three main ethnic minority groups were more likely to consult for blood disorders than white women. People from Pakistan/Bangladesh, men from India and Afro-Caribbean women were more likely to consult than white people for endocrine and nutritional disorders. Indian and Pakistani/Bangladeshi men were more likely to consult than white men for respiratory diseases, and people from Pakistan/Bangladesh for digestive illnesses and diseases of the skin. A higher proportion of Pakistani/Bangladeshi people and women from India also consulted more than white people for musculoskeletal conditions.

Among children there was no difference between those who were white and those of other ethnic groups in the proportion who consulted for all diseases and conditions, or for each category of severity except that more children from the Indian subcontinent consulted for minor ailments. For diseases in separate ICD chapters, white children were more likely to consult for nervous diseases than those of Afro-Caribbean origin and girls of Indian origin, and more likely than Pakistani/Bangladeshi children to consult for genitourinary conditions. Pakistani/Bangladeshi children were more likely than white children to consult for respiratory and digestive disorders. Pakistani/Bangladeshi children and Indian boys were more likely to consult for symptoms, signs and ill-defined conditions than white children.

There was no difference in the proportion of elderly white people who consulted compared with those in any other ethnic group for all diseases and conditions, each category of severity or for diseases in any individual ICD chapter.

Smoking

Among the study population aged over 16 years and over, 29 per cent said at interview that they smoked during the previous week, and 71 per cent that they did not. People who had smoked and temporarily stopped were therefore not counted as smokers, nor were ex-smokers.

People aged 16-64 years who smoked were in general more likely to consult than those who did not smoke, although there were some ICD chapters for which the situation was reversed. Regression analysis suggests that this was true for all diseases and conditions only for females, and that males aged 45-64 years who smoked were less likely to consult than those who did not smoke. Among elderly smokers the difference in the proportion who consulted compared with those who did not smoke was less, and elderly smoking men were less likely to consult for all diseases and conditions, and for intermediate and minor illnesses. Regression analysis suggests that both men and women aged 65 years and over who smoked were less likely to consult. For some ICD chapters the relationship between smokers and non-smokers among the elderly was different from that among younger adults.

Among those aged 16-64 years, people who smoked were more likely to consult for all diseases and conditions and for serious and intermediate categories of illness. A higher proportion of both men and women who smoked consulted for mental, digestive and musculoskeletal disorders, injury and poisoning, symptoms, signs and ill-defined conditions and reasons in the supplementary classification. Women smokers were also more likely to consult for infectious, nervous, respiratory, genitourinary and skin diseases. Both men and women who smoked were less likely than those who did not smoke to consult for circulatory disorders. Men who smoked were also less likely to consult for endocrine disorders.

In contrast to younger men, elderly men who smoked were less likely to consult for all diseases and conditions, and for intermediate and minor illnesses. There was no difference between men who smoked and those who did not for serious illnesses, or for women who did and did not smoke for all diseases and conditions and every category of severity. Like younger adults, elderly men and women who smoked were more likely than non-smokers to consult for mental disorders, although the difference was not so great. Women who smoked were more likely to consult for respiratory diseases, but there was no difference between male smokers and non-smokers. In contrast to younger adults, a smaller proportion of elderly people who smoked consulted for reasons in the supplementary classification than those who did not smoke. Men who smoked were less likely to consult for nervous, skin and musculoskeletal disorders and injury and poisoning than those who did not smoke, and elderly women who smoked were less likely to consult for genitourinary conditions.

Figure 4.10 Age-standardised patient consulting ratios for people aged 16-64 by ethnic group

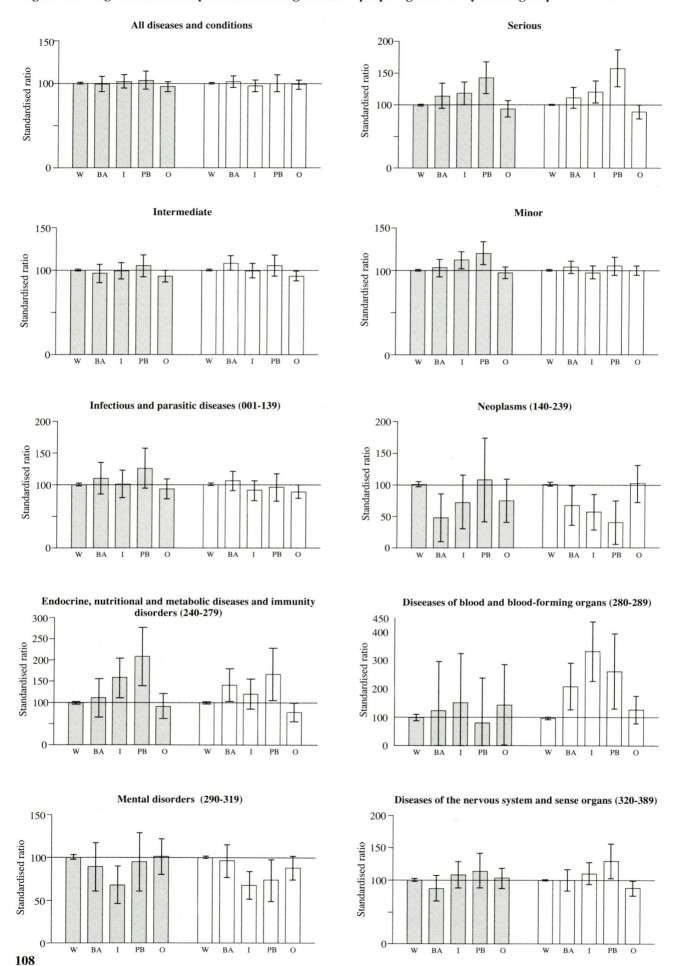

Figure 4.10 - continued

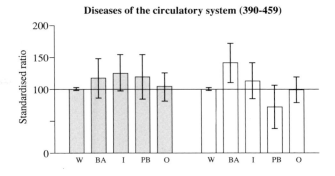

Diseases of the circulatory system (390-459)

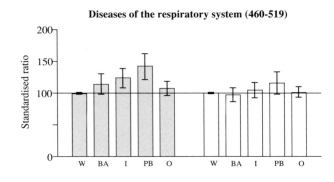

Diseases of the respiratory system (460-519)

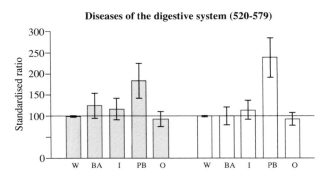

Diseases of the digestive system (520-579)

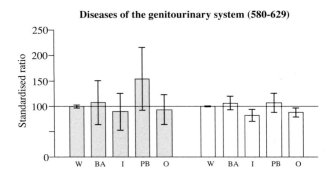

Diseases of the genitourinary system (580-629)

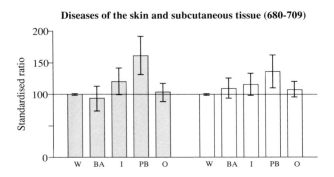

Diseases of the skin and subcutaneous tissue (680-709)

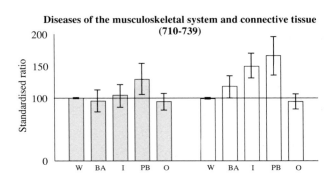

Diseases of the musculoskeletal system and connective tissue (710-739)

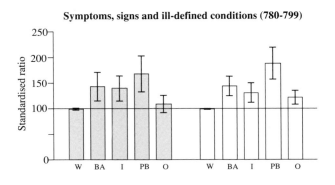

Symptoms, signs and ill-defined conditions (780-799)

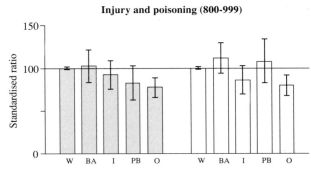

Injury and poisoning (800-999)

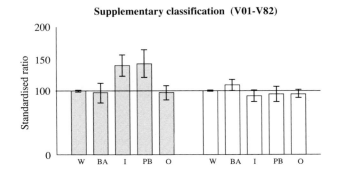

Supplementary classification (V01-V82)

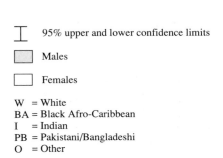

95% upper and lower confidence limits

Males

Females

W = White
BA = Black Afro-Caribbean
I = Indian
PB = Pakistani/Bangladeshi
O = Other

Figure 4.11 Age standardised patient consulting ratios for people aged 16-64 by smoking status

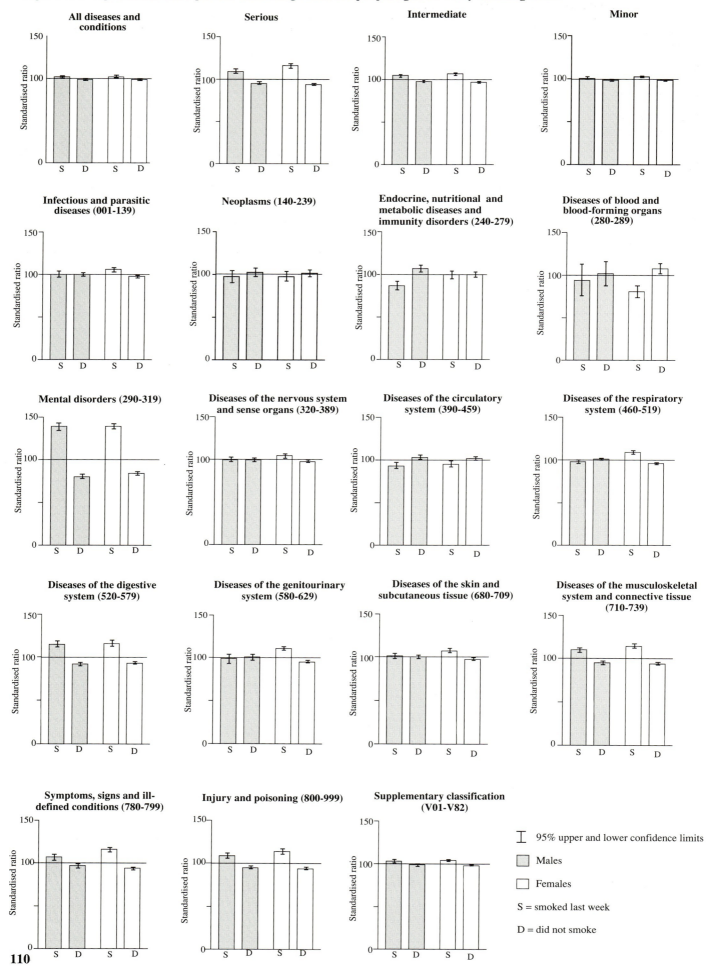

Table 4O ICD chapters for which people aged 16 and over were more likely to consult (lower SPCR confidence limit over 100), by whether they had smoked in the previous week

Whether smoked in previous week	I	II	III	IV	V	VI	VII	VIII	IX	X	XI	XII	XIII	XIV	XV	XVI	XVII	XVIII
Males aged 16-64																		
Smoked					✓				✓				✓			✓	✓	✓
Not smoked			✓				✓											
Females aged 16-64																		
Smoked	✓				✓	✓		✓	✓	✓		✓	✓			✓	✓	✓
Not smoked				✓														
Males aged 65 & over																		
Smoked					✓													
Not smoked			✓				✓											✓
Females aged 65 & over																		
Smoked					✓			✓										
Not smoked																		

5 Which patients consult: a multivariate analysis of socio-economic factors

5.1 Introduction

The previous chapter showed differences in consulting for people in different socio-economic and geographic categories. Each variable was considered in turn. It gave the proportions consulting in different categories, for example, social classes and employment status groups. It showed that generally there was the expected trend for people in Social Classes IV & V to consult more than those in Classes I & II. It also showed that people who were classified as long-term sick were much more likely than other employment status groups to consult. What the simple analysis cannot show is how much of the social class difference is associated with the higher proportions of long-term sick in the lower social classes. This chapter uses a well established multivariate analysis technique to estimate the effect of each variable while controlling for all the other variables. Unlike the previous chapter it does not give the proportion consulting in an identifiable group such as Social Class III M. Instead it gives an odds ratio which estimates how much greater or smaller consultation rates are in this group compared with a reference group when all the other factors in the model are accounted for. In general, the reference group is defined by those factors known to be related to low consultation rates such as Social Class I & II employed owner occupiers.

The model for 'explaining' patient consulting rates

The proportion of patients consulting for a given reason during the year in which the study took place is taken as the variable. Whether a patient consults in the year is related to *patient determined* need, supply factors and accessibility.

1. **Patient determined need** This is not directly measured in the study but is related to other factors such as age, sex, life events, environment and socio-economic characteristics;

2. **Supply** Factors relating to the health services available, which includes doctors, nurses, and ancillary staff per 10,000 patients, and other practice related variables. In the modelling presented here we have allowed for between-practice differences in patient consulting rates, which will reflect all these differences, but may also incorporate environmental and other factors relating to the practice, such as proximity of hospital outpatient departments, and the way in which different doctors label different diseases.

3. **Access to the practices** which includes crow-fly distances between practice and patient, and whether the patient lives in an urban or rural census enumeration district (ED).

4. **Other factors** which could influence the likelihood of consultation, e.g. number of days present in the study.

This chapter aims to describe one model and the results from it. But it also serves as an illustration of a type of analysis that can be carried out using data from the study. Other models and methodologies could be used. The regression equations are given in table 6A (p135). The detailed description of the data used and the statistical analysis are described at the end of the chapter.

Figure 5.1 summarises the model of the process leading to consulting a GP. The factors which affect consultations operate not only at the individual level but also at practice level and area level. The models allow for these different levels using data for *individuals* and a different value for each *practice* in the regression equations.

5.2 Results

The statistics arising from the analysis described above are presented here at two levels and in two sets of tables.

a) Tables 5L-5S give the results by reasons for consultation, including confidence intervals for the estimated odds ratios. All significance tests undertaken were two-tail tests. Although not shown in the tables, all these regressions included age, limiting long-term illness rate for the ED, distance from practice, latitude and longitude, and the number of days that the patient was in the study. It should be noted that the odds ratios given in tables 5L-5S are multiplicative, i.e. to calculate the odds ratios for a subgroup (such as Black, renting from local authority, etc) the odds ratios for each attribute should be multiplied together. Note also that the comparisons are made *within* each of the 64 disease/age/sex subgroups analysed. These tables are provided in detail so that readers can explore a wide range of hypotheses.

b) Tables 5A-5K in this chapter summarise the effects of a selection of socio-economic variables. These tables show odds ratios only, extracted from tables 5L-5S to show general patterns. They enable the reader to see more or less at a glance whether there is a general tendency for people in particular groups to have a raised or reduced risk of consultation for a range of reasons for consulting. The 5 per cent and 1 per cent significance levels are indicated in the tables. When interest lies in a particular value it is advisable to look also at the confidence intervals given in tables 5L-5S. If the confidence intervals

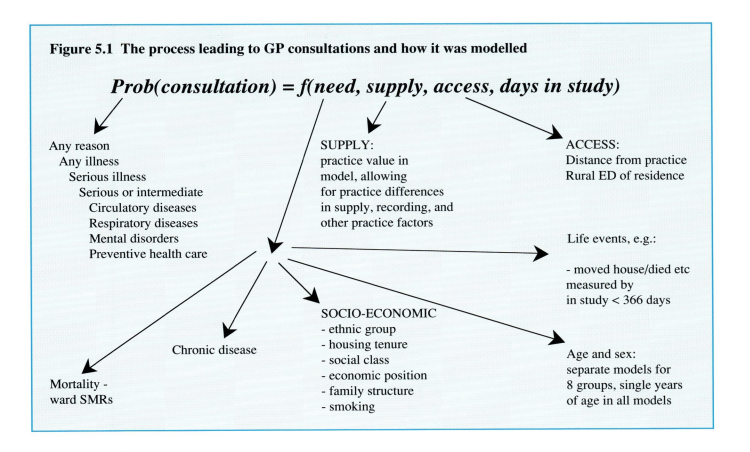

Figure 5.1 The process leading to GP consultations and how it was modelled

Prob(consultation) = f(need, supply, access, days in study)

Any reason
  Any illness
    Serious illness
      Serious or intermediate
        Circulatory diseases
        Respiratory diseases
        Mental disorders
        Preventive health care

Chronic disease

Mortality -
ward SMRs

SUPPLY:
practice value in
model, allowing
for practice differences
in supply, recording, and
other practice factors

SOCIO-ECONOMIC
- ethnic group
- housing tenure
- social class
- economic position
- family structure
- smoking

ACCESS:
Distance from practice
Rural ED of residence

Life events, e.g.:

- moved house/died etc
measured by
in study < 366 days

Age and sex:
separate models for
8 groups, single years
of age in all models

span the value 1.0 then the odds ratio for that particular group is not significantly different from that of the reference group. An odds ratio of 1.1 means that the group is approximately 10% more likely than the reference group to have consulted in the year. An odds ratio of 1.2 means 20% and so on. All relative risks are compared with the reference group described on page 119.

Social class (as defined by occupation)

The previous chapter used age and sex standardised ratios to compare consulting rates among different social groups. This simple analysis has been repeated for men and women aged 16-44 to create odds ratios. Table 5A compares these with odds ratios obtained from the more complex multivariate model.

To illustrate the effect of introducing more explanatory variables, take 'consulting for a serious illness' as an example. Among men aged 16-44 the relative risk of consulting compared with Social Classes I & II is 1.1 for Social Class III N, 1.3 for III M and 1.5 for Social Classes IV & V. These ratios suggest a clear gradient with men in Social Classes IV & V being 50% more likely than men in Social Classes I & II to consult for a serious illness during a year. When all the other variables in the model are included the gradient remains but is less strong. Taking all the other factors into account, men aged 16-44 in Social Classes IV & V are 20% more likely than their counterparts in Social Classes I & II to consult for a serious illness. Thus, other factors included in the model account for a large part of the observed differences between social classes.

Which ones are most important?

Study of subsequent tables standardised for all variables shows that men aged 16-44 who were local authority renters were 30 per cent more likely to consult for serious illness than owner occupiers. Unemployed men in this age group were 40% more likely. However, those classified as permanently sick were eight times more likely to have consulted for serious illness than the employed. Other studies have shown that renting, unemployment and being permanently sick are all more common among the manual class groups. Of all the factors included in the model used here, these are the ones that contribute to the steep social class gradient for serious illness in men aged 16-44. It must also be noted that the multivariate analysis tells us that there is a social class effect remaining once these variables are accounted for - that is, they do not account for *all* of the class gradient.

The next example discussed is the class gradient for women's consultation for mental disorders. The analysis that just standardises for age shows a gradient in odds ratios to 1.6 for women of 16-44 in Social Classes IV & V compared with Social Classes I & II. When the multivariate analysis is done, the gradient remains, but women in Classes IV & V are only 20% more likely to consult for mental disorders. The subsequent tables show that there are significantly raised odds ratios for women in the following groups - renters, unemployed, permanently sick, widowed, separated or divorced and smokers.

These findings help to explain why the differences between social classes are so large and the kinds of factors that contribute to the differences. However, it does not explain all

113

Table 5A Consulting rates, comparison of odds ratios from regression analysis including a) age and practice factors, b) all factors in the model - men and women aged 16-44, reasons for consulting and social class

Reason for consulting	Men aged 16-44				Women aged 16-44			
	Social class - odds ratios				Social class - odds ratios			
	I&II	IIIN	IIIM	IV&V	I & II	IIIN	IIIM	IV & V
Any reasons								
a) Age and practice standardised	1.0	1.1**	1.1**	1.4**	1.0	1.0	1.2**	1.1**
b) Standardised for everything	1.0	1.1**	1.1**	1.1**	1.0	1.0	1.0	1.0
Illness								
a)	1.0	1.1**	1.2**	1.2**	1.0	1.1 *	1.2**	1.2**
b)	1.0	1.1**	1.1**	1.1**	1.0	1.0	1.1*	1.0
Serious illness								
a)	1.0	1.1**	1.3**	1.5**	1.0	1.0	1.2**	1.3**
b)	1.0	1.1*	1.1**	1.2**	1.0	1.0	1.1**	1.1*
Serious/intermediate illness								
a)	1.0	1.1**	1.2**	1.3**	1.0	1.0	1.1**	1.2**
b)	1.0	1.1**	1.1**	1.2**	1.0	1.0	1.0	1.1*
Mental disorders								
a)	1.0	1.4**	1.3**	1.8**	1.0	1.2**	1.3**	1.6**
b)	1.0	1.3**	1.0	1.1	1.0	1.1	1.2**	1.2**
Circulatory								
a)	1.0	1.2**	1.1	1.2*	1.0	1.0	1.1 *	1.1
b)	1.0	1.2**	1.1	1.1	1.0	1.0	1.1	1.0
Respiratory								
a)	1.0	1.0	0.9**	1.0	1.0	1.0	1.1**	1.1**
b)	1.0	1.0	0.9**	0.9*	1.0	1.0	1.0*	1.0
Preventive health care								
a)	1.0	1.0	0.8**	0.8**	1.0	0.9**	1.0	0.9**
b)	1.0	1.0	0.9**	0.9**	1.0	1.0	0.9**	0.9**

* 5% significance level   ** 1% significance level

the difference and of course it cannot answer important questions about causality.

The rest of the chapter presents odds ratios for the main factors of interest and briefly describes their influence on the probability of consulting for a selection of reasons.

Table 5B gives the odds ratios for different social classes for all the age and sex groups. In Social Classes IV & V there were raised rates for serious illness in all age/sex groups apart from men aged 65 and over, and low rates for preventive health care. For mental disorders women in Social Classes IV & V had generally raised levels. Children in Social Class IIIM and girls in Social Class IIIN had raised consulting rates for all consultation categories apart from preventive health care. What is particularly striking about this table is that the odds ratios do not generally differ from 1 by a wide margin although there is a slight trend as you look from Social Classes I & II to Social Classes IV & V.

Housing tenure

Compared with owner occupiers, tenants of local authority accommodation who consulted for any reason had rates that were only raised in the 16-44 age group (Table 5C). However, the risk of consulting for serious illnesses was raised in all age groups. This also applies to respiratory and mental disorders. In contrast, rates for preventive health care were generally lower than those of owner occupier. Adults in 'other rented' accommodation had raised probabilities for consultation for serious illness and mental disorders. The findings for people living in communal establishments are heterogeneous. One finding worthy of note is the high relative risk of consulting for persons in the preventive health category among children. This was true for both sexes, but particularly girls.

Economic position

Unemployed adults had raised rates for all categories apart from the preventive health care and respiratory disorders. Children with unemployed parents had raised rates for mental disorders. Men aged 16-44 had double the patient consulting rate of employed men for mental disorders. The permanently sick, as would be expected, had very much higher rates. Children of permanently sick parents tended also to have raised rates, but had somewhat *lower* rates for preventive health care. (Table 5D).

Table 5B Social class, odds ratios for consulting compared to those in Social Classes I & II
NB the odds ratios are adjusted for all other variables in the regression

Sex	Age	Group	Any reason	Illness	Serious illness	Serious/ Intermediate	Mental disorders	Circulatory	Respiratory	Preventive health care
Females	0-15	IIIN	1.1	1.1**	1.1	1.1**	1.1	n/a	1.1	1.0
	0-15	IIIM	1.2**	1.2**	1.1	1.1**	1.1	n/a	1.1**	1.0
	0-15	IV&V	1.1	1.1**	1.1	1.1**	1.1	n/a	1.1**	1.0
	0-15	Other	0.9	0.9	0.8 *	1.0	1.2	n/a	1.0	1.0
Males	0-15	IIIN	1.0	1.0	1.0	1.0	1.1	n/a	1.1	1.0
	0-15	IIIM	1.1*	1.1**	1.1**	1.1**	1.2 *	n/a	1.1 *	1.0
	0-15	IV&V	1.1*	1.1 *	1.1	1.1 *	1.2 *	n/a	1.1 *	0.9
	0-15	Other	0.9	0.9	1.0	0.9 *	0.9	n/a	1.0	0.9 *
Females	16-44	IIIN	1.0	1.2	1.0	1.0	1.1	1.0	1.0	1.0
	16-44	IIIM	1.0	1.1 *	1.1 *	1.0	1.2**	1.1	1.0 *	0.9**
	16-44	IV&V	1.0	1.0	1.1**	1.1 *	1.2**	1.0	1.0	0.9**
	16-44	Other	0.7**	0.8**	0.9	0.8**	1.0	1.0	0.9**	0.8**
Males	16-44	IIIN	1.1**	1.1**	1.1*	1.1**	1.3**	1.2**	1.0	1.0
	16-44	IIIM	1.1**	1.1**	1.1**	1.1**	1.0	1.1	0.9**	0.9**
	16-44	IV&V	1.1**	1.1**	1.2**	1.2**	1.1	1.1	0.9 *	0.9**
	16-44	Other	0.6**	0.6**	0.8**	0.7**	0.9	0.8	0.7**	1.0
Females	45-64	IIIN	1.0	1.0	1.1 *	1.0	1.1	1.1 *	1.0	1.0
	45-64	IIIM	1.1*	1.2**	1.2**	1.2**	1.1**	1.3**	1.1**	1.0
	45-64	IV&V	1.0	1.1**	1.2**	1.1**	1.2**	1.2**	1.1**	0.9 *
	45-64	Other	0.9	0.9	1.1	0.9	1.3**	1.1	0.9	1.0
Males	45-64	IIIN	1.1	1.1	1.1 *	1.1	1.0	1.0	1.1	1.0
	45-64	IIIM	1.0	1.1	1.1**	1.1 *	0.9**	1.0	1.0	0.9**
	45-64	IV&V	1.1	1.1**	1.3**	1.1**	1.0	1.1**	1.0	0.9**
	45-64	Other	0.9**	0.9**	1.1**	0.9**	0.8**	1.1**	0.9**	1.0**
Females	65& over	IIIN	1.1	1.1	1.1	1.0	1.1 *	1.1 *	0.9	1.0
	65& over	IIIM	1.0	1.0	1.0	1.1	1.1	1.1 *	1.0	1.0
	65& over	IV&V	1.0	1.0	1.1 *	1.0	1.1	1.1	1.1 *	0.9**
	65& over	Other	0.7**	0.8**	0.9	0.8**	1.1	0.9	0.9 *	0.9**
Males	65& over	IIIN	1.0	1.0	1.0	0.9	1.0	1.0	1.0	1.0
	65& over	IIIM	1.0	1.0	1.1**	1.0	0.9	1.0	1.1	0.9 *
	65& over	IV&V	0.8**	0.9**	1.0	0.9**	0.8**	0.9	1.0	0.9**
	65& over	Other	0.8	0.9	1.0	0.9	1.0	0.8 *	1.1	0.8 *

* 5% significance level   ** 1% significance level

Table 5C Housing tenure, odds ratios for consulting, compared to owner occupiers
NB the odds ratios are adjusted for all other variables in the regression

Sex	Age	Group	Any Reason	Illness	Serious illness	Serious/ Intermediate	Mental disorders	Circulatory	Respiratory	Preventive health care
Females	0-15	Renting	1.0	1.1*	1.1*	1.1**	1.3**	n/a	1.1**	1.0
	16-44	local	1.2**	1.3**	1.4**	1.3**	1.4**	1.1	1.1**	0.9**
	45-64	authority	1.0	1.1	1.2**	1.1**	1.2**	1.2**	1.3**	0.9**
	65& over		1.0	1.1	1.2**	1.1**	1.2**	1.0	1.2**	0.9**
Males	0-15		1.0	1.0	1.1	1.0	1.1	n/a	1.1*	1.0
	16-44		1.1*	1.1**	1.3**	1.1**	1.3**	1.2*	1.1**	0.9*
	45-64		1.0	1.1	1.2**	1.1**	1.2**	1.1*	1.2**	1.0
	65& over		1.0	1.1	1.2**	1.1	1.2**	1.0	1.3**	0.9*
Females	0-15	Other	1.1	1.2**	1.0	1.0	1.2	n/a	1.0	1.1
	16-44	rented	1.0	1.1**	1.2**	1.1**	1.2**	1.1	1.0	1.0
	45-64		1.1	1.1	1.2**	1.0	1.2**	1.1	1.1	1.0
	65& over		1.1	1.1*	1.1*	1.1*	1.1*	1.0	1.1	1.0
Males	0-15		1.0	1.0	1.0	1.0	1.2	n/a	1.0	1.0
	16-44		1.1**	1.1**	1.2**	1.1**	1.4**	1.1	1.1**	1.0
	45-64		1.1**	1.1*	1.2**	1.1	1.2**	1.1	1.1	1.0
	65& over		1.2*	1.1	1.2**	1.1	1.1	1.1	1.1*	1.1
Females	0-15	Communal	1.8**	1.4	1.3	1.0	1.3	n/a	1.4*	9.1**
	16-44	estabs	0.3**	0.5**	0.9	0.5**	0.9	0.7	0.7**	0.4**
	45-64		0.5**	0.7	1.2	0.7	1.6*	1.0	0.7	0.9
	65& over		0.7	0.8	1.5*	0.9	2.1**	0.8	1.4	1.4
Males	0-15		1.2	1.0	1.3	1.0	1.5	n/a	0.9	4.8**
	16-44		0.5**	0.5**	0.8	0.6**	2.3**	0.7	0.5**	0.8*
	45-64		0.6**	0.5**	0.5**	0.6**	2.7**	0.4**	0.8	2.0**
	65& over		0.9	1.0	1.0	0.9	2.9**	0.5**	1.3	1.4*

* 5% significance level   ** 1% significance level

Table 5D Economic position† odds ratios for consulting, compared to full-time or part-time employment
NB the odds ratios are adjusted for all other variables in the regression

Sex	Age	Group	Any reason	Illness	Serious illness	Serious/ Intermediate	Mental disorders	Circulatory	Respiratory	Preventive health care
Females	0-15	Unemployed	1.0	1.0	0.9	1.0	1.1	n/a	1.0	1.0
	16-44		1.1	1.1*	1.3**	1.2**	1.4**	1.1	0.9*	1.0
	45-64		1.4**	1.4**	1.2	1.5**	1.5**	1.3**	0.9	1.0
Males	0-15		1.0	1.0	0.9	1.0	1.1	n/a	0.9	1.0
	16-44		1.1**	1.1**	1.4**	1.2**	2.0**	1.1	1.1*	1.0
	45-64		1.2**	1.2**	1.4**	1.3**	1.7**	1.1	1.0	1.0
Females	0-15	Student	1.0	0.9	0.9	0.8	1.9	n/a	1.0	1.0
	16-44		0.8**	0.9	1.0	0.9	1.0	0.9	1.0	0.7**
	45-64		0.8	0.7	1.2	0.8	1.1	0.2*	0.8	0.9
Males	0-15		1.0	1.0	0.9	1.1	1.2	n/a	0.8	0.8
	16-44		1.4**	1.3**	1.1	1.3**	1.2*	1.3	1.3**	1.2**
	45-64		1.6	2.1	1.7	1.1	1.0	0.7	0.9	0.5
Females	0-15	Permanently sick	1.2*	1.2*	1.3*	1.2*	1.0	n/a	1.1	0.9
	16-44		2.2**	2.9	5.0**	3.2**	4.0**	1.9**	1.3**	0.7**
	45-64		4.6**	4.1**	4.8**	4.7**	2.7**	2.2**	1.4**	1.3**
Males	0-15		1.2*	1.2*	1.0	1.2*	1.6*	n/a	1.2	0.9
	16-44		5.3**	4.8**	7.5**	6.0**	6.5**	3.0**	1.6**	1.3**
	45-64		7.9**	6.8**	6.9**	7.1**	3.8**	3.2**	1.9**	1.7**
Females	0-15	Other	1.0	1.0	1.0	0.9	1.0	n/a	1.0	0.9
	16-44		1.0	1.0	1.1**	1.1**	1.2**	1.3**	0.9**	1.2**
	45-64		0.9**	0.9**	1.2**	1.0	1.3**	1.3**	0.9**	1.0
Males	0-15		1.0	1.0	1.1	1.0	1.1	n/a	1.0	1.1
	16-44		1.4*	1.2	1.3	1.2	1.9**	1.5	1.0	1.5**
	45-64		1.4**	1.4**	1.7**	1.5**	1.6**	1.5**	1.1	1.3**

† For children aged 0-15 the economic position relates to the parent/guardian.
* 5% significance level   ** 1% significance level

Table 5E Summary of odds ratios for consulting by ethnic group, compared to white group.
NB the odds ratios are adjusted for all other variables in the regression.

Sex	Age	Group	Any reason	Illness	Serious illness	Serious/ Intermediate	Mental disorders	Circulatory	Respiratory	Preventive health care
Females	0-15	Black	1.0	0.9	1.3	0.8*	0.2*	n/a	1.1	1.2
	16-44		1.1	1.3*	1.1	1.2*	0.8	1.1	0.9	1.2
	45-64		1.0	1.1	1.1	1.3	1.1	1.6*	0.9	1.1
	65& over		1.1	1.3	0.6	1.1	1.6	1.4	0.9	0.9
Males	0-15		0.8	0.8	1.3	0.8*	0.7	n/a	1.1	1.2
	16-44		0.9	0.9	1.2	0.9	0.8	0.9	1.1	1.0
	45-64		1.2	1.1	1.0	1.1	0.7	1.3	1.3	1.2
	65& over		1.0	0.8	1.0	0.9	2.4**	0.9	0.9	1.1
Females	0-15	Indian subcontinent	1.6**	1.5**	1.0	1.1	0.7	n/a	1.6**	1.6**
	16-44		0.8	1.1	1.5**	1.2**	1.1	0.8	1.1	0.7**
	45-64		1.4	1.5*	2.1**	1.7**	1.0	0.7	1.8**	1.2
	65& over		0.5*	0.7	1.1	0.7	1.1	0.8	1.2	0.8
Males	0-15		1.5**	1.3**	1.3*	1.2*	1.3	n/a	1.7**	2.3**
	16-44		1.2*	1.1	1.5**	1.1	0.9	1.1	1.4**	1.9**
	45-64		0.9	1.0	1.4*	1.2	1.1	1.1	1.7**	1.6**
	65& over		0.7	0.7	1.3	0.9	0.9	0.9	1.0	2.1**
Females	0-15	Other	0.8*	0.8*	1.0	0.9	0.7	n/a	1.0	1.1
	16-44		0.8	0.9	0.7*	0.8**	0.8	1.0	1.1	0.8*
	45-64		0.7	0.7	1.3	0.9	0.9	1.2	0.7	0.9
	65& over		0.3**	0.3**	0.6	0.4**	0.7	0.5	0.9	0.7
Males	0-15		0.9	0.9	1.1	1.0	1.0	n/a	1.2*	1.2
	16-44		0.8*	0.9	0.8	0.8*	0.9	0.9	1.0	1.1
	45-64		0.7	0.7	1.0	0.9	0.7	1.2	1.1	1.2
	65& over		0.6	0.6	0.6	0.7	0.0	0.9	0.8	1.3

* 5% significance level   ** 1% significance level

Ethnic group

Table 5E explores the effect of ethnic group. The top part shows results for black people. There is no evidence of any general increased risk of having consulted during the year for any reason. However, black children and young adults were more likely to have consulted for a serious illness - for example, in age-group 0-15, the 'relative risk' (odds ratio) for a black child compared with a white child is 1.3 for serious illness, representing a 30 per cent excess risk. For mental disorders there was a general tendency for fewer black people to consult, except among the elderly where they were at much greater risk than the white reference population. Black women were more likely to consult for circulatory diseases, and almost all the age/sex groups had raised likelihoods of consultation for preventive health care. In general, patient consulting rates are higher for people from the Indian sub-continent ethnic group than for white people.

Family type

The results for different family types are shown in three tables for separate age-groups. table 5F gives the relative risk of consultation for children living with a sole adult. Girls living with a sole adult had higher consulting rates than those living with two or more adults, except for mental disorders and preventive health care. For boys there was little effect, except that they were more likely to consult for mental disorders.

Table 5G shows that widowed divorced and separated adults with and without dependent children generally had raised rates. Single people without dependent children generally had low rates for all categories of consultation apart from mental disorders, where men had 50 per cent higher rates and women aged 45-64 had 20 per cent higher rates.

Table 5F Living with sole adult, odds ratios for consulting children aged 0-15 compared to two adult families
NB the odds ratios are adjusted for all other variables in the regression.

Sex	Group	Any reason	Illness	Serious illness	Serious/ Intermediate	Mental disorders	Circulatory	Respiratory	Preventive health care
Females	Sole adult	1.1*	1.1*	1.1	1.1*	1.0	n/a	1.1	1.0
Males	family	1.0	1.0	1.0	1.0	1.3*	n/a	0.9	0.9

* 5% significance level

Table 5G Family type, odds ratios for consulting, compared to married/cohabiting with dependent children, adults aged 16-64
NB the odds ratios are adjusted for all other variables in the regression.

Sex	Age	Group	Any reason	Illness	Serious illness	Serious/ Intermediate	Mental disorders	Circulatory	Respiratory	Preventive health care
Females	16-44	Married/ cohab wo dependent children	1.0	1.0*	1.2**	1.0*	1.0	1.0	0.8**	1.1**
	45-64		1.1	1.1*	1.1	1.1*	1.1	1.2**	1.0	1.0
Males	16-44		0.9**	0.9**	1.1**	0.9*	1.1	1.1	0.8**	1.2**
	45-64		1.1*	1.0	1.1*	1.1*	1.0	1.2**	0.9*	1.3**
Females	16-44	Wid/sep/ div with dependent children	1.4**	1.4**	1.2**	1.3**	1.5*	1.1	1.2**	1.1*
	45-64		1.3*	1.4**	1.3**	1.3**	1.2	1.3	1.3**	1.0
Males	16-44		1.4**	1.4**	1.1	1.2*	2.4**	1.2	1.1	1.1
	45-64		1.2	1.2	1.2	1.3	1.7**	1.2	1.1	1.1
Females	16-44	Wid/sep/ div wo dependent children	1.3**	1.2**	1.1	1.2**	1.8**	1.0	1.1**	1.1*
	45-64		1.3**	1.3**	1.2**	1.3**	1.7**	1.2**	1.3**	1.0
Males	16-44		1.4**	1.4**	1.3**	1.4**	2.3**	1.0	1.0	1.0
	45-64		1.2**	1.2**	1.2**	1.3**	1.8**	1.3**	1.0	1.2**
Females	16-44	Single with dependent children	0.6**	0.8**	1.0	0.8**	1.0	1.0	0.9*	0.7**
	45-64		3.2*	1.7	1.4	1.1	0.4	1.4	1.7	1.4
Males	16-44		0.7**	0.8**	1.1	0.8**	1.1	0.9	0.8**	0.9
	45-64		1.7	1.4	1.7	1.4	1.2	1.2	1.0	1.3
Females	16-44	Single wo dep children	0.5**	0.6**	0.9**	0.7**	1.0	0.7**	0.9**	0.7*
	45-64		0.9	0.9	1.1	0.9	1.3*	1.2	0.8*	1.0
Males	16-44		0.8**	0.8**	1.0	0.8**	1.5**	1.0	0.8**	1.0
	45-64		0.8**	0.8**	0.9*	0.9	1.5**	1.1	0.7**	1.0

* 5% significance level ** 1% significance level

Among adults aged 65 and over (Table 5H), single people generally had lower rates for all consultation categories, apart from mental disorders. Those living alone were at 10 per cent higher risk than married/cohabiting people. The widowed, divorced and separated were at even higher risk of consulting for mental disorders, apart from women sharing with other adults.

Smoking

Whilst smoking is not a socio-economic variable it is a behaviour that varies significantly by social class - those in the manual groups smoking more than those in the non-manual classes. Many studies have shown that smoking reduces life expectancy. Generally, however, this does not appear to be related to high consulting rates, as can be seen from table 5I. Indeed, among men, apart from consulting for mental disorders, the risk of consulting during the year tended to be lower for smokers. Women smokers also had a raised risk of consultation for mental disorders. Smokers were less likely to consult for preventive health care than non-smokers, apart from women smokers aged 16-44, who were as likely to consult for preventive health care as non-smokers. However, our definition of not smoking includes only those who have not smoked in the week before interview and some may have stopped temporarily as a consequence of their illness. Women smokers were generally more likely to consult for serious illnesses and respiratory diseases than non-smokers.

Living in a rural area

Adults living in rural enumeration districts were some 10 per cent less likely to consult for 'any reason' than those who lived in urban areas, apart from men aged 65 and over. Consultation for preventive health care was lower among those aged 65 and over.

Limiting long-term illness

In the regression analysis, age-standardised limiting long-standing illness, standardised to a standard European population, were calculated for each age/sex group analysed, for each patient's enumeration district of residence. These were used as a proxy for the general chronic illness level of the locality. People living in areas with higher limiting long-standing illness rates were generally at higher risk of consulting (see table 6A - regression equations).

Table 5H Family type, odds ratios for consulting, compared to married/cohabiting, adults aged 65 and over
NB the odds ratios are adjusted for all other variables in the regression.

Sex	Age	Group	Any reason	Illness	Serious illness	Serious/ Intermediate	Mental disorders	Circulatory	Respiratory	Preventive health care
Females	65& over	Single, sharing with adult	0.7**	0.7**	0.8**	0.7**	1.0	0.8*	0.7**	0.8**
Males	65& over		0.5**	0.6**	0.8*	0.6**	0.9	0.7**	0.7**	0.7**
Females	65& over	Sep/wid/div, sharing with adult	0.9	1.0	1.1*	1.1	1.0	1.0	1.1**	0.8**
Males	65& over		0.9	1.0	1.1	1.0	1.4**	1.1	1.0	0.8**
Females	65& over	Single, lives alone	0.8**	0.8**	0.9**	0.8**	1.1	0.9	0.8**	0.8**
Males	65& over		0.8*	0.8	0.9	0.9	1.1	1.0	0.7**	0.9
Females	65& over	Sep/wid/div, lives alone	1.1*	1.1**	1.1*	1.1**	1.2**	1.0	1.1*	0.9
Males	65& over		0.9	1.0	1.0	1.0	1.4**	1.0	0.9	0.9*
Females	65& over	Not known	1.4	1.2	0.9	1.3	1.2	0.9	1.0	0.8
Males	65& over		0.8	0.9	1.1	1.0	1.0	1.4	1.1	0.8

* 5% significance level   ** 1% significance level

Table 5I   Smoking status, odds ratio for consulting, compared to non-smokers

Sex	Age	Group	Any reason	Illness	Serious illness	Serious/ Intermediate	Mental disorders	Circulatory	Respiratory	Preventive health care
Females	16-44	Smoker	1.2**	1.2**	1.2**	1.2**	1.5**	0.9	1.1	1.0
	45-64		0.9*	1.0	1.1*	1.0	1.4**	0.8**	1.2	0.8**
	65& over		0.8**	0.9**	1.0	0.9**	1.3**	0.8**	1.2**	0.8**
Males	16-44		1.0	1.0	1.0	1.1**	1.5**	0.9**	0.9	0.8**
	45-64		0.9**	0.9**	0.9**	0.9**	1.3**	0.8**	0.9	0.7**
	65& over		0.7**	0.8**	0.9**	0.8**	1.2**	0.7**	0.9	0.7**

* 5% significance level   ** 1% significance level

118

Table 5J Rurality, odds ratio for consulting, compared to people living in urban EDs

Sex	Age	Group	Any reason	Illness	Serious illness	Serious/ Intermediate	Mental disorders	Circulatory	Respiratory	Preventive health care
Females	0-15	Rural ED	1.0	1.0	1.0	1.0	0.7*	n/a	1.0	1.0
	16-44		0.9	1.0	1.0	1.0	0.9*	0.9	1.0	1.0
	45-64		0.9	0.9*	0.9	0.9*	0.9	1.0	0.9	1.1
	65& over		0.9*	0.9*	0.9	0.9**	1.0	1.0	0.9	0.9
Males	0-15		1.1	1.0	0.9	1.1	1.0	n/a	0.9*	1.0
	16-44		0.9**	0.9**	0.8**	0.9**	0.8**	1.0	0.9*	1.0
	45-64		0.9	1.0	0.9	1.0	0.8*	0.9	1.0	1.0
	65& over		1.0	1.0	1.0	0.9	0.9	0.9	1.0	0.9*

* 5% significance level   ** 1% significance level

Table 5K Odds ratios for consulting: In practice < 1 year, compared to in practice for full year
NB the odds ratios are adjusted for all other variables in the regression

Sex	Age	Group	Any reason	Illness	Serious illness	Serious/ Intermediate	Mental disorders	Circulatory	Respiratory	Preventive health care
Females	0-15	In	1.0	0.8**	1.2**	0.9**	1.5**	n/a	0.9**	2.1**
	16-44	practice	1.3**	1.1*	1.4**	1.1**	1.3**	1.2**	1.1**	1.9**
	45-64	< 1 year	1.9**	1.5**	1.9**	1.6**	1.7**	1.7**	1.2*	2.1**
	65& over		1.8**	1.9**	2.6**	1.9**	1.9**	2.1**	1.5**	1.2**
Males	0-15		1.0	0.8**	1.3**	0.8**	1.0	n/a	0.9**	2.3**
	16-44		2.0**	1.5**	1.7**	1.5**	1.9**	1.6**	1.3**	5.9**
	45-64		2.4**	1.6**	2.1**	1.6**	1.5**	1.6**	1.4**	3.6**
	65& over		1.8**	1.9**	2.8**	2.0**	2.4**	2.2**	1.7**	1.2**

* 5% significance level   ** 1% significance level

Distance from practice

Distance from the practice was generally a deterrent to consultation. The deterrent effect was less for the more serious illnesses.

Being in the practice for less than the whole study year

There are of course many reasons why patients were registered with practices for less than the whole study year. People who left the practice could have done so because they moved and/or changed doctors or died. Patients who joined the practice could have done so for many reasons and many practices like to see patients when they newly register. Thus it is not surprising that adults who had been in the practice for less than the full year had considerably higher consulting rates than those who had been with the practice throughout the study year. However, this was not true for children, except for serious illness and preventive health care, and for girls for mental disorders.

Between-practice differences

The regression equations allowed for practice differences. This was done by fitting a dummy variable for each practice. Models were fitted with and without practice variables, and chi-squared tests of between-practice differences were undertaken. In all models there were statistically significant between-practice differences. These differences were greatest by far for the preventive health care category, and least for mental disorders and serious illnesses.

Figure 5.2 illustrates the regression analysis results for the 16-44 age-group for patients consulting for 'any reason', 'serious illness' and 'mental disorders', as an illustration of how the information in tables 5L-5S can be used. It is immediately apparent, for example, that for this age-group there are greater social class differences for men than for women for 'any reason' and for 'serious illness', and that for men and women the patterns of mental illness are different.

5.3 Data available for analysis

a) Dependent variable - proportion of patients consulting in a year

The analysis was limited to describing the eight key measures of patient consulting rates described in figure 5.1. These were chosen to cover a range of morbidity, and preventive health care. The measures have been analysed for four age-groups for each gender separately: 0-15; 16-44; 45-64; 65 and over, since there are different patterns in patient consulting rates in these different age-groups. Patient consulting rates were chosen because they are the measures in the study which best approximate annual prevalence.

Figure 5.2 Comparison of odds ratios for men and women aged 16-44, relative to reference group*

Patients consulting - any reason

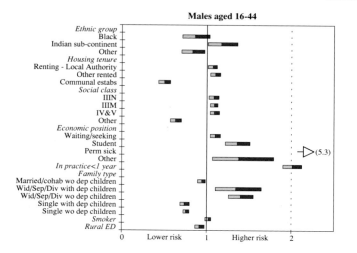

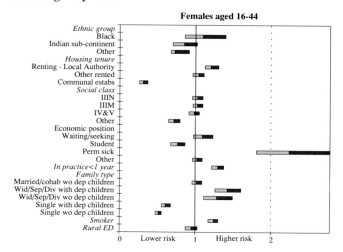

Patients consulting - serious illness

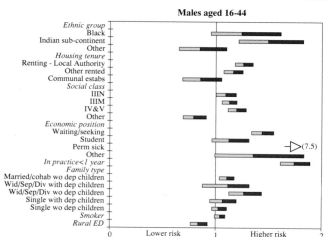

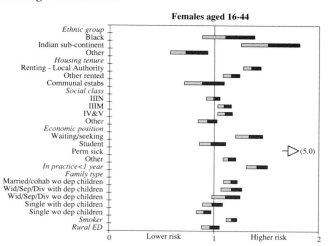

Patients consulting - mental disorders

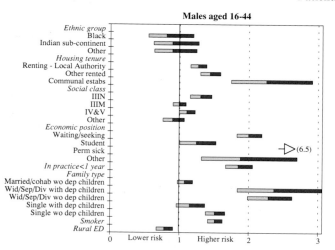

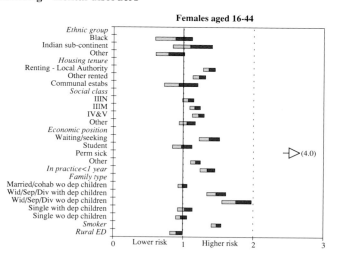

Note: bars show the 95% confidence interval. The mean (point estimate) is where the two shadings meet.

Individuals who were permanently sick were at considerably raised risk of consulting - where the intervals are off the scale this is indicated by an arrow and the estimated odds ratio is given.

What has been estimated in the above graphs is the ratio: odds of consulting in the group of interest divided by the odds of consulting in the reference group. Where the probability of consulting is small this approximates relative risk closely (eg serious illness, mental illness).

If the bar is clear of the vertical line at odds ratio = 1, then the result is statistically significant (*p*<0.05).

*   Reference group: white people of the same age/sex who were owner occupiers in Social Classes I & II, employed, in the practice for the full year, married/cohabiting with dependent children, non-smokers, living in urban enumeration districts.

b) Explanatory variables

The variables used in the model are defined below.

Individual patient data:

Age of patient — in single years. Separate models for age-groups 0-15, 16-44, 45-64, 65 and over. In each age/sex group 'mean age' was subtracted for the patient's age, and age, age^2, age^3 were fitted because the relationship between patient consulting rates and age is not linear (see figure 2.1, pp 25). Separate models were fitted for 4 broad age-groups 0-15, 16-44, 45-64, and 65 and over.

Sex — separate models were fitted for each gender, since socio-economic factors may act differently for the two sexes.

Ethnic group
1.* White — White
2. Black — Black Caribbean, Black African
3. Indian subcontinent — Indian, Pakistani, Bangladeshi
4. Other — Chinese, Sri Lankan, Other

Housing tenure
1.* Owner occupier — Buying, owns outright
2. Renting, local authority — Council, New Town
3. Renting other — With job, housing association, private furnished, private unfurnished
4. Communal estab. — Communal establishments

Social class
1.* I & II — Professional and managerial
2. IIIN — Skilled non-manual
3. IIIM — Skilled manual
4. IV & V — Semi-skilled and unskilled manual
5. Other — Armed forces, inadequately described, never worked, etc

NB For children, social class is that of parent. For married/cohabiting women, it is that of her partner.

Economic position last week
1.* Working — Working full-time or part-time
2. Waiting/ seeking — Waiting to start, seeking work
3. Student — Student
4. Perm. sick — Permanently sick
5. Other — Retired, home/family

NB For children, economic position is that of parent

Smoker (ages 16 and over only)
1. Smokes — Smoked in last week
2.* Does not smoke — Did not smoke in last week

Family structure - variables have been combined to form the following classifications

Ages 0-15
1. Single adult household
2.* Two or more adult household
3. Communal establishments (see Tenure above)

Ages 16-64
1.* Married/cohabiting with dependent children 0-15 (not sole adult in household)
2. Married/cohabiting without dependent children 0-15 (not sole adult in household)
3. Widowed/separated/divorced with dependent children 0-15
4. Widowed/separated/divorced without dependent children 0-15
5. Sole adult with dependent children 0-15
6. Sole adult without dependent children 0-15
7. Communal establishment (see Tenure - not asked about children)

Ages 65 and over
1.* Married/cohabiting (not sole adult in household)
2. Single but sharing with other adult
3. Separated/widowed/divorced, but sharing with other adult
4. Single, not sharing with other adult
5. Separated/widowed/divorced, not sharing with other adult
6. Communal establishments (see Tenure).

In practice less than 1 year
1.* In practice for whole of study year - 366 days
2. In practice less than 366 days

A patient would be in the study for less than a year if he/she were born, had died, or moved or changed GP during the year. This dummy variable allows for these events, which may significantly alter the likelihood of a consultation.

Days in the study (1 to 366)
The number of days for which the patient contributed to the study was directly taken into account by assuming that the proportion consulting is directly proportional to the days at risk.

Data based on the postcode of residence of the patient

Rural enumeration district
1.* Lives in urban enumeration district (ED)
2. Lives in rural enumeration district

This indicator was based on the postcode of residence for a patient, and enabled the enumeration district in which they lived to be identified, classified by the DoE and OPCS classification of urban EDs.

Distance to practice
Taken as the crow-fly distance between each patient's enumeration district of residence and the practice address

- to the nearest 100m. For regression purposes the mean distance in each age/sex group was subtracted and distance plus distance squared fitted, to allow for the possibility that the relationship with the probability of consultation might be non-linear.

Limiting long-term illness rate for enumeration district of residence (LLTI)

For the appropriate age/sex group (ie persons 0-15, males 16-44, 45-64, 65 and over) females 16-44, 45-64, 65 and over, a rate per 10,000 population age standardised to the European standard population was calculated. This was fitted as a continuous covariate in the regression models, as a proxy for individual limiting long-term illness, since no specific data on this characteristic were available from the MSGP4 survey.

Latitude/longitude of patient's enumeration district

These measurements were recorded to the nearest 100m and used in regression equations as continuous environmental covariates.

Data based on the practice serving the patients

Practice

There are a number of reasons, apart from differences in morbidity level, why the average patient consulting rate might differ between practices, even when all other socio-economic factors have been taken into account, for example, differences in supply of services, hours of availability, recording habits, etc. All models allowed for between-practice differences, by fitting a different value in the regression equation for each practice.

Other practice information was available, but for this chapter we were only concerned to adjust for practice differences, not to explain these. Models without the practice parameter were also fitted for comparison, to test whether there were statistically significant between-practice differences. These differences were generally statistically significant even when all other available data were adjusted for. The average travel to surgery distance for a practice in this study was less than 2 km, so practice populations are fairly localised when compared with hospital populations. By treating practice as a separate level within a multi-level model, our analysis is thus a *within-practice* analysis, ie, *we have removed the effect of between-practice variations from the data being analysed.* Because the number of patients within each practice is large (average 8,000), it is reasonable in our analyses to treat the effect of each practice as a fixed constant.

The standardised mortality ratios (SMRs) of electoral ward of residence (all causes, ages 0-64 and all ages) were tested in early exploratory models. However, they tended not to explain variations over and above those explained by other area variables, so have not been included.

5.4   Statistical analysis

The chosen approach was to use logistic regression, as provided in the Royal Statistical Society's GLIM4 analysis package[14] to predict the proportion of patients consulting, based on the socio-economic data available (see Box). A by-product of logistic regression is a set of 'relative risk' estimates for the socio-economic categories compared with a 'reference group'.* These estimates are 'odds ratios', being the ratio of the odds of consulting in the group of interest relative to the odds of consulting for the reference group. When the likelihood of consulting is small (say less than 10 per cent), then the odds ratio is a close approximation to the relative risk. We have chosen as our reference group those who are likely to be the most healthy. An ideal might be to improve the health of the other groups to the same level as the reference group. As far as possible the same explanatory variables have been included in all models.

5.5   Summary

This chapter describes a model and a multivariate analysis technique applied to the study data. It aims to quantify the independent effects of the many factors which are related to the prevalence of ill-health as measured by consultation

---

Logistic regression

Data that are concerned with the proportions (e.g. of patients consulting) have binomial errors. The old fashioned way of modelling these sorts of data was to use the percentage as response variable. However, there are three problems with this approach:

(i)   the variance is not normally distributed;

(ii)   the variance is not constant;

(iii)   by calculating the percentage we lose information regarding the size of the sample from which the proportion was estimated.

In logistic regression we use the number responding as the response variable, with the number at risk as the binomial denominator. GLIM then carries out a weighted regression, using the individual sample sizes as weights, and the logit link function to ensure linearity. The logit function takes care of the fact that proportions must lie between 0 and 1, and ensures that regression estimates of response proportions lie in the range 0 to 1. The logit transformation of probability p is $\log(p/1-p)$, and this is regressed as a linear combination of the explanatory variables, i.e. if p=probability of consulting, then $\log(p/(1-p))=\text{const} + b_1$. need $+ b_2$. supply + error.

---

*   The characteristics of the reference groups are marked with an asterisk in section 5.3. They comprise white owner occupiers in Social Classes I & II, in employment, not smoking, married/cohabiting, etc. All comparisons are made within the age/sex group being analysed, e.g. females 45-64.

during the practice year. To simplify interpretation we have chosen reference groups for comparisons. These groups have the characteristics which the previous chapter showed were related to the lowest consultation rates, that is, white owner occupiers in Social Classes I & II, in employment, not smoking, and so on.

Taking account of all other socio-economic factors the influence of social class was reduced. The clear trends seen in univariate analysis of health data did not hold systematically for each age and sex group. However, for consultation for all illnesses combined, almost all the age/sex groups in the manual social classes had a 10 per cent increased risk of consultation. In contrast, consultation for preventive reasons was 10 per cent less for the manual than the non-manual classes.

Other factors that tended to explain a higher rate of consultation were renting compared with owner occupation, being unemployed or permanently sick compared with being employed, etc. Being black or Asian was a significant factor particularly for serious and intermediate illness. Those who were widowed, divorced or separated had higher consulting rates generally than the married/cohabiting. There was a tendency for those living in rural areas to have lower consultation rates than those in urban areas.

Table 5L   Patients consulting for any reason: Odds ratios compared with reference group, for which ratio = 1 (see footnote)

Ages 0-15 / Ages 16-44

	Males Signif-icance	Males Odds ratio	Males 95% CI lower bd	Males 95% CI Upper bd	Females Signif-icance	Females Odds ratio	Females 95% CI Lower bd	Females 95% CI Upper bd
Ages 0-15								
Ethnic group								
Black		0.84	0.64	1.10		0.95	0.72	1.26
Indian sub-continent	**	1.46	1.17	1.81	**	1.63	1.29	2.07
Other		0.90	0.73	1.12		0.80	0.64	0.99
Housing tenure								
Renting-LA		0.96	0.90	1.04		1.04	0.97	1.13
Other rented		0.98	0.89	1.08		1.10	0.99	1.22
Communal estabs		1.24	0.95	1.61	**	1.81	1.20	2.72
Social class								
IIIN		0.99	0.91	1.07	*	1.12	1.02	1.22
IIIM	*	1.08	1.01	1.15	**	1.15	1.08	1.23
IV & V	*	1.08	1.00	1.16		1.08	1.00	1.17
Other		0.91	0.79	1.05		0.93	0.80	1.07
Economic position								
Waiting/seeking		0.97	0.89	1.07		1.00	0.91	1.10
Student		0.95	0.71	1.27		1.00	0.74	1.36
Perm sick	*	1.23	1.03	1.47		1.19	0.99	1.44
Other		1.02	0.91	1.14		1.02	0.90	1.15
In practice <1 year		0.97	0.89	1.05		1.01	0.93	1.10
Single adult in hhold		1.01	0.92	1.11	*	1.11	1.01	1.22
Rural enumeration district		1.07	0.97	1.19		1.05	0.94	1.16
Ages 16-44								
Ethnic group								
Black		0.86	0.71	1.03		1.10	0.86	1.40
Indian sub-continent	*	1.17	1.01			0.85	0.70	1.02
Other	*	0.83	0.70	0.97		0.83	0.68	1.02
Housing tenure								
Renting-LA	*	1.07	1.01	1.12	**	1.21	1.13	1.31
Other rented	**	1.10	1.04	1.16		1.04	0.96	1.11
Communal estabs	**	0.50	0.43	0.57	**	0.31	0.26	0.37
Social class								
IIIN	**	1.06	10.2	1.14		1.03	0.96	1.10
IIIM	**	1.09	1.04	1.13		1.03	0.97	1.10
IV & V	**	1.09	1.04	1.15		0.98	0.91	1.05
Other	**	0.63	0.57	0.70	**	0.72	0.65	0.80
Economic position								
Waiting/seeking	**	1.10	1.04	1.16		1.09	0.97	1.23
Student	**	1.36	1.22	1.51	**	0.76	0.67	0.86
Perm sick	**	5.33	4.56	6.24	**	2.24	1.81	2.78
Other	*	1.38	1.07	1.79		1.02	0.96	1.09
In practice<1 year	**	2.01	1.90	2.12	**	1.30	1.22	1.38
Family type								
Married/cohab no dependent children	**	0.94	0.89	0.98		1.02	0.96	1.09
Wid/sep/div with dep children	**	1.35	1.11	1.65	**	1.43	1.27	1.61
Wid/sep/div with no dep children	**	1.40	1.26	1.55	**	1.29	1.12	1.50
Single with dep children	**	0.74	0.69	0.80	**	0.61	0.56	0.68
Single no dep children	**	0.76	0.73	0.80	**	0.51	0.47	0.55
Smoker		1.02	0.98	1.05	**	1.24	1.17	1.30
Rural ED	**	0.92	0.87	0.98		0.95	0.87	1.03

Ages 45-64 / Ages 65 and over

	Males Signif-icance	Males Odds ratio	Males 95% CI lower bd	Males 95% CI Upper bd	Females Signif-icance	Females Odds ratio	Females 95% CI Lower bd	Females 95% CI Upper bd
Ages 45-64								
Ethnic group								
Black		1.16	0.80	1.67		0.97	0.62	1.51
Indian sub-continent		0.92	0.72	1.17		-1.44	0.97	2.14
Other		0.72	0.51	1.03		0.69	0.44	1.08
Housing tenure								
Renting-LA		1.04	0.96	1.13		0.97	0.89	1.07
Other rented	**	1.14	1.03	1.26		1.06	0.93	1.20
Communal estabs	**	0.58	0.39	0.85	**	0.53	0.35	0.79
Social class								
IIIN		1.05	0.97	1.14		0.98	0.89	1.07
IIIM		1.02	0.96	1.08	*	1.09	1.01	1.17
IV & V		1.06	0.99	1.13		1.03	0.94	1.12
Other	**	0.52	0.41	0.67		0.88	0.74	1.04
Economic position								
Waiting/seeking	**	1.21	1.10	1.33	**	1.35	1.08	1.69
Student		1.59	0.67	3.75		0.79	0.42	1.50
Perm sick	**	7.89	6.72	9.27	**	4.63	3.61	5.94
Other	**	1.42	1.30	1.55	**	0.86	0.81	0.92
In practice< 1 year	**	2.39	2.11	2.71	**	1.93	1.68	2.21
Family type								
Married/cohab no dependent children	*	1.07	1.00	1.14		1.07	0.97	1.17
Wid/sep/div with dep children		1.16	0.86	1.58	*	1.28	1.02	1.61
Wid/sep/div with no dep children	**	1.22	1.09	1.36	**	1.33	1.17	1.50
Single with dep children		1.66	0.88	3.12	*	3.23	1.01	10.38
Single no dep children	**	0.82	0.74	0.91		0.90	0.77	1.06
Smoker	**	0.86	0.82	0.90	*	0.94	0.88	1.00
Rural ED		0.93	0.86	1.02		0.91	0.82	1.01
Ages 65 and over								
Ethnic group								
Black		1.04	0.43	2.50		1.09	0.42	2.82
Indian sub-continent		0.74	0.43	1.27	*	0.53	0.32	0.87
Other		0.58	0.27	1.25	**	0.34	0.18	0.65
Housing tenure								
Renting-LA		1.04	0.94	1.15		1.01	0.93	1.10
Other rented	*	1.18	1.01	1.38		1.11	0.97	1.26
Communal estabs		0.94	0.60	1.48		0.74	0.47	1.16
Social class								
IIIN		0.98	0.85	1.12		1.08	0.97	1.21
IIIM		0.99	0.89	1.10		0.99	0.89	1.10
IV & V	**	0.82	0.73	0.91		1.02	0.92	1.13
Other		0.82	0.65	1.02	**	0.71	0.63	0.80
In practice<1 year	**	1.79	1.54	2.08	**	1.78	1.56	2.03
Living conditions								
Single sharing with adult	**	0.52	0.42	0.65	**	0.70	0.56	0.87
Sep/Wid/Div sharing with adult		0.91	0.76	1.08		0.90	0.81	1.01
Single, lives alone	*	0.79	0.64	0.98	**	0.75	0.64	0.88
Sep/wid/div, lives alone		0.91	0.81	1.02	*	1.10	1.01	1.20
Not known		0.83	0.50	1.36		1.44	0.91	2.27
Smoker	**	0.70	0.65	0.76	**	0.82	0.75	0.90
Rural ED		1.01	0.87	1.18	*	0.86	0.75	0.99

Notes: 1   Regressions also included age, distance from practice, limiting long-term illness rate for ED of residence.

2   Reference group is: white owner occupiers in social classes I& II, working full-time or part-time, in the study for the full year, and in an urban enumeration district. For adults the reference group members were also non-smokers who were married or cohabiting. For age group 16-64 they also had dependent children.

3   All comparisons are made within the age sex group.

Table 5M Patients consulting for illness: Odds ratios compared with reference group, for which ratio =1 (see footnote)

Ages 0-15

	Males Signif-icance	Males Odds ratio	Males 95% CI lower bd	Males 95% CI Upper bd	Females Signif-icance	Females Odds ratio	Females 95% CI Lower bd	Females 95% CI Upper bd
Ethnic group								
Black		0.82	0.64	1.06		0.85	0.66	1.10
Indian sub-continent	**	1.34	1.10	1.64	**	1.49	1.20	1.85
Other		0.92	0.75	1.12	*	0.80	0.65	0.98
Housing tenure								
Renting-LA		0.97	0.90	1.03	*	1.09	1.02	1.17
Other rented		0.95	0.87	1.04	**	1.15	1.05	1.27
Communal estabs		0.96	0.75	1.24		1.39	0.97	1.99
Social class								
IIIN		1.02	0.94	1.10	**	1.13	1.04	1.23
IIIM	**	1.08	1.02	1.15	**	1.15	1.08	1.22
IV & V	*	1.09	1.02	1.17	**	1.10	1.02	1.19
Other		0.93	0.81	1.05		0.95	0.83	1.08
Economic position								
Waiting/seeking		0.99	0.91	1.08		1.00	0.92	1.09
Student		0.98	0.75	1.29		0.95	0.72	1.25
Perm sick	*	1.23	1.03	1.46	*	1.20	1.01	1.44
Other		1.03	0.93	1.15		1.01	0.90	1.13
In practice <1 year	**	0.76	0.71	0.83	**	0.79	0.74	0.86
Single adult in hhold		1.02	0.94	1.11	*	1.12	1.02	1.22
Rural enumeration district		1.03	0.94	1.13		1.03	0.93	1.13

Ages 16-44

	Males Signif-icance	Males Odds ratio	Males 95% CI lower bd	Males 95% CI Upper bd	Females Signif-icance	Females Odds ratio	Females 95% CI Lower bd	Females 95% CI Upper bd
Ethnic group								
Black		0.86	0.72	1.03	*	1.27	1.04	1.56
Indian sub-continent		1.09	0.94	1.25		1.10	0.94	1.30
Other		0.85	0.73	1.00		0.90	0.76	1.07
Housing tenure								
Renting-LA	**	1.11	1.05	1.16	**	1.27	1.20	1.35
Other rented	**	1.12	1.07	1.18	**	1.09	1.03	1.15
Communal estabs	**	0.53	0.46	0.61	**	0.46	0.40	0.54
Social class								
IIIN	**	1.10	1.04	1.16		1.05	1.00	1.11
IIIM	**	1.11	1.07	1.16	*	1.06	1.01	1.11
IV & V	**	1.13	1.08	1.18		1.04	0.99	1.10
Other	**	0.65	0.59	0.71	**	0.80	0.73	0.87
Economic position								
Waiting/seeking	**	1.09	1.03	1.15	*	1.10	1.00	1.20
Student	**	1.31	1.18	1.45	*	0.91	0.82	1.20
Perm sick	**	4.85	4.19	5.61	**	2.94	2.43	3.56
Other		1.21	0.95	1.54		0.97	0.92	1.01
In practice<1 year	**	1.49	1.41	1.57	*	1.06	1.00	1.11
Family type								
Married/cohab no dependent children	**	0.91	0.87	0.95	*	0.95	0.90	1.00
Wid/sep/div with dep children	**	1.40	1.16	1.71	**	1.37	1.25	1.51
Wid/sep/div with no dep children	**	1.44	1.30	1.59	**	1.19	1.06	1.34
Single with dep children	**	0.75	0.69	0.81	**	0.77	0.71	0.84
Single no dep children	**	0.78	0.75	0.82	**	0.65	0.61	0.69
Smoker		1.03	1.00	1.06	**	1.24	1.20	1.30
Rural ED	**	0.91	0.85	0.96		0.95	0.89	1.02

Ages 45-64

	Males Signif-icance	Males Odds ratio	Males 95% CI lower bd	Males 95% CI Upper bd	Females Signif-icance	Females Odds ratio	Females 95% CI Lower bd	Females 95% CI Upper bd
Ethnic group								
Black		1.11	0.79	1.58		1.07	0.71	1.60
Indian sub-continent		0.95	0.75	1.20	*	1.54	1.08	2.20
Other		0.75	0.53	1.05		0.73	0.49	1.10
Housing tenure								
Renting-LA		1.07	0.99	1.15		1.07	0.99	1.17
Other rented	*	1.12	1.02	1.23		1.07	0.95	1.19
Communal estabs	**	0.53	0.37	0.76		0.70	0.47	1.02
Social class								
IIIN		1.08	1.00	1.17		1.01	0.93	1.10
IIIM		1.05	1.00	1.11	**	1.16	1.08	1.23
IV & V	**	1.12	1.05	1.20	**	1.13	1.05	1.22
Other	**	0.54	0.43	0.67		0.92	0.79	1.08
Economic position								
Waiting/seeking	**	1.23	1.13	1.35	**	1.39	1.14	1.70
Student		2.07	0.89	4.84		0.71	0.41	1.24
Perm sick	**	6.81	5.95	7.79	**	4.15	3.41	5.04
Other	**	1.41	1.29	1.53	**	0.88	0.83	0.93
In practice<1 year	**	1.62	1.45	1.81	**	1.50	1.33	1.69
Family type								
Married/cohab no dependent children		1.03	0.97	1.09	*	1.10	1.01	1.20
Wid/sep/div with dep children		1.22	0.91	1.63	**	1.38	1.12	1.70
Wid/sep/div with no dep children	**	1.22	1.10	1.35	**	1.34	1.20	1.50
Single with dep children		1.45	0.80	2.60		1.67	0.75	3.73
Single no dep children	**	0.83	0.75	0.92		0.92	0.79	1.06
Smoker	**	0.89	0.85	0.93		0.99	0.93	1.05
Rural ED		0.96	0.88	1.04	*	0.89	0.81	0.98

Ages 65 and over

	Males Signif-icance	Males Odds ratio	Males 95% CI lower bd	Males 95% CI Upper bd	Females Signif-icance	Females Odds ratio	Females 95% CI Lower bd	Females 95% CI Upper bd
Ethnic group								
Black		0.81	0.39	1.72		1.31	0.55	3.15
Indian sub-continent		0.69	0.42	1.13		0.74	0.45	1.21
Other		0.61	0.30	1.25	**	0.33	0.18	0.61
Housing tenure								
Renting-LA		1.08	0.98	1.18		1.07	0.99	1.15
Other rented		1.11	0.97	1.27	*	1.13	1.01	1.27
Communal estabs		0.96	0.65	1.42		0.84	0.56	1.26
Social class								
IIIN		0.96	0.85	1.09		1.08	0.98	1.19
IIIM		1.04	0.95	1.13		1.02	0.93	1.12
IV & V	**	0.85	0.77	0.94		1.04	0.95	1.14
Other		0.94	0.77	1.14	**	0.77	0.70	0.86
In practice<1 year	**	1.92	1.67	2.20	**	1.85	1.65	2.08
Living conditions								
Single sharing with adult	**	0.61	0.49	0.75	**	0.72	0.59	0.88
Sep/Wid/Div sharing with adult		1.00	0.85	1.17		0.97	0.87	1.07
Single, lives alone		0.84	0.69	1.01	**	0.78	0.68	0.90
Sep/wid/div, lives alone		0.97	0.87	1.07	**	1.14	1.06	1.24
Not known		0.87	0.57	1.35		1.22	0.81	1.85
Smoker	**	0.75	0.70	0.81	**	0.88	0.81	0.95
Rural ED		0.97	0.84	1.11		0.87	0.77	0.99

Notes:
1 Regressions also included age, distance from practice, limiting long-term illness rate for ED of residence.
2 Reference group is: white owner occupiers in social classes I& II, working full-time or part-time, in the study for the full year, and in an urban enumeration district. For adults the reference group members were also non-smokers who were married or cohabiting. For age group 16-64 they also had dependent children.
3 All comparisons are made within the age sex group.

Table 5N Consulting for serious illness: ratios compared with reference group, for which ratio =1 (see footnote)

Ages 0-15 and Ages 16-44

	Males Signif-icance	Males Odds ratio	Males 95% CI lower bd	Males 95% CI Upper bd	Females Signif-icance	Females Odds ratio	Females 95% CI Lower bd	Females 95% CI Upper bd
Ages 0-15								
Ethnic group								
Black		1.29	0.96	1.73		1.33	0.97	1.84
Indian sub-continent	*	1.32	1.03	1.71		0.97	0.71	1.33
Other		1.12	0.87	1.43		0.99	0.73	1.34
Housing tenure								
Renting-LA		1.08	0.99	1.17	*	1.11	1.00	1.22
Other rented		0.99	0.88	1.11		1.04	0.91	1.18
Communal estabs		1.26	0.85	1.87		1.26	0.73	2.20
Social class								
IIIN		1.01	0.92	1.12		1.05	0.94	1.18
IIIM	**	1.11	1.03	1.20		1.08	0.98	1.18
IV & V		1.08	0.99	1.19		1.06	0.96	1.18
Other		0.99	0.84	1.18	*	0.79	0.65	0.97
Economic position								
Waiting/seeking		0.93	0.84	1.04		0.93	0.83	1.06
Student		0.94	0.66	1,33		0.85	0.55	1.31
Perm sick		0.98	0.79	1.22	*	1.26	1.00	1.58
Other		1.05	0.92	1.20	**	0.99	0.85	1.15
In practice <1 year	**	1.33	1.20	1.47	**	1.21	1.07	1.37
Single adult in hhold		1.03	0.92	1.15		1.09	0.96	1.23
Rural enumeration district		0.89	0.76	1.01		0.98	0.85	1.13
Ages 16-44								
Ethnic group								
Black		1.24	0.95	1.61		1.10	0.88	1.38
Indian sub-continent	**	1.49	1.21	1.82	**	1.51	1.25	1.81
Other		0.85	0.65	1.10	*	0.73	0.58	0.94
Housing tenure								
Renting-LA	**	1.26	1.18	1.35	**	1.35	1.27	1.44
Other rented	**	1.16	1.07	1.25	**	1.16	1.08	1.24
Communal estabs		0.85	0.68	1.05		0.88	0.71	1.09
Social class								
IIIN	*	1.09	1.00	1.19		0.99	0.92	1.05
IIIM	**	1.13	1.06	1.20		1.09	1.03	1.16
IV & V	**	1.20	1.12	1.29	**	1.10	1.03	1.17
Other	**	0.79	0.69	0.91		0.94	0.85	1.03
Economic position								
Waiting/seeking	**	1.44	1.34	1.55	**	1.33	1.20	1.46
Student		1.12	0.96	1.31		0.97	0.86	1.11
Perm sick	**	7.50	6.70	8.40	**	4.99	4.40	5.66
Other	**	1.35	0.99	1.83	**	1.14	1.09	1.21
In practice<1 year	**	1.74	1.61	1.89	**	1.41	1.31	1.51
Family type								
Married/cohab no dependent children	**	1.11	1.04	1.18	**	1.16	1.09	1.22
Wid/sep/div with dep children		1.12	0.88	1.42	**	1.17	1.07	1.27
Wid/sep/div with no dep children	**	1.27	1.13	1.44		1.11	0.98	1.25
Single with dep children		1.07	0.95	1.20		0.98	0.89	1.08
Single no dep children		1.03	0.97	1.11	**	0.90	0.83	0.97
Smoker		1.04	0.99	1.09	**	1.17	1.12	1.22
Rural ED	**	0.84	0.77	0.93		0.96	0.88	1.05

Ages 45-64 and Ages 65 and over

	Males Signif-icance	Males Odds ratio	Males 95% CI lower bd	Males 95% CI Upper bd	Females Signif-icance	Females Odds ratio	Females 95% CI Lower bd	Females 95% CI Upper bd
Ages 45-64								
Ethnic group								
Black		1.04	0.74	1.46		1.08	0.78	1.50
Indian sub-continent	*	1.36	1.07	1.73	**	2.07	1.58	2.71
Other		1.02	0.70	1.50		1.33	0.92	1.92
Housing tenure								
Renting-LA	**	1.20	1.12	1.29	**	1.20	1.13	1.29
Other rented	**	1.21	1.10	1.33	**	1.17	1.07	1.29
Communal estabs	**	0.49	0.33	0.73		1.25	0.88	1.77
Social class								
IIIN	*	1.11	1.01	1.21	*	1.08	1.01	1.17
IIIM	**	1.14	1.07	1.21	**	1.23	1.16	1.31
IV & V	**	1.29	1.20	1.39	**	1.22	1.14	1.31
Other	**	0.70	0.57	0.86		1.07	0.94	1.22
Economic position								
Waiting/seeking	**	1.39	1.27	1.52		1.16	0.99	1.36
Student		1.71	0.70	4.16		1.24	0.70	2.21
Perm sick		6.92	6.35	7.54	**	4.80	4.31	5.34
Other	**	1.66	1.54	1.80	**	1.21	1.15	1.27
In practice<1 year	**	2.12	1.88	2.39	**	1.89	1.68	2.12
Family type								
Married/cohab no dependent children	*	1.08	1.00	1.16		1.09	1.00	1.19
Wid/sep/div with dep children		1.24	0.93	1.66	**	1.27	1.06	1.51
Wid/sep/div with no dep children	**	1.19	1.07	1.33	**	1.23	1.11	1.36
Single with dep children		1.69	0.96	2.98		1.42	0.80	2.53
Single no dep children	*	0.87	0.78	0.98	*	1.09	0.95	1.25
Smoker	**	0.88	0.83	0.92	*	1.05	1.00	1.11
Rural ED		0.93	0.85	1.03		0.93	0.85	1.01
Ages 65 and over								
Ethnic group								
Black		1.04	0.57	1.91		0.57	0.29	1.10
Indian sub-continent		1.26	0.81	1.97		1.07	0.69	1.66
Other		0.60	0.31	1.18		0.62	0.34	1.12
Housing tenure								
Renting-LA	**	1.16	1.08	1.24	**	1.18	1.12	1.25
Other rented	**	1.24	1.12	1.37	*	1.09	1.00	1.18
Communal estabs		1.00	0.74	1.37	*	1.46	1.05	2.03
Social class								
IIIN		1.03	0.94	1.13		1.07	0.99	1.15
IIIM	**	1.14	1.06	1.22		1.04	0.97	1.12
IV & V		1.00	0.92	1.08	*	1.08	1.01	1.16
Other		1.03	0.88	1.22		0.93	0.86	1.01
In practice<1 year	**	2.76	2.47	3.08	**	2.61	2.38	2.86
Living conditions								
Single sharing with adult	*	0.79	0.66	0.95	**	0.80	0.68	0.94
Sep/Wid/Div sharing with adult		1.05	0.93	1.19	*	1.08	1.00	1.17
Single, lives alone		0.88	0.75	1.02	**	0.86	0.76	0.96
Sep/wid/div, lives alone		0.96	0.88	1.04	*	1.07	1.01	1.14
Not known		1.08	0.77	1.52		0.85	0.61	1.19
Smoker	**	0.86	0.81	0.92		0.99	0.93	1.06
Rural ED		0.98	0.88	1.09		0.93	0.85	1.03

Notes: 1 Regressions also included age, distance from practice, limiting long-term illness rate for ED of residence.

2 Reference group is: white owner occupiers in social classes I & II, working full-time or part-time, in the study for the full year, and in an urban enumeration district. For adults the reference group members were also non-smokers who were married or cohabiting. For age group 16-64 they also had dependent children.

3 All comparisons are made within the age sex group.

Table 5O Patients consulting for serious or intermediate illness: Odds ratios compared with reference group, for which ratio =1 (see footnote)

Ages 0-15

	Males Signif-icance	Odds ratio	95% CI lower bd	Upper bd	Females Signif-icance	Odds ratio	95% CI Lower bd	Upper bd
Ethnic group								
Black	*	0.79	0.63	0.98	*	0.76	0.61	0.95
Indian sub-continent	*	1.25	1.05	1.49		1.09	0.91	1.30
Other		0.99	0.83	1.18		0.88	0.73	1.05
Housing tenure								
Renting-LA		0.99	0.93	1.05	**	1.13	1.06	1.20
Other rented		0.96	0.89	1.04		1.05	0.97	1.13
Communal estabs		1.04	0.81	1.32		1.02	0.74	1.41
Social class								
IIIN		1.01	0.94	1.08	**	1.13	1.05	1.21
IIIM	**	1.08	1.02	1.14	**	1.09	1.03	1.15
IV & V	*	1.08	1.01	1.14	**	1.11	1.04	1.18
Other	*	0.88	0.79	0.99		0.99	0.89	1.12
Economic position								
Waiting/seeking		0.99	0.92	1.07		0.95	0.88	1.03
Student		1.07	0.84	1.37		0.84	0.66	1.06
Perm sick	*	1.21	1.04	1.41	*	1.19	1.02	1.39
Other		1.04	0.95	1.14		0.94	0.86	1.04
In practice <1 year	**	0.85	0.79	0.91	**	0.89	0.83	0.95
Single adult in hhold		1.03	0.96	1.11	*	1.10	1.02	1.19
Rural enumeration district		1.06	0.98	1.16		1.01	0.93	1.10

Ages 16-44

	Males Signif-icance	Odds ratio	95% CI lower bd	Upper bd	Females Signif-icance	Odds ratio	95% CI Lower bd	Upper bd
Ethnic group								
Black		0.89	0.74	1.06	*	1.21	1.02	1.44
Indian sub-continent		1.12	0.98	1.29	**	1.24	1.07	1.43
Other	*	0.85	0.72	0.99	**	0.79	0.68	0.92
Housing tenure								
Renting-LA	**	1.11	1.06	1.17	**	1.26	1.22	1.35
Other rented	**	1.13	1.08	1.19	**	1.12	1.07	1.18
Communal estabs	**	0.59	0.51	0.68	**	0.52	0.45	0.60
Social class								
IIIN	**	1.10	1.04	1.16		1.03	0.98	1.08
IIIM	**	1.13	1.09	1.18		1.03	0.99	1.08
IV & V	**	1.17	1.12	1.23	*	1.05	1.01	1.11
Other	**	0.71	0.64	0.78	**	0.80	0.74	0.86
Economic position								
Waiting/seeking	**	1.18	1.12	1.24	**	1.19	1.10	1.29
Student	**	1.27	1.15	1.41		0.92	0.84	1.00
Perm sick	**	6.03	5.29	6.87	**	3.22	2.74	3.78
Other		1.20	0.96	1.49	**	1.07	1.02	1.11
In practice<1 year	**	1.51	1.43	1.59	**	1.13	1.08	1.18
Family type								
Married/cohab no dependent children	*	0.95	0.91	0.99	*	0.96	0.92	1.00
Wid/sep/div with dep children	*	1.21	1.01	1.44	**	1.26	1.16	1.36
Wid/sep/div with no dep children	**	1.40	1.28	1.53	**	1.19	1.08	1.32
Single with dep children	**	0.79	0.74	0.86	**	0.78	0.72	0.83
Single no dep children	**	0.85	0.81	0.89	**	0.68	0.65	0.72
Smoker	**	1.07	1.03	1.10	**	1.21	1.17	1.25
Rural ED	**	0.92	0.87	0.98		0.96	0.90	1.01

Ages 45-64

	Males Signif-icance	Odds ratio	95% CI lower bd	Upper bd	Females Signif-icance	Odds ratio	95% CI Lower bd	Upper bd
Ethnic group								
Black		1.15	0.83	1.59		1.26	0.89	1.80
Indian sub-continent		1.16	0.92	1.45	**	-1.75	1.29	2.37
Other		0.86	0.62	1.20		0.88	0.60	1.27
Housing tenure								
Renting-LA	**	1.13	1.05	1.21	**	1.14	1.06	1.22
Other rented		1.07	0.98	1.17		1.04	0.95	1.15
Communal estabs	**	0.59	0.42	0.84		0.72	0.51	1.03
Social class								
IIIN		1.06	0.98	1.15		1.03	0.96	1.11
IIIM	*	1.06	1.01	1.12	**	1.17	1.11	1.24
IV & V	**	1.11	1.04	1.18	**	1.12	1.05	1.20
Other	**	0.59	0.47	0.72		0.95	0.83	1.08
Economic position								
Waiting/seeking	**	1.26	1.16	1.37	**	1.46	1.23	1.72
Student		1.11	0.52	2.39		0.84	0.51	1.40
Perm sick	**	7.08	6.29	7.97	**	4.67	3.95	5.52
Other	**	1.48	1.37	1.60		0.98	0.93	1.03
In practice<1 year	**	1.59	1.43	1.78	**	1.55	1.39	1.73
Family type								
Married/cohab no dependent children	*	1.06	1.00	1.13	*	1.09	1.01	1.17
Wid/sep/div with dep children		1.31	1.00	1.72	**	1.30	1.09	1.55
Wid/sep/div with no dep children	**	1.29	1.17	1.43	**	1.29	1.17	1.42
Single with dep children		1.36	0.80	2.33		1.13	0.61	2.08
Single no dep children	*	0.88	0.80	0.97		0.91	0.80	1.03
Smoker	**	0.88	0.85	0.92		1.02	0.97	1.07
Rural ED		1.00	0.92	1.08	*	0.91	0.84	0.98

Ages 65 and over

	Males Signif-icance	Odds ratio	95% CI lower bd	Upper bd	Females Signif-icance	Odds ratio	95% CI Lower bd	Upper bd
Ethnic group								
Black		0.92	0.46	1.84		1.08	0.52	2.24
Indian sub-continent		0.86	0.54	1.37		0.74	0.47	1.16
Other		0.72	0.36	1.43	**	0.41	0.23	0.73
Housing tenure								
Renting-LA		1.08	1.00	1.17	**	1.12	1.04	1.19
Other rented		1.12	0.99	1.26	*	1.13	1.03	1.25
Communal estabs		0.92	0.65	1.30		0.90	0.63	1.31
Social class								
IIIN		0.94	0.84	1.05		1.04	0.96	1.14
IIIM		1.04	0.96	1.13		1.05	0.97	1.14
IV & V	**	0.87	0.79	0.95		1.03	0.95	1.12
Other		0.90	0.75	1.08	**	0.81	0.73	0.88
In practice<1 year	**	2.02	1.78	2.29	**	1.89	1.70	2.10
Living conditions								
Single sharing with adult	**	0.65	0.53	0.79	**	0.71	0.60	0.85
Sep/Wid/Div sharing with adult		1.01	0.88	1.17		1.07	0.97	1.17
Single, lives alone		0.94	0.79	1.12	**	0.84	0.74	0.96
Sep/wid/div, lives alone		0.97	0.88	1.06	**	1.12	1.05	1.20
Not known		1.02	0.69	1.51		1.25	0.86	1.83
Smoker	**	0.77	0.72	0.82	**	0.91	0.84	0.98
Rural ED		0.91	0.80	1.03	**	0.86	0.77	0.96

Notes: 1 Regressions also included age, distance from practice, limiting long-term illness rate for ED of residence.
2 Reference group is: white owner occupiers in social classes I& II, working full-time or part-time, in the study for the full year, and in an urban enumeration district. For adults the reference group members were also non-smokers who were married or cohabiting. For age group 16-64 they also had dependent children.
3 All comparisons are made within the age sex group.

Table 5P Patients consulting for mental disorders: Odds ratios compared with reference group, for which ratio =1 (see footnote)

Ages 0-15

	Males Signif-icance	Males Odds ratio	Males 95% CI lower bd	Males Upper bd	Females Signif-icance	Females Odds ratio	Females 95% CI Lower bd	Females Upper bd
Ethnic group								
Black		0.67	0.29	1.52	*	0.23	0.06	0.91
Indian sub-continent		1.25	0.67	2.34		0.71	0.33	1.55
Other		0.98	0.56	1.73		0.72	0.37	1.41
Housing tenure								
Renting-LA		1.15	0.96	1.38	**	1.30	1.07	1.59
Other rented		1.20	0.94	1.54		1.20	0.92	1.57
Communal estabs		1.48	0.66	3.32		1.29	0.45	3.70
Social class								
IIIN		1.11	0.88	1.40		1.06	0.83	1.37
IIIM	*	1.21	1.02	1.44		1.09	0.90	1.32
IV & V	*	1.24	1.02	1.52		1.14	0.92	1.42
Other		0.92	0.64	1.31		1.17	0.81	1.69
Economic position								
Waiting/seeking		1.12	0.89	1.40		1.13	0.89	1.44
Student		1.16	0.56	2.41		1.90	0.99	3.64
Perm sick	*	1.62	1.09	2.41		1.02	0.63	1.66
Other		1.08	0.82	1.42		1.01	0.74	1.38
In practice <1 year		0.98	0.77	1.26	**	1.46	1.14	1.86
Single adult in hhold	*	1.32	1.05	1.66		0.98	0.76	1.28
Rural enumeration district		0.98	0.73	1.31	*	0.70	0.50	0.99

Ages 16-44

	Males Signif-icance	Males Odds ratio	Males 95% CI lower bd	Males Upper bd	Females Signif-icance	Females Odds ratio	Females 95% CI Lower bd	Females Upper bd
Ethnic group								
Black		0.81	0.55	1.20		0.78	0.59	1.02
Indian sub-continent		0.89	0.62	1.27		1.09	0.84	1.40
Other		0.89	0.63	1.24		0.78	0.60	1.01
Housing tenure								
Renting-LA	**	1.27	1.16	1.39	**	1.36	1.28	1.45
Other rented	**	1.44	1.30	1.59	**	1.22	1.13	1.31
Communal estabs	**	2.25	1.74	2.91		0.93	0.72	1.20
Social class								
IIIN	**	1.30	1.15	1.46		1.06	0.98	1.14
IIIM		0.99	0.90	1.09	**	1.16	1.09	1.24
IV & V		1.10	0.99	1.22	**	1.21	1.12	1.29
Other		0.90	0.76	1.07		1.05	0.94	1.17
Economic position								
Waiting/seeking	**	2.00	1.83	2.19	**	1.36	1.22	1.51
Student	*	1.24	1.00	1.52		0.97	0.84	1.12
Perm sick	**	6.48	5.68	7.38	**	4.02	3.52	4.60
Other	**	1.88	1.32	2.70	**	1.17	1.10	1.24
In practice<1 year	**	1.85	1.67	2.06	**	1.34	1.24	1.45
Family type								
Married/cohab no dependent children		1.07	0.97	1.19		0.99	0.93	1.06
Wid/sep/div with dep children	**	2.37	1.84	3.06	**	1.47	1.34	1.61
Wid/sep/div with no dep children	**	2.29	1.99	2.63	**	1.75	1.55	1.97
Single with dep children		1.15	0.96	1.37		1.02	0.92	1.13
Single no dep children	**	1.51	1.38	1.66		0.97	0.90	1.06
Smoker	**	1.51	1.41	1.62	**	1.47	1.40	1.54
Rural ED	**	0.78	0.67	0.91	*	0.90	0.81	0.99

Ages 45-64

	Males Signif-icance	Males Odds ratio	Males 95% CI lower bd	Males Upper bd	Females Signif-icance	Females Odds ratio	Females 95% CI Lower bd	Females Upper bd
Ethnic group								
Black		0.67	0.35	1.27		1.14	0.75	1.73
Indian sub-continent		1.07	0.70	1.63		1.01	0.66	1.56
Other		0.66	0.33	1.30		0.91	0.55	1.51
Housing tenure								
Renting-LA	**	1.18	1.06	1.32	**	1.22	1.12	1.33
Other rented	**	1.24	1.07	1.43	**	1.20	1.06	1.35
Communal estabs	**	2.70	1.77	4.13	*	1.60	1.05	2.45
Social class								
IIIN		1.04	0.90	1.21		1.07	0.96	1.18
IIIM	**	0.88	0.79	0.97	**	1.14	1.05	1.24
IV & V		1.00	0.89	1.12	**	1.19	1.09	1.30
Other		0.84	0.64	1.10	**	1.26	1.07	1.49
Economic position								
Waiting/seeking	**	1.69	1.47	1.93	**	1.45	1.20	1.75
Student		1.04	0.24	4.46		1.11	0.54	2.28
Perm sick	**	3.84	3.43	4.30	**	2.68	2.38	3.02
Other	**	1.58	1.38	1.81	**	1.26	1.17	1.36
In practice<1 year	**	1.51	1.25	1.82	**	1.73	1.48	2.02
Family type								
Married/cohab no dependent children		1.04	0.93	1.17		1.06	0.95	1.19
Wid/sep/div with dep children	**	1.73	1.18	2.54		1.24	1.00	1.55
Wid/sep/div with no dep children	**	1.84	1.58	2.15	**	1.70	1.49	1.93
Single with dep children		1.23	0.52	2.92		0.39	0.14	1.10
Single no dep children	**	1.46	1.24	1.72	*	1.25	1.04	1.50
Smoker	**	1.32	1.22	1.43	**	1.41	1.32	1.50
Rural ED	*	0.82	0.70	0.97		0.89	0.79	1.01

Ages 65 and over

	Males Signif-icance	Males Odds ratio	Males 95% CI lower bd	Males Upper bd	Females Signif-icance	Females Odds ratio	Females 95% CI Lower bd	Females Upper bd
Ethnic group								
Black	*	2.41	1.00	5.78		1.58	0.69	3.61
Indian sub-continent		0.88	0.31	2.48		1.05	0.52	2.15
Other		0.02	0.00	2.95		0.70	0.25	1.98
Housing tenure								
Renting-LA	**	1.19	1.05	1.36	**	1.18	1.08	1.28
Other rented		1.14	0.94	1.38	*	1.13	1.00	1.28
Communal estabs	**	2.92	1.94	4.40	**	2.07	1.36	3.14
Social class								
IIIN		0.98	0.82	1.17	*	1.11	1.00	1.24
IIIM		0.92	0.81	1.05		1.06	0.96	1.18
IV & V	**	0.81	0.69	0.94		1.09	0.98	1.20
Other		1.00	0.74	1.33		1.11	0.99	1.25
In practice<1 year	**	2.45	2.06	2.91	**	1.90	1.68	2.15
Living conditions								
Single sharing with adult	**	0.93	0.63	1.36		0.97	0.75	1.24
Sep/Wid/Div sharing with adult	**	1.44	1.16	1.77		0.97	0.86	1.08
Single, lives alone		1.13	0.84	1.51		1.08	0.90	1.28
Sep/wid/div, lives alone	**	1.37	1.19	1.58	**	1.19	1.09	1.29
Not known		1.03	0.66	1.60		1.17	0.77	1.78
Smoker	**	1.21	1.08	1.35	**	1.25	1.14	1.37
Rural ED		0.90	0.72	1.12		0.96	0.82	1.11

Notes:
1 Regressions also included age, distance from practice, limiting long-term illness rate for ED of residence.
2 Reference group is: white owner occupiers in social classes I& II, working full-time or part-time, in the study for the full year, and in an urban enumeration district. For adults the reference group members were also non-smokers who were married or cohabiting. For age group 16-64 they also had dependent children.
3 All comparisons are made within the age sex group.

Table 5Q Patients consulting for Circulatory diseases: Odds ratios compared with reference group, for which ratio =1 (see footnote)

Ages 0-15 and Ages 16-44

	Males Signif-icance	Males Odds ratio	Males 95% CI lower bd	Males 95% CI Upper bd	Females Signif-icance	Females Odds ratio	Females 95% CI Lower bd	Females 95% CI Upper bd
Ages 0-15								
Ethnic group								
Black								
Indian sub-continent								
Other								
Housing tenure								
Renting-LA								
Other rented				NO CONVERGENCE				
Communal estabs				No model could be fitted for these ages				
Social class				Insufficient patients consulting?				
IIIN								
IIIM								
IV & V								
Other								
Economic position								
Waiting/seeking								
Student								
Perm sick								
Other								
In practice <1 year								
Single adult in hhold								
Rural enumeration district								
Ages 16-44								
Ethnic group								
Black		0.91	0.53	1.56		1.14	0.78	1.66
Indian sub-continent		1.15	0.79	1.67		0.78	0.55	1.10
Other		0.93	0.57	1.52		0.98	0.67	1.44
Housing tenure								
Renting-LA	*	1.15	1.00	1.31		1.07	0.96	1.19
Other rented		1.05	0.90	1.23		1.08	0.95	1.22
Communal estabs		0.73	0.45	1.20		0.67	0.42	1.07
Social class								
IIIN	**	1.22	1.05	1.42		1.03	0.92	1.16
IIIM		1.07	0.95	1.20		1.07	0.97	1.17
IV & V		1.08	0.95	1.24		1.04	0.93	1.16
Other		0.83	0.62	1.12		0.95	0.79	1.14
Economic position								
Waiting/seeking		1.10	0.94	1.28		1.14	0.94	1.38
Student		1.34	0.94	1.89		0.89	0.68	1.15
Perm sick	**	2.98	2.44	3.64	**	1.90	1.50	2.40
Other		1.47	0.89	2.44	**	1.33	1.22	1.45
In practice<1 year	**	1.56	1.32	1.84	**	1.23	1.08	1.41
Family type								
Married/cohab no dependent children		1.09	0.97	1.22		0.99	0.90	1.09
Wid/sep/div with dep children		1.24	0.84	1.85		1.06	0.92	1.24
Wid/sep/div with no dep children		1.04	0.83	1.30		0.95	0.77	1.17
Single with dep children		0.87	0.64	1.18		0.98	0.83	1.17
Single no dep children		1.03	0.90	1.17	**	0.74	0.64	0.85
Smoker	**	0.86	0.78	0.94		0.93	0.86	1.01
Rural ED		1.04	0.87	1.24		0.91	0.78	1.06

Ages 45-64 and Ages 65 and over

	Males Signif-icance	Males Odds ratio	Males 95% CI lower bd	Males 95% CI Upper bd	Females Signif-icance	Females Odds ratio	Females 95% CI Lower bd	Females 95% CI Upper bd
Ages 45-64								
Ethnic group								
Black		1.31	0.90	1.90	*	1.58	1.09	2.28
Indian sub-continent		1.14	0.87	1.50		-0.75	0.51	1.10
Other		1.17	0.76	1.80		1.20	0.77	1.88
Housing tenure								
Renting-LA	*	1.09	1.00	1.19	**	1.24	1.14	1.34
Other rented		1.08	0.96	1.21		1.07	0.95	1.21
Communal estabs	**	0.42	0.24	0.75		1.03	0.64	1.64
Social class								
IIIN		1.04	0.94	1.16	*	1.12	1.01	1.23
IIIM		1.02	0.95	1.09	**	1.28	1.18	1.38
IV & V	**	1.12	1.03	1.21	**	1.24	1.14	1.35
Other	**	0.64	0.51	0.81		1.10	0.94	1.29
Economic position								
Waiting/seeking		1.10	0.98	1.23	**	1.34	1.09	1.64
Student		0.70	0.16	3.03	*	0.16	0.03	0.83
Perm sick	**	3.22	2.94	3.51	**	2.23	1.98	2.52
Other	**	1.51	1.39	1.65	**	1.26	1.18	1.34
In practice<1 year	**	1.61	1.39	1.86	**	1.65	1.42	1.92
Family type								
Married/cohab no dependent children	**	1.18	1.08	1.29	**	1.23	1.09	1.39
Wid/sep/div with dep children		1.19	0.84	1.69	*	1.35	1.07	1.70
Wid/sep/div with no dep children	**	1.26	1.11	1.44	**	1.23	1.07	1.41
Single with dep children		1.18	0.58	2.39		1.44	0.70	2.96
Single no dep children		1.09	0.95	1.25		1.18	0.99	1.42
Smoker	**	0.75	0.71	0.80	**	0.75	0.70	0.80
Rural ED		0.91	0.81	1.01		1.02	0.91	1.14
Ages 65 and over								
Ethnic group								
Black		0.90	0.47	1.73		1.36	0.71	2.61
Indian sub-continent		0.90	0.56	1.46		0.80	0.50	1.29
Other		0.95	0.46	1.94		0.49	0.23	1.03
Housing tenure								
Renting-LA		1.02	0.95	1.10		1.04	0.98	1.10
Other rented		1.10	0.99	1.22		1.05	0.96	1.14
Communal estabs	**	0.53	0.37	0.75		0.76	0.53	1.09
Social class								
IIIN		0.98	0.89	1.09	*	1.10	1.02	1.18
IIIM		1.04	0.97	1.12	*	1.08	1.00	1.16
IV & V		0.94	0.86	1.02		1.07	1.00	1.15
Other	*	0.81	0.68	0.97		0.94	0.86	1.02
In practice<1 year	**	2.19	1.95	2.45	**	2.08	1.89	2.28
Living conditions								
Single sharing with adult	**	0.73	0.59	0.89	*	0.82	0.69	0.97
Sep/Wid/Div sharing with adult		1.12	0.99	1.27		1.02	0.94	1.11
Single, lives alone		0.96	0.81	1.13		0.94	0.83	1.06
Sep/wid/div, lives alone		1.00	0.92	1.08		1.03	0.97	1.10
Not known		1.43	0.96	2.12		0.94	0.66	1.36
Smoker	**	0.73	0.68	0.78	**	0.77	0.72	0.82
Rural ED		0.94	0.84	1.06		1.00	0.90	1.10

Notes:
1. Regressions also included age, distance from practice, limiting long-term illness rate for ED of residence.
2. Reference group is: white owner occupiers in social classes I& II, working full-time or part-time, in the study for the full year, and in an urban enumeration district. For adults the reference group members were also non-smokers who were married or cohabiting. For age group 16-64 they also had dependent children.
3. All comparisons are made within the age sex group.

Table 5R Patients consulting for respiratory diseases: Odds ratios compared with reference group, for which ratio =1 (see footnote)

Ages 0-15

	Males Signif-icance	Males Odds ratio	Males 95% CI lower bd	Males 95% CI Upper bd	Females Signif-icance	Females Odds ratio	Females 95% CI Lower bd	Females 95% CI Upper bd
Ethnic group								
Black		1.14	0.91	1.42		1.06	0.85	1.32
Indian sub-continent	**	1.68	1.41	2.00	**	1.62	1.36	1.94
Other	*	1.25	1.05	1.49		1.00	0.83	1.20
Housing tenure								
Renting-LA	*	1.07	1.01	1.14	**	1.09	1.03	1.16
Other rented		1.01	0.93	1.09		1.03	0.95	1.12
Communal estabs		0.86	0.65	1.13	*	1.43	1.03	1.99
Social class								
IIIN		1.06	0.98	1.13		1.07	1.00	1.15
IIIM	*	1.07	1.01	1.12	**	1.09	1.04	1.15
IV & V	*	1.08	1.02	1.15	**	1.14	1.07	1.21
Other		0.95	0.85	1.07		0.96	0.86	1.07
Economic position								
Waiting/seeking		0.93	0.86	1.00		0.95	0.88	1.02
Student		0.80	0.63	1.03		0.99	0.78	1.26
Perm sick		1.16	1.00	1.34		1.06	0.91	1.23
Other	**	1.03	0.94	1.13	**	1.03	0.90	1.13
In practice <1 year	**	0.86	0.80	0.92	**	0.87	0.81	0.94
Single adult in hhold		0.93	0.86	1.01		1.06	0.98	1.14
Rural enumeration district		0.90	0.83	0.98		1.01	0.93	1.10

Ages 16-44

	Males Signif-icance	Males Odds ratio	Males 95% CI lower bd	Males 95% CI Upper bd	Females Signif-icance	Females Odds ratio	Females 95% CI Lower bd	Females 95% CI Upper bd
Ethnic group								
Black		1.14	0.93	1.39		0.88	0.75	1.04
Indian sub-continent	**	1.36	1.17	1.58		1.12	0.97	1.30
Other		1.01	0.84	1.21		1.06	0.91	1.24
Housing tenure								
Renting-LA	**	1.12	1.06	1.18	**	1.13	1.08	1.18
Other rented	**	1.11	1.04	1.17		1.04	0.99	1.10
Communal estabs	**	0.54	0.46	0.63	**	0.67	0.58	0.78
Social class								
IIIN		1.01	0.95	1.08		1.01	0.96	1.06
IIIM	**	0.92	0.87	0.96	*	1.05	1.00	1.09
IV & V	*	0.94	0.89	0.99		1.04	1.00	1.09
Other	**	0.71	0.63	0.79	**	0.88	0.82	0.95
Economic position								
Waiting/seeking	*	1.06	1.00	1.13	*	0.92	0.85	0.99
Student	**	1.28	1.14	1.43		1.00	0.91	1.09
Perm sick	**	1.60	1.43	1.79	**	1.27	1.12	1.44
Other		1.04	0.81	1.34	**	0.91	0.88	0.95
In practice<1 year	**	1.34	1.26	1.43	**	1.07	1.02	1.13
Family type								
Married/cohab no dependent children	**	0.84	0.80	0.88	**	0.85	0.81	0.88
Wid/sep/div with dep children		1.13	0.93	1.37	**	1.20	1.12	1.29
Wid/sep/div with no dep children		0.98	0.89	1.09	**	1.14	1.03	1.25
Single with dep children	**	0.77	0.71	0.84	**	0.93	0.87	1.00
Single no dep children	**	0.78	0.74	0.82	**	0.86	0.81	0.90
Smoker	**	0.90	0.87	0.94	**	1.08	1.04	1.11
Rural ED	*	0.93	0.87	1.00		0.98	0.93	1.04

Ages 45-64

	Males Signif-icance	Males Odds ratio	Males 95% CI lower bd	Males 95% CI Upper bd	Females Signif-icance	Females Odds ratio	Females 95% CI Lower bd	Females 95% CI Upper bd
Ethnic group								
Black		1.25	0.90	1.76		0.90	0.65	1.25
Indian sub-continent	**	1.72	1.37	2.17	**	1.84	1.42	2.40
Other		1.10	0.76	1.60		0.73	0.49	1.09
Housing tenure								
Renting-LA	**	1.20	1.11	1.29	**	1.26	1.18	1.35
Other rented		1.06	0.96	1.17		1.09	1.00	1.20
Communal estabs		0.79	0.53	1.19		0.72	0.49	1.06
Social class								
IIIN		1.07	0.98	1.17		1.03	0.96	1.11
IIIM		0.99	0.93	1.05	**	1.15	1.08	1.22
IV & V		1.00	0.93	1.07	**	1.12	1.05	1.19
Other	**	0.63	0.50	0.79		0.94	0.82	1.07
Economic position								
Waiting/seeking		0.99	0.90	1.09		0.88	0.75	1.02
Student		0.91	0.34	2.43		0.76	0.43	1.36
Perm sick	**	1.89	1.74	2.06	**	1.37	1.23	1.52
Other		1.07	0.98	1.17	**	0.87	0.83	0.92
In practice<1 year	**	1.42	1.24	1.61	*	1.17	1.03	1.33
Family type								
Married/cohab no dependent children	*	0.91	0.85	0.98		1.02	0.94	1.10
Wid/sep/div with dep children		1.08	0.81	1.44	**	1.30	1.11	1.54
Wid/sep/div with no dep children		1.05	0.94	1.16	**	1.25	1.14	1.38
Single with dep children		1.02	0.56	1.83		1.68	0.98	2.88
Single no dep children	**	0.74	0.65	0.83	*	0.84	0.73	0.97
Smoker	**	0.88	0.83	0.93	**	1.16	1.10	1.22
Rural ED		1.03	0.94	1.13		0.93	0.86	1.02

Ages 65 and over

	Males Signif-icance	Males Odds ratio	Males 95% CI lower bd	Males 95% CI Upper bd	Females Signif-icance	Females Odds ratio	Females 95% CI Lower bd	Females 95% CI Upper bd
Ethnic group								
Black		0.92	0.47	1.77		0.88	0.44	1.76
Indian sub-continent		1.05	0.64	1.70		1.17	0.74	1.84
Other		0.76	0.37	1.54		0.94	0.50	1.78
Housing tenure								
Renting-LA	**	1.25	1.16	1.35	**	1.20	1.13	1.28
Other rented	*	1.14	1.02	1.27		1.07	0.98	1.17
Communal estabs		1.28	0.93	1.75		1.41	1.00	1.99
Social class								
IIIN		1.04	0.94	1.16		0.95	0.87	1.02
IIIM		1.07	0.99	1.15		0.96	0.89	1.04
IV & V		1.05	0.96	1.14	*	1.09	1.02	1.18
Other		1.07	0.90	1.27	*	0.91	0.83	0.99
In practice<1 year	**	1.65	1.47	1.86	**	1.52	1.38	1.68
Living conditions								
Single sharing with adult	**	0.65	0.52	0.81	**	0.71	0.59	0.86
Sep/Wid/Div sharing with adult		0.99	0.87	1.13	**	1.14	1.05	1.23
Single, lives alone	**	0.70	0.59	0.84	**	0.78	0.68	0.89
Sep/wid/div, lives alone		0.93	0.86	1.02	*	1.07	1.00	1.14
Not known		1.12	0.79	1.59		1.05	0.74	1.49
Smoker		0.95	0.88	1.01	**	1.23	1.15	1.31
Rural ED		1.00	0.89	1.12		0.93	0.84	1.04

Notes: 1 Regressions also included age, distance from practice, limiting long-term illness rate for ED of residence.

2 Reference group is: white owner occupiers in social classes I& II, working full-time or part-time, in the study for the full year, and in an urban enumeration district. For adults the reference group members were also non-smokers who were married or cohabiting. For age group 16-64 they also had dependent children.

3 All comparisons are made within the age sex group.

Table 5S Patients consulting for preventive health care: Odds ratios compared with reference group, for which ratio =1 (see footnote)

Ages 0-15 and Ages 16-44

	Males Signif-icance	Males Odds ratio	Males 95% CI lower bd	Males 95% CI Upper bd	Females Signif-icance	Females Odds ratio	Females 95% CI Lower bd	Females 95% CI Upper bd
Ages 0-15								
Ethnic group								
Black		1.16	0.86	1.58		1.23	0.94	1.62
Indian sub-continent	**	2.32	1.84	2.93	**	1.59	1.26	2.00
Other		1.17	0.92	1.49		1.12	0.88	1.42
Housing tenure								
Renting-LA		1.01	0.92	1.09		0.99	0.91	1.07
Other rented		1.04	0.94	1.16		1.06	0.96	1.18
Communal estabs	**	4.75	3.45	6.55	**	9.12	6.17	13.50
Social class								
IIIN		0.98	0.69	1.08		0.96	0.88	1.06
IIIM		1.02	0.95	1.10		1.01	0.94	1.08
IV & V		0.93	0.85	1.02		1.00	0.92	1.09
Other	*	0.85	0.73	1.00		0.96	0.84	1.11
Economic position								
Waiting/seeking		1.03	0.93	1.15		0.96	0.87	1.06
Student		0.84	0.59	1.18		0.98	0.72	1.32
Perm sick		0.90	0.71	1.15		0.94	0.76	1.15
Other		1.06	0.93	1.21		0.94	0.84	1.07
In practice <1 year	**	2.33	2.14	2.54	**	2.13	1.96	2.32
Single adult in hhold		0.94	0.84	1.06		1.01	0.91	1.12
Rural enumeration district		1.01	0.90	1.15		1.03	0.92	1.16
Ages 16-44								
Ethnic group								
Black		0.99	0.74	1.31		1.15	0.98	1.36
Indian sub-continent	**	1.88	1.55	2.27	**	0.74	0.64	0.85
Other		1.09	0.86	1.37	*	0.84	0.72	0.98
Housing tenure								
Renting-LA	*	0.90	0.83	0.98	**	0.94	0.90	0.98
Other rented		0.98	0.91	1.06		1.04	0.99	1.10
Communal estabs	*	0.77	0.63	0.96	**	0.42	0.36	0.48
Social class								
IIIN		1.02	0.95	1.11		0.97	0.93	1.02
IIIM	**	0.91	0.86	0.97	**	0.94	0.90	0.96
IV & V	**	0.90	0.84	0.97	**	0.92	0.88	0.96
Other		0.95	0.82	1.11	**	0.76	0.71	0.82
Economic position								
Waiting/seeking		1.02	0.93	1.11		0.96	0.89	1.04
Student	*	1.22	1.04	1.43	**	0.67	0.62	0.73
Perm sick	**	1.32	1.13	1.54	**	0.68	0.60	0.77
Other	**	1.51	1.12	2.05	**	1.22	1.18	1.27
In practice<1 year	**	5.92	5.56	6.30	**	1.90	1.81	1.99
Family type								
Married/cohab no dependent children	**	1.17	1.10	1.25	**	1.08	1.04	1.13
Wid/sep/div with dep children		1.06	0.82	1.37	*	1.08	1.00	1.16
Wid/sep/div with no dep children		1.00	0.87	1.14	*	1.11	1.00	1.22
Single with dep children		0.93	0.81	1.07	**	0.72	0.67	0.77
Single no dep children		1.04	0.97	1.11	**	0.65	0.62	0.69
Smoker	**	0.83	0.79	0.88		1.02	0.98	1.05
Rural ED		0.96	0.88	1.06		1.03	0.97	1.10

Ages 45-64 and Ages 65 and over

	Males Signif-icance	Males Odds ratio	Males 95% CI lower bd	Males 95% CI Upper bd	Females Signif-icance	Females Odds ratio	Females 95% CI Lower bd	Females 95% CI Upper bd
Ages 45-64								
Ethnic group								
Black		1.25	0.86	1.79		1.11	0.81	1.53
Indian sub-continent	**	1.58	1.23	2.04		1.19	0.91	1.57
Other		1.17	.078	1.75		0.93	0.64	1.35
Housing tenure								
Renting-LA		1.00	0.91	1.08	**	0.91	0.85	0.97
Other rented		1.03	0.93	1.14		1.01	0.92	1.11
Communal estabs	**	1.96	1.34	2.86		0.87	0.62	1.24
Social class								
IIIN		1.05	0.96	1.15		1.02	0.95	1.09
IIIM	**	0.90	0.84	0.96		1.01	0.95	1.07
IV & V	**	0.87	0.80	0.94	*	0.93	0.88	1.00
Other	**	0.67	0.53	0.84		0.98	9.86	1.12
Economic position								
Waiting/seeking		1.01	0.91	1.12		1.01	0.86	1.18
Student		0.49	0.16	1.54		0.90	0.53	1.55
Perm sick	**	1.65	1.51	1.81	**	1.30	1.17	1.45
Other	**	1.26	1.15	1.37		1.01	0.96	1.07
In practice<1 year	**	3.60	3.21	4.04	**	2.09	1.87	2.34
Family type								
Married/cohab no dependent children	**	1.31	1.21	1.42		1.05	0.97	1.13
Wid/sep/div with dep children		1.12	0.80	1.56		1.04	0.88	1.24
Wid/sep/div with no dep children	**	1.22	1.08	1.37		1.04	0.95	1.15
Single with dep children		1.27	0.66	2.46		1.38	0.79	2.42
Single no dep children		1.04	0.91	1.18		0.97	0.85	1.10
Smoker	**	0.72	0.68	0.77	**	0.84	0.80	0.88
Rural ED		1.01	0.92	1.11		1.07	0.99	1.17
Ages 65 and over								
Ethnic group								
Black		1.07	0.56	2.08		0.87	0.46	1.67
Indian sub-continent	**	2.15	1.34	3.45		0.82	0.50	1.33
Other		1.28	0.65	2.52		0.68	0.35	1.32
Housing tenure								
Renting-LA	*	0.91	0.84	0.98	**	0.91	0.86	0.97
Other rented		1.10	0.99	1.23		0.98	0.90	1.07
Communal estabs	*	1.43	1.04	1.98		1.40	1.00	1.97
Social class								
IIIN		0.97	0.88	1.07		1.00	0.93	1.08
IIIM	*	0.92	0.86	0.99		0.95	0.89	1.02
IV & V	**	0.87	0.80	0.95	**	0.89	0.83	0.96
Other	*	0.80	0.68	0.96	**	0.85	0.79	0.93
In practice<1 year	**	1.20	1.07	1.35	**	1.24	1.12	1.36
Living conditions								
Single sharing with adult	**	0.65	0.53	0.80	*	0.84	0.71	0.99
Sep/Wid/Div sharing with adult	**	0.80	0.70	0.91	**	0.81	0.75	0.88
Single, lives alone		0.88	0.75	1.05	**	0.80	0.71	0.90
Sep/wid/div, lives alone	*	0.90	0.83	0.98		0.95	0.89	1.01
Not known		0.84	0.59	1.20		0.81	0.57	1.14
Smoker	**	0.73	0.68	0.78	**	0.83	0.78	0.89
Rural ED	*	0.89	0.79	1.00		0.93	0.84	1.03

Notes: 1 Regressions also included age, distance from practice, limiting long-term illness rate for ED of residence.

2 Reference group is: white owner occupiers in social classes I& II, working full-time or part-time, in the study for the full year, and in an urban enumeration district. For adults the reference group members were also non-smokers who were married or cohabiting. For age group 16-64 they also had dependent children.

3 All comparisons are made within the age sex group.

6 Estimating morbidity levels for small areas

6.1 Introduction

In addition to national morbidity estimates there is a need for small area estimates to answer questions such as: How many patients suffering from serious illness are there likely to be in my FHSA or DHA? GP fundholding practices need to be able to estimate their likely prescribing and hospitalisation needs. Small area statistics are also needed to compare areas with each other and the national average. Local data are available on the population and its demographic and socio-economic characteristics. Information on morbidity is usually only available at national level, from surveys such as the Health Survey, the General Household Survey and the MSGP surveys. National surveys do not generally answer local questions because the sample size is usually too small to produce reliable estimates, and often the small area of interest will not even have been included in the survey sample. If local surveys cannot be mounted, an alternative is to apply national survey results to the local population to obtain estimates. It is a straightforward matter to apply national age/sex rates to the local population distribution and obtain estimates of the expected local consulting rates. However, this simple approach does not allow for other differences from the national population, such as unemployment, the mix of ethnic groups or social classes. The purpose of this chapter is to illustrate what can be done with the regression results presented in the previous chapter, which take into consideration a wide range of socio-economic characteristics.

As an example the analysis presented here takes one age group (ages 16-44) and one dependent variable. This is serious illness, that is, patients consulting for a condition that is 'life threatening, requiring major surgery or intensive care, or having the potential for serious complications or recurring disability'. Maps showing the distribution of estimated serious illness rates are shown for men and women aged 16-44. The regression coefficients derived from the models of morbidity in the previous chapter apply to individual patients. The approach in this chapter is to apply these coefficients to data from individual census records, rather than use aggregate tables for small areas. Previous synthetic estimates in the UK have been based on aggregated data for enumeration districts or larger areas. One problem with using data at area level is the 'ecological fallacy' - relationships that hold at area level might not necessarily hold at individual area, and false associations can be found. It has been shown that if a model is not correctly specified biased estimates can result (Conner et al.[15]).

6.2 Method

The individual census records used as the basis for estimates were the 1991 census Sample of Anonymised Records (SARs - see Box, p 134). This sample comprises two per cent of the total population of England and Wales. They were grouped into 253 areas corresponding to county districts. (See Annex A.) For each of the one million individuals we calculated the probability of consulting for serious illness using the regression equations given in table 6A. The method used is described in the previous chapter (see Box on logistic regression). The expected number of people consulting were then estimated for each area by summing probabilities. The proportion of patients consulting was then derived for each area. Separate estimates were produced for men and women in households and in communal establishments and combined to provide estimates for men and women aged 16-44.

6.3 Regression equations used for estimates (table 6A)

The regression equations on which the estimates were based were those presented in the previous chapter with one small modification. The coefficients of the 'practice effects' could clearly not be used with the census data, and estimates would have to be based on the average practice effect. Latitude and longitude variables were highly correlated with the 'practice'

What are synthetic estimates?

Synthetic estimation techniques synthesise survey data with other data for small areas to provide local estimates with greater precision. For example, OPCS has combined Labour Force Survey data with 1981 Census data to produce synthetic small area estimates of the population in different ethnic groups.[16] In the USA the National Centre for Health Statistics[17] has obtained estimates of long and short term physical disabilities, based on the National Health Interview Survey. The use of synthetic estimates to meet government and local needs and the methodology has been reviewed for OPCS in New Methodology Series No.18.[18]

All synthetic estimation techniques are based on some model assumption, either implicitly or explicitly. They use the whole national dataset of the survey to produce estimates of how the variable of interest relates to other characteristics of individuals in the sample and to characteristics of the areas in which they live. The local information is then combined with the national estimates to produce estimates for local areas throughout the country. Synthetic estimates essentially consist of national survey data applied to local areas in this way. The synthetic estimate is the value that would be expected if the assumptions underlying a model were true.

variables: leaving 'practice' out of the regression equations resulted in large changes in the 'latitude' and 'longitude' regression coefficients. Since it was not possible to reliably estimate what the effects of latitude and longitude should be for an 'average practice', the estimates presented here were based on models that *excluded* latitude and longitude — it was felt to be more important to include 'practice' in all models. The other variables in the models did not have coefficients that changed much whether or not practice was included in the models. Using the equations in table 6A it is possible to calculate the probability (p) of a person consulting as follows: Add the constant to the coefficients corresponding to the person's characteristics, e.g. age, Indian subcontinent, together with the adjustment for time at risk in the study and an adjustment for average practice. The results is $x=\log(p/(1-p))$. To calculate p the transformation $p=\exp(p)/(1-\exp(p))$ is used.

In the regression models, only patients from whom socio-economic data were collected could be used in the analyses, some 85 per cent of all MSGP4 patients. These patients, not surprisingly, tended to have higher consultation rates overall than those from whom no socio-economic data were collected, since for example it was easier to collect information from patients or their relatives in contact with the surgery, and indeed some patients on the GPs' lists had moved away, died, or registered with a different GP ('ghost patients'). Our analyses thus excluded all ghost patients (currently estimated at 5 per cent of GPs' lists nationally), and some non-consulters who could not be interviewed. The general MSGP4 rates tables would include all patients on the GPs' lists, and hence show slightly lower patient-consulting rates due to higher denominator figures.

6.4 Data used for estimates

The MSGP4 social enquiry questionnaire was designed to correspond to census questions. The census form was completed by one individual in each household, whereas the MSGP4 information was collected by an interviewer. This methodological difference may have a small effect on comparability. For the variables that were available at individual level in both the MSGP4 study and the census, the coefficients from the regression equation were applied directly to the census data according to the characteristics of the individual. For example, the probability of consulting for unemployed individuals in the study was applied to unemployed people in the census. There were a number of MSGP4 variables that did not correspond exactly with census variables, and a best approximation was made. Details are given in Annex B.

6.5 Results

Figure 6.1 shows the distribution of estimated rates of patients consulting for serious illnesses by area, for men and women aged 16-44. For men aged 16-44 the expected proportion consulting for serious illness in a year varied from 10% to 15% between areas. The corresponding range for women in this age-group was 13%-18%. It can be seen that men have lower estimated rates than women, consistent with the findings for MSGP4 patients generally (see fig 2.3). There is only a slight overlap in the distributions for men and women, which are both skewed to the right, i.e. there are a relatively small number of areas with much higher rates than the rest. Figures 6.2 and 6.3 provide maps showing the proportion consulting for serious illness for men and women aged 16-44, respectively. Table 6B lists the areas which came in the top

Figure 6.1   Distribution of estimated proportion consulting for serious illnesses in the study year for men and women aged 16-44, by area

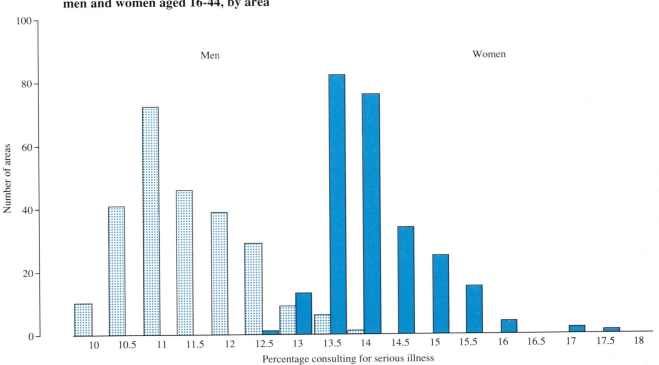

133

and bottom groups for either female or male rates as shown on the maps. It also shows the standardised mortality ratios per million population for the same area. The estimated proportions consulting for serious illness have been rounded to the nearest 0.5 per cent, while mortality ratios have been rounded to the nearest whole number.

In order to do some cross validation of the results the estimates of proportions of patients consulting for serious illness are compared by area for men and women using a scatter plot (fig 6.4). Male and female probabilities were derived separately from different regression equations. There is a close relationship ($r=0.81$) which is not quite linear. Women's rates are relatively higher than men's rates in the areas with highest rates, the most unusual district being Blaenau Gwent & Islwyn. This had the highest women's rates, but ranked 11th in the country for men's consulting rates.

Comparisons were also made between estimates of serious illness and age-standardised mortality ratios. Rates of patients consulting for serious illness for ages 16-44 years were compared by district with standardised mortality ratios for ages 15-64 (to allow a further 20-year period for mortality) using 1990-92 mortality data and population estimates. While an exact relationship would be unlikely, since not all serious illness results in death, some relationship might reasonably be expected. Figure 6.5 shows the relationship for men, and figure 6.6 that for women. There was a stronger relationship for men ($r=0.81$) than for women ($r=0.73$), which to some extent may reflect the fact that women's consulting rates are higher than those for men. For women there were three

outlying districts: Tower Hamlets, Blaenau Gwent & Islwyn, and Cynon Valley & Rhondda. These had the highest predicted serious illness rates but standardised mortality ratios only 10 to 20 per cent above the average, which for England and Wales was 100. These simple cross validations provide confidence that the estimates may be predicting real differences in morbidity.

6.6 Potential for future analysis

This chapter has taken just one measure — percentage consulting for serious illness, in one age group — to illustrate a method of estimating consultation at local level. But the MSGP4 survey provides a wide variety of information which has potential usefulness for the NHS. For example, it provides rates for consultation and patients consulting by diagnosis or combination of diagnoses, referral rates, home visit rates, new episode rates, and consulting information for the period up to 12 months before death. The survey also includes information about the organisation and resources available to the practices, which makes it possible to identify the effects of availability of resources on consultation rates, and so obtain a measure of service use that has been adjusted for the level of resources available. OPCS is in the course of producing a range of synthetic estimates for other categories described in Chapter 5, and these will be made available on floppy discs.

6.7 Summary

This chapter has described a method of combining data from the MSGP4 and the 1991 census to produce small area estimates of the proportion of 16-44 years olds who consulted for serious illness during a year. The method could be used to produce further estimates of other measures of morbidity in general practice for other age groups.

The estimates take into account the socio-economic make up of county districts as well as age/sex structure. Table 6C summarises the findings by comparing for six districts, estimates derived using a simple and the more complex method described.

The six districts were chosen from the ranked list summarised in table 6B. A district in the north/western part of England and Wales and one in the south/eastern part were chosen from the top, middle and bottom of the ranked list. As can be seen, the estimates using only age and sex distribution vary little. For men the proportion who consulted for serious illness was 10.6 or 10.7. For women it varied from 13.7 to 13.9. When the multivariate method was used, greater variability was to be seen. There was the greatest difference between the two methods in the districts with the highest estimated consultation rates — using the multivariate method. They tend to be the districts with high proportions of renters, unemployed and permanently sick and have high SMRs. Thus, the multivariate estimating method used here is likely to produce a more realistic estimate of consultation than the simple method based on age and sex distribution alone.

Table 6A Regression equations used for synthetic estimates - probability of consulting for serious illness
The equation estimates log $(p/(1p))$ where p = probability of consulting

Model term	Men 16-44		Women 16-44	
	estimate	s.e.	estimate	s.e.
Constant	- 8.344000	0.086880*	- 8.117000	0.074380
Age				
Age - mean age	0.023640	0.003883	0.025840	0.003337*
(Age - mean age) squared	0.000712	0.000226*	0.000329	0.000205
(Age - mean age) cubed	- 0.000022	0.000028	- 0.000054	0.000025*
Ethnic group				
Black	0.212400	0.133700	0.097550	0.113000
Indian subcontinent	0.397800	0.103500*	0.407500	0.094520*
Other	- 0.167400	0.134800	- 0.309300	0.124400*
Tenure				
Renting local authority	0.233400	0.035130	0.301600	0.030580
Renting other	0.148400	0.039480*	0.144400	0.034280
Communal establishment	- 0.163800	0.109600	- 0.120700	0.108400
Social class				
IIIN	0.087040	0.043530*	- 0.013590	0.033530
IIIM	0.119400	0.032230*	0.088290	0.028780*
IV & V	0.181800	0.037140*	0.095030	0.032250
Other	- 0.231400	0.070900*	- 0.066450	0.051030
Economic position				
Unemployed	0.363900	0.037250*	0.281600	0.049570*
Student	0.117400	0.078650	- 0.026360	0.064140
Permanently sick	2,015000	0.057920*	1.607000	0.064150*
Other	0.300000	0.156700	0.134100	0.026590
In practice <1 year	0.555600	0.040490*	0.340100	0.035880*
Family type				
Married/cohabiting without children	0.100800	0.033650*	0.144600	0.028840*
Widowed/separated/divorced with children	0.110500	0.124000	0.153700	0.045420*
Widowed/separated/divorced without children	0.241300	0.062840*	0.102400	0.061970
Single with children	0.064850	0.061450	- 0.019670	0.047740
Single without children	0.033400	0.034980	- 0.106200	0.037900*
Smoker	0.040690	0.025410	0.156700	0.022500*
Distance to practice				
Distance - mean distance	0.030370	0.010750*	- 0.001003	0.009458
(Distance - mean distance) squared	- 0.000872	0.000931	0.000634	0.000816
Lives in rural ED	- 0.712300	0.049470*	- 0.043600	0.043290
Limiting long-term illness rate/10,000	0.000063	0.000030*	0.000132	0.000030*
58 individual practice parameters, suppressed for confidentiality reasons				
Adjustment for offset**	5.902633		5,902633	
Adjustment (average practice)***	- 0.039340		0.011330	

Notes

Men 16-44: mean age = 30.13, mean distance to practice = 1.858Km, n = 77,133 observations

Women 16-44: mean age = 30.08, mean distance to practice = 1.849km, n = 87,837 observations

*   Denotes $p<0.05$ for significance test that coefficient = 0

**   Days in study was an offset. Log (366) has to be added in order to predict ratios for patients consulting *per year*

***   This is a constant that needs to be added corresponding to the average 'practice effect'

To calculate the probability of consulting (p), add the following: constant, coefficients corresponding to the patient's characteristics, and finally the adjustments for offset, and for average practice. This gives x = log $(p/(1 - p))$.

To calculate p, use the following equation: p = exp $(x)/(1+\exp(x))$

Figure 6.2 Estimated proportions of men aged 16-44 who consulted for serious illness during the study year, by area

Key: percentage of consulting

- 13.0 - 14.3
- 12.0 - 12.9
- 11.0 - 11.9
- 10.5 - 10.9
- 10 - 10.4

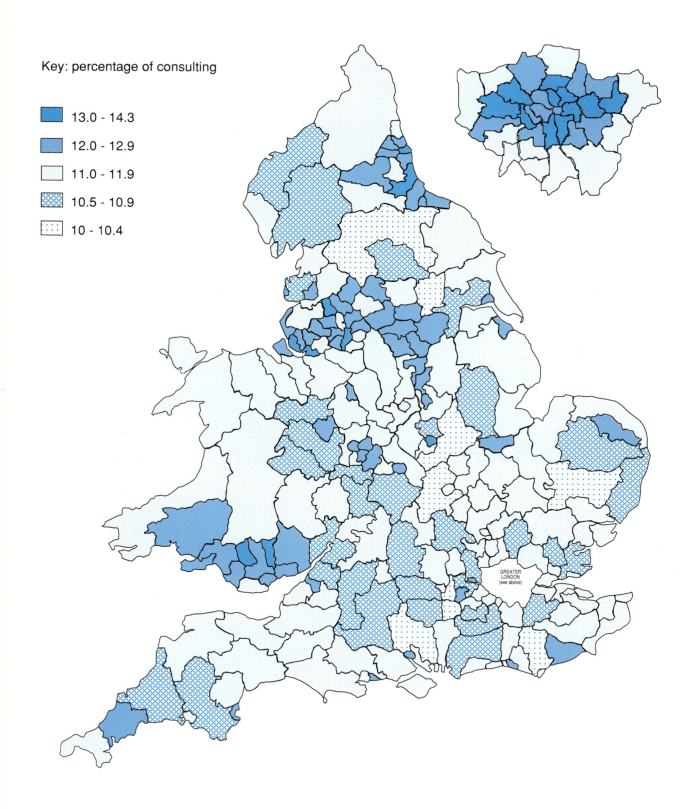

Figure 6.3 Estimated proportions of women aged 16-44 who consulted for serious illness during the study year, by area

Key: percentage consulting

- 15.5 - 17.6
- 14.5 - 15.4
- 14.0 - 14.4
- 13.5 - 13.9
- 13.0 - 13.4

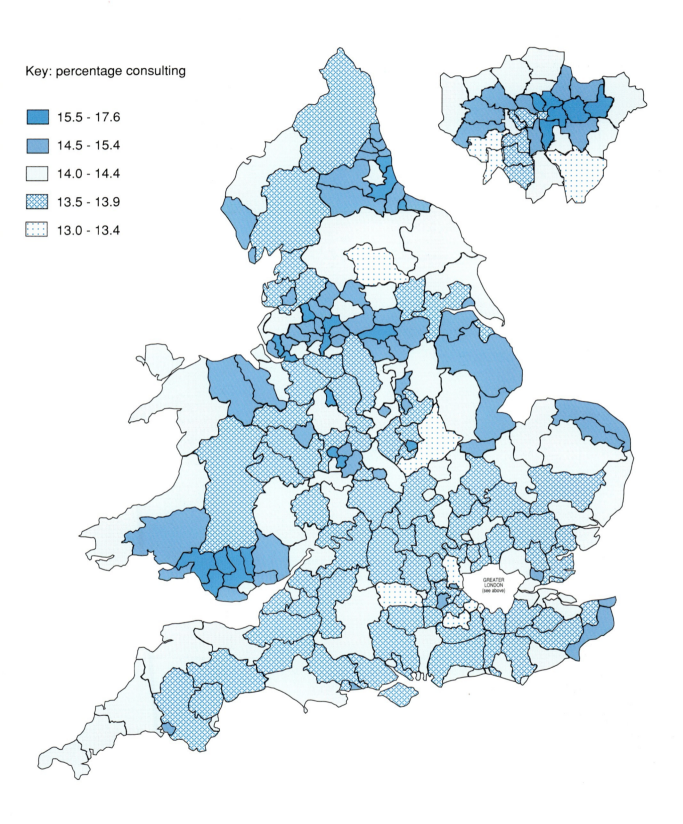

GREATER
LONDON
(see above)

Figure 6.4   Estimated proportions of men and women aged 16-44 consulting for serious illness, by area

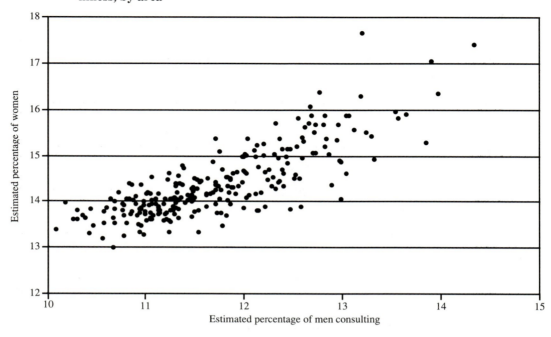

Figure 6.5   Comparison of the estimated proportion of men aged 16-44 consulting for serious illness with SMRs for men aged 15-64, by area

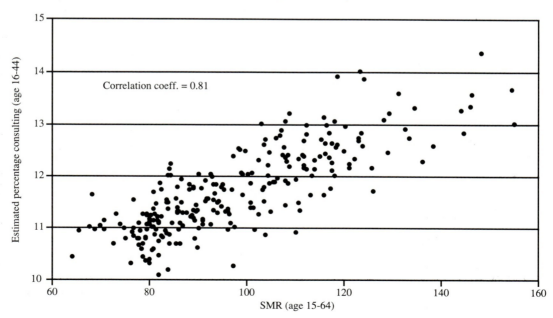

Figure 6.6 Comparison of the estimated proportion of women aged 16-44 consulting for serious illness with SMRs for women aged 15-64, by area

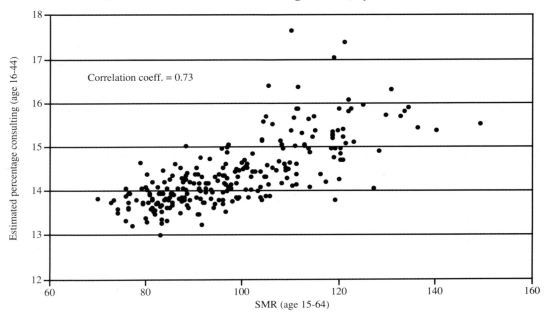

Correlation coeff. = 0.73

Table 6B Estimated proportion rates of men and women aged 16-44 who consulted for serious illness during the study years
Areas in the highest and lowest categories.

		Percentage consulting for serious illness		Category for maps*		1990-92** Age-standardised mortality ratios	
		Men	Women	Men	Women	Men 15-64	Women 15-64
Highest estimated serious illness							
003	Hackney LB	13.5	16.0	5	5	133	131
006	Islington LB	13.0	15.5	5	5	106	144
008	Lambeth LB	13.5	15.0	5	4	128	146
010	Newham LB	14.0	16.5	5	5	111	123
011	SouthwarkLB	13.5	16.0	5	5	125	146
012	Tower Hamlets LB	14.5	17.5	5	5	121	148
014	Barking and Dagenham LB	13.0	15.5	5	5	104	116
035	Manchester MCD	13.5	16.0	5	5	134	154
037	Rochdale MCD	12.5	15.5	4	5	133	123
043	Knowsley MCD	12.5	16.0	4	5	122	123
044	Liverpool MCD	13.5	15.5	5	4	136	134
048	Barnsley MCD	12.5	16.0	4	5	122	108
055	South Tyneside MCD	14.0	15.5	5	4	119	124
056	Sunderland MCD	13.0	16.0	4	5	122	123
060	Sandwell MCD	12.5	15.5	4	5	114	117
063	Wolverhampton MCD	13.0	15.5	4	5	115	112
091	Halton CD	13.0	15.5	4	5	111	116
096	Middlesbrough CD	12.5	15.5	4	5	149	133
121	Easington CD, Sedgefield CD	13.0	16.5	5	5	131	129
171	Blackburn CD	13.0	16.0	5	5	120	128
184	Leicester CD	13.0	16.0	4	5	112	118
219	Stoke-on-Trent CD	12.5	15.5	4	5	130	122
242	Blaenau Gwent CD, Islwyn CD	13.0	17.5	5	5	110	109
246	Cynon Valley CD, Rhondda CD	14.0	17.0	5	5	119	119
247	Merthyr Tydfil CD, Rhymney Valley CD, Taff-Ely CD	12.5	16.0	4	5	111	104
248	Ogwr CD	12.5	15.5	4	5	105	112
252	Lliw Valley CD, Neath CD, Port Talbot CD	13.0	16.5	4	5	105	107
Lowest estimated serious illness rates							
018	Bromley LB	11.0	13.5	3	1	83	79
027	Kingston upon Thames LB	11.5	13.5	3	1	84	86
030	Richmond upon Thames LB	12.0	13.5	3	1	82	89
077	Newbury CD	10.5	13.0	2	1	83	84
080	Wokingham CD	10.5	13.5	1	1	80	64
082	Chiltern CD, South Bucks CD	11.0	13.5	2	1	76	69
125	Wealden CD	10.5	13.5	1	2	83	80
141	Hart CD, Rushmoor CD	10.5	13.5	1	2	82	79
145	Test Valley CD, Winchester CD	10.5	14.0	1	2	78	76
182	Harborough CD, Melton CD, Rutland CD	10.0	13.5	1	1	80	82
193	Daventry CD, S Northamptonshire CD	10.5	13.5	1	2	81	80
198	Craven CD, Hambleton CD, Richmondshire CD	10.0	14.0	1	3	92	84
200	Harrogate CD	11.0	13.0	2	1	92	89
201	Selby CD, York CD	10.5	13.5	1	2	94	97
221	Forest Heath CD, Mid Suffolk CD, St Edmunds CD	10.5	14.0	1	2	87	79
223	Elmbridge CD, Epsom & Ewell CD	11.0	13.5	3	1	83	75
224	Guildford CD	10.5	13.0	2	1	77	81

* Key as for Figures 6.2 and 6.3   ** England and Wales = 100

Table 6C Comparison of expected percentage of patients aged 16-44 consulting for serious illness, based on age and sex alone, compared with estimates based on multivariate regression analysis

	Men Age & Sex	Multivariate	Women Age & Sex	Multivariate
Tower Hamlets	10.6	14.5	13.7	17.5
Cynon Valley/ Rhondda	10.6	14.0	13.7	17.0
Alnwick	10.6	11.5	13.9	14.5
Canterbury	10.6	11.5	13.7	13.5
Wealden	10.7	10.5	13.9	13.5
Harborough/ Melton/Rutland	10.7	10.0	13.8	13.5

ANNEX A

County Districts as used to form areas for the analysis of the census sample of anonymised records

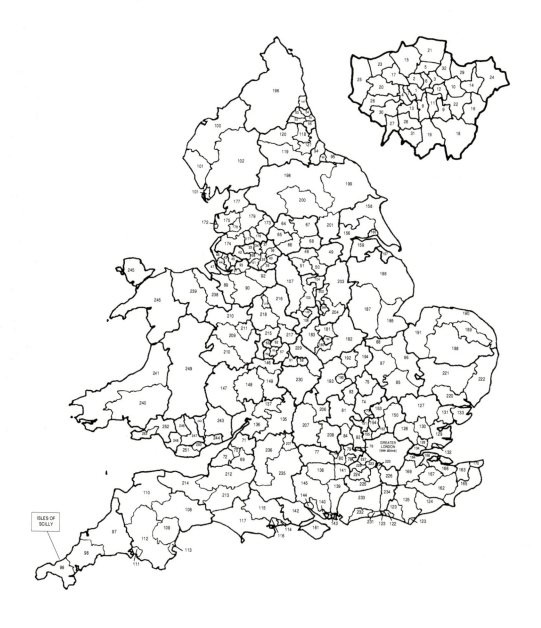

Key: SAR areas

Local authorities/London boroughs

Inner London
1 City of London; City of Westminister
2 Camden
3 Hackney
4 Hammersmith and Fulham
5 Haringey
6 Islington
7 Kensington and Chelsea
8 Lambeth
9 Lewisham
10 Newham
11 Southwark
12 Tower Hamlets
13 Wandsworth

Outer London
14 Barking and Dagenham
15 Barnet
16 Bexley
17 Brent
18 Bromley
19 Croydon
20 Ealing
21 Enfield
22 Greenwich
23 Harrow
24 Havering
25 Hillingdon
26 Hounslow
27 Kingston upon Thames
28 Merton
29 Redbridge
30 Richmond upon Thames
31 Sutton
32 Waltham Forest

Greater Manchester
33 Bolton
34 Bury
35 Manchester
36 Oldham
37 Rochdale
38 Salford
39 Stockport
40 Tameside
41 Trafford
42 Wigan

Merseyside
43 Knowsley
44 Liverpool
45 St Helens
46 Sefton
47 Wirral

South Yorkshire
48 Barnsley
49 Doncaster
50 Rotherham
51 Sheffield

Tyne and Wear
52 Gateshead
53 Newcastle upon Tyne
54 North Tyneside
55 South Tyneside
56 Sunderland

West Midlands
57 Birmingham
58 Coventry
59 Dudley
60 Sandwell
61 Solihull
62 Walsall
63 Wolverhampton

West Yorkshire
64 Bradford
65 Calderdale
66 Kirklees
67 Leeds
68 Wakefield

Avon
69 Bath; Kingswood; Wansdyke
70 Bristol
71 Northavon
72 Woodspring

Bedfordshire
73 Luton
74 Mid Bedfordshire; South Bedfordshire
75 North Bedfordshire

Berkshire
76 Bracknell Forest; Slough
77 Newbury
78 Reading
79 Windsor & Maidenhead
80 Wokingham

Buckinghamshire
81 Aylesbury Vale
82 Chiltern
83 Milton Keynes
84 Wycombe

Cambridgeshire
85 Cambridge; South Cambridgeshire
86 East Cambridgeshire; Fenland
87 Huntingdonshire
88 Peterborough

Cheshire
89 Chester; Ellesmere Port and Neston
90 Congleton; Crewe and Nantwich; Vale Royal
91 Halton
92 Macclesfield
93 Warrington

Cleveland
94 Hartlepool; Stockton-on-Tees
95 Langbaurgh-on-Tees
96 Middlesbrough

Cornwall & Isles of Scilly
97 Caradon; North Cornwall
98 Carrick; Restormel
99 Kerrier; Penwith; Isles of Scilly

Cumbria
100 Allerdale; Carlisle
101 Barrow-in-Furness Copeland
102 Eden; South Lakeland

Derbyshire
103 Amber Valley; North East Derbyshire
104 Bolsover; Chesterfield
105 Derby
106 Erewash; South Derbyshire
107 High Peak; The Derbyshire Dales

Devon
108 East Devon; Mid Devon
109 Exeter; Teignbridge
110 North Devon; Torridge
111 Plymouth
112 South Ham; West Devon
113 Torbay

Dorset
114 Bournemouth
115 Christchurch; East Dorset North Dorset
116 Poole
117 Purbeck; West Dorset; Weymouth and Portland

Durham
118 Chester-le-Street; Durham
119 Darlington; Teesdale
120 Derwentside; Wear Valley
121 Easington; Sedgefield

East Sussex
122 Brighton
123 Eastbourne; Hove; Lewes
124 Hastings; Rother
125 Wealdon

Essex
126 Basildon
127 Braintree; Uttlesford
128 Brentwood; Epping Forest; Harlow
129 Castle Point; Maldon; Rochford
130 Chelmsford
131 Colchester
132 Southend-on-Sea
133 Tendring
134 Thurrock

Gloucestershire
135 Cheltenham; Cotswold
136 Forest of Dean; Stroud
137 Gloucester; Tewkes'bury

Hampshire
138 Basingstoke & Deane
139 East Hampshire; Havant
140 Eastleigh; Fareham; Gosport
141 Hart; Rushmoor
142 New Forest
143 Portsmouth
144 Southampton
145 Test Valley; Winchester

Hereford and Worcester
146 Bromsgrove; Wyre Forest
147 Hereford; Leominster; South Herefordshire
148 Malvern Hills; Worcester
149 Redditch; Wychavon

Hertfordshire
150 Broxbourne; East Hertfordshire
151 Dacorum
152 Hertsmere; Welwyn Hatfield
153 North Hertfordshire; Stevenage
154 St Albans
155 Three Rivers; Watford

Humberside
156 Beverley; Boothferry
157 Cleethorpes; Great Grimsby
158 East Yorkshire; Holderness
159 Glanford; Scunthorpe
160 Kingston-upon-Hull

Isle of Wight
161 Medina; South Wight

Kent
162 Ashford; Tunbridge Wells
163 Canterbury
164 Dartford; Gravesham
165 Dover; Shepway
166 Gillingham; Swale
167 Maidstone
168 Rochester upon Medway
169 Sevenoaks; Tonbridge & Malling
170 Thanet

Lancashire
171 Blackburn
172 Blackpool
173 Burnley; Pendle
174 Chorley; West Lancashire
175 Fylde; Wyre
176 Hyndburn; Rossendale
177 Lancaster
178 Preston
179 Ribble Valley; South Ribble

Leicestershire
180 Blaby; Oadby & Wigston
181 Charnwood
182 Harborough; Melton; Rutland
183 Hinckley & Bosworth; North West Leicestershire
184 Leicester

Lincolnshire
185 Boston; South Holland
186 East Lindsey; Lincoln; West Lindsey
187 North Kesteven; South Kesteven

Norfolk
188 Breckland; South Norfolk
189 Broadland; Norwich
190 Great Yarmouth
191 Kings Lynn & West Norfolk

Northamptonshire
192 Corby; Kettering
193 Daventry; South Northamptonshire
194 East Northamptonshire; Wellingborough
195 Northampton

Northumberland
196 Alnwick; Berwick-upon-Tweed; Castle Morpeth; Tynedale
197 Blyth Valley, Wansbeck

North Yorkshire
198 Craven; Hambleton; Richmondshire
199 Ryedale; Scarborough
200 Harrogate
201 Selby; York

Nottinghamshire
202 Ashfield; Mansfield
203 Bassetlaw; Newark & Sherwood
204 Broxtowe; Gedling; Rushcliffe
205 Nottingham

Oxfordshire
206 Cherwell
207 Oxford; Vale of White Horse; West Oxfordshire
208 South Oxfordshire

Shropshire
209 Bridgnorth; Shrewsbury & Atcham
210 North Shropshire; Oswestry; South Shropshire
211 The Wrekin

Somerset
212 Mendip; Sedgemoor
213 South Somerset
214 Taunton Deane; West Somerset

Staffordshire
215 Cannock Chase; South Staffordshire
216 East Staffordshire; Staffordshire Moorlands
217 Lichfield; Tamworth
218 Newcastle-under-Lyme; Stafford
219 Stoke-on-Trent

Suffolk
220 Babergh; Ipswich
221 Forest Heath; Mid Suffolk; St Edmundsbury
222 Suffolk Coastal; Waveney

Surrey
223 Elmbridge; Epsom & Ewell
224 Guildford
225 Mole Valley; Waverley;
226 Reigate & Banstead; Tandridge
227 Runnymede; Spelthorne
228 Surrey Heath; Woking

Warwickshire
229 North Warwickshire; Nuneaton & Bedworth; Rugby
230 Stratford-on-Avon; Warwick

West Sussex
231 Adur; Worthing
232 Arun
233 Chichester; Horsham
234 Crawley; Mid Sussex

Wiltshire
235 Kennet; Salisbury
236 North Wiltshire; West Wiltshire
237 Thamesdown

Clwyd
238 Alyn & Deeside; Delyn; Wrexham Maelor
239 Colwyn; Glyndwr; Rhuddlan

Dyfed
240 Carmarthen; Dinefwr; Llanelli
241 Ceredigion; Preseli Pembrokeshire; South Pembrokeshire

Gwent
242 Blaenau Gwent; Islwyn
243 Monmouth; Torfean
244 Newport

Gwynedd
245 Aberconwy; Arfon; Dwyfor; Meirionnydd; Ynys Mon - Isle of Anglesey

Mid Glamorgan
246 Cynon Valley; Rhondda
247 Merthyr Tydfil; Rhymney Valley; Taff-Ely
248 Ogwr

Powys
249 Brecknock; Montgomeryshire; Radnorshire

South Glamorgan
250 Cardiff
251 Vale of Glamorgan

West Glamorgan
252 Lliw Valley; Neath; Port Talbot
253 Swansea

ANNEX B

Assumptions made in approximating census variables to match MSGP4 variables

Social class in MSGP4 was that of the husband for married and cohabiting women, otherwise their own social class. From the census, only 'own' and 'head of household' social class were available. We used 'own social class' for men, and 'head of household social class' for women. The census had more 'missing' social class data than MSGP4 (including armed forces, home/family, and more usually 'not worked in past 10 years'). To increase comparability between the two sources the following imputations were made for the Census data. For men where own social class was missing, head of household social class was used. For women where head of household social class was missing, own social class was used. The remaining Census 'missing' social class data were treated as equivalent to the MSGP4 'other' category.

Family type was not available in MSGP4 for those living in communal establishments, hence separate estimates were made for those who lived in communal establishments and those who did not. The separate estimates were later combined for purposes of tabulation and mapping.

Limiting long-term illness was available for the census individuals but not for MSGP4 patients, so it had been fitted in the MSGP4 regressions as an area-of-residence parameter, for small areas (EDs, which have an average of 200 households in each). Thus when applying the regression coefficients to individuals in the census it was also used as an area effect, using an average for the county district as the level applying to all residents of the area.

Smoking data were available for the MSGP4 patients but not in the census and were dealt with by fitting a constant effect for each age/sex group in the district. GHS age/sex specific smoking rates for ll standard regions in 1992 were used for all districts within their boundaries. For a small number of districts in the South East the district boundary cut across Regional boundaries, and in these cases the district was given the values of the most appropriate region.

No census data were available to cover the different 'practice effects', so a national practice level constant was used corresponding to the average MSGP4 doctor.

The census variable 'moved address within the previous 12 months' was used as the proxy for the MSGP4 variable 'In practice for less than 366 days'. Not being in the practice for the full year was due to being born, dying, moving house, or changing GP. The census variable chosen was the only similar measure. In order to test its validity a small study was undertaken on the 65 county districts in the MSGP4 study from which more than 200 men and women aged 16-44 had been sampled. For each of these the proportion changing address within a year was calculated from the census data and compared with the proportion in that practice for less than the full year, analyzing men and women separately. In both cases the correlation was 0.5, which increased to 0.6 when one unusual county district sample with a high student population was excluded. There were large variations in moving (range 8-22 per cent) and being in the practice for less than the full year (range 5-38 per cent) in our (non-random) sample of 65 county districts. Other Census measures of migration were also tested (eg moving more than 5 km), but these had lower correlations than the one originally tested. It was thus decided that the census variable did capture a large proportion of what the MSGP4 was measuring, and was thus usable for synthetic estimates. The alternative would have been to assume that there were no variations by area in the proportion of people with the practice for the full year, which in view of the observed variations did not seem reasonable.

The approach to the data not available at individual level in both samples can be summarised as follows:

Fit constant for entire country district:

Smoking: used average rates for standard regions plus an expansion of the South East to differentiate inner and outer London for ages 16-44, calculated from 1992 GHS.

Living in rural areas: For each age/sex group we used the proportion of residents in the SAR area who were living in rural EDs as classified by the Department of Environment at the time of the 1991 Census.

Limiting long-term illness: used age standardised limiting long-term illness rate for ages 16-44 for SAR areas.

Fit constant for whole country:

Distance to practice: national average distance to practice for ages 16-44 and specific sex.

Practice effect: the average effect for the study was applied.

Fit on basis of proxy variable for each individual in the census (sample of anonymised records)

In practice less than 366 days: used the Census proportion who changed address within the previous 12 months.

Detailed tables

List of detailed tables

Table 1 Study population - person years at risk: age, sex and broad geographical region

Broad geographical region	Persons, by age group								
	Total	0-4	5-15	16-24	25-44	45-64	65-74	75-84	85 and over
All practices	**468,042**	32,133	65,019	59,713	143,714	99,118	38,235	23,351	6,759
North	**146,082**	9,524	20,417	17,335	43,035	32,853	13,097	7,678	2,144
Midlands and Wales	**151,492**	10,205	21,762	20,286	46,551	30,846	11,995	7,591	2,256
South	**170,467**	12,404	22,841	22,093	54,128	35,419	13,143	8,082	2,358

Table 2 Study population - person years at risk: age, sex and tenure

Tenure	Persons, by age group								
	Total	0-4	5-15	16-24	25-44	45-64	65-74	75-84	85 and over
Owner occupied	**280,752**	19,300	41,258	29,404	87,100	67,784	22,161	11,370	2,374
Council house	**73,728**	7,068	12,498	8,924	17,648	12,359	8,676	5,412	1,143
Other rented	**37,311**	3,035	4,307	7,990	11,237	5,533	2,570	2,147	493
Communal	**6,968**	21	532	2,216	675	347	494	1,332	1,350
Not stated	**69,282**	2,709	6,424	11,180	27,053	13,095	4,334	3,089	1,398

Table 3 Study population - person years at risk: age, sex and urban/rural place of residence

Urban/rural	Persons, by age group								
	Total	0-4	5-15	16-24	25-44	45-64	65-74	75-84	85 and over
Urban	**401,601**	27,898	56,118	51,039	123,485	83,917	33,082	20,251	5,811
Rural	**56,343**	3,326	7,500	7,355	16,926	13,362	4,471	2,624	779
Not stated	**10,098**	909	1,401	1,319	3,303	1,839	682	476	169

Table 4 Study population - person years at risk: age, sex and ethnic group

Ethnic group	Persons, by age group								
	Total	0-4	5-15	16-24	25-44	45-64	65-74	75-84	85 and over
White	**387,691**	28,123	56,009	46,985	112,955	84,513	33,603	20,165	5,336
Black Afro-Caribbean	**2,341**	230	447	341	867	369	67	17	5
Indian	**2,497**	196	473	326	911	448	106	31	6
Pakistani/Bangladeshi	**1,627**	197	452	275	422	247	25	7	2
Other	**2,845**	397	654	381	1,018	309	56	26	4
Not stated	**71,040**	2,991	6,984	11,405	27,539	13,233	4,378	3,106	1,405

By age-group and sex

0-4		5-15		16-24		25-44		45-64		65-74		75-84		85 and over	
Male	Female	Male	Female	Male	Female	Male	Female	Male	Female	Male	Female	Male	Female	Male	Female
16,457	15,677	33,318	31,702	29,753	29,960	72,124	71,589	50,015	49,103	17,144	21,090	8,733	14,618	1,683	5,076
4,876	4,647	10,390	10,026	8,813	8,522	21,563	21,472	16,353	16,500	5,810	7,287	2,873	4,805	492	1,652
5,224	4,982	11,074	10,688	10,078	10,208	23,168	23,383	15,693	15,153	5,329	6,666	2,787	4,804	567	1,690
6,356	6,048	11,854	10,987	10,863	11,230	21,394	26,735	17,970	17,449	6,006	7,137	3,073	5,009	624	1,734

By age-group and sex

0-4		5-15		16-24		25-44		45-64		65-74		75-84		85 and over	
Male	Female	Male	Female	Male	Female	Male	Female	Male	Female	Male	Female	Male	Female	Male	Female
9,975	9,325	21,015	20,243	14,754	14,650	41,284	45,816	33,451	34,333	10,311	11,850	4,640	6,730	683	1,691
3,596	3,472	6,386	6,113	4,120	4,804	7,959	9,688	5,745	6,614	3,562	5,114	1,929	3,483	279	864
1,495	1,540	2,162	2,145	3,493	4,496	5,342	5,895	2,841	2,692	1,078	1,491	731	1,416	131	362
10	11	374	158	1,016	1,200	456	219	170	177	193	301	324	1,008	199	1,151
1,381	1,328	3,380	3,043	6,370	4,809	17,082	9,971	7,808	5,286	2,000	2,334	1,109	1,981	391	1,007

By age-group and sex

0-4		5-15		16-24		25-44		45-64		65-74		75-84		85 and over	
Male	Female	Male	Female	Male	Female	Male	Female	Male	Female	Male	Female	Male	Female	Male	Female
14,284	13,613	28,693	27,425	25,291	25,748	61,876	61,609	42,208	41,709	14,698	18,384	7,511	12,740	1,413	4,398
1,725	1,600	3,885	3,615	3,844	3,511	8,534	8,392	6,846	6,516	2,146	2,324	1,050	1,574	226	553
447	464	739	663	619	701	1,714	1,588	962	878	300	382	172	304	44	125

By age-group and sex

0-4		5-15		16-24		25-44		45-64		65-74		75-84		85 and over	
Male	Female	Male	Female	Male	Female	Male	Female	Male	Female	Male	Female	Male	Female	Male	Female
14,396	13,727	28,607	27,402	22,640	24,345	53,297	59,658	41,388	43,125	14,985	18,619	7,594	12,571	1,286	4,051
109	121	223	224	144	197	378	489	184	184	40	27	4	13	-	5
93	103	258	215	166	160	437	474	252	196	47	59	11	20	3	3
99	97	221	231	134	141	225	197	163	84	19	6	4	3	1	1
219	178	330	324	189	191	489	529	166	143	28	28	9	17	2	2
1,540	1,451	3,678	3,306	6,479	4,926	17,297	10,242	7,862	5,370	2,027	2,351	1,112	1,994	391	1,014

Table 5   Study population - person years at risk:
age, sex and marital status

Marital status	Persons, by age group								
	Total	0-4	5-15	16-24	25-44	45-64	65-74	75-84	85 and over
Single	**168,119**	29,457	58,652	43,750	26,687	5,466	2,028	1,515	564
Married	**188,110**	-	-	4,615	81,590	69,943	22,580	8,525	857
Widowed/divorced	**42,941**	-	-	243	8,507	10,711	9,314	10,224	3,942
Not stated	**68,873**	2,677	6,367	11,105	26,929	12,998	4,313	3,087	1,396

Table 6   Study population aged 16 and over - person years at risk:
age, sex and cohabiting status

Cohabiting status	Persons, by age-group						
	Total	16-24	25-44	45-64	65-74	75-84	85 and over
Single	**67,358**	39,397	19,162	4,809	1,945	1,486	559
Married/cohabiting	**200,798**	8,779	89,201	70,824	22,621	8,513	860
Separated/widowed/divorced not cohabiting	**42,904**	431	8,422	10,487	9,356	10,265	3,943
Not stated	**59,829**	11,105	26,929	12,998	4,313	3,087	1,396

Table 7   Study population - person years at risk:
age, sex and social class (as defined by occupation)*

Social class*	Persons, by age group								
	Total	0-4	5-15	16-24	25-44	45-64	65-74	75-84	85 and over
I and II	**121,495**	9,574	19,878	5,660	41,642	30,365	8,954	4,473	950
IIIN	**52,129**	3,449	6,609	8,835	15,094	9,442	4,831	3,107	761
IIIM	**115,042**	9,072	17,906	9,779	35,588	27,037	9,884	4,864	912
IV & V	**79,477**	5,849	11,426	9,591	20,882	17,237	8,297	4,945	1,250
Other	**30,219**	1,478	2,265	14,705	3,496	1,979	1,943	2,870	1,484
Not known	**69,680**	2,711	6,935	11,142	27,011	13,059	4,327	3,093	1,401

* Social class for children is social class of parent; social class of married/cohabiting women is that of partner.

Table 8   Study population aged 16 and over - person years at risk:
age, sex and smoking status

Smoking status	Persons, by age-group						
	Total	16-24	25-44	45-64	65-74	75-84	85 and over
Smoked in last week	**89,035**	14,639	37,704	26,033	7,520	2,784	356
Did not smoke	**221,231**	33,494	78,901	60,017	26,383	17,450	4,986
Not stated	**60,623**	11,580	27,108	13,068	4,332	3,117	1,417

By age-group and sex

0-4		5-15		16-24		25-44		45-64		65-74		75-84		85 and over	
Male	Female	Male	Female	Male	Female	Male	Female	Male	Female	Male	Female	Male	Female	Male	Female
15,088	14,368	29,969	28,683	22,020	21,730	15,370	11,317	3,334	2,132	912	1,116	426	1,089	72	493
-	-	-	-	1,336	3,278	37,006	44,584	35,566	34,377	12,175	10,405	5,086	3,439	558	299
-	-	-	-	65	178	2,748	5,760	3,367	7,345	2,063	7,250	2,116	8,108	662	3,280
1,368	1,309	3,348	3,019	6,332	4,774	17,000	9,929	7,749	5,249	1,994	2,319	1,106	1,982	391	1,004

By age-group and sex

16-24		25-44		45-64		65-74		75-84		85 and over	
Male	Female	Male	Female	Male	Female	Male	Female	Male	Female	Male	Female
20,441	18,956	11,409	7,753	2,890	1,919	861	1,084	408	1,077	70	490
2,886	5,894	41,153	48,048	36,237	34,587	12,242	10,379	5,106	3,407	563	297
95	336	2,562	5,860	3,139	7,348	2,047	7,308	2,114	8,152	658	3,285
6,332	4,774	17,000	9,929	7,749	5,249	1,994	2,319	1,106	1,982	391	1,004

By age-group and sex

0-4		5-15		16-24		25-44		45-64		65-74		75-84		85 and over	
Male	Female	Male	Female	Male	Female	Male	Female	Male	Female	Male	Female	Male	Female	Male	Female
4,946	4,628	10,138	9,740	2,441	3,219	19,473	22,169	15,296	15,068	4,354	4,600	2,105	2,368	354	596
1,736	1,713	3,366	3,243	2,685	6,151	5,884	9,210	3,730	5,712	1,519	3,312	826	2,281	139	622
4,679	4,394	9,196	8,710	6,170	3,609	18,523	17,065	14,387	12,650	5,453	4,431	2,633	2,231	420	492
2,983	2,866	5,762	5,665	4,990	4,601	10,209	10,673	8,265	8,972	3,458	4,839	1,719	3,225	296	954
730	747	1,117	1,148	7,137	7,569	1,038	2,458	590	1,389	372	1,570	346	2,524	84	1,400
1,383	1,328	3,739	3,196	6,331	4,811	16,997	10,015	7,747	5,312	1,989	2,338	1,104	1,989	391	1,011

By age-group and sex

16-24		25-44		45-64		65-74		75-84		85 and over	
Male	Female	Male	Female	Male	Female	Male	Female	Male	Female	Male	Female
7,171	7,468	19,264	18,441	14,173	11,859	3,893	3,627	1,588	1,196	196	160
16,013	17,481	35,720	43,182	28,039	31,978	11,247	15,136	6,030	11,420	1,092	3,893
6,569	5,011	17,141	9,967	7,803	5,265	2,005	2,328	1,115	2,002	395	1,022

**Table 9   Study population aged 16 and over - person years at risk:
age, sex and household composition**

Household composition	Persons, by age-group						
	Total	16-24	25-44	45-64	65-74	75-84	85 and over
Living alone*	**34,152**	1,554	7,031	7,623	7,869	7,862	2,213
Not living alone	**336,737**	58,158	136,683	91,495	30,366	15,489	4,545
All adults	**370,889**	59,713	143,714	99,118	38,235	23,351	6,759
Sole adult with children	**5,398**	910	4,071	370	22	20	6
Children in household†							
None	**271,770**	44,173	73,683	86,550	37,595	23,074	6,695
Under 5 years only	**25,680**	5,004	19,235	1,260	136	38	8
5-15 years only	**54,922**	8,990	34,828	10,474	405	182	44
Under 5 years and 5-15 years	**18,517**	1,546	15,967	834	100	57	12

Footnotes
* If sole adult and no children stated, included in 'living alone'.
† If no children in household stated, included in 'none'.

**Table 10   Study population aged 16 and over - person years at risk:
age, sex and economic position last week**

Economic position last week	Persons, by age-group						
	Total	16-24	25-44	45-64	65-74	75-84	85 and over
Working full time	**139,612**	25,206	71,619	42,097	593	81	16
Working part time	**34,243**	1,956	18,136	12,791	1,140	202	19
Waiting/seeking work	**15,107**	4,737	6,710	3,641	15	3	-
Long-term sick	**8,963**	464	2,455	5,515	356	118	54
Home/family	**34,332**	3,172	16,451	9,222	2,878	1,997	613
Other	**74,502**	10,619	1,345	11,883	28,131	17,865	4,659
Not stated	**64,130**	13,559	26,998	13,968	5,122	3,086	1,397

**Table 11   Study population aged 16 and over - person years at risk:
age, sex and economic position one year ago**

Economic position 1 year ago	Persons, by age-group						
	Total	16-24	25-44	45-64	65-74	75-84	85 and over
Working full time	**148,078**	25,372	75,773	45,652	1,167	97	17
Working part time	**33,626**	1,521	17,374	13,261	1,268	189	13
Waiting/seeking work	**8,607**	2,412	3,937	2,214	40	2	2
Long-term sick	**8,375**	417	2,216	5,094	472	122	53
Home/family	**33,319**	2,625	15,880	9,327	2,878	1,996	613
Other	**78,484**	16,053	1,340	10,486	28,087	17,857	4,661
Not stated	**60,400**	11,312	27,194	13,084	4,323	3,089	1,398

Series MB5 no.3 Study population

Study population

By age-group and sex

16-24		25-44		45-64		65-74		75-84		85 and over	
Male	Female	Male	Female	Male	Female	Male	Female	Male	Female	Male	Female
760	794	4,071	2,960	3,075	4,548	1,949	5,921	1,668	6,194	415	1,798
28,993	29,165	68,053	68,630	46,940	44,555	15,196	15,170	7,066	8,424	1,268	3,277
29,753	29,960	72,124	71,589	50,015	49,103	17,144	21,090	8,733	14,618	1,683	5,076
40	870	304	3,767	100	270	6	16	6	14	1	5
23,030	21,142	41,989	31,694	42,452	44,098	16,854	20,741	8,625	14,448	1,667	5,028
1,326	3,678	8,978	10,257	720	540	70	66	15	23	1	7
4,777	4,213	14,148	20,680	6,255	4,219	185	220	67	115	10	33
620	926	7,010	8,958	588	246	36	64	26	31	4	8

By age-group and sex

16-24		25-44		45-64		65-74		75-84		85 and over	
Male	Female	Male	Female	Male	Female	Male	Female	Male	Female	Male	Female
13,261	11,945	47,181	24,438	30,057	12,041	427	165	58	23	12	4
439	1,517	642	17,494	1,033	11,758	547	593	110	92	4	15
3,125	1,613	4,964	1,746	2,809	832	9	6	1	2	-	-
265	199	1,458	997	3,691	1,825	213	143	46	72	7	48
33	3,139	246	16,205	200	9,022	19	2,859	7	1,990	3	610
5,021	5,597	592	753	4,461	7,422	13,128	15,003	7,409	10,456	1,268	3,391
7,609	5,950	17,042	9,956	7,764	6,204	2,801	2,321	1,103	1,983	390	1,008

By age-group and sex

16-24		25-44		45-64		65-74		75-84		85 and over	
Male	Female	Male	Female	Male	Female	Male	Female	Male	Female	Male	Female
13,373	11,999	49,483	26,290	32,364	13,287	940	226	68	29	12	5
313	1,208	466	16,908	875	12,386	628	640	108	82	3	11
1,652	760	2,926	1,011	1,744	469	35	5	-	2	1	1
235	182	1,289	927	3,343	1,752	329	144	50	72	6	48
22	2,604	209	15,671	173	9,154	24	2,854	8	1,988	1	612
7,763	8,290	575	765	3,721	6,765	13,193	14,893	7,397	10,460	1,271	3,391
6,396	4,916	17,176	10,018	7,795	5,289	1,996	2,327	1,104	1,985	390	1,008

Table 12 Study population aged 16-64 - person years at risk:
      age, sex and occupation

| | Persons, by age-group | | | | By age-group and sex | | | | | |
| | Total | 16-24 | 25-44 | 45-64 | 16-24 | | 25-44 | | 45-64 | |
					Male	Female	Male	Female	Male	Female
1 a) Corporate managers & administrators	**16,095**	924	8,658	6,512	406	518	5,597	3,062	4,999	1,513
b) Managers/proprietors in agriculture and services	**11,578**	1,068	5,766	4,745	480	588	3,041	2,725	2,706	2,039
2 a) Science & engineering professionals	**5,514**	424	3,037	2,053	336	88	2,605	432	1,961	92
b) Health professionals	**1,510**	50	980	480	19	32	561	419	354	126
c) Teaching professionals	**9,414**	208	4,880	4,325	46	163	1,515	3,365	1,605	2,721
d) Other professional occupations	**5,497**	368	3,182	1,947	194	174	1,942	1,240	1,272	675
3 a) Science & engineering associate professionals	**4,093**	691	2,382	1,020	530	161	1,735	647	777	243
b) Health associate professionals	**6,592**	673	3,939	1,980	80	593	451	3,488	210	1,770
c) Other associate professional occupations	**7,786**	935	4,325	2,526	462	474	2,227	2,098	1,580	946
4 a) Clerical occupations	**27,893**	5,779	13,719	8,395	1,942	3,837	3,524	10,195	2,395	6,000
b) Secretarial occupations	**11,988**	1,908	5,797	4,283	24	1,884	65	5,732	69	4,213
5 a) Skilled construction trades	**6,636**	1,169	3,207	2,,260	1,132	37	3,139	68	2,235	25
b) Skilled engineering trades	**10,059**	1,525	4,864	3,670	1,457	69	4,689	175	3,581	89
c) Other skilled trades	**18,681**	3,793	8,568	6,320	2,937	856	6,405	2,163	4,351	1,969
6 a) Protective service occupations	**3,474**	484	1,876	1,114	398	87	1,580	296	1,000	114
b) Personal service occupations	**18,102**	4,170	8,488	5,444	846	3,324	1,241	7,247	886	4,558
7 a) Buyers, brokers and sales reps	**3,525**	394	1,909	1,222	239	155	1,271	637	959	263
b) Other sales occupations	**13,672**	3,015	6,307	4,350	875	2,140	906	5,400	490	3,860
8 a) Industrial plant and machine operators, assemblers	**15,772**	2,493	7,167	6,112	1,461	1,032	4,152	3,015	3,567	2,545
b) Drivers and mobile machine operators	**8,165**	715	3,858	3,592	657	58	3,599	260	3,460	132
9 a) Other occupations in agriculture, forestry and fishing	**1,462**	340	570	551	204	136	325	245	301	251
b) Other elementary occupations	**20,040**	2,770	8,373	8,897	1,760	1,011	3,669	4,704	3,025	5,871
Not stated/other	**74,996**	25,816	31,860	17,320	13,271	12,545	17,884	13,976	8,232	9,088

Table 13 Study population of married/cohabiting women aged 16 and over - person years at risk: age and economic position of partner last week

Economic position of partner last week	Total	16-24	25-44	45-64	65-74	75-84	85 and over
Working full time	**70,507**	4,728	42,708	22,395	604	69	3
Working part time	**1,853**	70	446	977	314	46	1
Waiting/seeking work	**5,764**	861	3,274	1,565	61	3	-
Long-term sick	**3,396**	51	805	2,311	206	22	-
Home/family	**298**	25	145	110	13	4	1
Other	**20,076**	68	382	7,016	9,111	3,217	283
Not stated	**718**	91	288	213	71	47	8

Table 14 Study population of married/cohabiting women aged 16 and over - person years at risk: age and economic position of partner one year ago

Economic position of partner 1 year ago	Total	16-24	25-44	45-64	65-74	75-84	85 and over
Working full time	**74,609**	5,119	44,454	24,217	750	68	1
Working part time	**1,585**	53	321	840	325	45	1
Waiting/seeking work	**3,165**	470	1,760	889	44	2	-
Long-term sick	**3,079**	41	710	2,107	201	21	-
Home/family	**268**	17	141	95	12	3	1
Other	**19,155**	96	349	6,226	8,978	3,223	284
Not stated	**750**	97	315	214	69	46	9

Table 15 Study population of married/cohabiting women aged 16 and over - person years at risk: age and own social class (as defined by occupation)

Own social class	Total	16-24	25-44	45-64	65-74	75-84	85 and over
I & II	**25,310**	947	14,083	8,182	1,580	479	39
IIIN	**35,194**	2,403	17,560	11,450	2,920	811	50
IIIM	**7,859**	565	3,195	2,664	1,031	370	33
IV & V	**24,936**	1,403	10,215	9,284	3,064	893	77
Other	**9,288**	572	2,984	2,997	1,782	855	98
Not known	**25**	3	10	9	2	-	-

Table 16 Study population aged 0-15 - person years at risk:
age, sex and household composition

Household composition	Persons, by age-group			By age-group and sex			
	Total	0-4	5-15	0-4		5-15	
				Male	Female	Male	Female
Living with sole adult	**10,191**	3,197	6,993	1,644	1,553	3,524	3,469
Not living with sole adult	**77,340**	26,228	51,112	13,430	12,799	26,059	25,053
Not applicable/not stated	**9,622**	2,708	6,914	1,383	1,325	3,735	3,180

Table 17 Study population aged 0-15 - person years at risk:
age, sex and economic position of parent/guardian last week

Economic position of parent/guardian last week	Persons, by age-group			By age-group and sex			
	Total	0-4	5-15	0-4		5-15	
				Male	Female	Male	Female
Working full time	**66,900**	22,241	44,659	11,410	10,831	22,856	21,803
Working part time	**3,307**	742	2,565	373	370	1,288	1,277
Waiting/seeking work	**7,816**	2,848	4,969	1,467	1,381	2,459	2,509
Long term sick	**1,617**	324	1,293	161	163	652	641
Home/family	**6,909**	2,988	3,921	1,530	1,458	1,988	1,933
Other	**898**	254	644	119	135	319	325
Not stated	**9,705**	2,736	6,969	1,397	1,339	3,755	3,213

Table 18 Study population aged 0-15 - person years at risk:
age, sex and economic position of parent/guardian one year ago

Economic position of parent/guardian 1 year ago	Persons, by age-group			By age-group and sex			
	Total	0-4	5-15	0-4		5-15	
				Male	Female	Male	Female
Working full time	**70,864**	23,859	47,005	12,228	11,631	24,037	22,967
Working part time	**3,197**	705	2,492	370	335	1,244	1,248
Waiting/seeking work	**4,565**	1,558	3,008	816	742	1,499	1,509
Long term sick	**1,438**	287	1,151	146	141	583	568
Home/family	**6,473**	2,719	3,755	1,383	1,335	1,890	1,865
Other	**857**	252	604	112	140	285	319
Not stated	**9,759**	2,754	7,005	1,401	1,353	3,780	3,226

Table 19 Patients consulting - rates per 10,000 person years at risk:
ICD chapter and category of severity by age and sex

Disease group	Persons, by age group								
	Total	0-4	5-15	16-24	25-44	45-64	65-74	75-84	85 and over
All diseases and conditions (I-XVIII)	7,803	10,221	7,234	7,572	7,357	7,610	8,271	9,050	9,193
Serious	1,984	1,289	985	966	1,246	2,625	4,258	5,304	5,843
Intermediate	5,385	7,624	4,950	5,014	4,947	5,269	5,999	6,365	6,328
Minor	6,169	9,042	5,191	6,192	5,931	5,886	6,151	7,215	7,388
All illnesses (I-XVII)	7,270	9,481	6,938	6,907	6,707	7,162	7,905	8,534	8,745
I Infectious and parasitic diseases (001-139)	1,399	3,648	1,888	1,602	1,298	789	776	794	906
Serious	9	15	6	5	9	12	9	17	19
Intermediate	1,154	3,277	1,511	1,332	1,064	604	612	668	766
Minor	297	570	483	330	275	198	173	128	130
II Neoplasms (140-239)	239	54	88	133	218	317	452	555	524
Serious	90	5	4	7	25	130	300	433	436
Intermediate	155	50	84	127	195	198	171	144	99
Minor	-	-	-	-	-	-	-	-	-
III Endocrine, nutritional and metabolic diseases and immunity disorders (240-279)	377	60	43	120	277	682	907	776	633
Serious	185	11	12	36	93	306	575	603	497
Intermediate	205	49	31	87	191	407	367	194	149
Minor	-	-	-	-	-	-	-	-	-
IV Diseases of blood and blood-forming organs (280-289)	97	58	56	55	74	88	182	327	408
Serious	8	7	8	5	5	7	18	16	15
Intermediate	90	51	48	50	68	81	165	311	395
Minor	-	-	-	-	-	-	-	-	-
V Mental disorders (290-319)	728	228	194	611	824	946	919	1,154	1,484
Serious	113	1	4	65	103	136	161	389	771
Intermediate	520	143	152	452	624	700	627	637	608
Minor	159	88	42	137	172	201	222	241	287
VI Diseases of the nervous system and sense organs (320-389)	1,732	4,252	1,881	1,067	1,258	1,549	2,078	2,460	2,505
Serious	199	32	41	78	125	241	478	794	877
Intermediate	964	2,963	1,426	594	656	728	880	918	913
Minor	793	2,014	599	484	610	764	1,033	1,167	1,230
VII Diseases of the circulatory system (390-459)	931	19	26	146	376	1,488	3,035	3,556	3,570
Serious	367	6	6	20	49	482	1,303	2,027	2,662
Intermediate	640	10	10	116	324	1,107	2,081	2,017	1,274
Minor	17	4	10	11	10	15	34	67	105
VIII Diseases of the respiratory system (460-519)	3,070	6,471	3,680	3,120	2,546	2,405	2,817	2,970	3,273
Serious	579	968	785	468	358	485	846	949	1,003
Intermediate	1,284	2,548	1,457	1,281	998	1,056	1,346	1,537	1,832
Minor	1,957	5,234	2,446	2,020	1,680	1,388	1,349	1,240	1,252
IX Diseases of the digestive system (520-579)	866	834	306	632	791	1,038	1,405	1,653	1,804
Serious	229	60	33	103	199	351	469	514	521
Intermediate	378	545	189	303	337	417	545	610	611
Minor	359	270	96	272	331	413	616	785	940
X Diseases of the genitourinary system (580-629)	1,133	570	453	1,279	1,431	1,327	928	1,074	1,237
Serious	31	6	8	33	32	35	49	50	83
Intermediate	813	410	321	954	1,059	771	796	982	1,126
Minor	409	176	147	428	516	685	142	95	114
XI Complications of pregnancy, childbirth and the puerperium (630-679)	108	7	5	247	240	5	2	1	3
Serious	19	-	1	42	42	1	-	-	1
Intermediate	94	7	4	221	210	2	1	0	1
Minor	5	0	0	7	11	2	1	0	-

By age-group and sex

Total		0-4		5-15		16-24		25-44		45-64		65-74		75-84		85 and over	
Male	Female	Male	Female	Male	Female	Male	Female	Male	Female	Male	Female	Male	Female	Male	Female	Male	Female
6,999	8,575	10,245	10,197	7,026	7,452	6,192	8,942	6,072	8,651	6,922	8,310	8,127	8,389	9,001	9,079	9,086	9,228
1,841	2,121	1,489	1,079	1,113	851	879	1,053	1,077	1,417	2,491	2,761	4,330	4,199	5,429	5,229	6,192	5,727
4,626	6,113	7,678	7,567	4,742	5,168	3,904	6,116	3,759	6,145	4,571	5,981	5,666	6,270	6,033	6,564	6,139	6,391
5,179	7,118	9,126	8,953	4,907	5,489	4,361	8,011	4,388	7,485	5,024	6,764	5,909	6,348	7,138	7,262	7,369	7,394
6,613	7,901	9,546	9,411	6,786	7,098	5,928	7,879	5,678	7,743	6,514	7,821	7,743	8,037	8,418	8,604	8,658	8,773
1,137	1,650	3,601	3,697	1,767	2,016	1,073	2,128	847	1,752	607	976	682	853	711	843	814	936
-	-	16	14	8	4	5	4	7	10	12	11	12	7	27	10	6	24
-	-	3,214	3,343	1,418	1,608	810	1,851	590	1,542	406	806	482	718	564	730	701	788
1,188	1,722	578	561	438	530	298	360	280	270	207	188	209	145	140	120	113	136
190	286	49	60	83	92	87	179	137	300	242	393	481	429	680	480	701	465
-	-	4	6	3	5	6	8	17	34	101	160	336	271	571	351	612	378
195	293	46	54	80	88	81	172	121	269	148	248	169	174	136	149	107	97
-	-	-	-	-	-	-	-	-	-	-	-	-	-	-	-	-	-
305	446	63	57	36	50	56	184	197	357	591	774	837	964	764	783	695	613
-	-	12	11	10	14	28	44	59	127	246	367	495	641	548	636	487	500
313	464	52	46	26	37	29	145	141	242	363	451	370	366	229	173	220	126
-	-	-	-	-	-	-	-	-	-	-	-	-	-	-	-	-	-
49	143	61	55	51	62	9	100	13	135	41	136	151	207	240	379	357	426
-	-	10	4	9	8	3	6	3	7	7	8	14	21	18	15	30	10
49	144	52	51	42	55	6	93	10	128	34	129	138	187	223	364	333	416
-	-	-	-	-	-	-	-	-	-	-	-	-	-	-	-	-	-
503	944	256	199	196	192	400	819	533	1,117	681	1,216	632	1,152	814	1,357	1,290	1,549
-	-	1	1	5	3	69	61	86	119	104	169	106	205	311	435	677	802
-	-	166	119	159	144	287	616	391	860	504	900	432	785	417	769	511	640
541	1,033	93	83	34	50	74	199	101	244	128	275	149	282	163	288	238	303
1,538	1,919	4,305	4,197	1,762	2,007	817	1,316	975	1,543	1,339	1,763	2,039	2,111	2,533	2,416	2,526	2,498
-	-	33	41	41	41	70	86	99	150	215	268	451	499	808	786	891	873
-	-	3,023	2,900	1,345	1,512	412	775	433	880	546	914	769	971	847	960	856	932
1,731	2,171	2,041	1,986	537	665	400	567	536	685	725	803	1,122	960	1,309	1,082	1,278	1,214
839	1,020	19	19	25	27	102	191	310	443	1,500	1,477	3,136	2,952	3,516	3,580	3,768	3,505
-	-	6	6	5	6	12	28	49	48	614	348	1,631	1,037	2,332	1,844	3,048	2,534
-	-	10	9	10	11	83	150	263	386	1,011	1,205	1,901	2,227	1,691	2,212	1,070	1,342
930	1,114	4	4	10	10	8	14	5	16	14	16	38	30	79	60	101	106
2,722	3,404	6,643	6,290	3,552	3,814	2,524	3,712	1,956	3,140	1,979	2,838	2,743	2,877	3,192	2,837	3,714	3,127
-	-	1,110	820	895	670	434	502	311	406	453	517	958	754	1,193	804	1,498	839
-	-	2,707	2,381	1,327	1,595	1,031	1,529	782	1,215	884	1,230	1,349	1,344	1,714	1,432	2,092	1,746
3,388	4,233	5,311	5,154	2,326	2,572	1,526	2,510	1,186	2,177	1,031	1,752	1,167	1,496	1,153	1,292	1,272	1,245
757	971	870	796	299	314	444	819	645	938	943	1,134	1,410	1,400	1,693	1,629	2,056	1,720
-	-	78	40	37	30	98	107	206	193	368	333	538	412	627	446	677	469
-	-	570	519	191	186	231	375	282	392	375	460	516	569	558	642	618	609
842	1,084	264	276	81	111	148	396	218	446	325	504	585	642	782	787	1,064	898
359	1,876	656	480	310	604	189	2,362	250	2,621	337	2,335	647	1,157	894	1,182	1,087	1,287
-	-	8	4	7	10	10	55	23	41	35	34	59	41	63	42	131	67
-	-	366	457	206	443	157	1,746	205	1,920	292	1,259	581	971	831	1,073	981	1,174
373	2,097	321	23	114	182	26	827	29	1,008	21	1,362	31	232	33	133	24	144
-	211	-	15	-	10	-	492	-	482	-	9	-	4	-	1	-	4
-	-	-	-	-	1	-	84	-	85	-	1	-	-	-	-	-	2
-	-	-	14	-	8	-	441	-	423	-	4	-	1	-	1	-	2
-	231	-	1	-	1	-	14	-	21	-	4	-	2	-	1	-	-

159

Table 19 - *continued*

Disease group	Persons, by age group								
	Total	0-4	5-15	16-24	25-44	45-64	65-74	75-84	85 and over
XII Diseases of the skin and subcutaneous tissue (680-709)	1,455	2,715	1,418	1,697	1,288	1,177	1,387	1,472	1,613
Serious	-	-	-	-	-	-	-	-	-
Intermediate	1,100	2,295	1,014	1,339	950	852	1,044	1,110	1,235
Minor	455	602	498	477	421	407	451	473	506
XIII Diseases of the musculoskeletal system and connective tissue (710-739)	1,521	161	489	842	1,393	2,354	2,702	2,945	2,811
Serious	534	5	16	80	272	986	1,457	1,707	1,709
Intermediate	931	102	375	629	1,007	1,396	1,280	1,314	1,127
Minor	275	57	115	180	252	383	496	523	487
XIV Congenital anomalies (740-759)	53	217	59	33	34	42	46	46	44
Serious	29	129	37	17	14	21	30	30	36
Intermediate	24	93	23	16	20	21	16	17	9
Minor	-	-	-	-	-	-	-	-	-
XV Certain conditions originating in the perinatal period (760-779)	13	173	0	2	2	0	-	3	-
Serious	3	40	0	0	1	0	-	3	-
Intermediate	10	136	0	2	1	0	-	-	-
Minor	-	-	-	-	-	-	-	-	-
XVI Symptoms, signs and ill-defined conditions (780-799)	1,510	2,721	1,363	1,246	1,195	1,403	1,855	2,359	2,900
Serious	7	1	0	-	1	4	23	47	98
Intermediate	216	710	248	146	141	142	211	336	460
Minor	1,357	2,230	1,173	1,146	1,093	1,305	1,708	2,123	2,563
XVII Injury and poisoning (800-999)	1,390	1,293	1,375	1,518	1,375	1,306	1,293	1,632	2,132
Serious	61	66	50	69	48	50	64	119	286
Intermediate	358	472	394	371	310	302	370	500	654
Minor	1,070	854	1,031	1,190	1,098	1,036	955	1,190	1,523
XVIII Supplementary classification of factors influencing health status and contact with health services (VO1-V82)	3,348	5,313	1,140	3,746	3,525	3,254	3,380	4,724	4,402
Serious	-	-	-	-	-	-	-	-	-
Intermediate	-	-	-	-	-	-	-	-	-
Minor	3,348	5,313	1,140	3,746	3,525	3,254	3,380	4,724	4,402

By age-group and sex

Total		0-4		5-15		16-24		25-44		45-64		65-74		75-84		85 and over	
Male	Female	Male	Female	Male	Female	Male	Female	Male	Female	Male	Female	Male	Female	Male	Female	Male	Female
1,271	1,631	2,674	2,758	1,301	1,541	1,413	1,979	1,013	1,566	1,023	1,333	1,329	1,435	1,434	1,495	1,474	1,659
-	-	-	-	-	-	-	-	-	-	-	-	-	-	-	-	-	-
-	-	2,257	2,334	906	1,128	1,091	1,585	735	1,167	759	946	1,025	1,060	1,092	1,121	1,034	1,302
1,354	1,747	594	610	478	520	419	535	337	506	330	485	404	489	444	490	541	495
1,295	1,738	185	135	466	513	724	960	1,222	1,566	2,054	2,660	2,362	2,979	2,469	3,229	2,329	2,971
-	-	6	3	13	19	79	82	238	307	839	1,136	1,195	1,669	1,294	1,954	1,200	1,878
-	-	115	88	357	393	545	713	899	1,116	1,239	1,557	1,150	1,386	1,154	1,410	1,076	1,145
1,458	2,010	67	46	111	119	135	225	192	313	297	470	437	543	487	545	493	485
54	52	265	167	71	46	27	40	29	40	35	48	41	49	34	53	36	47
-	-	177	79	52	21	17	18	13	16	18	23	24	35	21	35	30	37
55	53	93	92	20	26	10	23	16	24	17	25	17	14	15	18	6	10
-	-	-	-	-	-	-	-	-	-	-	-	-	-	-	-	-	-
12	13	168	179	0	0	-	4	0	3	-	1	-	-	3	3	-	-
-	-	47	33	-	0	-	1	0	1	-	1	-	-	3	3	-	-
13	14	125	148	0	-	-	4	-	2	-	0	-	-	-	-	-	-
-	-	-	-	-	-	-	-	-	-	-	-	-	-	-	-	-	-
1,218	1,791	2,734	2,708	1,269	1,461	800	1,689	816	1,577	1,129	1,683	1,659	2,014	2,228	2,437	2,918	2,894
-	-	-	1	1	-	-	-	1	1	4	4	30	17	62	38	125	89
-	-	696	724	242	255	119	174	104	179	118	166	228	198	405	295	553	429
1,273	1,874	2,268	2,190	1,076	1,274	707	1,582	735	1,453	1,038	1,578	1,482	1,891	1,908	2,252	2,496	2,585
1,356	1,423	1,370	1,212	1,480	1,264	1,642	1,396	1,368	1,382	1,169	1,445	1,076	1,470	1,308	1,827	1,830	2,232
-	-	66	66	61	39	98	40	60	37	48	53	38	85	61	155	155	329
-	-	537	405	479	303	466	276	327	293	286	319	326	405	387	568	648	656
1,457	1,520	884	823	1,066	995	1,226	1,155	1,073	1,124	905	1,170	781	1,096	971	1,321	1,331	1,586
2,301	4,353	5,313	5,313	884	1,409	1,256	6,219	1,801	5,262	2,710	3,809	3,367	3,390	4,833	4,659	4,617	4,330
-	-	-	-	-	-	-	-	-	-	-	-	-	-	-	-	-	-
-	-	-	-	-	-	-	-	-	-	-	-	-	-	-	-	-	-
2,301	4,353	5,313	5,313	884	1,409	1,256	6,219	1,801	5,262	2,710	3,809	3,367	3,390	4,833	4,659	4,617	4,330

Patients consulting

**Table 20   Patients consulting - rates per 10,000 person years at risk:
disease related groups by age and sex**

Disease group	Persons, by age group								
	Total	0-4	5-15	16-24	25-44	45-64	65-74	75-84	85 and over
Intestinal infectious diseases (001-009)	404	1,851	388	372	293	209	240	319	439
Tuberculosis (010-018)	2	-	0	1	1	3	4	4	1
Zoonotic bacterial diseases (020-027)	0	0	1	-	0	0	-	-	-
Other bacterial diseases (030-041)	19	59	32	15	13	14	12	16	19
Poliomyelitis and other non-arthropod-borne viral diseases of central nervous system (045-049)	1	2	2	1	2	1	0	-	-
Viral diseases accompanied by exanthem (050-057)	231	841	313	198	167	130	175	176	170
Arthropod-borne viral diseases (060-066)	0	-	-	-	0	-	-	-	-
Other diseases due to viruses and Chlamydiae (070-079)	298	633	783	390	202	110	79	66	55
Rickettsioses and other arthropod- borne diseases (080-088)	1	1	0	0	1	1	1	-	1
Syphilis and other venereal diseases (090-099)	6	2	1	16	8	4	4	1	3
Other spirochaetal diseases (100-104)	0	1	1	0	0	1	0	1	-
Mycoses (110-118)	473	659	278	668	645	327	281	222	197
Helminthiases (120-129)	42	167	135	25	23	5	2	1	4
Other infectious and parasitic diseases (130-136)	87	226	199	97	67	32	16	27	50
Late effects of infectious and parasitic diseases (137-139)	0	0	0	-	0	1	-	1	-
Malignant neoplasm of lip, oral cavity and pharynx (140-149)	1	-	-	-	0	2	4	5	3
Malignant neoplasm of digestive organs and peritoneum (150-159)	13	-	0	0	1	15	48	84	86
Malignant neoplasm of respiratory and intrathoracic organs (160-165)	8	-	-	0	0	13	33	36	30
Malignant neoplasm of bone, connective tissue, skin and breast (170-175)	26	0	1	2	9	44	75	110	121
Malignant neoplasm of genitourinary organs (179-189)	17	1	1	1	5	22	54	98	86
Malignant neoplasm of other and unspecified sites (190-199)	17	1	0	0	4	24	62	81	89
Malignant neoplasm of lymphatic and haematopoietic tissue (200-208)	5	2	1	2	2	7	19	21	13
Benign neoplasms (210-229)	126	40	64	112	167	162	120	81	41
Carcinoma in situ (230-234)	6	-	-	1	2	7	21	31	31
Neoplasms of uncertain behaviour (235-238)	5	1	1	3	4	8	12	13	15
Neoplasms of unspecified nature (239)	29	10	20	15	29	36	49	56	46
Disorders of thyroid gland (240-246)	66	2	3	13	45	112	185	168	189
Diseases of other endocrine glands (250-259)	122	3	12	30	59	197	386	421	265
Nutritional deficiencies (260-269)	3	2	2	1	1	3	9	14	19
Other metabolic disorders and immunity disorders (270-279)	200	53	26	78	178	403	372	205	182
Diseases of blood and blood-forming organs (280-289)	97	58	56	55	74	88	182	327	408
Organic psychotic conditions (290-294)	31	0	0	4	6	13	51	257	629
Other psychoses (295-299)	77	0	2	46	84	123	114	143	163
Neurotic disorders, personality disorders and other nonpsychotic mental disorders (300-316)	649	228	191	572	762	852	800	836	839
Mental retardation (317-319)	3	1	1	7	3	3	2	-	1
Inflammatory diseases of the central nervous system (320-326)	3	5	2	1	3	4	1	3	-
Hereditary and degenerative diseases of the central nervous system (330-337)	34	4	6	8	12	36	106	185	222
Other disorders of the central nervous system (340-349)	166	25	125	200	211	189	123	107	95
Disorders of the peripheral nervous system (350-359)	45	1	4	14	47	80	72	85	46
Disorders of the eye and adnexa (360-379)	637	1,980	522	335	392	535	914	1,179	1,283
Diseases of the ear and mastoid process (380-389)	1,012	2,933	1,356	570	683	833	1,065	1,193	1,169
Acute rheumatic fever (390-392)	0	-	0	0	0	0	0	-	-
Chronic rheumatic heart disease (393-398)	5	0	0	-	1	10	18	14	10
Hypertensive disease (401-405)	419	1	1	11	101	811	1,642	1,426	663
Ischaemic heart disease (410-414)	170	0	0	1	16	288	687	765	667
Diseases of pulmonary circulation (415417)	7	-	0	1	3	9	20	33	25
Other forms of heart disease (420-429)	134	6	3	9	15	100	423	964	1,648
Cerebrovascular disease (430-438)	66	-	0	2	4	60	220	465	729
Diseases of arteries, arterioles and capillaries (440-448)	55	4	10	14	18	70	192	245	203
Diseases of veins and lymphatics, and other diseases of circulatory system (451-459)	232	7	11	109	229	332	484	572	521
Acute respiratory infections (460-466)	2,420	6,082	2,861	2,371	1,948	1,829	2,082	2,207	2,539
Other diseases of upper respiratory tract (470-478)	430	328	641	607	441	311	322	225	136
Pneumonia and influenza (480-487)	234	239	187	235	236	230	226	304	473

By age-group and sex

Total		0-4		5-15		16-24		25-44		45-64		65-74		75-84		85 and over	
Male	Female	Male	Female	Male	Female	Male	Female	Male	Female	Male	Female	Male	Female	Male	Female	Male	Female
366	442	1,876	1,825	391	385	284	459	240	345	164	255	185	285	246	363	362	465
2	1	-	-	0	1	1	1	1	1	3	2	7	2	8	1	-	2
0	0	1	-	1	0	-	-	0	-	0	0	-	-	-	-	-	-
16	22	52	67	26	37	13	18	8	18	13	16	12	12	24	12	-	26
1	2	2	1	2	1	2	1	1	3	0	2	1	-	-	-	-	-
193	268	826	858	294	332	133	262	111	224	90	170	149	197	161	185	196	162
-	0	-	-	-	-	-	-	-	0	-	-	-	-	-	-	-	-
281	314	663	601	745	822	319	460	170	234	100	121	80	78	56	71	65	51
1	1	1	-	1	-	-	0	1	1	1	1	2	-	-	-	6	-
9	3	2	1	1	1	24	8	12	5	6	2	2	5	2	1	-	4
0	1	1	1	1	0	0	-	-	1	0	1	-	0	2	-	-	-
287	652	578	742	246	312	281	1,053	294	999	232	424	272	288	220	224	178	203
33	50	142	193	106	165	17	32	14	33	5	6	1	2	1	1	-	6
70	103	221	232	151	250	76	118	48	87	23	42	13	19	21	31	30	57
0	0	1	-	0	-	-	-	0	1	1	0	-	-	-	1	-	-
1	1	-	-	-	-	-	-	0	0	2	2	6	3	7	3	-	4
15	11	-	-	-	0	-	0	1	1	18	12	66	33	121	61	113	77
11	5	-	-	-	-	0	-	1	0	16	10	52	17	66	18	71	16
9	42	-	1	1	1	1	2	3	15	11	77	33	110	68	135	48	146
21	14	-	2	-	3	0	1	5	5	19	26	78	35	196	40	232	37
16	17	1	1	0	0	1	-	3	5	22	25	68	57	106	66	125	77
6	5	2	2	1	1	2	2	2	2	7	7	26	13	26	18	24	10
91	159	37	43	61	68	71	153	104	231	121	203	114	124	68	89	36	43
4	7	-	-	-	-	0	1	0	4	4	9	24	18	29	33	42	28
5	5	1	1	2	1	3	2	4	4	7	9	17	9	18	10	12	16
23	35	9	11	20	20	10	20	18	39	28	44	50	49	58	54	59	41
17	114	2	2	1	6	3	23	10	80	26	200	55	291	56	235	107	217
124	120	2	4	11	13	28	33	54	65	222	171	432	349	479	386	327	244
2	4	2	2	2	3	0	1	1	2	2	4	8	9	13	15	18	20
171	229	57	48	23	28	26	130	137	220	360	446	374	370	235	187	261	156
49	143	61	55	51	62	9	100	13	135	41	136	151	207	240	379	357	426
22	40	-	1	1	-	4	4	7	6	14	12	45	55	219	280	582	644
54	99	1	-	3	2	40	51	61	108	90	156	64	154	103	167	125	175
444	845	256	199	192	189	365	777	482	1,045	604	1,104	547	1,005	551	1,007	725	877
3	2	1	-	1	1	7	7	4	3	3	2	-	3	-	-	-	2
3	3	5	4	2	1	2	1	3	3	3	4	1	1	3	2	-	-
30	39	5	3	7	6	6	10	9	15	33	38	107	106	224	161	190	232
107	222	24	25	115	135	116	283	114	308	118	261	100	142	104	108	89	97
32	57	1	1	5	3	9	20	28	67	58	102	68	76	84	86	42	47
534	735	1,994	1,965	485	560	255	414	288	495	410	662	761	1,037	1,079	1,239	1,194	1,312
969	1,053	3,003	2,859	1,263	1,454	463	677	586	782	805	862	1,193	961	1,339	1,105	1,307	1,123
0	0	-	-	-	0	0	-	0	0	0	-	-	-	0	-	-	-
3	6	-	1	0	-	-	-	1	0	6	14	15	20	16	12	6	12
357	479	1	1	2	1	9	13	103	99	762	861	1,482	1,773	1,124	1,606	505	715
204	137	-	1	0	-	1	0	23	9	397	176	920	498	915	675	879	597
6	7	-	-	1	-	0	2	1	4	10	9	25	16	41	28	48	18
121	146	6	5	4	2	7	10	15	14	113	87	496	363	1,047	915	1,807	1,596
64	68	-	-	0	-	2	3	3	4	72	46	272	177	546	417	749	723
59	51	4	4	8	12	7	21	11	25	87	53	263	135	321	200	273	179
181	282	7	7	10	11	76	143	163	295	276	389	449	513	531	596	475	536
2,053	2,772	6,191	5,966	2,620	3,115	1,784	2,954	1,389	2,511	1,413	2,253	1,936	2,201	2,268	2,170	2,716	2,480
398	460	349	306	697	581	529	684	354	528	265	359	313	330	243	215	190	118
211	256	259	217	183	190	200	270	206	266	195	266	217	233	311	299	582	437

Patients consulting

163

Table 20 - *continued*

Disease group	Persons, by age group								
	Total	0-4	5-15	16-24	25-44	45-64	65-74	75-84	85 and over
Chronic obstructive pulmonary disease and allied conditions (490-496)	**538**	938	771	449	329	447	779	809	676
Pneumoconioses and other lung diseases due to external agents (500-508)	**1**	-	0	-	0	1	4	4	1
Other diseases of respiratory system (510-519)	**34**	38	10	23	28	39	60	78	80
Diseases of oral cavity, salivary glands and jaws (520-529)	**155**	344	121	153	150	145	139	122	104
Diseases of oesophagus, stomach and duodenum (530-537)	**353**	80	53	210	334	519	698	710	613
Appendicitis (540-543)	**10**	1	20	20	10	4	2	1	-
Hernia of abdominal cavity (550-553)	**70**	70	9	11	34	101	192	237	194
Noninfective enteritis and colitis (555-558)	**34**	43	13	25	36	41	42	44	44
Other diseases of intestines and peritoneum (560-569)	**293**	329	98	237	265	291	446	673	957
Other diseases of digestive system (570-579)	**43**	11	3	16	33	66	93	120	152
Nephritis, nephrotic syndrome and nephrosis (580-589)	**9**	3	2	3	4	9	25	34	67
Other diseases of urinary system (590- 599)	**397**	246	177	424	394	391	572	747	962
Diseases of male genital organs (600-608)	**97**	263	101	54	75	81	127	123	70
Disorders of breast (610-611)	**99**	13	40	87	168	113	47	31	15
Inflammatory disease of female pelvic organs (614-616)	**105**	51	32	183	175	64	43	48	55
Other disorders of female genital tract (617-629)	**574**	12	120	727	840	831	207	201	200
Pregnancy with abortive outcome (630-639)	**25**	0	2	66	53	1	-	-	-
Complications mainly related to pregnancy (640-648)	**47**	-	2	119	101	1	-	-	1
Normal delivery, and other indications for care in pregnancy, labour and delivery (650-659)	**29**	2	1	66	67	0	-	-	-
Complications occurring mainly in the course of labour and delivery (660-669)	**12**	5	0	24	29	0	-	-	-
Complications of the puerperium (670-676)	**18**	0	1	25	47	3	2	1	1
Infections of skin and subcutaneous tissue (680-686)	**348**	580	427	337	306	279	316	394	522
Other inflammatory conditions of skin and subcutaneous tissue (690-698)	**760**	2,098	626	705	638	633	770	715	725
Other diseases of skin and subcutaneous tissue (700-709)	**488**	295	489	832	463	373	458	530	592
Arthropathies and related disorders (710-719)	**612**	49	168	253	374	970	1,442	1,789	1,815
Dorsopathies (720-724)	**591**	28	108	340	674	950	866	821	721
Rheumatism, excluding the back (725-729)	**490**	52	159	267	461	804	827	827	661
Osteopathies, chondropathies and acquired musculoskeletal deformities (730-739)	**65**	37	82	44	39	71	109	140	155
Congenital anomalies (740-759)	**53**	217	59	33	34	42	46	46	44
Certain conditions originating in the perinatal period (760-779)	**13**	173	0	2	2	0	-	3	-
Symptoms, signs and ill-defined conditions (780-789)	**1,387**	2,524	1,273	1,166	1,096	1,264	1,698	2,175	2,580
Nonspecific abnormal findings (790-796)	**144**	297	116	100	115	169	183	143	102
Ill-defined and unknown causes of morbidity and mortality (797-799)	**32**	14	8	14	18	25	55	138	411
Fracture of skull (800-804)	**7**	4	8	16	8	4	3	4	10
Fracture of spine and trunk (805-809)	**17**	1	2	10	15	22	29	48	81
Fracture of upper limb (810-819)	**47**	25	71	58	37	35	51	73	99
Fracture of lower limb (820-829)	**40**	13	25	42	33	39	49	87	235
Dislocation (830-839)	**14**	11	11	20	5	11	11	17	16
Sprains and strains of joints and adjacent muscles (840-848)	**550**	94	407	656	677	622	455	419	385
Intracranial injury, excluding those with skull fracture (850-854)	**23**	78	48	27	11	9	8	15	21
Internal injury of chest, abdomen and pelvis (860-869)	**1**	1	1	2	2	2	2	2	-
Open wound of head, neck and trunk (870-879)	**52**	178	89	47	29	26	28	53	136
Open wound of upper limb (880-887)	**57**	41	54	81	55	53	49	57	81
Open wound of lower limb (890-897)	**34**	23	52	29	19	24	54	104	98
Injury to blood vessels (900-904)	**1**	-	0	1	0	1	1	1	-
Late effects of injuries, poisonings, toxic effects and other external causes (905-909)	**3**	2	2	3	2	3	4	3	7
Superficial injury (910-919)	**154**	208	216	150	119	125	150	218	290
Contusion with intact skin surface (920-924)	**124**	131	167	139	96	93	123	203	334
Crushing injury (925-929)	**7**	16	10	11	6	6	2	3	1
Effects of foreign body entering through orifice (930-939)	**22**	43	24	21	26	18	15	9	12
Burns (940-949)	**26**	68	20	29	22	19	22	27	43
Injury to nerves and spinal cord (950-957)	**6**	9	2	6	7	7	5	7	1

Patients consulting

By age-group and sex

Total		0-4		5-15		16-24		25-44		45-64		65-74		75-84		85 and over	
Male	Female	Male	Female	Male	Female	Male	Female	Male	Female	Male	Female	Male	Female	Male	Female	Male	Female
553	524	1,075	794	876	661	417	480	285	374	417	479	886	691	1,032	676	1,105	534
1	0	-	-	0	0	-	-	0	0	2	0	6	1	9	1	6	-
31	37	43	33	10	11	19	27	22	35	34	44	62	59	97	66	107	71
129	181	351	337	110	132	107	199	114	185	111	179	120	155	103	133	83	110
339	367	82	77	57	48	201	220	325	343	504	535	726	675	712	709	677	591
9	10	1	1	21	20	17	24	8	12	4	5	2	1	-	2	-	-
89	51	94	44	14	4	19	4	44	23	134	68	254	141	352	168	327	150
30	38	42	44	14	12	21	29	29	42	37	44	44	41	38	48	36	47
200	383	335	323	86	111	97	375	147	384	205	378	374	504	633	697	1,004	942
36	50	10	13	5	2	11	21	26	40	55	78	92	94	131	114	196	138
10	8	5	1	2	1	3	2	4	4	11	7	30	20	44	28	119	49
157	628	149	347	78	281	63	782	99	691	176	611	383	725	603	833	767	1,026
197	-	513	-	197	-	108	-	149	-	161	-	284	-	329	-	279	-
13	181	7	20	41	38	19	155	5	333	8	220	7	80	10	43	18	14
0	206	-	104	-	65	-	364	0	351	-	128	-	77	-	76	-	73
0	1,125	-	25	-	247	-	1,450	-	1,686	0	1,677	-	375	-	322	-	266
-	49	-	1	-	4	-	131	-	107	-	2	-	-	-	-	-	-
-	91	-	-	-	4	-	238	-	202	-	1	-	-	-	-	-	2
-	58	-	4	-	1	-	132	-	135	-	0	-	-	-	-	-	-
-	24	-	9	-	0	-	48	-	58	-	1	-	-	-	-	-	-
-	36	-	1	-	2	-	50	-	94	-	5	-	4	-	1	-	2
327	369	625	533	435	420	308	366	274	337	252	308	286	339	344	423	398	563
636	879	2,017	2,183	521	737	452	956	475	802	542	725	750	787	719	713	666	745
424	549	294	296	449	531	786	879	348	579	315	432	442	471	530	529	624	581
477	742	57	40	150	188	241	265	324	424	788	1,156	1,153	1,677	1,320	2,069	1,319	1,980
508	670	30	25	95	121	268	412	574	774	848	1,054	779	936	734	873	683	733
434	544	63	40	155	164	221	312	408	514	710	901	785	861	824	829	671	658
47	81	41	33	93	71	39	48	29	50	44	98	59	149	62	186	71	183
54	52	265	167	71	46	27	40	29	40	35	48	41	49	34	53	36	47
12	13	168	179	0	0	-	4	0	3	-	1	-	-	3	3	-	-
1,112	1,652	2,535	2,513	1,182	1,368	747	1,582	744	1,450	995	1,537	1,513	1,848	2,045	2,252	2,531	2,597
119	168	303	290	103	129	57	143	78	153	151	187	158	204	129	150	125	95
25	39	13	16	10	7	8	19	12	24	21	29	51	58	148	133	475	390
10	5	4	4	9	7	25	6	12	4	4	3	2	4	1	6	6	12
17	16	1	1	3	1	12	7	21	9	24	20	27	30	33	57	48	93
51	43	23	27	86	55	90	26	52	21	27	43	22	75	26	101	59	112
39	41	13	13	32	16	62	22	43	23	36	42	22	71	33	118	119	274
15	12	7	15	10	13	25	16	19	11	12	10	10	12	11	21	18	16
550	549	98	89	412	401	708	604	703	651	574	670	377	517	377	445	333	402
25	20	77	80	64	32	30	24	11	12	7	10	6	10	14	15	18	22
2	1	1	1	2	1	1	2	2	1	2	1	3	1	2	1	-	-
66	38	222	133	119	57	70	24	41	18	28	24	28	28	50	55	137	136
73	41	44	38	70	38	123	40	70	41	63	43	65	36	62	53	119	69
30	38	26	20	65	38	39	19	18	19	18	31	29	73	40	143	48	114
0	1	-	-	1	-	0	1	0	0	0	2	1	1	1	1	-	-
3	2	2	1	4	1	4	2	3	1	3	2	5	4	2	3	-	10
145	162	213	202	235	197	162	138	113	124	102	149	117	178	169	248	267	297
116	132	137	125	190	142	149	130	94	98	76	111	79	158	135	243	303	345
10	5	23	8	11	9	15	6	9	3	8	3	2	2	2	3	6	-
26	19	42	45	25	22	26	16	28	23	22	13	21	10	14	7	24	8
23	29	70	65	19	21	27	31	19	25	14	24	15	28	23	29	24	49
7	5	13	6	2	3	6	5	8	5	8	7	6	5	8	6	-	2

Table 20 - *continued*

Disease group	Persons, by age group								
	Total	0-4	5-15	16-24	25-44	45-64	65-74	75-84	85 and over
Certain traumatic complications and unspecified injuries (958-959)	**47**	30	54	64	46	38	41	51	93
Poisoning by drugs, medicaments and biological substances (960-979)	**2**	5	1	3	2	2	3	6	9
Toxic effects of substances chiefly nonmedicinal as to source (980-989)	**6**	3	6	9	6	5	5	5	6
Other and unspecified effects of external causes (990-995)	**309**	451	305	302	261	264	316	489	726
Complications of surgical and medical care not elsewhere classified (996-999)	**46**	25	17	32	57	52	60	77	64
Persons with potential health hazards related to communicable diseases (V01-V07)	**1,380**	4,546	790	567	798	1,247	2,435	2,805	2,604
Persons encountering health services in circumstances related to reproduction and development (V20-V28)	**967**	1,838	81	2,598	1,567	78	3	1	1
Persons encountering health services for specific procedures and aftercare (V50-V59)	**0**	-	-	-	0	0	-	1	1
Persons encountering health services in other circumstances (V60-V68)	**613**	74	55	616	814	1,046	364	325	271
Persons without reported diagnosis encountered during examination and investigation of individuals and populations (V70-V82)	**1,210**	223	267	1,182	1,377	1,559	1,117	2,599	2,290

By age-group and sex

Total		0-4		5-15		16-24		25-44		45-64		65-74		75-84		85 and over	
Male	Female	Male	Female	Male	Female	Male	Female	Male	Female	Male	Female	Male	Female	Male	Female	Male	Female
51	43	30	29	62	47	84	44	54	38	37	40	33	47	33	62	89	95
2	3	4	5	0	1	2		1	2	1	2	3	3	3	7	12	8
5	6	5	2	7	5	7	10	4	7	5	4	3	7	3	6	18	2
247	368	470	431	294	317	241	362	194	329	188	341	255	367	364	564	576	776
41	51	35	13	17	16	22	42	37	76	49	56	71	51	112	55	131	41
1,228	1,526	4,555	4,537	586	1,005	447	687	653	945	1,088	1,409	2,417	2,451	3,000	2,688	2,734	2,561
154	1,747	1,804	1,875	10	155	10	5,169	64	3,080	8	150	3	3	1	1	-	2
0	0	-	-	-	-	-	-	-	0	-	0	-	-	1	1	6	-
621	604	78	69	48	62	521	710	756	872	1,154	937	473	275	344	313	362	240
681	1,718	215	231	272	263	394	1,964	557	2,203	955	2,174	1,002	1,211	2,583	2,609	2,365	2,266

Patients consulting

**Table 21 Patients consulting - rates per 10,000 person years at risk:
first 3 ICD digits by age and sex**

Disease group	Persons, by age group								
	Total	0-4	5-15	16-24	25-44	45-64	65-74	75-84	85 and over
Cholera (001)	0	1	-	-	-	-	-	-	-
Typhoid and paratyphoid fevers (002)	0	-	-	1	-	0	-	-	-
Other salmonella infections (003)	3	8	1	3	4	4	1	2	4
Shigellosis (004)	2	6	4	0	1	0	1	-	-
Other food poisoning (bacterial) (005)	2	1	1	2	3	2	2	1	1
Amoebiasis (006)	0	-	-	0	0	0	0	-	-
Other protozoal intestinal diseases (007)	1	4	1	1	1	1	-	-	-
Intestinal infections due to other organisms (008)	7	21	6	7	6	5	5	5	4
Ill-defined intestinal infections (009)	394	1,827	379	362	281	201	234	313	435
Primary tuberculous infection (010)	0	-	-	-	0	-	0	-	-
Pulmonary tuberculosis (011)	1	-	0	0	1	2	4	2	1
Other respiratory tuberculosis (012)	0	-	-	-	0	0	-	-	-
Tuberculosis of meninges and central nervous system (013)	0	-	-	0	0	0	-	-	-
Tuberculosis of bones and joints (015)	0	-	-	0	0	0	-	-	-
Tuberculosis of genitourinary system (016)	0	-	-	-	-	0	-	1	-
Tuberculosis of other organs (017)	0	-	0	0	0	0	-	0	-
Miliary tuberculosis (018)	0	-	-	-	-	-	-	0	-
Anthrax (022)	0	-	-	-	-	0	-	-	-
Brucellosis (023)	0	-	-	-	-	0	-	-	-
Other zoonotic bacterial diseases (027)	0	0	1	-	0	-	-	-	-
Leprosy (030)	0	-	-	0	-	-	-	-	-
Diseases due to other mycobacteria (031)	0	-	0	-	0	-	1	-	-
Diphtheria (032)	0	-	0	-	-	-	-	-	-
Whooping cough (033)	1	12	4	0	0	-	-	-	-
Streptococcal sore throat and scarlatina (034)	10	34	23	11	6	3	2	2	1
Erysipelas (035)	3	3	1	2	2	5	7	4	4
Meningococcal infection (036)	1	2	1	0	1	0	-	0	-
Tetanus (037)	1	-	0	0	0	1	0	1	1
Septicaemia (038)	1	2	0	0	0	1	2	7	12
Actinomycotic infections (039)	1	-	0	0	1	1	-	-	-
Other bacterial diseases (040)	0	-	-	0	0	0	-	-	-
Bacterial infection in conditions classified elsewhere and of unspecified site (041)	2	7	2	2	1	2	1	2	-
Acute poliomyelitis (045)	0	-	-	-	0	0	-	-	-
Slow virus infection of central nervous system (046)	0	-	-	0	0	-	-	-	-
Meningitis due to enterovirus (047)	0	1	0	1	1	0	-	-	-
Other non-arthropod-borne viral diseases of central nervous system (049)	1	1	1	1	1	1	0	-	-
Cowpox and paravaccinia (051)	0	0	0	-	0	0	-	-	-
Chickenpox (052)	70	470	151	54	30	4	1	3	-
Herpes zoster (053)	49	10	27	24	29	63	119	138	146
Herpes simplex (054)	81	80	77	108	102	62	55	34	24
Measles (055)	4	42	4	1	0	0	-	-	-
Rubella (056)	7	56	15	4	1	0	0	0	-
Other viral exanthemata (057)	24	212	44	8	7	2	1	2	-
Mosquito-borne viral encephalitis (062)	0	-	-	-	0	-	-	-	-
Viral hepatitis (070)	4	1	6	5	5	3	2	2	1
Rabies (071)	0	-	-	-	0	-	-	-	-
Mumps (072)	4	23	10	2	1	1	1	1	1
Ornithosis (073)	0	-	-	-	0	0	-	-	-
Specific diseases due to Coxsackie virus (074)	10	86	10	5	5	3	1	0	3
Infectious mononucleosis (075)	11	3	16	46	7	1	1	-	-
Trachoma (076)	0	-	-	-	-	0	-	-	-
Other diseases of conjunctiva due to viruses and Chlamydiae (077)	0	0	0	0	0	-	-	0	-
Other diseases due to viruses and Chlamydiae (078)	205	204	635	283	141	76	55	42	22
Viral infection in conditions classified elsewhere and of unspecified site (079)	69	331	120	53	45	28	21	20	27
Other rickettsioses (083)	0	-	0	-	0	-	-	-	-
Malaria (084)	1	1	0	0	1	1	1	-	1
Relapsing fever (087)	0	-	-	-	0	0	0	-	-

By age-group and sex

Total		0-4		5-15		16-24		25-44		45-64		65-74		75-84		85 and over	
Male	Female	Male	Female	Male	Female	Male	Female	Male	Female	Male	Female	Male	Female	Male	Female	Male	Female
-	0	-	1	-	-	-	-	-	-	-	-	-	-	-	-	-	-
-	0	-	-	-	-	-	1	-	-	-	0	-	-	-	-	-	-
3	3	6	10	1	1	4	2	5	3	3	4	1	2	3	1	12	2
1	2	5	6	4	5	-	1	1	2	0	0	1	0	-	-	-	-
2	2	1	1	1	1	2	2	3	3	2	1	1	4	-	2	6	-
0	0	-	-	-	-	0	0	-	0	0	1	-	0	-	-	-	-
1	1	4	4	2	1	0	2	1	1	1	1	-	-	-	-	-	-
7	7	18	23	9	3	6	8	6	7	5	6	5	4	6	5	6	4
356	431	1,853	1,799	379	378	276	447	230	333	157	246	179	279	242	356	357	461
0	0	-	-	-	-	-	-	-	0	-	-	1	-	-	-	-	-
1	1	-	-	0	-	-	0	1	1	3	1	6	2	5	1	-	2
-	0	-	-	-	-	-	-	-	0	-	0	-	-	-	-	-	-
0	0	-	-	-	-	0	-	-	0	0	-	-	-	-	-	-	-
0	0	-	-	-	-	-	0	0	-	0	0	-	-	-	-	-	-
0	-	-	-	-	-	-	-	-	-	0	-	-	-	2	-	-	-
0	0	-	-	1	0	0	0	0	0	-	0	-	-	-	-	1	-
0	-	-	-	-	-	-	-	-	-	-	-	-	-	1	-	-	-
-	0	-	-	-	-	-	0	-	-	-	-	-	0	-	-	-	-
0	0	-	-	0	-	-	-	-	0	-	-	1	0	-	-	-	-
0	-	-	-	0	-	-	-	0	-	-	-	-	-	-	-	-	-
1	2	9	15	3	5	-	0	0	1	-	-	-	-	-	-	-	-
8	11	30	38	19	27	8	13	4	9	2	3	1	2	1	2	-	2
3	3	3	3	-	2	2	1	1	3	5	5	6	7	8	2	-	6
1	0	2	2	1	0	0	0	1	0	0	0	-	-	-	1	-	-
1	1	-	-	0	-	0	-	0	0	1	1	-	0	1	1	-	2
1	1	1	2	0	-	1	-	0	0	2	1	2	2	14	3	-	16
0	1	-	-	0	1	-	0	0	2	1	2	-	-	-	-	-	-
0	0	-	-	-	-	-	0	0	0	0	0	-	-	-	-	-	-
2	3	7	7	2	3	1	2	0	3	2	2	2	0	-	3	-	-
0	0	-	-	-	-	-	0	0	-	0	-	-	-	-	-	-	-
0	0	-	-	-	-	0	-	0	0	-	-	-	-	-	-	-	-
0	1	1	-	0	0	1	1	0	1	-	0	-	-	-	-	-	-
1	1	1	1	2	1	1	0	0	1	0	1	1	-	-	-	-	-
0	0	-	1	0	0	-	-	0	-	0	-	-	-	-	-	-	-
72	69	466	473	151	150	49	59	29	30	4	4	-	2	2	4	-	-
41	56	9	11	26	28	23	25	27	31	53	74	99	135	132	142	160	142
50	111	75	85	62	93	56	160	51	154	33	91	48	60	26	38	36	20
4	3	42	41	5	4	1	1	0	0	0	0	-	-	-	-	-	-
6	7	55	57	13	16	1	7	1	2	0	-	-	0	1	-	-	-
24	25	208	216	42	45	4	12	5	8	2	2	1	1	1	2	-	-
-	0	-	-	-	-	-	-	-	0	-	-	-	-	-	-	-	-
5	3	2	1	8	5	7	3	7	3	3	2	2	1	1	2	-	2
-	0	-	-	-	-	-	-	-	0	-	-	-	-	-	-	-	-
4	4	30	16	9	10	2	2	1	1	0	1	-	1	-	1	-	2
-	0	-	-	-	-	-	-	-	0	-	0	-	-	-	-	-	-
11	9	105	66	11	9	4	7	4	5	2	3	-	1	-	1	6	2
10	12	5	1	15	18	37	55	7	7	1	1	-	1	-	-	-	-
0	-	-	-	-	-	-	-	-	-	0	-	-	-	-	-	-	-
0	0	-	1	-	1	-	0	0	-	-	-	-	-	-	-	1	-
195	214	199	209	604	667	242	323	123	159	74	79	61	51	40	44	42	16
61	77	346	316	112	128	30	77	30	60	20	35	17	24	15	23	18	30
0	-	-	-	0	-	-	-	-	0	-	-	-	-	-	-	-	-
1	1	1	-	0	-	-	-	0	0	1	1	1	1	-	-	6	-
0	0	-	-	-	-	-	-	-	-	0	-	0	1	-	-	-	-

169

Table 21 - *continued*

Disease group	Persons, by age group								
	Total	0-4	5-15	16-24	25-44	45-64	65-74	75-84	85 and over
Congenital syphilis (090)	0	0	-	-	-	0	-	-	-
Neurosyphilis (094)	0	-	-	-	-	0	-	-	1
Other and unspecified syphilis (097)	0	-	-	0	0	-	-	-	-
Gonococcal infections (098)	1	0	-	2	1	-	0	0	1
Other venereal diseases (099)	5	1	1	14	7	3	3	1	-
Leptospirosis (100)	0	-	-	0	0	0	-	-	-
Vincent's angina (101)	0	1	1	-	0	1	0	0	-
Yaws (102)	0	-	-	-	-	-	-	0	-
Dermatophytosis (110)	151	109	189	167	162	142	135	82	59
Dermatomycosis, other and unspecified (111)	18	7	16	35	24	10	10	7	1
Candidiasis (112)	313	546	76	483	474	180	140	137	136
Other mycoses (117)	0	1	0	0	0	1	0	0	-
Echinococcosis (122)	0	-	-	0	0	0	-	-	-
Other cestode infection (123)	0	0	0	0	0	-	-	-	-
Filarial infection and dracontiasis (125)	0	1	0	0	0	0	-	-	-
Other intestinal helminthiases (127)	41	163	132	24	23	5	2	1	4
Other and unspecified helminthiases (128)	1	3	2	1	0	-	-	-	-
Toxoplasmosis (130)	0	-	-	-	0	-	0	-	-
Trichomoniasis (131)	3	-	0	4	6	3	1	-	-
Pediculosis and phthirus infestation (132)	32	82	114	27	20	3	1	3	6
Acariasis (133)	34	49	58	57	30	17	8	17	44
Sarcoidosis (135)	1	-	-	0	2	2	2	1	-
Other and unspecified infectious and parasitic diseases (136)	17	97	29	10	10	8	4	7	-
Late effects of acute poliomyelitis (138)	0	0	-	-	0	1	-	1	-
Late effects of other infectious and parasitic diseases (139)	0	-	0	-	-	0	-	-	-
Malignant neoplasm of lip (140)	0	-	-	-	-	-	-	0	-
Malignant neoplasm of tongue (141)	0	-	-	-	-	1	2	1	-
Malignant neoplasm of major salivary glands (142)	0	-	-	-	-	1	1	2	1
Malignant neoplasm of gum (143)	0	-	-	-	0	0	1	1	1
Malignant neoplasm of floor of mouth (144)	0	-	-	-	0	0	-	-	-
Malignant neoplasm of other and unspecified parts of mouth (145)	0	-	-	-	0	0	0	-	-
Malignant neoplasm of oropharynx (146)	0	-	-	-	-	0	0	0	-
Malignant neoplasm of nasopharynx (147)	0	-	-	-	-	0	0	-	-
Malignant neoplasm of other and ill-defined sites within the lip, oral cavity and pharynx (149)	0	-	-	-	-	0	1	-	-
Malignant neoplasm of oesophagus (150)	2	-	-	-	0	2	7	11	12
Malignant neoplasm of stomach (151)	2	-	-	-	-	2	10	19	15
Malignant neoplasm of small intestine, including duodenum (152)	0	-	-	-	-	-	0	-	-
Malignant neoplasm of colon (153)	5	-	0	0	0	7	18	32	33
Malignant neoplasm of rectum, rectosigmoid junction and anus (154)	3	-	-	-	0	3	10	17	21
Malignant neoplasm of liver and intrahepatic bile ducts (155)	0	-	-	-	0	0	0	0	1
Malignant neoplasm of gallbladder and extrahepatic bile ducts (156)	0	-	-	-	-	0	-	1	-
Malignant neoplasm of pancreas (157)	1	-	-	-	-	1	3	6	6
Malignant neoplasm of other and ill-defined sites within the digestive organs and peritoneum (159)	0	-	-	-	-	0	0	-	-
Malignant neoplasm of nasal cavities, middle ear and accessory sinuses (160)	0	-	-	-	-	-	-	0	-
Malignant neoplasm of larynx (161)	1	-	-	-	0	2	3	2	-
Malignant neoplasm of trachea, bronchus and lung (162)	7	-	-	0	0	11	29	33	30
Malignant neoplasm of pleura (163)	0	-	-	-	-	-	0	-	-
Malignant neoplasm of thymus, heart and mediastinum (164)	0	-	-	-	-	-	0	-	-
Malignant neoplasm of bone and articular cartilage (170)	0	0	0	-	0	0	1	1	-
Malignant neoplasm of connective and other soft tissue (171)	0	-	0	0	-	0	0	0	-
Malignant melanoma of skin (172)	2	-	0	1	2	4	4	4	6
Other malignant neoplasm of skin (173)	7	-	-	0	1	9	25	49	50
Malignant neoplasm of female breast (174)	15	-	-	-	5	30	45	55	65
Malignant neoplasm of male breast (175)	0	-	-	-	-	-	1	1	-

Patients consulting

By age-group and sex

Total		0-4		5-15		16-24		25-44		45-64		65-74		75-84		85 and over	
Male	Female	Male	Female	Male	Female	Male	Female	Male	Female	Male	Female	Male	Female	Male	Female	Male	Female
0	0	-	1	-	-	-	-	-	-	0	-	-	-	-	-	-	-
0	0	-	-	-	-	-	-	-	-	0	0	-	-	-	-	-	2
0	-	-	-	-	-	0	-	0	-	-	-	-	-	-	-	-	-
1	1	1	-	-	-	2	1	1	1	-	-	-	0	1	-	-	2
8	3	2	-	1	1	22	6	11	4	5	1	2	4	1	1	-	-
0	0	-	-	-	-	0	-	-	0	-	0	-	-	-	-	-	-
0	1	1	1	1	0	-	-	-	-	1	0	1	-	0	1	-	-
0	-	-	-	-	-	-	-	-	-	-	-	-	-	1	-	-	-
177	126	119	99	202	175	182	152	197	126	163	121	173	104	105	68	71	55
17	19	9	6	14	18	27	42	22	25	11	10	13	7	5	8	-	2
97	521	452	644	31	123	76	887	81	870	60	302	90	181	116	150	107	146
0	1	1	1	-	1	0	0	0	0	0	1	-	0	-	1	-	-
-	0	-	-	-	-	-	0	-	0	-	0	-	-	-	-	-	-
0	0	-	1	1	-	-	0	-	0	-	-	-	-	-	-	-	-
0	0	1	-	0	0	-	0	-	0	0	-	-	-	-	-	-	-
32	49	139	188	103	163	17	31	13	33	5	5	1	2	1	1	-	6
1	1	2	4	2	3	1	0	0	0	-	-	-	-	-	-	-	-
0	0	-	-	-	-	-	-	0	0	-	-	-	0	-	-	-	-
1	6	-	-	-	1	1	7	1	11	0	5	-	1	-	-	-	-
22	42	64	102	71	159	21	33	12	28	2	3	-	2	2	3	-	8
29	38	50	47	51	66	45	69	24	35	13	21	8	8	15	18	30	49
1	1	-	-	-	-	0	0	2	2	1	3	1	2	-	1	-	-
18	17	108	86	31	27	8	11	8	11	6	10	4	4	3	9	-	-
0	0	1	-	-	-	-	-	0	1	1	0	-	-	-	1	-	-
0	0	-	-	0	-	-	-	-	-	-	0	-	-	-	-	-	-
0	-	-	-	-	-	-	-	-	-	-	-	-	-	1	-	-	-
0	0	-	-	-	-	-	-	-	-	1	0	3	1	-	1	-	-
0	0	-	-	-	-	-	-	-	-	1	0	1	0	3	1	-	2
0	0	-	-	-	-	-	-	0	-	-	0	1	0	2	-	-	2
0	0	-	-	-	-	-	-	0	-	-	0	-	-	-	-	-	-
0	0	-	-	-	-	-	-	0	0	-	-	0	-	-	-	-	-
0	0	-	-	-	-	-	-	-	-	0	0	1	-	-	1	-	-
-	0	-	-	-	-	-	-	-	-	-	0	-	0	-	-	-	-
0	0	-	-	-	-	-	-	-	-	0	0	1	-	-	-	-	-
2	1	-	-	-	-	-	-	0	-	2	1	10	5	22	4	18	10
3	2	-	-	-	-	-	-	-	-	4	1	16	5	30	12	36	8
0	-	-	-	-	-	-	-	-	-	-	-	1	-	-	-	-	-
5	5	-	-	-	0	-	0	0	0	7	6	23	14	35	29	24	35
3	2	-	-	-	-	-	-	0	0	4	3	14	7	30	10	30	18
0	0	-	-	-	-	-	-	-	0	0	0	1	-	1	-	-	2
0	0	-	-	-	-	-	-	-	-	0	0	-	-	1	1	-	-
1	1	-	-	-	-	-	-	-	-	1	0	3	3	5	6	6	6
0	0	-	-	-	-	-	-	-	-	0	-	-	0	-	-	-	-
-	0	-	-	-	-	-	-	-	-	-	-	-	-	-	1	-	-
1	0	-	-	-	-	-	-	0	0	3	1	6	1	6	-	-	-
9	5	-	-	-	0	-	0	0	0	14	9	45	15	61	17	71	16
-	0	-	-	-	-	-	-	-	-	-	-	-	0	-	-	-	-
0	-	-	-	-	-	-	-	-	-	-	-	1	-	-	-	-	-
0	0	-	1	0	0	-	-	0	0	0	0	2	1	2	-	-	-
0	0	-	-	-	0	0	-	-	-	-	0	-	0	-	1	-	-
2	3	-	-	1	-	1	2	2	3	3	6	4	4	7	2	-	8
7	8	-	-	-	-	0	-	1	1	9	10	26	24	56	44	48	51
-	30	-	-	-	-	-	-	-	10	-	61	-	81	-	88	-	87
0	-	-	-	-	-	-	-	-	-	-	-	2	-	2	-	-	-

Table 21 - *continued*

Disease group	Persons, by age group								
	Total	0-4	5-15	16-24	25-44	45-64	65-74	75-84	85 and over
Malignant neoplasm of uterus, part unspecified (179)	0	-	-	-	-	1	2	1	3
Malignant neoplasm of cervix uteri (180)	2	-	-	-	2	3	3	4	3
Malignant neoplasm of body of uterus (182)	1	-	-	-	0	2	6	5	1
Malignant neoplasm of ovary and other uterine adnexa (183)	2	1	1	1	1	6	4	4	7
Malignant neoplasm of other and unspecified female genital organs(184)	0	-	-	-	0	0	1	2	-
Malignant neoplasm of prostate (185)	6	-	-	-	-	3	20	51	38
Malignant neoplasm of testis (186)	1	-	-	0	2	2	1	0	-
Malignant neoplasm of penis and other male genital organs (187)	0	-	-	-	-	0	1	0	-
Malignant neoplasm of bladder (188)	4	-	-	-	0	3	14	26	31
Malignant neoplasm of kidney and other and unspecified urinary organs (189)	1	-	-	-	0	2	5	6	1
Malignant neoplasm of eye (190)	0	0	-	-	0	-	0	-	-
Malignant neoplasm of brain (191)	1	-	0	0	1	2	3	2	-
Malignant neoplasm of other and unspecified parts of nervous system (192)	0	-	-	-	-	0	0	-	-
Malignant neoplasm of thyroid gland (193)	1	-	-	-	1	1	1	1	-
Malignant neoplasm of other endocrine glands and related structures (194)	0	-	-	-	-	-	-	0	-
Malignant neoplasm of other and ill-defined sites (195)	8	-	-	0	1	11	30	43	53
Secondary and unspecified malignant neoplasm of lymph nodes (196)	0	-	-	-	0	1	2	1	1
Secondary malignant neoplasm of respiratory and digestive systems (197)	2	0	0	-	0	3	9	10	7
Secondary malignant neoplasm of other specified sites (198)	4	-	-	-	1	5	14	17	16
Malignant neoplasm without specification of site (199)	2	-	-	-	0	2	6	9	10
Lymphosarcoma and reticulosarcoma (200)	0	-	-	-	0	0	0	0	1
Hodgkin's disease (201)	0	-	0	0	0	1	1	1	-
Other malignant neoplasm of lymphoid and histiocytic tissue (202)	1	0	0	1	0	1	2	0	-
Multiple myeloma and immunoproliferative neoplasms (203)	1	-	-	-	0	1	3	6	1
Lymphoid leukaemia (204)	1	1	0	0	0	2	5	7	4
Myeloid leukaemia (205)	1	-	-	0	0	1	3	1	-
Monocytic leukaemia (206)	0	-	-	-	-	0	-	0	1
Other specified leukaemia (207)	0	1	-	0	0	-	1	0	1
Leukaemia of unspecified cell type (208)	1	-	-	1	0	2	4	5	3
Benign neoplasm of lip, oral cavity and pharynx (210)	1	0	0	2	1	2	2	3	-
Benign neoplasm of other parts of digestive system (211)	1	1	0	0	1	2	2	3	1
Benign neoplasm of respiratory and intrathoracic organs (212)	0	-	-	-	0	1	0	0	-
Benign neoplasm of bone and articular cartilage (213)	1	1	1	2	1	2	1	-	-
Lipoma (214)	21	4	3	13	29	34	25	16	9
Other benign neoplasm of connective and other soft tissue (215)	3	1	1	3	5	4	2	1	-
Benign neoplasm of skin (216)	75	21	53	79	96	87	73	45	22
Benign neoplasm of breast (217)	7	0	0	7	14	6	1	0	-
Uterine leiomyoma (218)	6	-	-	0	11	14	0	0	1
Other benign neoplasm of uterus (219)	0	-	-	-	0	0	0	-	-
Benign neoplasm of ovary (220)	1	-	-	1	1	1	1	1	-
Benign neoplasm of other female genital organs (221)	0	0	-	0	1	0	0	0	-
Benign neoplasm of male genital organs (222)	1	-	-	0	1	1	2	0	-
Benign neoplasm of kidney and other urinary organs (223)	1	-	-	0	0	1	2	4	-
Benign neoplasm of eye (224)	0	-	-	0	0	1	1	-	-
Benign neoplasm of brain and other parts of nervous system (225)	1	-	0	0	1	2	3	1	-
Benign neoplasm of thyroid gland (226)	1	-	0	0	1	2	0	0	1
Benign neoplasm of other endocrine glands and related structures (227)	0	-	-	0	0	0	-	-	-
Haemangioma and lymphangioma, any site (228)	4	11	4	3	4	4	3	3	3
Benign neoplasm of other and unspecified sites (229)	2	1	1	2	2	2	3	1	3
Carcinoma in situ of digestive organs (230)	2	-	-	0	0	2	7	15	13
Carcinoma in situ of respiratory system (231)	1	-	-	-	-	1	4	3	1
Carcinoma in situ of skin (232)	0	-	-	-	-	0	0	3	-
Carcinoma in situ of breast and genitourinary system (233)	3	-	-	0	2	4	9	9	16
Carcinoma in situ of other and unspecified sites (234)	0	-	-	-	-	0	1	3	-

By age-group and sex

Total		0-4		5-15		16-24		25-44		45-64		65-74		75-84		85 and over	
Male	Female	Male	Female	Male	Female	Male	Female	Male	Female	Male	Female	Male	Female	Male	Female	Male	Female
-	1	-	-	-	-	-	-	-	-	-	1	-	3	-	2	-	4
-	3	-	-	-	-	-	-	-	3	-	5	-	5	-	7	-	4
-	2	-	-	-	-	-	-	-	0	-	4	-	11	-	8	-	2
-	4	-	2	-	3	-	1	-	1	-	11	-	7	-	6	-	10
-	1	-	-	-	-	-	-	-	0	-	0	-	2	-	3	-	-
11	-	-	-	-	-	-	-	-	-	7	-	45	-	137	-	155	-
3	-	-	-	-	-	0	-	5	-	5	-	1	-	1	-	-	-
0	-	-	-	-	-	-	-	-	-	0	-	2	-	1	-	-	-
6	2	-	-	-	-	-	-	0	-	5	1	27	3	50	12	71	18
1	1	-	-	-	-	-	-	0	-	2	2	3	7	10	3	6	-
0	0	-	1	-	-	-	-	0	0	-	-	1	-	-	-	-	-
1	1	-	-	0	-	0	-	1	1	2	2	3	3	2	2	-	-
0	0	-	-	-	-	-	-	-	-	0	0	-	0	-	-	-	-
0	1	-	-	-	-	-	-	0	1	1	2	1	1	-	2	-	-
0	-	-	-	-	-	-	-	-	-	-	-	-	-	1	-	-	-
8	8	-	-	-	-	0	-	1	1	12	9	34	27	58	34	59	51
0	1	-	-	-	-	-	-	0	-	0	1	1	2	1	1	-	2
2	2	1	-	-	0	-	-	0	1	3	3	9	8	17	6	18	4
3	4	-	-	-	-	-	-	0	1	3	8	13	14	24	13	36	10
1	2	-	-	-	-	-	-	0	0	2	2	6	5	8	9	12	10
0	0	-	-	-	-	-	-	0	-	0	0	1	-	1	-	-	2
1	0	-	-	0	-	0	0	1	0	1	0	2	0	1	1	-	-
1	1	-	1	0	0	1	1	-	0	1	1	3	1	-	1	-	-
1	1	-	-	-	-	-	-	0	1	2	4	3	7	6	-	-	-
2	1	2	1	0	0	0	-	0	0	2	1	8	3	10	5	12	2
0	1	-	-	-	-	-	-	0	0	1	0	1	3	2	1	1	-
0	0	-	-	-	-	-	-	-	-	0	-	-	-	-	1	-	2
0	0	1	1	-	-	-	-	0	0	-	-	1	-	-	1	6	-
1	1	-	-	-	-	1	0	0	1	1	2	3	4	10	1	-	4
2	1	1	-	1	-	2	1	2	1	2	2	2	2	2	3	-	-
1	1	-	1	-	0	-	0	1	1	3	2	2	2	5	2	-	2
0	0	-	-	-	-	-	0	-	0	1	1	1	-	-	-	1	-
1	1	1	1	2	0	2	2	1	2	0	3	1	0	-	-	-	-
22	21	3	4	4	3	14	12	32	25	33	35	17	31	11	19	6	10
3	4	2	1	1	1	2	5	4	7	4	4	1	2	-	1	-	-
55	95	21	21	50	57	47	111	58	135	70	104	75	71	40	47	18	24
0	13	1	-	-	1	0	14	-	27	0	12	-	2	-	1	-	-
-	13	-	-	-	-	-	0	-	22	-	28	-	0	-	1	-	2
-	0	-	-	-	-	-	-	-	0	-	1	-	0	-	-	-	-
-	1	-	-	-	-	-	1	-	2	-	1	-	1	-	1	-	-
-	1	-	1	-	-	-	0	-	2	-	1	-	0	-	1	-	-
1	-	-	-	-	-	1	-	1	-	1	-	4	-	1	-	-	-
1	1	-	-	-	-	0	-	0	0	1	1	2	2	6	3	-	-
0	0	-	-	-	-	0	-	1	0	1	1	1	1	-	-	-	-
1	1	-	-	-	1	-	1	1	2	2	2	3	3	3	1	1	-
0	1	-	-	-	0	-	0	0	2	0	3	-	0	-	1	-	2
0	0	-	-	-	-	0	-	0	0	-	-	-	-	-	-	-	-
3	5	7	15	3	4	1	4	3	5	3	5	5	2	-	5	12	-
2	2	2	-	1	1	2	2	2	1	2	2	1	4	1	1	-	4
2	2	-	-	-	-	0	-	0	0	2	2	9	4	15	14	18	12
1	0	-	-	-	-	-	-	-	-	2	-	5	3	6	1	6	-
0	0	-	-	-	-	-	-	-	-	0	0	-	0	1	3	-	-
1	5	-	-	-	-	1	0	4	1	7	8	10	2	12	18	16	-
0	0	-	-	-	-	-	-	-	-	-	0	2	0	5	1	-	-

Patients consulting

Table 21 - *continued*

Disease group	Persons, by age group								
	Total	0-4	5-15	16-24	25-44	45-64	65-74	75-84	85 and over
Neoplasm of uncertain behaviour of digestive and respiratory systems (235)	1	0	-	0	0	2	2	2	1
Neoplasm of uncertain behaviour of genitourinary organs (236)	1	-	-	1	0	1	2	1	1
Neoplasm of uncertain behaviour of endocrine glands and nervous system (237)	1	1	1	1	1	2	1	1	-
Neoplasm of uncertain behaviour of other and unspecified sites and tissues (238)	3	-	0	0	2	4	7	9	13
Neoplasm of unspecified nature (239)	29	10	20	15	29	36	49	56	46
Simple and unspecified goitre (240)	4	1	1	4	5	6	5	2	4
Nontoxic nodular goitre (241)	2	-	-	0	3	4	1	3	4
Thyrotoxicosis with or without goitre (242)	9	-	-	2	9	14	22	20	15
Congenital hypothyroidism (243)	1	1	1	1	1	1	0	-	-
Acquired hypothyroidism (244)	50	0	2	6	27	87	154	146	167
Thyroiditis (245)	1	-	0	0	2	2	3	1	-
Other disorders of thyroid (246)	2	-	-	1	2	3	4	2	3
Diabetes mellitus (250)	111	1	8	20	41	186	378	412	260
Other disorders of pancreatic internal secretion (251)	5	1	1	3	4	6	9	16	6
Disorders of parathyroid gland (252)	1	-	-	0	0	1	3	2	1
Disorders of the pituitary gland and its hypothalamic control (253)	1	-	1	0	2	2	1	2	3
Disorders of adrenal glands (255)	1	1	0	0	1	1	1	2	1
Ovarian dysfunction (256)	6	-	0	8	12	5	-	-	-
Testicular dysfunction (257)	0	-	0	1	0	0	-	-	-
Polyglandular dysfunction and related disorders (258)	0	-	-	-	0	-	-	-	-
Other endocrine disorders (259)	1	0	2	0	1	0	1	-	-
Nutritional marasmus (261)	0	0	-	-	-	-	1	0	1
Vitamin A deficiency (264)	0	0	0	-	-	-	1	-	-
Thiamine and niacin deficiency states (265)	0	-	-	-	0	0	1	0	-
Deficiency of B-complex components (266)	2	0	0	0	0	3	5	12	15
Ascorbic acid deficiency (267)	0	-	-	-	0	-	0	-	1
Vitamin D deficiency (268)	0	0	0	0	0	-	0	-	-
Other nutritional deficiencies (269)	1	1	2	-	1	0	2	1	1
Disorders of amino-acid transport and metabolism (270)	0	1	1	0	0	0	1	-	-
Disorders of carbohydrate transport and metabolism (271)	3	35	0	0	0	0	-	1	1
Disorders of lipoid metabolism (272)	61	0	2	5	39	172	128	15	-
Disorders of plasma protein metabolism (273)	0	-	-	-	0	0	1	0	4
Gout (274)	40	-	0	1	24	73	117	110	99
Disorders of mineral metabolism (275)	2	1	0	0	1	3	6	5	1
Disorders of fluid, electrolyte, and acid-base balance (276)	16	6	1	6	15	23	27	35	67
Other and unspecified disorders of metabolism (277)	3	6	4	4	2	2	2	1	1
Obesity and other hyperalimentation (278)	82	4	18	61	102	142	103	39	9
Disorders involving the immune mechanism (279)	0	1	-	-	0	0	0	0	-
Iron deficiency anaemias (280)	54	20	10	35	53	51	87	178	246
Other deficiency anaemias (281)	16	1	0	2	5	19	54	94	101
Hereditary haemolytic anaemias (282)	1	1	2	1	1	1	1	1	-
Acquired haemolytic anaemias (283)	0	1	0	1	0	0	1	0	1
Aplastic anaemia (284)	0	-	-	-	0	0	1	1	1
Other and unspecified anaemias (285)	14	7	3	10	11	13	29	48	59
Coagulation defects (286)	1	2	0	-	0	0	2	-	-
Purpura and other haemorrhagic conditions (287)	5	4	6	3	3	4	12	14	12
Diseases of white blood cells (288)	1	0	0	1	0	1	1	0	-
Other diseases of blood and blood-forming organs (289)	9	24	35	4	2	3	3	5	4
Senile and presenile organic psychotic conditions (290)	18	0	-	-	0	4	26	176	434
Alcoholic psychoses (291)	1	-	-	1	2	3	2	-	4
Drug psychoses (292)	2	-	-	3	2	2	3	1	4
Transient organic psychotic conditions (293)	10	-	0	1	2	4	20	80	197
Other organic psychotic conditions (chronic) (294)	2	-	-	0	1	1	1	18	38

Patients consulting

By age-group and sex

Total		0-4		5-15		16-24		25-44		45-64		65-74		75-84		85 and over	
Male	Female	Male	Female	Male	Female	Male	Female	Male	Female	Male	Female	Male	Female	Male	Female	Male	Female
1	1	-	1	-	-	0	0	-	0	2	1	4	1	5	1	-	2
1	0	-	-	-	-	1	1	1	0	1	1	3	0	2	-	6	-
2	1	1	1	1	1	1	1	1	1	2	1	1	1	3	-	-	-
2	3	-	-	1	-	0	-	2	2	2	5	8	6	8	9	12	14
23	35	9	11	20	20	10	20	18	39	28	44	50	49	58	54	59	41
1	7	1	1	0	1	-	9	1	10	1	11	2	7	1	3	-	6
0	4	-	-	-	-	-	1	0	5	1	8	1	1	1	4	6	4
3	15	-	-	-	-	1	4	2	16	5	23	10	31	6	28	18	14
0	1	1	1	1	1	1	1	0	1	-	1	-	0	-	-	-	-
12	86	-	1	-	4	1	11	6	48	19	156	42	245	48	204	89	193
0	2	-	-	-	1	-	1	0	3	0	4	1	4	-	1	-	-
1	3	-	-	-	-	0	1	1	3	1	5	-	8	1	3	-	4
119	102	1	1	8	7	24	15	49	34	217	154	428	337	475	374	327	238
4	5	1	1	0	1	3	3	3	4	6	6	8	10	10	19	12	4
0	1	-	-	-	-	0	-	0	0	-	3	1	5	-	3	-	2
1	1	-	-	1	1	0	-	2	2	2	1	1	1	2	1	-	4
0	1	-	1	-	1	0	-	1	1	0	1	1	1	-	3	-	2
0	11	-	-	-	1	0	15	0	25	-	10	-	-	-	-	-	-
1	-	-	-	1	-	1	-	1	-	1	-	-	-	-	-	-	-
-	0	-	-	-	-	-	-	-	0	-	-	-	-	-	-	-	-
1	1	-	1	1	3	0	0	1	1	0	0	1	-	-	-	-	-
0	0	1	-	-	-	-	-	-	-	-	-	-	1	1	-	-	2
-	0	-	1	-	0	-	-	-	-	-	-	-	1	-	-	-	-
0	0	-	-	-	-	-	-	0	-	-	0	1	0	-	1	-	-
1	3	1	-	-	0	-	1	-	1	2	3	5	5	11	12	18	14
0	0	-	-	-	-	-	-	-	0	-	-	1	-	-	-	-	2
0	0	-	1	-	0	0	-	0	0	-	-	-	0	-	-	-	-
1	1	1	1	2	2	-	-	0	1	-	0	2	2	-	2	-	2
0	0	1	1	1	-	0	0	0	0	0	0	-	1	-	-	-	-
3	2	38	31	1	-	-	0	0	1	0	0	-	-	-	2	-	2
61	60	1	-	1	2	5	6	53	25	164	181	99	151	11	18	-	-
0	0	-	-	-	-	-	-	-	0	0	-	1	-	-	1	18	-
64	16	-	-	1	-	1	2	43	4	125	21	197	53	180	68	178	73
1	2	1	-	0	0	0	0	0	1	2	3	6	6	1	7	-	2
5	26	8	4	1	1	0	11	1	28	5	42	17	36	23	42	65	67
3	3	5	7	4	3	5	3	2	2	2	1	2	2	1	1	-	2
38	125	4	4	14	22	15	107	41	163	72	213	62	135	21	51	-	12
0	0	1	1	-	-	-	-	-	0	0	0	1	-	-	1	-	-
20	87	22	18	9	11	2	68	4	101	17	86	70	101	121	212	184	266
11	22	1	1	-	0	0	3	3	8	11	26	48	59	79	103	113	97
1	1	-	1	2	2	1	1	1	1	1	1	-	1	1	1	-	-
0	0	1	-	0	-	1	0	-	0	0	0	1	2	1	-	-	2
0	0	-	-	-	-	-	-	-	0	0	0	1	1	1	1	-	2
5	22	9	5	2	5	1	19	1	20	4	21	22	35	25	61	30	69
1	1	2	1	1	0	-	-	0	0	0	1	1	2	-	-	-	-
4	6	6	2	6	5	1	4	1	4	4	4	10	13	15	13	30	6
0	1	-	1	-	1	0	1	0	1	1	1	1	1	-	1	-	-
8	9	21	27	31	39	3	5	2	2	3	2	5	2	8	3	6	4
11	25	-	1	-	-	-	-	-	0	4	3	22	29	139	198	404	443
2	1	-	-	-	-	0	1	3	1	4	1	3	2	-	-	6	4
1	2	-	-	-	-	4	1	2	2	1	3	1	4	1	1	-	6
8	12	-	-	1	-	0	2	1	2	5	2	20	20	80	79	196	197
1	3	-	-	-	-	-	0	1	0	0	2	-	2	15	21	30	41

Table 21 - *continued*

Disease group	Persons, by age group								
	Total	0-4	5-15	16-24	25-44	45-64	65-74	75-84	85 and over
Schizophrenic psychoses (295)	11	-	0	6	14	21	13	9	7
Affective psychoses (296)	58	-	1	34	62	94	92	110	129
Paranoid states (297)	4	-	-	3	3	6	7	15	24
Other nonorganic psychoses (298)	4	-	-	3	5	5	4	12	7
Psychoses with origin specific to childhood (299)	0	0	1	1	1	-	-	-	-
Neurotic disorders (300)	344	15	51	322	434	475	437	409	355
Personality disorders (301)	15	1	1	14	18	20	15	24	28
Sexual deviations and disorders (302)	15	-	-	11	17	31	22	3	1
Alcohol dependence syndrome (303)	13	-	-	4	22	22	8	6	1
Drug dependence (304)	19	-	1	21	25	24	28	19	15
Nondependent abuse of drugs (305)	17	-	2	17	25	26	12	6	6
Physiological malfunction arising from mental factors (306)	11	4	8	15	12	11	9	12	7
Special symptoms or syndromes not elsewhere classified (307)	97	107	62	85	87	108	129	144	219
Acute reaction to stress (308)	26	1	3	29	44	33	15	8	3
Adjustment reaction (309)	36	-	2	17	36	53	77	83	59
Specific nonpsychotic mental disorders following organic brain damage (310)	5	1	2	5	3	5	9	21	16
Depressive disorder, not elsewhere classified (311)	110	0	6	78	141	159	138	171	179
Disturbance of conduct not elsewhere classified (312)	14	41	42	11	5	3	3	13	37
Disturbance of emotions specific to childhood and adolescence (313)	1	4	6	2	0	0	-	-	-
Hyperkinetic syndrome of childhood (314)	1	11	3	-	-	-	-	-	-
Specific delays in development (315)	5	51	10	1	0	0	0	0	-
Mild mental retardation (317)	1	-	0	1	1	0	0	-	-
Other specified mental retardation (318)	1	-	1	4	1	1	1	-	1
Unspecified mental retardation (319)	1	1	0	2	1	2	0	-	-
Bacterial meningitis (320)	0	2	0	0	0	0	-	0	-
Meningitis of unspecified cause (322)	1	3	1	1	1	1	0	-	-
Encephalitis, myelitis and encephalomyelitis (323)	1	-	0	1	2	2	1	1	-
Intracranial and intraspinal abscess (324)	0	-	0	0	0	0	-	-	-
Phlebitis and thrombophlebitis of intracranial venous sinuses (325)	0	-	-	-	0	0	0	1	-
Cerebral degenerations usually manifest in childhood (330)	0	2	0	0	0	0	-	1	-
Other cerebral degenerations (331)	5	0	0	0	0	2	12	43	68
Parkinson's disease (332)	15	-	-	0	1	12	56	113	135
Other extrapyramidal disease and abnormal movement disorders (333)	12	2	6	8	9	18	31	21	22
Spinocerebellar disease (334)	1	-	0	-	1	1	2	3	-
Anterior horn cell disease (335)	1	-	-	-	0	1	3	3	1
Other diseases of spinal cord (336)	1	-	-	-	1	1	4	3	-
Disorders of autonomic nervous system (337)	0	-	-	-	0	1	1	0	-
Multiple sclerosis (340)	7	-	-	1	10	15	9	2	-
Other demyelinating diseases of central nervous system (341)	0	-	-	0	0	0	0	-	-
Hemiplegia (342)	4	0	0	1	1	4	11	21	43
Infantile cerebral palsy (343)	1	5	2	2	1	1	0	1	-
Other paralytic syndromes (344)	1	0	0	1	1	2	3	3	4
Epilepsy (345)	36	16	24	45	37	38	41	42	34
Migraine (346)	115	3	99	150	158	126	58	36	13
Cataplexy and narcolepsy (347)	0	-	-	0	0	0	0	-	-
Other conditions of brain (348)	2	0	0	1	2	3	1	2	1
Other and unspecified disorders of the nervous system (349)	1	-	0	0	1	2	1	1	-
Trigeminal nerve disorders (350)	9	1	1	3	7	16	21	26	16
Facial nerve disorders (351)	4	0	1	2	4	6	8	7	6
Disorders of other cranial nerves (352)	0	-	-	-	0	0	0	1	-
Nerve root and plexus disorders (353)	2	-	0	1	3	5	3	4	1
Mononeuritis of upper limb and mononeuritis multiplex (354)	21	-	0	7	27	37	25	27	16
Mononeuritis of lower limb (355)	3	-	0	1	3	6	4	6	1
Hereditary and idiopathic peripheral neuropathy (356)	1	-	-	-	0	2	2	4	1
Inflammatory and toxic neuropathy (357)	3	-	-	1	2	5	6	8	1
Myoneural disorders (358)	1	-	-	0	0	1	3	2	-
Muscular dystrophies and other myopathies (359)	1	0	1	0	1	3	2	1	1

Patients consulting

By age-group and sex

Total		0-4		5-15		16-24		25-44		45-64		65-74		75-84		85 and over	
Male	Female	Male	Female	Male	Female	Male	Female	Male	Female	Male	Female	Male	Female	Male	Female	Male	Female
13	10	-	-	0	-	8	3	19	9	22	21	10	15	3	12	12	6
35	80	-	-	2	1	25	44	35	90	62	126	48	128	80	127	107	136
4	5	-	-	-	-	5	2	4	2	4	7	4	9	9	18	12	28
3	5	-	-	-	-	2	3	4	7	4	6	2	5	14	10	-	10
1	0	1	-	1	0	1	0	1	0	-	-	-	-	-	-	-	-
202	481	16	15	37	66	181	462	243	627	298	656	257	582	244	508	226	398
13	16	-	1	2	1	17	11	17	19	16	24	13	17	10	33	24	30
23	8	-	-	-	-	11	11	17	18	56	6	48	1	9	-	-	2
20	6	-	-	-	-	7	2	33	10	35	10	8	9	6	5	-	2
19	19	-	-	1	2	34	8	30	20	16	32	10	43	11	23	12	16
20	13	-	-	2	2	21	12	29	21	30	21	19	7	10	3	12	4
7	14	3	4	4	11	9	20	7	17	8	14	9	9	9	13	-	10
68	125	106	107	67	57	47	124	50	123	74	142	100	152	98	171	160	238
18	35	1	-	2	5	16	42	29	58	24	42	6	22	2	12	6	2
17	55	-	-	2	2	7	28	16	56	23	84	40	107	56	99	71	55
4	5	1	-	2	2	6	4	3	2	4	5	10	8	18	23	12	18
61	158	1	-	3	8	37	119	67	215	99	221	94	174	112	207	190	175
17	10	54	27	53	29	15	6	7	4	3	2	2	4	15	12	65	28
1	2	2	6	5	8	1	3	-	0	-	0	-	-	-	-	-	-
2	0	17	5	5	1	-	-	-	-	-	-	-	-	-	-	-	-
7	4	63	38	14	6	1	2	1	-	0	1	1	-	-	1	-	-
1	1	-	-	-	0	1	2	1	1	0	0	-	0	-	-	-	-
1	1	-	-	0	1	4	3	2	1	1	1	-	2	-	-	-	2
1	1	1	-	0	-	2	2	1	1	2	1	-	0	-	-	-	-
0	0	2	2	-	0	-	0	0	0	0	0	-	-	-	1	-	-
1	1	4	3	1	0	1	-	1	1	1	1	-	0	-	-	-	-
1	1	-	-	1	0	0	1	2	2	2	2	1	-	1	1	-	-
0	0	-	-	-	0	0	-	0	0	0	-	-	-	-	-	-	-
0	0	-	-	-	-	-	-	0	0	-	0	-	0	2	1	-	-
0	0	2	1	1	-	1	-	-	0	0	-	-	-	1	1	-	-
3	6	1	-	0	-	0	-	0	0	2	2	12	11	40	44	36	79
15	15	-	-	-	-	0	-	1	1	14	9	64	51	149	91	155	128
9	16	3	1	5	6	5	10	6	13	13	23	23	37	24	18	-	30
1	1	-	-	0	-	-	-	1	1	1	1	2	1	3	3	-	-
1	1	-	-	-	-	-	-	1	0	1	1	2	3	5	2	-	2
1	1	-	-	-	-	-	-	1	1	2	1	5	3	6	2	-	-
0	0	-	-	-	-	-	-	0	0	0	1	1	-	-	1	-	-
5	10	-	-	-	-	1	2	6	14	11	20	6	11	5	1	-	-
0	0	-	-	-	-	0	-	0	0	-	0	1	-	-	-	-	-
4	4	-	1	0	0	0	1	1	1	5	2	14	9	22	21	42	43
2	1	7	3	1	2	1	3	2	1	1	1	1	-	1	1	-	-
2	1	-	1	0	-	2	-	2	1	2	1	3	2	3	2	6	4
35	36	15	18	25	24	45	45	36	38	40	36	38	43	46	40	30	35
58	169	4	3	89	109	67	233	65	251	56	197	36	75	24	42	6	16
0	0	-	-	-	-	0	-	0	0	0	0	-	0	-	-	-	-
1	2	1	-	0	1	-	1	1	3	2	4	1	1	1	2	6	-
1	1	-	-	0	-	0	0	1	2	2	1	2	1	2	-	-	-
6	12	1	1	1	0	2	3	4	10	11	21	15	27	21	29	12	18
4	4	1	-	1	2	1	3	4	4	6	6	7	9	11	4	-	8
0	0	-	-	-	-	-	-	-	-	0	-	0	1	-	1	1	-
2	3	-	-	-	0	1	1	2	4	4	5	2	3	6	3	-	2
11	30	-	-	-	0	2	11	12	42	21	54	23	26	23	29	18	16
3	3	-	-	0	0	2	1	3	3	5	7	3	4	6	6	6	-
1	1	-	-	-	-	-	-	0	0	2	1	1	2	7	3	6	-
3	2	-	-	-	-	1	0	2	1	4	5	9	4	7	9	-	2
1	1	-	-	-	-	-	1	0	1	1	1	4	2	3	1	-	-
1	1	-	1	2	1	-	0	1	2	3	2	2	1	-	2	-	2

Table 21 - *continued*

Disease group	Persons, by age group								
	Total	0-4	5-15	16-24	25-44	45-64	65-74	75-84	85 and over
Disorders of the globe (360)	0	0	-	0	0	0	-	0	3
Retinal detachments and defects (361)	2	-	0	1	1	4	6	5	-
Other retinal disorders (362)	12	0	1	1	3	12	38	71	102
Chorioretinal inflammations and scars and other disorders of choroid (363)	1	-	0	0	1	2	1	1	1
Disorders of iris and ciliary body (364)	5	1	1	4	5	7	5	8	4
Glaucoma (365)	21	-	0	-	3	29	77	123	118
Cataract (366)	34	1	1	1	1	19	127	283	342
Disorders of refraction and accommodation (367)	4	7	5	3	3	4	4	4	1
Visual disturbances (368)	21	7	16	9	14	24	48	55	62
Blindness and low vision (369)	8	3	2	2	3	5	18	50	104
Keratitis (370)	6	-	1	4	5	9	10	11	9
Corneal opacity and other disorders of cornea (371)	3	0	0	2	2	5	3	7	4
Disorders of conjunctiva (372)	415	1,833	389	228	259	302	419	430	505
Inflammation of eyelids (373)	81	78	87	72	73	79	104	106	80
Other disorders of eyelids (374)	13	9	5	5	9	16	23	46	62
Disorders of lacrimal system (375)	28	18	4	3	10	36	99	108	104
Disorders of the orbit (376)	2	3	2	1	2	2	3	3	6
Disorders of optic nerve and visual pathways (377)	1	1	0	0	1	2	2	1	-
Strabismus and other disorders of binocular eye movements (378)	9	70	15	3	2	2	2	2	-
Other disorders of eye (379)	19	11	7	9	15	27	46	39	22
Disorders of external ear (380)	409	218	235	263	371	506	683	802	777
Nonsuppurative otitis media and Eustachian tube disorders (381)	346	1,899	757	181	168	119	88	53	36
Suppurative and unspecified otitis media (382)	164	1,033	355	68	64	47	44	30	21
Mastoiditis and related conditions (383)	1	1	1	1	1	2	1	2	-
Other disorders of tympanic membrane (384)	9	18	13	7	9	8	8	9	4
Other disorders of middle ear and mastoid (385)	1	0	0	0	1	1	2	2	1
Vertiginous syndromes and other disorders of vestibular system (386)	73	2	8	30	62	117	165	174	154
Otosclerosis (387)	1	-	0	0	1	1	1	-	-
Other disorders of ear (388)	115	271	199	66	75	92	116	121	145
Deafness (389)	43	50	41	13	21	44	82	139	197
Rheumatic fever without mention of heart involvement (390)	0	-	0	0	0	-	0	-	-
Rheumatic fever with heart involvement (391)	0	-	-	-	-	0	-	-	-
Rheumatic chorea (392)	0	-	-	-	0	-	-	-	-
Diseases of mitral valve (394)	3	-	0	-	0	6	12	9	4
Diseases of aortic valve (395)	1	0	-	-	0	2	3	3	3
Diseases of mitral and aortic valves (396)	0	-	-	-	0	1	2	-	3
Diseases of other endocardial structures (397)	0	-	-	-	-	0	-	-	-
Other rheumatic heart disease (398)	1	-	-	-	-	2	2	3	1
Essential hypertension (401)	412	1	1	9	97	796	1,623	1,406	651
Hypertensive heart disease (402)	7	-	0	1	2	16	22	25	10
Hypertensive renal disease (403)	1	-	0	-	1	2	3	1	-
Hypertensive heart and renal disease (404)	0	-	-	-	-	0	0	-	-
Secondary hypertension (405)	2	0	0	1	2	4	3	3	1
Acute myocardial infarction (410)	29	-	-	0	4	47	110	143	126
Other acute and subacute forms of ischaemic heart disease (411)	1	-	-	-	0	2	2	5	4
Old myocardial infarction (412)	6	-	-	-	1	12	25	17	10
Angina pectoris (413)	114	0	-	0	10	196	461	511	399
Other forms of chronic ischaemic heart disease (414)	47	-	0	0	5	82	185	201	198
Acute pulmonary heart disease (415)	5	-	-	1	2	8	16	28	22
Chronic pulmonary heart disease (416)	1	-	0	0	0	1	4	6	3
Other diseases of pulmonary circulation (417)	0	-	0	-	0	-	-	1	-

By age-group and sex

Total		0-4		5-15		16-24		25-44		45-64		65-74		75-84		85 and over	
Male	Female	Male	Female	Male	Female	Male	Female	Male	Female	Male	Female	Male	Female	Male	Female	Male	Female
0	0	1	-	-	0	0	0	0	1	0	0	-	-	-	1	6	2
2	2	-	-	0	-	1	1	1	1	5	4	7	6	6	5	-	-
9	14	-	1	0	1	1	-	2	3	12	11	31	43	66	74	107	100
1	1	-	-	-	0	-	0	1	0	2	1	2	-	2	1	6	-
4	5	1	1	1	1	4	4	5	5	5	8	3	8	9	8	6	4
19	23	-	-	-	0	-	-	3	2	29	30	79	75	127	120	149	108
25	43	1	1	0	1	2	1	2	1	19	19	107	144	251	303	333	345
4	4	7	6	6	4	3	4	3	3	4	4	2	5	7	2	-	2
20	22	7	6	17	15	12	6	12	16	26	23	44	52	61	52	30	73
6	10	2	4	1	3	3	2	3	3	4	6	19	18	47	51	83	110
6	5	-	-	1	2	6	2	6	5	7	11	13	7	9	12	30	2
3	3	1	-	0	1	2	2	2	3	5	4	5	1	8	6	-	6
355	473	1,856	1,809	367	412	163	293	184	334	217	390	337	486	381	459	398	540
62	99	73	84	73	101	53	90	51	96	60	98	85	120	88	117	59	87
11	15	10	8	4	6	3	7	6	11	12	21	22	24	63	36	95	51
16	40	15	21	4	3	2	4	5	16	18	54	64	128	77	127	77	112
2	3	5	2	2	3	1	1	2	3	1	3	3	3	-	5	6	6
1	1	2	1	1	-	0	0	1	2	1	2	2	2	-	1	-	-
9	8	71	69	15	15	2	4	2	3	1	2	2	2	2	1	-	-
15	23	12	10	8	6	8	9	13	18	19	35	36	54	33	42	36	18
419	400	230	205	198	273	242	285	368	375	541	471	851	546	1,005	681	927	727
325	366	1,924	1,872	722	794	126	235	122	215	88	150	82	92	44	59	12	43
165	163	1,087	976	355	355	55	81	52	76	37	57	35	51	33	28	6	26
1	1	1	1	1	1	1	1	1	1	1	2	1	2	-	3	-	-
9	10	19	17	13	14	7	7	7	10	7	9	9	6	6	11	6	4
1	1	1	-	0	0	0	-	2	1	1	1	2	2	2	2	-	2
49	96	2	1	8	9	19	41	34	90	83	153	132	191	149	189	155	154
0	1	-	-	1	-	-	0	0	1	1	1	-	2	-	-	-	-
94	135	264	278	147	253	45	88	49	101	85	99	121	112	100	134	119	154
45	42	59	40	43	39	10	17	19	23	55	34	100	68	147	135	244	181
0	0	-	-	-	0	0	-	-	0	-	-	-	-	0	-	-	-
0	-	-	-	-	-	-	-	-	-	0	-	-	-	-	-	-	-
0	-	-	-	-	-	-	-	0	-	-	-	-	-	-	-	-	-
2	4	-	-	0	-	-	-	0	0	3	10	9	15	9	8	6	4
1	1	-	1	-	-	-	-	0	-	2	2	4	1	5	2	-	4
0	1	-	-	-	-	-	-	0	-	1	1	1	2	-	-	-	4
0	-	-	-	-	-	-	-	-	-	0	-	-	-	-	-	-	-
0	1	-	-	-	-	-	-	-	-	1	3	2	1	2	3	-	2
349	472	1	1	1	1	9	10	99	95	743	849	1,458	1,757	1,108	1,584	493	703
7	7	-	-	0	-	-	1	2	2	17	14	24	21	22	27	6	12
1	1	-	-	0	0	-	-	1	2	3	1	3	2	1	1	-	-
0	0	-	-	-	-	-	-	-	-	0	-	-	0	-	-	-	-
2	2	-	1	-	0	0	2	1	2	4	3	3	2	1	4	6	-
38	20	-	-	-	-	0	-	6	1	73	20	158	71	188	117	166	112
1	1	-	-	-	-	-	-	0	0	4	1	2	3	8	3	12	2
9	3	-	-	-	-	-	-	2	0	20	4	40	14	34	7	18	8
130	98	-	1	-	-	0	0	14	7	257	133	580	364	586	466	505	364
62	33	-	-	0	-	0	-	8	2	122	43	275	111	262	165	273	173
5	6	-	-	-	-	2	1	4	4	8	7	19	13	32	25	36	18
1	1	-	-	0	-	0	-	-	0	1	1	6	3	10	3	12	-
0	0	-	-	0	-	-	-	0	0	-	-	-	-	2	-	-	-

Patients consulting

Table 21 - *continued*

Disease group	Persons, by age group								
	Total	0-4	5-15	16-24	25-44	45-64	65-74	75-84	85 and over
Acute pericarditis (420)	1	-	0	1	0	2	1	2	1
Acute and subacute endocarditis (421)	0	-	-	-	0	1	1	1	1
Acute myocarditis (422)	0	-	-	0	-	-	-	-	-
Other diseases of pericardium (423)	0	1	-	-	0	0	1	0	-
Other diseases of endocardium (424)	6	2	1	1	1	8	22	21	34
Cardiomyopathy (425)	2	-	0	0	1	5	4	4	-
Conduction disorders (426)	2	1	0	1	1	3	6	14	19
Cardiac dysrhythmias (427)	45	2	1	5	10	47	152	284	315
Heart failure (428)	89	2	0	1	1	42	273	741	1,403
Ill-defined descriptions and complications of heart disease (429)	1	-	0	1	0	1	1	4	7
Subarachnoid haemorrhage (430)	1	-	-	1	1	3	3	-	-
Intracerebral haemorrhage (431)	2	-	-	0	0	3	6	4	15
Other and unspecified intracranial haemorrhage (432)	0	-	0	0	-	1	1	1	3
Occlusion and stenosis of precerebral arteries (433)	2	-	-	-	0	3	7	12	12
Occlusion of cerebral arteries (434)	3	-	-	0	0	3	10	16	19
Transient cerebral ischaemia (435)	30	-	-	1	1	23	101	234	321
Acute but ill-defined cerebrovascular disease (436)	27	-	-	0	1	22	91	194	336
Other and ill-defined cerebrovascular disease (437)	7	-	-	-	0	7	21	50	80
Late effects of cerebrovascular disease (438)	1	-	-	-	0	1	2	3	6
Atherosclerosis (440)	2	-	-	-	0	2	8	19	22
Aortic aneurysm (441)	3	-	-	-	0	3	12	21	18
Other aneurysm (442)	0	-	-	-	0	1	1	4	3
Other peripheral vascular disease (443)	40	1	2	7	11	56	152	178	136
Arterial embolism and thrombosis (444)	1	-	-	-	0	1	4	7	7
Polyarteritis nodosa and allied conditions (446)	3	-	-	0	1	3	14	18	21
Other disorders of arteries and arterioles (447)	0	-	-	1	-	0	1	2	-
Diseases of capillaries (448)	6	4	8	6	6	5	4	5	1
Phlebitis and thrombophlebitis (451)	24	-	1	6	13	40	67	98	53
Other venous embolism and thrombosis (453)	4	-	0	0	1	6	12	15	12
Varicose veins of lower extremities (454)	89	1	1	22	63	141	233	279	241
Haemorrhoids (455)	103	4	4	73	145	135	148	127	99
Varicose veins of other sites (456)	2	-	1	2	3	2	3	2	1
Noninfective disorders of lymphatic channels (457)	2	1	2	2	3	3	3	3	6
Hypotension (458)	11	-	2	5	4	11	30	62	104
Other disorders of circulatory system (459)	4	2	0	1	2	7	13	15	18
Acute nasopharyngitis (common cold) (460)	320	1,967	412	199	156	140	168	164	216
Acute sinusitis (461)	250	19	118	262	362	303	204	120	87
Acute pharyngitis (462)	409	460	630	629	420	259	196	157	112
Acute tonsillitis (463)	407	1,006	951	678	312	89	38	30	15
Acute laryngitis and tracheitis (464)	140	430	119	104	120	132	119	100	81
Acute upper respiratory infections of multiple or unspecified site (465)	772	3,103	1,002	600	496	490	556	628	735
Acute bronchitis and bronchiolitis (466)	719	1,578	422	430	494	762	1,142	1,346	1,669
Deflected nasal septum (470)	5	-	3	12	6	5	4	2	1
Nasal polyps (471)	8	1	3	5	7	15	16	9	3
Chronic pharyngitis and nasopharyngitis (472)	101	147	91	70	87	109	152	113	80
Chronic sinusitis (473)	25	0	8	23	33	34	29	19	7
Chronic disease of tonsils and adenoids (474)	8	24	21	13	4	2	1	1	-
Peritonsillar abscess (475)	3	1	2	7	4	1	2	-	-
Chronic laryngitis and laryngotracheitis (476)	4	1	2	2	3	7	7	5	3
Allergic rhinitis (477)	283	155	522	489	302	147	113	78	40
Other diseases of upper respiratory tract (478)	9	9	8	7	9	9	13	7	6
Viral pneumonia (480)	2	4	1	0	1	1	2	5	9
Pneumococcal pneumonia (481)	6	9	5	1	4	6	12	22	30
Other bacterial pneumonia (482)	2	3	1	2	1	2	5	9	13
Pneumonia due to other specified organism (483)	0	-	0	1	0	0	0	0	-
Bronchopneumonia, organism unspecified (485)	12	7	3	1	2	6	23	72	231
Pneumonia, organism unspecified (486)	10	15	5	4	4	10	20	32	53
Influenza (487)	205	202	172	227	224	209	168	178	160

By age-group and sex

Total		0-4		5-15		16-24		25-44		45-64		65-74		75-84		85 and over	
Male	Female	Male	Female	Male	Female	Male	Female	Male	Female	Male	Female	Male	Female	Male	Female	Male	Female
1	0	-	-	0	0	1	0	1	0	2	1	3	-	2	1	6	-
1	0	-	-	-	-	-	-	1	-	1	0	2	1	1	1	6	-
0	-	-	-	-	-	0	-	-	-	-	-	-	-	1	-	-	-
0	0	1	1	-	-	-	-	0	-	0	-	1	0	1	-	-	-
6	6	2	1	1	1	1	1	1	2	9	8	24	20	26	18	48	30
2	1	-	-	0	0	-	1	1	0	7	3	6	3	6	3	-	-
3	2	1	-	1	-	1	1	1	0	3	2	10	3	24	8	24	18
41	48	2	2	2	-	3	6	9	11	53	41	176	132	293	278	279	327
77	101	2	1	0	0	-	1	1	1	47	38	323	233	799	706	1,575	1,346
1	1	-	-	-	-	0	1	1	0	2	1	2	1	5	3	6	8
1	1	-	-	-	-	1	1	1	1	2	4	3	2	-	-	-	-
2	1	-	-	-	-	0	0	0	-	4	2	8	4	3	5	18	14
0	0	-	-	0	-	-	-	0	-	1	0	2	-	2	1	-	4
1	2	-	-	-	-	-	-	0	-	3	3	6	9	8	14	6	14
3	2	-	-	-	-	0	0	-	-	4	2	15	6	25	10	30	16
28	31	-	-	-	-	0	1	1	2	24	21	125	81	283	205	380	301
26	27	-	-	-	-	0	-	1	1	30	14	117	70	219	179	368	325
7	7	-	-	-	-	-	-	0	0	10	4	24	19	61	43	53	89
1	1	-	-	-	-	-	-	0	-	1	0	1	2	6	2	6	6
3	2	-	-	-	-	-	-	0	0	3	1	12	4	29	13	36	18
5	1	-	-	-	-	-	-	0	0	5	2	22	3	44	7	24	16
0	1	-	-	-	-	-	-	0	-	0	1	1	1	6	3	6	2
45	34	1	1	0	4	3	12	6	15	74	37	218	100	230	147	202	114
1	1	-	-	-	-	-	-	0	0	1	1	6	3	9	5	6	8
2	5	-	-	-	-	1	-	1	1	2	4	6	19	15	19	12	24
0	0	-	-	-	-	1	0	-	-	0	0	-	1	1	2	-	-
4	7	4	4	7	9	4	9	3	9	3	7	3	5	2	7	-	2
17	32	-	-	0	1	3	8	7	18	29	52	61	72	77	111	18	65
3	5	-	-	0	-	1	-	2	1	4	8	10	14	10	17	-	16
58	119	1	1	1	1	10	33	31	96	97	186	197	263	232	307	232	244
92	114	5	3	3	6	51	94	116	173	134	137	159	140	143	118	125	91
3	1	-	-	2	-	4	-	3	2	3	1	4	3	5	1	-	2
2	3	1	1	1	2	2	2	3	2	3	4	2	3	1	3	-	8
10	13	-	-	2	1	4	5	2	7	12	10	35	26	77	53	101	104
3	6	1	3	1	-	0	2	1	3	5	9	8	16	9	18	12	20
290	349	1,966	1,967	386	440	134	265	105	207	110	171	153	181	159	167	178	229
159	338	19	19	104	132	171	352	213	512	177	431	147	250	92	138	59	97
322	491	451	469	521	745	449	807	299	541	199	320	162	224	142	166	83	122
347	466	1,074	935	799	1,110	503	852	224	401	62	117	36	40	30	29	12	16
104	174	500	357	115	122	53	155	60	180	74	192	85	146	81	112	59	89
667	873	3,119	3,085	945	1,063	430	768	335	658	366	616	489	610	577	658	832	703
643	792	1,664	1,488	440	402	358	502	374	615	632	894	1,148	1,136	1,521	1,242	1,913	1,588
8	3	-	-	4	2	17	6	9	4	7	3	5	3	5	-	-	2
11	5	1	1	5	2	6	3	9	5	21	8	24	10	15	5	6	2
91	110	136	158	96	85	61	78	68	107	94	124	156	149	127	105	107	71
18	31	-	1	8	7	16	30	23	42	25	44	20	37	10	25	12	6
6	10	24	23	19	24	4	21	3	5	1	2	-	2	1	1	-	-
3	3	1	1	2	1	9	6	4	4	1	1	2	1	-	-	-	-
3	5	1	1	1	3	2	3	2	4	5	9	9	6	6	5	-	4
265	301	187	121	576	465	421	555	240	366	119	175	101	123	89	72	59	33
8	9	10	8	9	7	7	6	8	10	7	11	11	14	6	8	18	2
2	1	5	3	1	2	0	-	1	1	1	1	3	1	6	4	6	10
7	6	11	6	6	4	1	0	3	4	6	5	14	11	27	18	53	22
3	2	3	3	2	0	1	2	1	2	3	1	8	3	11	8	24	10
0	0	-	-	-	0	1	1	1	0	0	0	-	0	1	-	-	-
10	13	8	7	4	2	1	1	3	1	7	5	25	21	82	65	244	227
11	9	17	13	7	3	4	4	5	4	11	9	26	16	44	25	89	41
181	228	216	188	164	180	193	262	194	255	172	248	148	185	156	191	190	150

Patients consulting

181

Table 21 - *continued*

Disease group	Persons, by age group								
	Total	0-4	5-15	16-24	25-44	45-64	65-74	75-84	85 and over
Bronchitis, not specified as acute or chronic (490)	46	96	18	18	26	48	90	125	206
Chronic bronchitis (491)	45	5	3	6	8	65	193	204	124
Emphysema (492)	8	-	-	-	1	13	36	35	24
Asthma (493)	425	861	755	428	296	300	394	343	203
Bronchiectasis (494)	5	1	0	1	3	11	13	14	13
Extrinsic allergic alveolitis (495)	0	-	0	-	0	1	2	1	3
Chronic airways obsruction, not elsewhere classified (496)	48	1	0	-	3	69	209	242	195
Coalworkers' pneumoconiosis (500)	0	-	-	-	-	-	1	1	-
Asbestosis (501)	0	-	-	-	0	1	2	1	-
Pneumoconiosis due to other silica or silicates (502)	0	-	-	-	-	0	0	-	-
Pneumoconiosis due to other inorganic dust (503)	0	-	0	-	-	-	0	-	-
Pneumoconiosis, unspecified (505)	0	-	-	-	-	-	0	-	-
Respiratory conditions due to chemical fumes and vapours (506)	0	-	-	-	0	0	0	-	-
Pneumonitis due to solids and liquids (507)	0	-	-	-	0	-	1	1	1
Respiratory conditions due to other and unspecified external agents (508)	0	-	-	-	-	0	-	-	-
Empyema (510)	0	-	-	0	0	1	1	1	1
Pleurisy (511)	19	1	3	13	19	25	36	46	47
Pneumothorax (512)	2	-	0	3	2	1	2	2	4
Abscess of lung and mediastinum (513)	0	-	-	-	0	-	-	-	-
Pulmonary congestion and hypostasis (514)	1	-	-	0	0	1	2	8	18
Postinflammatory pulmonary fibrosis (515)	0	-	-	-	-	-	-	-	1
Other alveolar and parietoalveolar pneumopathy (516)	2	1	0	-	0	3	7	13	3
Other diseases of lung (518)	0	0	-	-	-	1	1	-	-
Other diseases of respiratory system (519)	10	36	7	8	7	8	12	9	6
Disorders of tooth development and eruption (520)	5	67	0	0	0	0	-	-	-
Diseases of hard tissues of teeth (521)	13	122	4	6	5	5	5	3	1
Diseases of pulp and periapical tissues (522)	34	7	23	36	48	41	21	10	7
Gingival and periodontal diseases (523)	8	15	5	9	9	8	7	5	7
Dentofacial anomalies, including malocclusion (524)	14	1	7	23	19	14	9	8	4
Other diseases and conditions of the teeth and supporting structures (525)	2	-	1	4	2	1	2	2	6
Diseases of the jaws (526)	1	0	0	1	0	1	1	-	-
Diseases of the salivary glands (527)	9	4	6	6	9	13	7	12	10
Diseases of the oral soft tissues, excluding lesions specific for gingiva and tongue (528)	65	127	73	68	52	54	75	66	52
Diseases and other conditions of the tongue (529)	10	10	6	5	9	11	16	21	16
Diseases of oesophagus (530)	103	27	5	42	90	162	234	223	178
Gastric ulcer (531)	6	-	-	1	4	10	16	26	33
Duodenal ulcer (532)	33	-	0	9	34	64	66	50	36
Peptic ulcer, site unspecified (533)	13	-	0	6	13	22	20	27	19
Gastritis and duodenitis (535)	74	45	36	73	77	88	93	113	111
Disorders of function of stomach (536)	153	4	13	90	143	226	331	334	269
Other disorders of stomach and duodenum (537)	0	3	0	0	-	1	1	1	1
Acute appendicitis (540)	4	0	8	7	4	2	1	1	-
Appendicitis, unqualified (541)	5	0	12	13	5	2	1	0	-
Other appendicitis (542)	1	0	1	1	1	0	0	-	-
Other diseases of appendix (543)	0	-	0	-	0	-	-	-	-
Inguinal hernia (550)	31	30	6	8	14	45	76	110	93
Other hernia of abdominal cavity, with gangrene (551)	0	-	-	-	-	-	0	-	-
Other hernia of abdominal cavity with obstruction, without mention of gangrene (552)	0	0	-	-	0	0	1	2	4
Other hernia of abdominal cavity without mention of obstruction or gangrene (553)	39	42	3	4	19	57	115	128	98
Regional enteritis (555)	7	1	1	7	9	9	7	8	9
Idiopathic proctocolitis (556)	10	1	0	3	12	17	15	15	16
Vascular insufficiency of intestine (557)	0	-	-	-	-	0	2	1	3
Other noninfective gastroenteritis and colitis (558)	17	41	11	15	15	17	19	20	19

By age-group and sex

Total		0-4		5-15		16-24		25-44		45-64		65-74		75-84		85 and over	
Male	Female	Male	Female	Male	Female	Male	Female	Male	Female	Male	Female	Male	Female	Male	Female	Male	Female
41	51	103	87	20	16	18	17	19	32	39	57	92	89	124	127	232	197
54	37	5	4	2	4	5	6	6	9	73	57	270	130	319	135	279	73
11	5	-	-	-	-	-	-	1	1	17	9	55	20	61	19	83	4
429	422	994	722	860	645	396	459	258	334	260	342	372	412	360	334	267	181
4	6	1	1	0	0	1	1	2	4	7	14	12	14	15	14	24	10
0	1	-	-	0	-	-	-	0	0	1	1	1	2	1	1	-	4
57	38	1	-	0	1	-	-	3	4	80	58	299	137	363	170	374	136
0	-	-	-	-	-	-	-	-	-	-	-	2	-	3	-	-	-
1	-	-	-	-	-	-	-	0	-	1	-	3	-	3	-	-	-
0	-	-	-	-	-	-	-	-	-	0	-	1	-	-	-	-	-
0	0	-	-	0	0	-	-	-	-	-	-	-	0	-	-	-	-
0	-	-	-	-	-	-	-	-	-	-	-	1	-	-	-	-	-
0	-	-	-	-	-	-	-	0	-	0	-	1	-	-	-	-	-
0	0	-	-	-	-	-	-	-	0	-	-	-	1	2	1	6	-
0	0	-	-	-	-	-	-	-	-	0	0	-	-	-	-	-	-
0	0	-	-	-	-	-	0	0	0	1	0	1	0	2	1	-	2
15	23	-	1	3	3	8	17	13	24	20	30	36	37	54	41	65	41
2	1	-	-	0	-	-	5	1	3	2	2	3	1	5	1	6	4
0	0	-	-	-	-	-	-	-	0	0	-	-	-	-	-	-	-
1	1	-	-	-	-	0	-	-	0	1	1	2	3	11	6	18	18
0	-	-	-	-	-	-	-	-	-	-	-	-	-	-	-	6	-
2	2	1	1	-	0	-	-	0	0	4	2	9	5	18	10	6	2
0	0	-	1	-	-	-	-	-	-	1	0	1	1	-	-	-	-
9	10	42	31	6	8	7	8	6	9	6	9	11	13	9	8	6	6
5	5	64	70	0	-	1	0	0	0	0	-	-	-	-	-	-	-
3	12	139	104	2	5	2	9	4	6	4	5	5	6	6	1	-	2
31	37	9	6	25	20	30	42	40	57	38	44	23	19	13	9	12	6
7	10	16	14	5	6	7	11	6	12	7	10	6	8	3	6	-	10
8	19	-	1	5	8	13	32	11	27	8	21	3	13	9	7	12	2
1	2	-	-	1	1	1	6	2	3	1	2	2	2	3	1	-	8
0	1	1	-	-	0	1	1	0	1	1	1	2	1	-	-	-	-
7	11	4	4	5	7	5	6	8	10	8	18	6	8	6	16	12	10
51	78	119	136	64	82	45	90	39	65	38	69	66	82	52	75	36	57
7	12	9	11	5	6	6	5	7	11	8	15	10	22	16	23	12	18
89	116	30	24	5	5	36	49	80	101	139	185	216	248	205	233	202	169
7	6	-	-	-	-	2	1	5	3	12	8	17	16	30	24	24	35
46	21	-	-	0	-	14	4	49	18	85	42	96	42	69	38	42	33
16	10	-	-	0	1	8	5	16	10	28	16	26	16	38	21	12	22
70	78	45	46	40	31	69	77	72	82	82	93	92	93	109	116	101	114
143	162	4	5	13	12	87	94	133	153	214	239	349	317	338	332	321	252
1	0	3	3	0	-	0	-	-	-	1	0	1	-	1	1	6	-
3	4	1	-	8	8	4	10	3	5	2	2	1	0	-	1	-	-
5	6	1	-	12	12	12	14	4	6	1	3	1	1	-	1	-	-
1	1	-	1	1	0	1	1	1	1	1	0	-	-	0	-	-	-
0	0	-	-	1	-	-	-	0	0	-	-	-	-	-	-	-	-
57	6	52	7	10	2	14	2	25	3	83	7	156	10	262	18	267	35
-	0	-	-	-	-	-	-	-	-	-	-	-	0	-	-	-	-
0	0	1	-	-	-	-	-	0	0	0	0	1	1	1	2	-	6
33	44	47	37	4	2	5	2	19	19	52	62	97	130	94	148	59	110
5	8	1	1	2	1	5	8	7	10	5	12	6	7	7	9	12	8
9	11	-	1	0	-	2	5	10	15	17	17	16	14	14	16	18	16
0	0	-	-	-	-	-	-	-	-	0	-	2	1	2	1	-	4
16	19	41	42	12	11	13	17	12	18	16	18	20	18	16	23	18	20

Table 21 - *continued*

Disease group	Persons, by age group								
	Total	0-4	5-15	16-24	25-44	45-64	65-74	75-84	85 and over
Intestinal obstruction without mention of hernia (560)	6	3	0	1	2	7	13	26	56
Diverticula of intestine (562)	22	-	0	0	3	31	84	120	135
Functional digestive disorders, not elsewhere classified (564)	211	258	78	183	194	196	298	477	709
Anal fissure and fistula (565)	26	51	12	35	34	21	11	14	10
Abscess of anal and rectal regions (566)	7	3	2	6	10	9	4	4	-
Peritonitis (567)	0	-	0	-	1	0	1	-	1
Other disorders of peritoneum (568)	1	0	0	0	1	1	1	1	1
Other disorders of intestine (569)	34	25	8	20	30	39	62	84	120
Acute and subacute necrosis of liver (570)	0	0	0	1	0	0	0	-	-
Chronic liver disease and cirrhosis (571)	5	-	-	0	4	10	10	6	-
Liver abscess and sequelae of chronic liver disease (572)	0	-	-	-	0	1	1	0	-
Other disorders of liver (573)	0	-	-	-	0	1	1	1	-
Cholelithiasis (574)	11	-	0	4	9	21	23	21	15
Other disorders of gallbladder (575)	10	-	-	3	9	18	21	18	21
Other disorders of biliary tract (576)	3	0	0	0	1	4	7	13	22
Diseases of pancreas (577)	2	-	0	1	2	4	6	8	6
Gastrointestinal haemorrhage (578)	12	4	1	6	7	11	27	55	92
Intestinal malabsorption (579)	3	6	1	2	3	4	5	5	4
Acute glomerulonephritis (580)	0	1	1	1	0	0	1	-	-
Nephrotic syndrome (581)	1	2	1	1	1	1	2	2	-
Chronic glomerulonephritis (582)	0	-	-	0	0	1	1	0	-
Nephritis and nephropathy, not specified as acute or chronic (583)	0	-	0	0	0	0	0	0	-
Acute renal failure (584)	1	-	-	0	0	2	5	6	7
Chronic renal failure (585)	4	-	-	1	2	5	14	19	44
Renal failure, unspecified (586)	1	1	-	-	0	1	3	6	15
Renal sclerosis, unspecified (587)	0	0	-	-	-	-	-	-	-
Disorders resulting from impaired renal function (588)	0	-	-	0	-	-	0	-	-
Infections of kidney (590)	14	0	5	26	19	13	10	10	9
Hydronephrosis (591)	1	2	0	1	1	1	2	0	4
Calculus of kidney and ureter (592)	7	0	1	4	8	12	8	6	4
Other disorders of kidney and ureter (593)	1	5	2	1	1	2	2	2	-
Calculus of lower urinary tract (594)	1	-	0	0	0	1	4	1	1
Cystitis (595)	110	24	31	134	124	122	153	170	166
Other disorders of bladder (596)	6	-	1	2	4	9	19	18	13
Urethritis, not sexually transmitted, and urethral syndrome (597)	2	1	1	2	3	4	1	2	1
Urethral stricture (598)	2	-	1	-	1	2	5	5	6
Other disorders of urethra and urinary tract (599)	280	219	143	284	259	258	412	591	809
Hyperplasia of prostate (600)	13	-	-	-	0	21	61	68	37
Inflammatory diseases of prostate (601)	4	-	-	1	4	7	9	13	4
Other disorders of prostate (602)	0	-	-	-	-	0	0	2	-
Hydrocele (603)	6	26	4	3	2	5	9	11	10
Orchitis and epididymitis (604)	15	1	3	13	25	16	16	9	3
Redundant prepuce and phimosis (605)	14	77	33	8	4	4	3	5	7
Infertility, male (606)	3	-	-	1	8	1	0	-	-
Disorders of penis (607)	32	167	60	16	16	14	18	14	7
Other disorders of male genital organs (608)	14	4	9	14	18	17	18	8	1
Benign mammary dysplasias (610)	18	1	3	16	34	22	3	2	-
Other disorders of breast (611)	83	13	37	73	139	93	44	29	15
Inflammatory disease of ovary, fallopian tube, pelvic cellular tissue and peritoneum (614)	31	0	1	80	64	7	0	1	-
Inflammatory diseases of uterus, except cervix (615)	4	-	-	8	9	1	-	0	-
Inflammatory disease of cervix, vagina and vulva (616)	72	50	32	102	108	56	42	46	55

By age-group and sex

Total		0-4		5-15		16-24		25-44		45-64		65-74		75-84		85 and over	
Male	Female	Male	Female	Male	Female	Male	Female	Male	Female	Male	Female	Male	Female	Male	Female	Male	Female
5	6	4	2	0	0	0	1	2	3	6	8	15	12	27	25	83	47
13	31	-	-	-	0	-	0	3	4	18	43	61	103	79	145	95	148
130	290	254	262	63	94	63	303	85	303	116	278	248	339	471	480	767	690
22	31	53	49	12	11	17	53	23	45	22	21	13	9	18	11	18	8
10	4	5	1	2	1	7	4	13	6	14	5	9	0	7	2	-	-
0	1	-	-	-	0	-	-	1	1	0	1	1	1	-	-	-	2
0	1	1	-	0	1	-	0	0	2	0	2	1	1	-	2	-	2
30	38	29	21	10	6	13	27	27	33	40	39	53	70	72	92	113	122
0	0	-	1	0	-	1	0	0	-	0	-	1	-	-	-	-	-
5	4	-	-	-	-	1	-	6	2	11	10	11	9	6	6	-	-
0	0	-	-	-	-	-	-	0	0	1	1	1	0	-	1	-	-
0	0	-	-	-	-	-	-	0	-	1	0	1	1	-	1	-	-
5	17	-	-	0	-	0	7	2	16	10	32	18	28	18	23	12	16
5	14	-	-	-	-	1	5	3	15	11	25	13	27	21	17	24	20
3	3	1	-	-	0	-	1	1	1	4	4	9	4	18	10	36	18
3	2	-	-	0	-	0	1	3	1	5	2	5	6	11	6	-	8
14	10	4	5	2	1	7	4	9	5	14	8	37	19	68	48	131	79
2	4	5	7	2	1	1	4	2	4	2	5	3	7	1	7	-	6
0	0	1	1	1	0	1	0	0	1	0	0	-	1	-	-	-	-
1	1	3	-	2	1	-	1	1	1	2	0	2	1	2	2	-	-
1	0	-	-	-	-	0	0	0	0	1	1	2	-	1	-	-	-
0	0	-	-	-	0	-	0	1	0	1	0	-	0	-	1	-	-
2	1	-	-	-	-	1	-	0	0	2	1	6	4	8	5	12	6
4	4	-	-	-	-	1	-	2	2	5	5	17	12	24	16	65	37
1	1	1	-	-	-	-	-	0	0	1	1	5	2	8	5	42	6
-	0	-	1	-	-	-	-	-	-	-	-	-	-	-	-	-	-
0	0	-	-	-	-	0	-	-	-	-	-	-	0	-	-	-	-
5	23	-	1	3	8	3	49	7	31	6	19	9	12	7	12	-	12
1	1	3	2	1	-	-	1	1	1	1	1	3	1	-	1	12	2
9	4	-	1	1	0	3	4	11	5	17	8	12	6	11	3	-	6
2	1	5	4	2	2	-	1	1	1	2	1	1	2	3	1	-	-
1	0	-	-	0	-	0	0	1	0	1	0	6	2	2	-	-	2
14	203	5	43	6	56	6	262	10	240	20	225	36	249	42	246	71	197
5	7	-	-	-	1	1	2	3	5	6	12	22	17	25	14	18	12
3	2	2	-	2	1	1	3	3	2	4	3	1	1	6	-	-	2
3	0	-	-	2	-	-	-	1	0	3	1	10	0	13	1	18	2
125	430	135	307	66	224	49	517	69	451	131	387	316	491	528	629	683	851
28	-	-	-	-	-	-	-	1	-	41	-	136	-	182	-	149	-
9	-	-	-	-	-	2	-	8	-	14	-	20	-	34	-	18	-
0	-	-	-	-	-	-	-	-	-	1	-	1	-	6	-	-	-
12	-	52	-	7	-	5	-	5	-	9	-	20	-	30	-	42	-
30	-	2	-	5	-	26	-	49	-	32	-	35	-	24	-	12	-
28	-	151	-	65	-	16	-	9	-	7	-	8	-	14	-	30	-
6	-	-	-	-	-	2	-	16	-	2	-	1	-	-	-	-	-
66	-	327	-	117	-	31	-	33	-	28	-	41	-	37	-	30	-
29	-	7	-	17	-	27	-	35	-	33	-	40	-	22	-	6	-
1	35	-	1	2	4	1	32	0	68	1	44	-	6	-	3	-	-
13	150	7	18	40	34	18	127	4	274	7	180	7	75	10	40	18	14
-	62	-	1	-	1	-	159	-	129	-	14	-	0	-	1	-	-
-	8	-	-	-	-	-	16	-	18	-	2	-	-	-	1	-	-
-	142	-	103	-	65	-	204	-	217	-	113	-	77	-	74	-	73

Table 21 - *continued*

Disease group	Persons, by age group								
	Total	0-4	5-15	16-24	25-44	45-64	65-74	75-84	85 and over
Endometriosis (617)	6	-	-	6	14	3	0	-	-
Genital prolapse (618)	23	-	0	1	10	36	68	106	84
Fistulae involving female genital tract (619)	0	-	-	-	0	0	1	1	3
Noninflammatory disorders of ovary, fallopian tube and broad ligament (620)	5	-	0	6	8	5	1	3	1
Disorders of uterus, not elsewhere classified (621)	2	0	-	2	4	4	1	0	-
Noninflammatory disorders of cervix (622)	11	-	0	12	19	17	4	3	-
Noninflammatory disorders of vagina (623)	33	9	9	57	55	22	13	11	30
Noninflammatory disorders of vulva and perineum (624)	2	1	1	1	4	2	3	4	4
Pain and other symptoms associated with female genital organs (625)	142	-	61	239	275	73	18	18	21
Disorders of menstruation and other abnormal bleeding from female genital tract (626)	229	1	56	454	428	149	2	2	-
Menopausal and postmenopausal disorders (627)	167	1	-	1	85	604	109	66	80
Infertility, female (628)	16	-	-	17	44	1	-	-	-
Other disorders of female genital organs (629)	0	-	0	0	-	0	-	-	-
Hydatidiform mole (630)	0	-	-	1	1	0	-	-	-
Other abnormal product of conception (631)	1	0	0	0	2	0	-	-	-
Missed abortion (632)	2	-	0	5	6	-	-	-	-
Ectopic pregnancy (633)	3	-	0	7	7	-	-	-	-
Spontaneous abortion (634)	15	-	0	36	32	1	-	-	-
Legally induced abortion (635)	5	-	1	18	8	0	-	-	-
Unspecified abortion (637)	0	-	-	1	0	-	-	-	-
Failed attempted abortion (638)	0	-	-	0	-	-	-	-	-
Complications following abortion and ectopic and molar pregnancies (639)	0	-	-	1	1	-	-	-	-
Haemorrhage in early pregnancy (640)	21	-	1	53	46	0	-	-	-
Antepartum haemorrhage, abruptio placentae, and placenta praevia (641)	2	-	-	4	5	-	-	-	-
Hypertension complicating pregnancy, childbirth and the puerperium (642)	3	-	-	6	6	0	-	-	-
Excessive vomiting in pregnancy (643)	8	-	0	25	16	0	-	-	-
Early or threatened labour (644)	2	-	-	7	3	-	-	-	-
Prolonged pregnancy (645)	0	-	-	1	0	-	-	-	-
Other complications of pregnancy, not elsewhere classified (646)	10	-	1	29	21	0	-	-	1
Infective and parasitic conditions in the mother classifiable elsewhere but complicating pregnancy, childbirth and the puerperium (647)	0	-	-	0	0	-	-	-	-
Other current conditions in the mother classifiable elsewhere but complicating pregnancy, childbirth and the puerperium (648)	5	-	0	10	11	-	-	-	-
Delivery in a completely normal case (650)	25	1	1	55	58	-	-	-	-
Multiple gestation (651)	1	-	-	2	3	-	-	-	-
Malposition and malpresentation of fetus (652)	1	-	-	3	3	-	-	-	-
Disproportion (653)	0	-	-	1	0	-	-	-	-
Abnormality of organs and soft tissues of pelvis (654)	0	0	-	-	0	0	-	-	-
Known or suspected fetal abnormality affecting management of mother (655)	0	-	-	1	0	-	-	-	-
Other fetal and placental problems affecting management of mother (656)	2	1	-	5	3	-	-	-	-
Polyhydramnios (657)	0	-	-	0	1	-	-	-	-
Other problems associated with amniotic cavity and membranes (658)	0	-	-	1	0	-	-	-	-
Other indications for care or intervention related to labour and delivery and not elsewhere classified (659)	0	-	-	1	0	-	-	-	-
Obstructed labour (660)	0	-	-	0	0	-	-	-	-
Abnormality of forces of labour (661)	0	-	-	1	0	-	-	-	-
Long labour (662)	0	-	-	0	0	-	-	-	-
Umbilical cord complications (663)	0	4	-	0	0	-	-	-	-
Trauma to perineum and vulva during delivery (664)	1	0	-	2	2	-	-	-	-
Other obstetrical trauma (665)	0	-	-	1	0	0	-	-	-
Postpartum haemorrhage (666)	2	-	-	5	6	-	-	-	-
Retained placenta or membranes, without haemorrhage (667)	1	-	-	2	3	0	-	-	-
Other complications of labour and delivery, not elsewhere classified (669)	7	1	0	14	17	0	-	-	-

By age-group and sex

| Total | | 0-4 | | 5-15 | | 16-24 | | 25-44 | | 45-64 | | 65-74 | | 75-84 | | 85 and over | |
Male	Female	Male	Female	Male	Female	Male	Female	Male	Female	Male	Female	Male	Female	Male	Female	Male	Female
-	11	-	-	-	-	-	11	-	28	-	7	-	0	-	-	-	-
-	45	-	-	-	0	-	1	-	20	-	73	-	123	-	169	-	112
-	1	-	-	-	-	-	-	-	0	-	1	-	2	-	2	-	4
-	9	-	-	-	0	-	13	-	16	-	9	-	1	-	4	-	2
-	5	-	1	-	-	-	4	-	8	-	9	-	1	-	1	-	-
-	22	-	-	-	0	-	25	-	38	-	35	-	8	-	5	-	-
-	64	-	18	-	19	-	114	-	111	-	45	-	23	-	18	-	39
-	5	-	3	-	2	-	3	-	7	-	4	-	5	-	6	-	6
-	278	-	-	-	126	-	476	-	553	-	148	-	32	-	29	-	28
0	449	-	2	-	115	-	905	-	859	0	301	-	4	-	3	-	-
-	328	-	-	-	-	-	1	-	170	-	1,219	-	197	-	106	-	106
-	31	-	-	-	-	-	33	-	89	-	1	-	-	-	-	-	-
-	0	-	-	-	0	-	0	-	-	-	0	-	-	-	-	-	-
-	1	-	-	-	-	-	1	-	1	-	0	-	-	-	-	-	-
-	1	-	1	-	1	-	1	-	3	-	0	-	-	-	-	-	-
-	5	-	-	-	1	-	11	-	11	-	-	-	-	-	-	-	-
-	6	-	-	-	0	-	13	-	14	-	-	-	-	-	-	-	-
-	29	-	-	-	0	-	71	-	65	-	1	-	-	-	-	-	-
-	10	-	-	-	2	-	36	-	16	-	0	-	-	-	-	-	-
-	0	-	-	-	-	-	2	-	1	-	-	-	-	-	-	-	-
-	0	-	-	-	-	-	1	-	-	-	-	-	-	-	-	-	-
-	1	-	-	-	-	-	2	-	2	-	-	-	-	-	-	-	-
-	41	-	-	-	2	-	105	-	93	-	1	-	-	-	-	-	-
-	4	-	-	-	-	-	8	-	9	-	-	-	-	-	-	-	-
-	5	-	-	-	-	-	12	-	12	-	0	-	-	-	-	-	-
-	16	-	-	-	0	-	49	-	33	-	0	-	-	-	-	-	-
-	3	-	-	-	-	-	13	-	5	-	-	-	-	-	-	-	-
-	0	-	-	-	-	-	1	-	0	-	-	-	-	-	-	-	-
-	21	-	-	-	1	-	59	-	43	-	0	-	-	-	-	-	2
-	0	-	-	-	-	-	1	-	1	-	-	-	-	-	-	-	-
-	10	-	-	-	0	-	21	-	23	-	-	-	-	-	-	-	-
-	49	-	3	-	1	-	110	-	117	-	-	-	-	-	-	-	-
-	2	-	-	-	-	-	4	-	5	-	-	-	-	-	-	-	-
-	3	-	-	-	-	-	6	-	7	-	-	-	-	-	-	-	-
-	0	-	-	-	-	-	1	-	0	-	-	-	-	-	-	-	-
-	0	-	1	-	-	-	-	-	0	-	0	-	-	-	-	-	-
-	0	-	-	-	-	-	2	-	1	-	-	-	-	-	-	-	-
-	3	-	1	-	-	-	9	-	6	-	-	-	-	-	-	-	-
-	1	-	-	-	-	-	1	-	1	-	-	-	-	-	-	-	-
-	0	-	-	-	-	-	2	-	1	-	-	-	-	-	-	-	-
-	0	-	-	-	-	-	1	-	0	-	-	-	-	-	-	-	-
-	0	-	-	-	-	-	0	-	0	-	-	-	-	-	-	-	-
-	0	-	-	-	-	-	2	-	1	-	-	-	-	-	-	-	-
-	0	-	-	-	-	-	1	-	1	-	-	-	-	-	-	-	-
0	1	1	7	-	-	-	1	-	0	-	-	-	-	-	-	-	-
-	2	-	1	-	-	-	5	-	5	-	-	-	-	-	-	-	-
-	0	-	-	-	-	-	1	-	1	-	0	-	-	-	-	-	-
-	5	-	-	-	-	-	10	-	12	-	-	-	-	-	-	-	-
-	2	-	-	-	-	-	4	-	6	-	0	-	-	-	-	-	-
-	14	-	1	-	0	-	27	-	34	-	0	-	-	-	-	-	-

Table 21 - *continued*

Disease group	Persons, by age group								
	Total	0-4	5-15	16-24	25-44	45-64	65-74	75-84	85 and over
Major puerperal infection (670)	1	-	-	2	2	-	-	-	1
Venous complications in pregnancy and the puerperium (671)	4	-	0	6	9	0	1	0	-
Pyrexia of unknown origin during the puerperium (672)	0	-	0	-	0	-	-	-	-
Other and unspecified complications of the puerperium, not elsewhere classified (674)	1	-	-	2	3	-	-	-	-
Infections of the breast and nipple associated with childbirth (675)	9	-	-	11	23	0	-	-	-
Other disorders of the breast associated with childbirth, and disorders of lactation (676)	5	0	0	7	11	2	1	0	-
Carbuncle and furuncle (680)	60	34	44	82	81	54	41	32	21
Cellulitis and abscess of finger and toe (681)	61	113	93	46	46	54	61	65	77
Other cellulitis and abscess (682)	105	55	57	75	96	116	158	231	348
Acute lymphadenitis (683)	19	41	34	27	18	8	4	3	6
Impetigo (684)	66	284	165	64	28	17	20	21	19
Pilonidal cyst (685)	6	3	1	17	8	3	1	1	-
Other local infections of skin and subcutaneous tissue (686)	44	70	47	38	41	39	43	57	77
Erythematosquamous dermatosis (690)	79	163	64	71	75	66	97	87	67
Atopic dermatitis and related conditions (691)	303	1,602	297	252	186	166	199	175	169
Contact dermatitis and other eczema (692)	203	371	178	247	193	166	195	173	161
Dermatitis due to substances taken internally (693)	1	3	1	1	1	2	2	3	1
Bullous dermatoses (694)	2	1	2	1	1	2	5	8	12
Erythematous conditions (695)	67	54	19	37	62	91	118	113	136
Psoriasis and similar disorders (696)	73	20	58	86	85	77	80	55	33
Lichen (697)	5	1	1	3	4	7	8	9	3
Pruritus and related conditions (698)	79	45	37	47	71	100	136	149	191
Corns and callosities (700)	16	2	7	11	13	18	36	47	47
Other hypertrophic and atrophic conditions of skin (701)	10	5	10	10	8	9	13	23	12
Other dermatoses (702)	39	3	6	8	18	64	122	139	99
Diseases of nail (703)	61	34	103	108	41	47	50	56	55
Diseases of hair and hair follicles (704)	40	31	28	58	57	32	23	15	7
Disorders of sweat glands (705)	23	24	20	32	30	18	11	5	7
Diseases of sebaceous glands (706)	203	36	217	549	219	106	83	69	49
Chronic ulcer of skin (707)	20	1	1	2	3	17	58	137	281
Urticaria (708)	71	137	98	71	65	54	58	47	41
Other disorders of skin and subcutaneous tissue (709)	21	26	19	20	23	21	22	15	13
Diffuse diseases of connective tissue (710)	4	-	0	1	3	7	7	5	3
Arthropathy associated with infections (711)	1	1	0	1	2	1	2	2	7
Crystal arthropathies (712)	0	-	-	-	-	0	-	-	-
Rheumatoid arthritis and other inflammatory polyarthropathies (714)	38	1	3	6	21	71	111	101	71
Osteoarthrosis and allied disorders (715)	315	1	1	10	69	559	1,038	1,370	1,444
Other and unspecified arthropathies (716)	23	1	3	10	24	40	36	41	34
Internal derangement of knee (717)	32	-	41	60	39	26	13	6	1
Other derangement of joint (718)	3	1	2	5	4	2	3	2	1
Other and unspecified disorder of joint (719)	241	45	124	171	235	344	351	405	376
Ankylosing spondylitis and other inflammatory spondylopathies (720)	10	-	1	5	14	19	9	11	3
Spondylosis and allied disorders (721)	119	-	0	10	73	266	292	241	197
Intervertebral disc disorders (722)	39	-	1	14	51	74	48	34	19
Other disorders of cervical region (723)	91	18	48	64	127	117	84	72	65
Other and unspecified disorders of back (724)	372	9	59	257	452	556	495	517	481
Polymyalgia rheumatica (725)	11	-	-	-	1	9	41	87	50
Peripheral enthesopathies and allied syndromes (726)	194	2	42	75	196	391	269	224	138
Other disorders of synovium, tendon and bursa (727)	82	10	32	72	92	119	106	83	75
Disorders of muscle, ligament and fascia (728)	40	6	17	23	32	67	78	63	61
Other disorders of soft tissues (729)	190	35	70	103	161	268	390	422	370

By age-group and sex

Total		0-4		5-15		16-24		25-44		45-64		65-74		75-84		85 and over	
Male	Female	Male	Female	Male	Female	Male	Female	Male	Female	Male	Female	Male	Female	Male	Female	Male	Female
-	2	-	-	-	-	-	4	-	4	-	-	-	-	-	-	-	2
-	7	-	-	-	0	-	11	-	19	-	0	-	1	-	1	-	-
-	0	-	-	-	0	-	-	-	1	-	-	-	-	-	-	-	-
-	3	-	-	-	-	-	4	-	7	-	-	-	-	-	-	-	-
-	17	-	-	-	-	-	21	-	46	-	0	-	-	-	-	-	-
-	9	-	1	-	1	-	14	-	21	-	4	-	2	-	1	-	-
56	64	35	33	46	42	70	93	73	88	49	60	43	40	30	33	18	22
60	63	125	100	94	91	50	42	42	50	45	63	57	64	61	67	89	73
93	116	60	50	60	55	70	81	90	103	109	122	137	175	181	261	214	392
16	22	54	28	31	37	19	36	12	25	4	11	3	5	2	3	6	6
67	64	294	275	173	156	55	73	25	31	16	18	20	19	24	18	36	14
8	4	2	3	1	0	22	13	11	5	3	2	2	-	1	1	-	-
39	50	84	55	43	52	32	44	32	50	34	43	35	49	56	58	65	81
77	82	172	153	52	75	56	85	70	80	67	65	115	81	102	78	48	73
264	341	1,514	1,694	254	343	149	355	133	240	144	189	218	183	205	157	166	169
160	244	375	366	150	206	154	340	126	259	134	199	189	200	181	169	155	164
1	2	4	2	1	1	1	0	-	1	1	3	1	2	1	5	-	2
2	3	1	1	2	1	1	1	1	2	1	3	6	5	7	8	18	10
50	83	49	59	17	22	27	47	47	78	71	112	89	142	89	128	71	158
67	79	24	15	47	70	62	110	77	93	79	76	80	80	56	55	53	26
4	5	2	1	1	2	2	4	3	5	8	7	9	7	7	10	-	4
54	102	29	62	23	51	26	68	46	97	74	127	113	155	127	161	178	195
12	21	3	2	2	12	7	15	9	16	13	24	33	39	45	48	42	49
7	12	7	4	8	12	7	14	4	11	7	12	11	14	24	23	12	12
36	43	4	1	7	5	6	9	13	24	60	68	131	114	158	127	125	91
69	53	41	27	111	96	143	74	49	33	42	52	52	48	70	48	77	47
33	48	30	32	24	32	44	71	46	69	24	40	15	29	8	18	12	6
17	29	17	32	17	22	16	47	20	40	16	21	9	13	3	5	6	8
182	224	39	32	188	248	535	562	159	279	99	114	88	79	88	57	59	45
16	25	1	1	2	0	2	2	3	2	16	18	58	59	121	146	267	286
51	91	125	149	88	109	40	102	38	93	32	77	45	69	27	58	30	45
18	25	32	21	17	21	15	25	17	29	16	26	18	25	9	18	18	12
1	6	-	-	-	0	1	2	1	6	4	10	3	10	2	6	-	4
1	1	2	1	1	-	1	1	2	2	1	1	1	3	2	1	6	8
-	0	-	-	-	-	-	-	-	-	-	0	-	-	-	-	-	-
22	53	1	1	1	5	2	9	12	29	48	96	71	144	52	131	18	89
228	398	1	-	1	1	11	9	55	82	466	654	818	1,217	1,017	1,581	1,022	1,584
18	29	1	1	2	3	7	13	18	30	32	48	33	39	24	51	30	35
36	29	-	-	29	55	59	60	51	28	31	21	17	9	7	5	6	-
4	2	1	1	1	2	6	3	5	3	3	2	3	3	1	2	-	2
200	281	51	38	118	130	162	180	201	270	271	419	289	401	316	458	333	390
9	11	-	-	1	1	5	6	11	16	17	21	10	8	14	9	6	2
98	139	-	-	-	1	10	11	53	94	234	299	269	311	211	259	143	215
39	39	-	-	1	2	13	15	55	47	72	75	44	52	31	36	18	20
73	109	17	20	48	47	48	80	92	163	95	140	76	91	66	75	77	61
323	418	13	5	46	73	201	313	403	502	500	613	436	543	458	552	487	479
6	15	-	-	-	-	-	-	1	1	3	15	24	55	78	92	36	55
191	196	2	1	39	46	71	79	199	193	375	407	278	262	239	215	184	122
62	100	12	9	26	38	46	97	71	113	91	147	85	124	71	90	36	89
43	37	9	3	19	15	25	22	31	33	72	62	98	61	84	51	71	57
152	225	42	28	71	68	83	123	122	199	208	329	352	421	401	434	380	366

Table 21 - *continued*

Disease group	Persons, by age group								
	Total	0-4	5-15	16-24	25-44	45-64	65-74	75-84	85 and over
Osteomyelitis, periostitis and other infections involving bone (730)	2	1	1	1	1	2	4	3	3
Osteitis deformans and osteopathies associated with other disorders classified elsewhere (731)	2	-	0	-	-	2	7	15	18
Osteochondropathies (732)	9	1	49	7	2	1	0	0	-
Other disorders of bone and cartilage (733)	29	1	7	21	22	37	63	85	108
Flat foot (734)	4	11	9	3	2	3	4	5	3
Acquired deformities of toe (735)	11	14	9	6	6	17	18	21	10
Other acquired deformities of limbs (736)	4	7	4	3	2	5	5	4	4
Curvature of spine (737)	3	1	4	3	3	4	5	6	7
Other acquired deformity (738)	1	1	1	2	1	1	3	3	1
Spina bifida (741)	0	1	0	2	0	0	-	-	1
Other congenital anamolies of nervous system (742)	0	2	-	1	0	0	1	-	-
Congenital anomalies of eye (743)	3	17	1	1	1	2	2	6	9
Congenital anomalies of ear, face and neck (744)	2	6	5	2	1	1	-	1	1
Bulbus cordis anomalies and anomalies of cardiac septal closure (745)	2	17	3	2	0	1	1	1	-
Other congenital anomalies of heart (746)	1	3	1	1	1	1	1	2	-
Other congenital anomalies of ciculatory system (747)	1	3	0	1	0	1	1	1	-
Congenital anomalies of respiratory system (748)	0	1	-	0	-	0	0	-	-
Cleft palate and cleft lip (749)	0	2	0	0	0	-	1	-	-
Other congenital anomalies of upper alimentary tract (750)	5	19	1	1	1	4	16	13	18
Other congenital anomalies of digestive system (751)	1	3	1	0	0	1	1	2	6
Congenital anomalies of genital organs (752)	7	49	18	3	1	1	1	0	-
Congenital anomalies of urinary system (753)	1	5	1	1	2	1	-	-	-
Certain congenital musculoskeletal deformities (754)	6	39	10	4	3	2	2	2	-
Other congenital anomalies of limbs (755)	2	10	3	2	1	2	1	3	3
Other congenital musculoskeletal anomalies (756)	4	7	2	2	4	5	5	2	1
Congenital anomalies of the integument (757)	15	33	9	9	16	19	13	13	4
Chromosomal anomalies (758)	1	5	1	2	1	1	-	-	-
Other and unspecified congenital anomalies (759)	1	4	2	2	1	1	1	-	-
Fetus or newborn affected by maternal complications of pregnancy (761)	0	-	-	0	0	-	-	-	-
Fetus or newborn affected by complications of placenta, cord and membranes (762)	0	6	-	-	0	-	-	-	-
Fetus or newborn affected by other complications of labour and delivery (763)	0	-	-	-	0	-	-	-	-
Slow fetal growth and fetal malnutrition (764)	0	0	-	0	0	-	-	-	-
Disorders relating to short gestation and unspecified low birthweight (765)	1	9	-	-	-	-	-	-	-
Disorders relating to long gestation and high birthweight (766)	0	-	-	-	0	-	-	-	-
Birth trauma (767)	0	1	-	0	-	-	-	-	-
Intrauterine hypoxia and birth asphyxia (768)	0	1	-	-	0	-	-	-	-
Respiratory distress syndrome (769)	0	2	-	-	-	-	-	-	-
Other respiratory conditions of fetus and newborn (770)	0	6	-	-	0	-	-	0	-
Infections specific to the perinatal period (771)	9	127	0	1	0	0	-	1	-
Fetal and neonatal haemorrhage (772)	0	0	-	0	0	-	-	1	-
Haemolytic disease of fetus or newborn, due to isoimmunization (773)	0	0	-	-	-	-	-	0	-
Other perinatal jaundice (774)	1	9	-	-	-	-	-	0	-
Endocrine and metabolic disturbances specific to the fetus and newborn (775)	0	1	-	-	-	-	-	-	-
Conditions involving the integument and temperature regulation of fetus and newborn (778)	0	1	-	-	0	-	-	-	-
Other and ill-defined conditions originating in the perinatal period (779)	1	16	-	1	0	-	-	-	-

By age-group and sex

Total		0-4		5-15		16-24		25-44		45-64		65-74		75-84		85 and over	
Male	Female	Male	Female	Male	Female	Male	Female	Male	Female	Male	Female	Male	Female	Male	Female	Male	Female
2	1	1	1	1	1	1	0	1	1	3	1	6	3	-	5	-	4
2	2	-	-	-	0	-	-	-	-	3	1	7	8	11	18	30	14
11	6	1	1	63	35	8	6	2	2	1	1	1	-	-	1	-	-
14	44	1	1	7	8	17	24	15	30	16	57	23	95	15	127	24	136
4	4	13	10	9	9	2	3	2	2	3	3	3	5	10	2	-	4
6	16	15	13	7	11	2	9	3	10	8	25	8	25	13	25	-	14
4	4	8	6	3	4	2	3	3	2	5	5	5	6	8	2	6	4
3	4	1	1	4	3	3	3	2	3	4	4	5	6	2	9	6	8
2	1	2	1	1	1	3	0	1	1	1	1	2	4	3	2	6	-
0	1	1	1	-	0	1	2	0	0	0	1	-	-	-	-	-	2
0	0	4	1	-	-	-	1	0	0	0	-	-	1	-	-	-	-
2	3	18	17	0	2	0	1	1	1	0	3	2	2	6	7	-	12
2	2	6	6	4	7	1	3	1	2	1	1	-	-	2	1	-	2
2	2	15	19	4	3	2	1	0	1	0	1	1	0	-	1	-	-
1	1	4	3	2	0	1	2	1	1	1	1	1	1	3	1	-	-
1	1	3	3	-	0	1	1	1	0	1	1	1	1	-	1	-	-
0	0	1	1	-	-	0	-	-	-	0	0	-	0	-	-	-	-
0	0	2	3	0	0	0	-	0	-	-	-	-	1	-	-	-	-
5	5	27	11	2	0	0	1	2	1	4	4	15	17	8	16	18	18
1	1	4	2	1	1	-	0	0	0	-	1	1	1	2	2	6	6
13	1	94	3	35	1	2	3	1	0	1	0	1	0	-	1	-	-
1	1	9	2	0	1	0	2	1	2	1	2	-	-	-	-	-	-
6	6	38	40	9	10	4	4	2	4	1	3	2	1	3	1	-	-
2	3	10	10	3	3	1	3	1	1	2	2	1	1	1	3	-	4
3	4	10	4	2	3	2	3	3	4	5	5	3	6	-	3	6	-
13	18	27	40	7	12	6	12	12	20	16	21	13	13	9	15	6	4
1	2	2	7	1	2	2	1	2	1	1	1	-	-	-	-	-	-
1	1	4	4	2	2	1	2	1	1	1	1	1	0	-	-	-	-
-	0	-	-	-	-	-	0	-	0	-	-	-	-	-	-	-	-
1	0	11	1	-	-	-	-	-	0	-	-	-	-	-	-	-	-
-	0	-	-	-	-	-	-	-	0	-	-	-	-	-	-	-	-
0	0	1	-	-	-	-	1	-	0	-	-	-	-	-	-	-	-
0	1	7	11	-	-	-	-	-	-	-	-	-	-	-	-	-	-
-	0	-	-	-	-	-	-	-	0	-	-	-	-	-	-	-	-
0	0	1	2	-	-	-	0	-	-	-	-	-	-	-	-	-	-
0	0	1	-	-	-	-	-	-	0	-	-	-	-	-	-	-	-
0	0	2	1	-	-	-	-	-	-	-	-	-	-	-	-	-	-
1	0	8	4	-	-	-	-	-	0	-	-	-	-	1	-	-	-
8	10	112	142	0	0	-	1	0	1	-	1	-	-	1	1	-	-
0	0	-	1	-	-	-	0	-	0	-	-	-	-	1	1	-	-
-	0	-	1	-	-	-	-	-	-	-	-	-	-	-	1	-	-
1	0	12	5	-	-	-	-	-	-	-	-	-	-	-	1	-	-
0	-	1	-	-	-	-	-	-	-	-	-	-	-	-	-	-	-
0	0	1	1	-	-	-	-	-	0	-	-	-	-	-	-	-	-
1	1	18	13	-	-	-	2	-	1	-	-	-	-	-	-	-	-

Table 21- *continued*

Disease group	Persons, by age group								
	Total	0-4	5-15	16-24	25-44	45-64	65-74	75-84	85 and over
General symptoms (780)	293	374	133	198	224	318	472	715	889
Symptoms involving nervous and musculoskeletal systems (781)	15	23	9	11	9	16	32	38	31
Symptoms involving skin and other integumentary tissue (782)	217	528	193	162	155	184	254	372	510
Symptoms concerning nutrition, metabolism and development (783)	43	137	28	44	25	29	60	72	96
Symptoms involving head and neck (784)	179	93	222	221	168	167	163	208	204
Symptoms involving cardiovascular system (785)	61	115	52	55	52	54	79	82	64
Symptoms involving respiratory system and other chest symptoms (786)	366	1,096	345	203	235	344	473	514	531
Symptoms involving digestive system (787)	102	262	67	87	72	78	137	196	262
Symptoms involving urinary system (788)	81	104	78	48	55	70	124	221	280
Other symptoms involving abdomen and pelvis (789)	266	294	305	316	260	206	263	282	330
Nonspecific findings on examination of blood (790)	70	285	106	57	45	40	39	42	38
Nonspecific findings on examination of urine (791)	10	2	3	6	9	15	19	21	22
Nonspecific abnormal findings in other body substances (792)	13	8	5	22	20	10	5	3	3
Nonspecific abnormal findings on radiological and other examinatiion of body structure (793)	1	1	0	1	1	3	3	2	-
Nonspecific abnormal results of function studies (794)	3	1	1	1	2	6	8	7	4
Nonspecific abnormal histological and immunological findings (795)	4	0	0	6	8	2	1	1	1
Other nonspecific abnormal findings (796)	43	-	0	8	31	95	109	66	34
Senility without mention of psychosis (797)	6	-	-	-	0	0	4	39	259
Sudden death, cause unknown (798)	6	0	0	-	1	4	21	44	98
Other ill-defined and unknown causes of morbidity and mortality (799)	20	14	8	14	17	20	31	57	62
Fracture of vault of skull (800)	0	2	0	-	0	0	-	-	-
Fracture of base of skull (801)	0	-	-	0	0	0	0	-	-
Fracture of face bones (802)	6	1	6	14	7	3	2	4	6
Other and unqualified skull fractures (803)	1	1	1	1	1	1	1	0	4
Multiple fractures involving skull or face with other bones (804)	0	0	0	0	0	-	1	-	-
Fracture of vertebral column without mention of spinal cord lesion (805)	4	-	0	3	3	4	5	14	24
Fracture of vertebral column with spinal cord lesion (806)	0	-	-	0	0	0	-	0	1
Fracture of rib(s), sternum, larynx and trachea (807)	11	1	2	6	11	17	21	26	38
Fracture of pelvis (808)	2	0	0	1	1	1	3	9	19
Ill-defined fractures of trunk (809)	0	-	-	-	-	0	-	-	-
Fracture of clavicle (810)	4	7	8	6	3	2	4	2	9
Fracture of scapula (811)	0	-	-	1		0	1	0	-
Fracture of humerus (812)	5	3	6	3	2	4	12	14	27
Fracture of radius and ulna (813)	19	13	30	15	11	16	25	42	55
Fracture of carpal bone(s) (814)	5	0	4	8	6	4	3	4	3
Fracture of metacarpal bone(s) (815)	7	0	9	17	7	3	2	6	1
Fracture of one or more phalanges of hand (816)	7	1	14	10	7	5	4	3	1
Multiple fractures of hand bones (817)	0	-	-	0	-	-	-	-	-
Ill-defined fractures of upper limb (818)	0	-	-	0	0	1	1	2	3
Multiple fractures involving both upper limbs, and upper limb with rib(s) and sternum (819)	0	-	-	-	0	1	1	1	-
Fracture of neck of femur (820)	7	-	-	0	0	3	15	46	167
Fracture of other and unspecified parts of femur (821)	3	1	2	2	2	2	5	14	43
Fracture of patella (822)	2	0	2	2	1	2	2	3	3
Fracture of tibia and fibula (823)	7	7	6	12	8	7	4	3	13
Fracture of ankle (824)	7	0	2	11	7	9	11	10	4
Fracture of one or more tarsal and metatarsal bones (825)	7	3	7	5	7	9	7	4	1
Fracture of one or more phalanges of foot (826)	5	1	5	8	6	6	3	2	3
Other, multiple and ill-defined fractures of lower limb (827)	0	-	-	0	0	0	0	0	-
Multiple fractures involving both lower limbs, lower with upper limb, and lower limb(s) with rib(s) and sternum (828)	0	-	-	-	0	0	-	-	-
Fracture of unspecified bones (829)	2	1	2	3	2	2	3	4	6

By age-group and sex

Total		0-4		5-15		16-24		25-44		45-64		65-74		75-84		85 and over	
Male	Female	Male	Female	Male	Female	Male	Female	Male	Female	Male	Female	Male	Female	Male	Female	Male	Female
208	374	372	376	118	149	118	277	136	312	230	408	362	561	581	796	856	900
13	18	19	27	10	8	9	13	8	11	14	17	23	40	42	36	24	33
161	271	525	531	173	214	92	232	98	213	125	244	198	299	254	442	416	542
34	51	137	137	27	28	28	61	12	38	21	37	57	62	76	69	89	99
138	219	101	85	216	229	136	306	112	224	122	213	145	178	195	216	190	209
48	73	133	95	56	48	46	64	34	71	34	74	56	98	58	96	24	77
339	392	1,114	1,077	327	364	165	241	202	268	309	379	459	484	519	512	630	498
73	129	270	253	68	66	37	137	33	110	52	104	117	154	177	207	279	256
74	87	83	125	71	85	38	57	43	67	63	78	149	103	307	170	398	240
185	345	307	281	260	351	149	481	139	381	150	263	225	294	268	290	261	353
63	77	295	276	98	115	46	67	33	58	32	48	31	46	37	45	30	41
9	11	1	3	3	3	3	10	5	12	16	13	24	15	27	18	30	20
1	24	4	12	1	9	1	43	1	39	2	19	1	9	-	5	-	4
1	2	1	1	0	0	0	1	0	1	2	5	2	4	2	2	-	-
3	3	1	-	0	2	0	1	3	1	6	5	9	8	7	8	-	6
0	8	1	-	-	1	0	12	0	17	-	4	1	1	-	2	6	-
42	45	-	-	0	-	6	11	36	27	95	95	90	123	56	73	59	26
4	8	-	-	-	-	-	-	-	0	0	0	3	4	38	39	297	246
6	6	-	1	1	-	-	-	0	1	4	4	27	16	60	35	125	89
14	25	13	15	9	7	8	19	11	23	16	25	22	38	50	62	53	65
0	0	1	2	0	0	-	-	1	0	0	-	-	-	-	-	-	-
0	-	-	-	-	-	0	-	0	-	0	-	1	-	-	-	-	-
8	4	1	1	7	6	23	6	10	4	3	3	-	4	1	5	6	6
1	0	1	-	2	0	2	1	1	1	1	-	1	-	-	1	-	6
0	0	-	1	-	0	0	-	0	-	-	-	1	-	-	-	-	-
3	4	-	-	0	-	3	2	3	3	3	4	3	6	7	18	6	30
0	0	-	-	-	-	0	-	0	-	0	0	-	-	-	1	-	2
13	10	1	1	2	1	7	4	16	5	19	15	23	19	24	27	30	41
1	2	1	-	0	0	1	1	1	1	1	0	1	4	2	13	12	22
-	0	-	-	-	-	-	-	-	-	-	0	-	-	-	-	-	-
5	3	7	8	11	4	9	2	4	2	1	2	3	4	2	2	12	8
0	0	-	-	-	-	0	1	1	0	0	-	-	1	-	1	-	-
3	7	2	4	6	6	4	1	2	2	2	7	3	19	5	20	12	32
16	21	12	14	35	26	23	8	14	8	10	22	7	40	9	62	24	65
6	4	1	-	5	3	10	5	8	4	3	5	3	2	2	5	6	2
11	3	-	1	14	3	31	3	12	3	4	3	2	3	6	7	-	2
9	5	1	1	15	12	14	6	11	3	6	4	2	5	2	3	-	2
0	-	-	-	-	-	0	-	-	-	-	-	-	-	-	-	-	-
1	0	-	-	-	-	1	-	1	0	0	1	-	1	2	2	6	2
1	0	-	-	-	-	-	-	1	0	1	0	1	1	-	1	-	-
2	11	-	-	-	-	0	-	1	0	2	3	5	23	18	63	89	193
3	4	1	1	2	1	4	-	2	1	3	2	3	6	5	20	18	51
2	2	-	1	3	0	3	1	2	1	2	1	1	2	-	5	-	4
10	5	7	6	6	5	19	5	12	3	7	7	3	5	-	4	-	18
8	7	-	1	4	1	17	4	9	4	9	10	2	18	5	14	6	4
7	6	4	1	10	4	6	4	9	6	8	10	4	9	2	5	-	2
5	5	1	1	6	4	11	6	6	5	4	8	2	5	-	3	-	4
0	0	-	-	-	-	1	-	1	0	1	-	-	0	1	-	-	-
0	0	-	-	-	-	-	-	0	0	-	0	-	-	-	-	-	-
2	2	-	3	2	1	4	2	3	2	2	2	2	4	2	5	6	6

Table 21 - *continued*

Disease group	Persons, by age group								
	Total	0-4	5-15	16-24	25-44	45-64	65-74	75-84	85 and over
Dislocation of jaw (830)	0	-	-	1	0	0	0	0	-
Dislocation of shoulder (831)	4	1	1	8	4	2	4	7	10
Dislocation of elbow (832)	1	7	1	1	0	1	0	-	1
Dislocation of wrist (833)	0	-	1	1	0	0	-	0	1
Dislocation of finger (834)	2	1	2	2	2	2	1	3	1
Dislocation of hip (835)	1	1	0	1	0	0	2	1	1
Dislocation of knee (836)	3	-	3	6	4	2	2	1	-
Dislocation of ankle (837)	1	-	1	0	1	0	1	0	1
Dislocation of foot (838)	0	-	1	0	0	0	1	1	-
Other, multiple and ill-defined dislocations (839)	2	0	1	1	3	2	2	3	-
Sprains and strains of shoulder and upper arm (840)	49	8	16	45	60	69	54	51	47
Sprains and strains of elbow and forearm (841)	13	16	15	12	14	16	7	5	3
Sprains and strains of wrist and hand (842)	42	12	73	59	41	33	29	31	37
Sprains and strains of hip and thigh (843)	34	8	32	34	35	41	35	45	41
Sprains and strains of knee and leg (844)	80	12	79	114	92	84	60	46	34
Sprains and strains of ankle and foot (845)	90	29	123	122	89	81	86	64	50
Sprains and strains of sacroiliac region (846)	44	-	5	32	65	68	43	30	28
Sprains and strains of other and unspecified parts of back (847)	168	5	53	224	247	193	101	102	93
Other and ill-defined sprains and strains (848)	65	4	36	67	79	79	66	69	77
Concussion (850)	12	38	26	16	6	4	4	9	13
Cerebral laceration and contusion (851)	0	2	1	0	0	0	-	1	-
Subarachnoid, subdural and extradural haemorrhage, following injury (852)	0	0	-	0	0	0	-	1	-
Intracranial injury of other and unspecified nature (854)	10	40	22	11	5	4	5	4	7
Traumatic pneumothorax and haemothorax (860)	0	-	0	1	0	0	-	0	-
Injury to heart and lung (861)	0	0	-	-	-	-	-	0	-
Injury to other and unspecified intrathoracic organs (862)	0	-	-	0	0	0	0	-	-
Injury to gastrointestinal tract (863)	0	0	1	0	0	0	1	-	-
Injury to spleen (865)	0	-	-	0	0	-	-	-	-
Injury to kidney (866)	0	-	0	0	0	-	-	-	-
Injury to pelvic organs (867)	0	-	-	0	1	0	1	-	-
Internal injury to unspecified or ill-defined organs (869)	0	-	-	0	0	1	0	1	-
Open wound of ocular adnexa (870)	2	4	3	2	2	2	1	1	-
Open wound of eyeball (871)	3	2	3	3	4	3	2	0	-
Open wound of ear (872)	2	4	6	3	1	1	1	0	1
Other open wound of head (873)	39	159	67	33	18	17	22	42	123
Open wound of neck (874)	0	1	0	1	0	0	-	-	-
Open wound of chest (wall) (875)	0	-	0	1	0	-	-	-	1
Open wound of back (876)	0	1	1	0	0	0	-	-	-
Open wound of buttock (877)	0	-	1	0	0	0	0	-	3
Open wound of genital organs (external), including traumatic amputation (878)	2	4	5	3	1	1	1	2	1
Open wound of other and unspecified sites, except limbs (879)	3	5	4	3	2	2	1	7	6
Open wound of shoulder and upper arm (880)	3	1	2	4	3	2	2	4	3
Open wound of elbow, forearm and wrist (881)	9	2	13	13	7	5	6	25	44
Open wound of hand except finger(s) alone (882)	12	8	11	22	11	10	9	8	13
Open wound of finger(s) (883)	32	30	27	42	34	35	30	19	22
Multiple and unspecified open wounds of upper limb (884)	1	-	0	1	1	0	2	2	4
Traumatic amputation of thumb (complete) (partial) (885)	0	-	-	0	0	-	-	-	-
Traumatic amputation of other finger(s) (complete) (partial) (886)	0	-	0	0	1	1	1	-	-
Traumatic amputation of arm and hand (complete) (partial) (887)	0	-	-	-	-	0	-	0	-
Open wound of hip and thigh (890)	1	1	4	2	1	1	1	1	1
Open wound of knee, leg (except thigh) and ankle (891)	21	7	31	15	9	14	38	83	78
Open wound of foot except toe(s) alone (892)	7	7	11	8	6	4	6	6	4
Open wound of toe(s) (893)	4	8	5	2	2	4	5	10	6
Multiple and unspecified open wound of lower limb (894)	2	-	2	2	1	2	4	7	9
Traumatic amputation of toe(s) (complete) (partial) (895)	0	-	-	-	0	0	0	-	-
Traumatic amputation of foot (complete) (partial) (896)	0	-	0	-	0	-	0	-	-
Traumatic amputation of leg(s) (complete) (partial) (897)	0	-	-	-	0	0	-	0	-

Patients consulting

By age-group and sex

Total		0-4		5-15		16-24		25-44		45-64		65-74		75-84		85 and over	
Male	Female	Male	Female	Male	Female	Male	Female	Male	Female	Male	Female	Male	Female	Male	Female	Male	Female
0	0	-	-	-	-	-	1	0	1	0	0	1	-	-	1	-	-
4	3	-	1	1	2	12	4	5	2	2	2	3	4	2	10	12	10
1	1	4	11	1	-	1	1	0	0	1	0	-	0	-	-	-	2
0	1	-	-	0	1	0	1	0	0	-	1	-	-	-	1	-	2
2	2	1	1	3	2	2	2	3	1	2	2	1	1	5	1	-	2
1	0	1	1	0	-	1	1	-	0	1	-	3	0	1	1	-	2
4	3	-	-	2	4	6	5	5	3	3	1	1	2	1	1	-	-
1	1	-	-	1	2	0	-	1	1	-	1	1	1	-	1	6	-
0	0	-	-	0	1	0	-	0	0	-	0	1	1	-	1	-	-
2	2	1	-	2	1	2	1	3	2	3	2	1	2	2	3	-	-
50	49	6	10	15	17	48	43	63	58	70	67	44	62	56	48	30	53
14	12	12	20	13	16	14	9	17	12	17	15	8	5	3	5	-	4
39	46	12	12	73	72	62	55	38	43	21	45	18	38	19	38	48	33
39	30	10	6	41	22	44	24	41	29	41	42	35	35	52	40	42	41
91	70	12	13	81	76	138	91	112	72	88	81	66	55	32	55	-	45
84	95	38	20	115	130	139	104	90	89	59	102	50	116	44	76	30	57
37	51	-	-	4	5	26	37	53	77	58	78	38	46	27	32	24	30
168	167	6	4	54	52	221	227	251	243	190	195	87	112	94	107	119	85
64	66	3	4	40	31	76	58	85	73	67	90	48	81	62	73	53	85
13	11	39	37	37	15	16	16	5	7	4	5	2	5	8	9	12	14
0	0	2	2	1	0	0	0	0	0	0	1	-	-	1	1	-	-
0	0	1	-	-	-	0	-	0	-	0	0	-	-	1	1	-	-
11	9	36	43	27	16	13	8	5	5	3	4	4	5	3	5	6	8
0	0	-	-	0	-	1	0	-	0	0	-	-	-	-	1	-	-
-	0	-	1	-	-	-	-	-	-	-	-	-	-	-	1	-	-
0	0	-	-	-	-	-	0	0	0	0	-	1	-	-	-	-	-
0	0	1	-	1	1	-	0	0	0	0	0	1	1	-	-	-	-
0	0	-	-	-	-	0	-	1	0	-	-	-	-	-	-	-	-
0	0	-	-	1	-	0	0	0	-	-	-	-	-	-	-	-	-
0	0	-	-	-	-	-	-	0	0	1	0	-	1	-	-	-	-
1	0	-	-	-	-	0	-	1	0	1	1	1	-	2	-	-	-
3	1	4	4	3	2	3	-	4	1	3	1	1	1	3	-	-	-
4	2	1	3	4	2	4	1	6	2	3	2	2	2	-	1	-	-
2	2	5	2	6	3	3	3	2	1	0	1	2	1	1	-	-	2
51	28	202	114	94	40	49	16	25	11	19	15	22	22	39	44	125	122
1	0	2	-	0	0	1	0	0	0	0	0	-	-	-	-	-	-
0	0	-	-	1	0	2	-	-	0	-	-	-	-	-	-	-	2
0	0	-	1	1	-	0	-	-	0	0	0	-	-	-	-	-	-
1	0	-	-	2	1	0	0	0	0	0	-	1	-	-	-	6	2
2	2	3	6	5	4	4	2	2	1	0	1	1	1	3	1	6	-
3	2	7	3	6	3	4	1	2	2	1	3	1	0	5	9	-	8
3	2	1	1	4	1	4	3	3	2	2	2	1	3	3	4	-	4
12	7	3	1	18	8	20	6	10	4	5	5	5	7	27	23	59	39
17	8	9	8	15	7	35	10	14	9	14	7	16	3	13	5	24	10
41	24	31	28	33	21	64	21	41	26	41	28	41	20	21	18	42	16
1	1	-	-	1	0	2	1	0	1	0	0	2	2	1	2	12	2
0	-	-	-	-	-	0	-	0	-	-	-	-	-	-	-	-	-
1	0	-	-	0	0	0	-	1	0	1	0	1	1	-	-	-	-
0	-	-	-	-	-	-	-	-	-	0	-	-	-	1	-	-	-
2	1	1	1	5	2	4	0	2	0	1	0	1	0	1	1	-	2
16	25	7	6	39	22	21	9	9	9	10	19	14	58	26	117	30	95
7	7	9	6	14	8	10	7	5	7	3	5	6	6	5	6	12	2
4	4	10	7	4	5	2	2	2	2	3	4	7	3	8	11	6	6
2	3	-	-	3	2	1	2	1	1	2	2	2	7	2	10	-	12
0	0	-	-	-	-	-	-	0	-	0	0	-	-	-	-	-	-
0	0	-	-	-	0	-	-	0	-	-	-	-	0	-	-	-	-
0	0	-	-	-	-	-	-	-	-	0	0	0	-	-	-	1	-

Table 21 - *continued*

Disease group	Persons, by age group								
	Total	0-4	5-15	16-24	25-44	45-64	65-74	75-84	85 and over
Injury to blood vessels of head and neck (900)	0	-	0	-	-	-	-	-	-
Injury to blood vessels of abdomen and pelvis (902)	0	-	0	0	0	-	-	0	-
Injury to blood vessels of upper extremity (903)	0	-	-	0	-	0	0	-	-
Injury to blood vessels of lower extremity and unspecified sites (904)	0	-	-	0	0	1	1	0	-
Late effects of musculoskeletal and connective tissue injuries (905)	0	-	0	0	0	1	1	-	1
Late effects of injuries to skin and subcutaneous tissues (906)	0	-	0	0	0	0	1	0	1
Late effects of injuries to the nervous system (907)	1	1	0	1	1	1	2	1	1
Late effects of other and unspecified external causes (909)	1	1	1	2	1	1	1	1	3
Superficial injury of face, neck and scalp except eye (910)	21	73	36	17	10	10	16	31	55
Superficial injury of trunk (911)	14	10	20	15	11	12	15	25	38
Superficial injury of shoulder and upper arm (912)	9	5	12	12	8	6	9	17	25
Superficial injury of elbow, forearm and wrist (913)	3	1	4	2	2	2	4	6	9
Superficial injury of hand(s) except finger(s) alone (914)	20	31	30	23	16	17	15	16	30
Superficial injury of finger(s) (915)	4	6	4	3	3	5	5	6	3
Superficial injury of hip, thigh, leg and ankle (916)	32	18	37	29	23	30	44	79	93
Superficial injury of foot and toe(s) (917)	22	23	38	25	18	17	22	17	22
Superficial injury of eye and adnexa (918)	10	12	11	7	12	10	6	6	-
Superficial injury of other, multiple and unspecified sites (919)	24	35	34	23	20	20	18	30	36
Contusion of face, scalp, and neck except eye(s) (920)	19	68	33	19	9	7	13	26	43
Contusion of eye and adnexa (921)	7	10	12	10	5	3	6	11	19
Contusion of trunk (922)	24	8	18	20	22	24	29	47	112
Contusion of upper limb (923)	28	22	47	35	22	20	24	44	53
Contusion of lower limb and of other and unspecified sites (924)	51	25	62	60	42	43	55	87	127
Crushing injury of face, scalp and neck (925)	0	-	0	0	0	-	-	-	-
Crushing injury of trunk (926)	0	1	1	-	0	0	-	0	-
Crushing injury of upper limb (927)	4	12	7	6	3	3	2	2	1
Crushing injury of lower limb (928)	2	3	2	4	2	2	1	0	-
Crushing injury of multiple and unspecified sites (929)	0	1	0	1	1	1	-	-	-
Foreign body on external eye (930)	12	8	8	14	16	12	10	5	7
Foreign body in ear (931)	4	13	11	1	2	2	3	3	1
Foreign body in nose (932)	1	15	2	-	-	-	-	-	-
Foreign body in pharynx and larynx (933)	1	1	0	1	1	1	1	2	-
Foreign body in trachea, bronchus and lung (934)	0	-	-	-	0	0	-	-	-
Foreign body in mouth, oesophagus and stomach (935)	1	3	1	1	0	1	1	-	3
Foreign body in intestine and colon (936)	0	-	0	0	-	-	-	-	-
Foreign body in anus and rectum (937)	0	-	-	-	0	-	-	-	-
Foreign body in digestive system, unspecified (938)	0	3	0	0	0	0	-	-	-
Foreign body in genitourinary tract (939)	2	0	0	3	5	2	-	-	-
Burn confined to eye and adnexa (940)	0	1	1	1	1	1	0	-	-
Burn of face, head and neck (941)	2	6	2	4	2	1	1	0	1
Burn of trunk (942)	2	7	2	1	1	2	3	3	4
Burn of upper limb, except wrist and hand (943)	4	8	2	5	4	3	4	4	4
Burn of wrist(s) and hand(s) (944)	8	22	6	9	7	6	6	8	9
Burn of lower limb(s) (945)	6	13	5	6	4	4	6	10	21
Burns of multiple specified sites (946)	0	-	0	0	0	0	-	0	-
Burn of internal organs (947)	0	-	0	1	0	1	0	-	1
Burns classified according to extent of body surface involved (948)	1	2	0	1	1	1	1	-	-
Burn, unspecified (949)	2	9	1	3	2	2	1	2	6
Injury to other cranial nerve(s) (951)	0	-	-	0	0	0	1	0	-
Spinal cord lesion without evidence of spinal bone injury (952)	0	-	-	-	-	0	1	0	-
Injury to nerve roots and spinal plexus (953)	1	-	0	0	1	1	1	1	-
Injury to other nerve(s) of trunk excluding shoulder and pelvic girdles (954)	0	-	-	0	0	-	-	-	-
Injury to peripheral nerve(s) of shoulder girdle and upper limb (955)	2	-	1	2	3	3	2	2	-
Injury to peripheral nerve(s) of pelvic girdle and lower limb (956)	1	-	-	0	1	1	1	2	-
Injury to other and unspecified nerves (957)	2	9	2	3	2	1	1	1	1

Patients consulting

By age-group and sex

Total		0-4		5-15		16-24		25-44		45-64		65-74		75-84		85 and over	
Male	Female	Male	Female	Male	Female	Male	Female	Male	Female	Male	Female	Male	Female	Male	Female	Male	Female
0	-	-	-	0	-	-	-	-	-	-	-	-	-	-	-	-	-
0	-	-	-	0	-	0	-	0	-	-	-	-	-	1	-	-	-
-	0	-	-	-	-	-	0	-	-	-	0	-	0	-	-	-	-
0	1	-	-	-	-	-	0	-	0	0	2	1	0	-	1	-	-
0	0	-	-	0	-	1	-	-	-	0	1	0	1	0	-	-	2
0	0	-	-	0	1	0	-	1	0	0	0	1	1	-	1	-	2
1	1	1	1	1	-	2	-	1	0	1	1	2	2	2	1	-	2
1	1	1	-	2	0	1	2	1	1	1	1	2	0	-	2	-	4
20	21	74	71	42	29	18	16	9	10	7	13	9	22	30	32	42	59
14	15	9	11	22	17	15	14	12	10	10	14	1	19	26	24	59	32
9	9	2	7	13	10	14	10	8	7	5	7	5	11	11	21	6	32
3	2	1	1	5	3	3	2	2	1	2	2	5	4	7	5	18	6
24	17	32	29	36	24	30	17	20	12	18	17	19	13	21	14	48	24
4	4	7	6	3	4	3	3	3	3	5	4	6	4	8	4	12	-
24	40	21	15	37	37	34	25	17	29	18	41	19	65	40	103	65	102
21	24	23	22	37	39	25	24	16	19	14	21	22	23	11	21	12	26
11	8	13	10	14	8	9	4	13	12	11	9	9	3	6	6	-	-
20	27	36	33	35	33	18	28	16	24	15	25	14	21	18	38	24	39
18	19	74	61	42	24	19	19	8	10	4	9	5	20	9	36	30	47
6	8	9	11	14	10	9	11	5	5	3	4	2	9	7	13	12	22
22	25	9	8	19	16	22	18	23	21	22	25	19	37	31	57	125	108
29	28	26	19	50	44	38	32	24	20	19	20	20	28	38	48	65	49
44	57	22	27	73	50	67	53	37	47	30	57	34	72	54	106	77	144
0	0	-	-	0	-	0	0	-	0	-	-	-	-	-	-	-	-
1	0	2	-	1	0	-	-	1	0	0	-	-	-	-	1	-	-
6	3	17	6	7	6	9	3	5	2	4	2	1	2	2	1	6	-
3	1	4	3	2	3	4	3	3	1	4	1	1	0	-	1	-	-
1	0	1	-	-	0	2	0	1	0	1	0	-	-	-	-	-	-
18	6	10	5	10	7	23	5	24	8	18	6	15	6	7	3	18	4
4	4	12	13	11	11	1	1	2	3	2	2	4	3	6	1	6	-
1	2	11	20	2	2	-	-	-	-	-	-	-	-	-	-	-	-
1	2	-	2	1	0	1	2	1	2	1	1	1	1	1	3	-	-
0	0	-	-	-	-	-	-	-	-	0	0	-	-	-	-	-	-
1	1	5	2	1	1	0	1	0	1	1	0	1	-	-	-	-	4
0	0	-	-	-	-	-	-	-	0	-	-	-	-	-	-	-	-
0	-	-	-	-	-	-	-	0	-	-	-	-	-	-	-	-	-
0	0	3	3	0	1	-	1	0	0	0	0	0	-	-	-	-	-
0	5	1	-	0	1	-	6	-	10	0	3	-	-	-	-	-	-
1	0	-	1	1	1	1	0	1	1	1	0	1	-	-	-	-	-
2	2	9	3	1	3	4	3	2	2	1	1	2	1	-	1	-	2
2	2	9	5	2	3	1	1	1	2	1	2	1	5	2	3	6	4
3	5	7	10	2	1	4	5	3	5	2	4	2	5	2	5	6	4
7	9	24	20	8	5	8	9	6	7	4	8	3	8	6	10	6	10
5	7	12	15	6	5	7	5	4	5	2	6	5	7	10	10	12	24
0	0	-	-	-	-	0	0	0	0	-	0	-	-	-	-	1	-
0	0	-	-	-	-	0	1	0	1	0	0	1	1	-	-	-	2
1	1	2	3	0	1	-	2	1	0	0	1	1	1	-	-	-	-
2	3	10	8	1	1	2	4	1	3	1	2	2	1	2	1	6	6
0	0	-	-	-	-	-	-	0	1	0	0	1	-	1	-	1	-
0	0	-	-	-	-	-	-	-	-	0	0	1	0	1	0	-	-
1	1	-	-	-	-	0	-	1	1	1	1	1	1	-	2	-	-
0	0	-	-	-	-	-	-	0	0	-	-	-	-	-	-	-	-
3	1	-	-	1	1	2	1	4	2	3	2	3	1	3	1	-	-
1	1	-	-	-	-	1	-	1	1	1	2	1	1	2	2	-	-
3	2	13	6	2	2	4	2	2	1	2	1	1	1	1	1	-	2

Table 21 - *continued*

Disease group	Persons, by age group								
	Total	0-4	5-15	16-24	25-44	45-64	65-74	75-84	85 and over
Certain early complications of trauma (958)	3	1	3	3	3	3	4	4	13
Injury, other and unspecified (959)	44	29	52	61	43	36	36	48	80
Poisoning by antibiotics (960)	0	-	-	0	0	0	0	1	-
Poisoning by other anti-infectives (961)	0	-	-	-	-	0	1	0	3
Poisoning by hormones and synthetic substitutes (962)	0	1	-	-	0	-	-	-	-
Poisoning by primarily systemic agents (963)	0	-	-	0	0	-	-	-	-
Poisoning by agents primarily affecting blood constituents (964)	0	0	-	-	-	-	-	-	-
Poisoning by analgesics, antipyretics and antirheumatics (965)	0	0	0	1	0	-	1	-	-
Poisoning by anticonvulsants and anti-Parkinsonism drugs (966)	0	-	-	-	-	0	-	-	-
Poisoning by sedatives and hypnotics (967)	0	-	-	-	-	0	-	-	-
Poisoning by psychotropic agents (969)	0	-	-	1	-	0	-	-	-
Poisoning by agents primarily affecting the cardiovascular system (972)	0	-	-	-	0	0	1	3	4
Poisoning by water, mineral and uric acid metabolism drugs (974)	0	-	-	-	-	-	-	-	1
Poisoning by other and unspecified drugs and medicaments (977)	1	2	0	1	1	0	1	1	-
Poisoning by bacterial vaccines (978)	0	0	0	0	0	-	-	-	-
Poisoning by other vaccines and biological substances (979)	0	1	-	-	0	0	-	-	-
Toxic effect of alcohol (980)	1	-	0	1	1	1	-	-	-
Toxic effect of petroleum products (981)	0	-	-	0	-	-	-	-	-
Toxic effect of solvents other than petroleum-based (982)	0	-	1	1	0	0	-	-	-
Toxic effect of corrosive aromatics, acids and caustic alkalis (983)	0	1	-	-	0	-	-	-	-
Toxic effect of lead and its compounds (including fumes) (984)	0	-	-	0	0	0	-	-	-
Toxic effect of other metals (985)	0	-	0	1	0	-	-	-	-
Toxic effect of carbon monoxide (986)	0	0	-	0	0	0	0	-	-
Toxic effect of other gases, fumes or vapours (987)	0	-	0	1	0	0	0	0	1
Toxic effect of noxious substances eaten as food (988)	1	1	1	1	2	1	1	2	3
Toxic effect of other substances, chiefly nonmedicinal as to source (989)	2	2	3	4	2	2	4	3	1
Effects of radiation, unspecified (990)	0	-	-	-	0	1	1	0	-
Effects of reduced temperature (991)	8	4	9	6	6	7	17	17	25
Effects of heat and light (992)	1	3	1	1	2	1	2	2	1
Effects of air pressure (993)	1	-	1	1	1	1	0	-	-
Effects of other external causes (994)	5	9	6	2	3	4	7	6	1
Certain adverse effects not elsewhere classified (995)	294	437	288	292	251	250	291	466	698
Complications peculiar to certain specified procedures (996)	3	1	0	2	2	2	5	20	31
Complications affecting specified body systems, not elsewhere classified (997)	0	-	0	-	0	1	1	0	1
Other complications of procedures, not elsewhere classified (998)	41	15	16	30	53	49	53	55	30
Complications of medical care, not elsewhere classified (999)	2	9	1	1	1	1	1	2	3
Contact with or exposure to communicable diseases (V01)	15	37	28	14	19	5	2	0	1
Carrier or suspected carrier of infectious diseases (V02)	1	1	1	1	2	1	-	0	1
Need for prophylactic vaccination and inoculation against bacterial diseases (V03)	428	203	240	339	498	583	498	343	210
Need for prophylactic vaccination and inoculation against certain viral diseases (V04)	688	268	364	221	315	749	2,097	2,581	2,455
Need for other prophylactic vaccination and inoculation against single diseases (V05)	15	4	4	23	24	16	3	2	-
Need for prophylactic vaccination and inoculation against combinations of diseases (V06)	375	4,466	245	61	56	38	18	8	1
Need for isolation and other prophylactic measures (V07)	48	8	22	57	63	71	31	6	-
Health supervision of infant or child (V20)	128	1,830	10	1	1	-	0	-	-
Normal pregnancy (V22)	147	1	4	343	332	2	-	-	-
Supervision of high-risk pregnancy (V23)	2	-	-	6	5	0	-	-	-
Postpartum care and examination (V24)	100	9	2	214	235	1	0	0	-
Contraceptive management (V25)	728	3	68	2,365	1,303	76	2	0	1
Procreative management (V26)	9	1	1	26	19	0	0	-	-
Attention to artificial openings (V55)	0	-	-	-	0	0	-	1	1

By age-group and sex

Total		0-4		5-15		16-24		25-44		45-64		65-74		75-84		85 and over	
Male	Female	Male	Female	Male	Female	Male	Female	Male	Female	Male	Female	Male	Female	Male	Female	Male	Female
4	3	1	1	3	2	5	2	3	2	3	3	5	4	5	3	24	10
48	41	30	29	59	45	79	42	50	36	34	37	27	44	29	59	65	85
0	0	-	-	-	-	-	0	-	0	0	0	-	0	-	2	-	-
0	0	-	-	-	-	-	-	-	-	0	0	1	0	-	1	6	2
0	0	1	1	-	-	-	-	0	-	-	-	-	-	-	-	-	-
0	0	-	-	-	-	-	1	0	-	-	-	-	-	-	-	-	-
-	0	-	1	-	-	-	-	-	-	-	-	-	-	-	-	-	-
0	0	-	1	-	0	1	1	0	0	-	-	1	1	-	-	-	-
-	0	-	-	-	-	-	-	-	-	-	0	-	-	-	-	-	-
-	0	-	-	-	-	-	-	-	-	-	0	-	-	-	-	-	-
0	0	-	-	-	-	1	0	-	-	-	1	-	-	-	-	-	-
0	1	-	-	-	-	-	-	0	0	0	0	1	0	2	4	-	6
0	-	-	-	-	-	-	-	-	-	-	-	-	-	-	-	6	-
1	1	2	3	0	-	0	1	1	1	-	1	2	1	1	1	-	-
-	0	-	1	-	1	-	0	-	0	-	-	-	-	-	-	-	-
0	0	1	-	-	-	-	-	-	0	-	0	-	-	-	-	-	-
1	0	-	-	1	0	1	0	1	1	2	-	-	-	-	-	-	-
0	-	-	-	-	-	0	-	-	-	-	-	-	-	-	-	-	-
0	0	-	-	1	0	1	1	1	0	-	0	-	-	-	-	-	-
0	0	1	-	-	-	-	-	0	0	-	-	-	-	-	-	-	-
0	0	-	-	-	-	0	-	0	-	-	0	-	-	-	-	-	-
-	0	-	-	-	0	-	1	-	0	-	-	-	-	-	-	-	-
0	0	1	-	-	-	-	0	0	0	0	0	-	0	-	-	-	-
1	0	-	-	1	-	2	1	0	0	0	0	-	0	1	-	6	-
1	2	1	1	1	1	1	2	1	3	1	1	1	0	1	2	12	-
2	3	2	1	4	3	2	5	1	3	1	2	2	5	1	4	-	2
0	0	-	-	-	-	-	-	0	-	0	1	1	1	1	1	-	-
5	12	4	4	4	15	1	12	1	11	5	10	17	18	18	16	42	20
1	2	2	3	2	1	1	1	1	2	1	1	2	1	1	2	-	2
1	1	-	-	2	1	1	1	1	1	1	0	1	-	-	-	-	-
3	6	10	9	6	6	1	3	2	4	2	7	4	9	6	7	-	2
237	349	456	417	280	296	238	345	189	312	179	322	232	339	340	541	535	753
4	3	-	1	-	0	2	2	0	4	2	2	9	2	38	9	113	4
0	0	-	-	-	0	-	-	0	0	2	1	1	1	-	1	-	2
35	46	24	5	17	14	20	39	36	70	45	52	61	47	73	44	18	33
1	2	11	7	0	1	0	1	1	2	1	1	-	1	1	2	6	2
14	16	34	40	26	31	11	16	16	21	6	5	3	1	-	1	-	2
1	1	1	1	2	1	1	2	2	2	1	1	-	-	-	1	-	2
385	469	208	196	240	240	284	395	426	570	509	658	501	495	363	331	267	191
568	803	272	264	156	582	172	269	257	373	656	844	2,072	2,118	2,773	2,467	2,514	2,435
12	18	2	6	3	4	14	32	21	27	13	20	3	4	2	2	-	-
384	367	4,478	4,453	239	251	50	71	40	71	31	45	17	19	7	8	-	2
44	52	7	10	23	21	40	73	57	70	69	74	29	32	7	5	-	-
131	125	1,797	1,866	9	12	1	1	1	2	-	-	1	-	-	-	-	-
0	287	1	2	-	9	-	683	0	666	0	3	-	-	-	-	-	-
-	5	-	-	-	-	-	11	-	11	-	0	-	-	-	-	-	-
1	196	8	10	-	3	-	427	0	471	0	1	-	0	-	1	-	-
21	1,406	3	4	1	138	7	4,707	56	2,559	7	147	2	2	1	-	-	2
3	16	1	-	-	1	2	49	7	31	0	0	-	-	-	-	-	-
0	0	-	-	-	-	-	-	0	-	0	-	-	-	1	1	6	-

Patients consulting

199

Table 21 - *continued*

Disease group	Persons, by age group								
	Total	0-4	5-15	16-24	25-44	45-64	65-74	75-84	85 and over
Housing, household and economic circumstances (V60)	10	8	1	18	11	7	9	21	22
Other family circumstances (V61)	84	16	12	63	108	106	114	146	96
Other psychosocial circumstances (V62)	13	-	3	21	19	15	4	9	18
Other persons seeking consultation without complaint or sickness (V65)	42	34	25	55	46	47	39	35	30
Encounters for administrative purposes (V68)	480	16	15	473	656	902	203	123	112
General medical examination (V70)	419	57	153	353	365	384	249	2,115	2,015
Special investigations and examinations (V72)	62	2	7	149	102	43	10	10	4
Special screening examination for viral diseases (V73)	35	1	11	102	63	5	2	0	1
Special screening examination for bacterial and spirochaetal diseases (V74)	1	2	0	2	1	0	0	0	-
Special screening examination for other infectious diseases (V75)	1	1	1	2	2	0	0	1	-
Special screening for malignant neoplasms (V76)	420	-	3	529	681	627	118	15	7
Special screening for endocrine, nutritional, metabolic and immunity disorders (V77)	141	3	10	61	144	291	225	127	59
Special screening for disorders of blood and blood-forming organs (V78)	12	2	2	15	14	12	14	21	16
Special screening for mental disorders and developmental handicaps (V79)	8	86	1	1	2	3	2	1	3
Special screening for neurological, eye and ear diseases (V80)	10	10	4	2	3	10	42	40	34
Special screening for cardiovascular, respiratory and genitourinary diseases (V81)	278	45	76	156	238	448	564	517	317
Special screening for other conditions (V82)	14	17	6	12	14	17	16	15	4

By age-group and sex

Total		0-4		5-15		16-24		25-44		45-64		65-74		75-84		85 and over	
Male	Female	Male	Female	Male	Female	Male	Female	Male	Female	Male	Female	Male	Female	Male	Female	Male	Female
5	15	9	8	2	0	4	32	6	17	6	9	7	10	6	30	30	20
42	125	14	18	8	16	12	113	49	168	54	159	69	151	124	159	149	79
13	13	-	-	4	3	18	24	19	19	16	14	2	5	8	9	24	16
33	51	42	26	21	29	37	72	32	60	36	58	34	42	29	38	24	32
541	423	14	17	14	15	456	490	669	644	1,066	735	364	72	181	88	155	99
326	507	62	52	157	149	241	464	262	469	326	443	243	254	2,116	2,114	2,026	2,012
2	119	1	4	2	11	1	295	2	204	3	83	-	18	8	12	-	6
9	61	2	1	9	13	20	184	11	116	5	5	3	1	1	-	-	2
1	1	1	2	-	1	2	1	1	1	0	0	1	-	1	-	-	-
1	1	2	-	2	1	2	3	1	2	0	0	1	-	1	1	-	-
1	823	-	-	-	7	1	1,053	1	1,366	1	1,264	5	211	3	22	-	10
126	155	2	3	10	9	44	78	129	160	259	324	211	237	136	122	89	49
6	17	2	2	2	3	5	24	6	23	9	15	10	17	13	26	18	16
8	8	81	91	2	0	1	1	2	2	2	3	2	2	-	1	6	2
9	11	7	12	5	3	2	1	2	4	9	10	41	43	45	37	48	30
240	314	46	43	84	67	94	219	187	289	415	483	558	569	510	521	315	317
10	18	12	24	6	6	5	20	8	21	15	20	18	14	15	16	6	4

Patients consulting

201

**Table 22   New and first ever episodes - rates per 10,000 years at risk:
first 3 ICD digits by age and sex**

Disease Group	Persons, by age group								
	Total	0-4	5-15	16-24	25-44	45-64	65-74	75-84	85 and over
Cholera (001)	0	1	-	-	-	-	-	-	-
Typhoid and paratyphoid fevers (002)	0	-	-	0	-	0	-	-	-
Other salmonella infections (003)	2	5	1	2	3	3	1	2	1
Shigellosis (004)	1	6	3	0	1	0	1	-	-
Other food poisoning (bacterial) (005)	2	1	1	2	3	2	2	1	1
Amoebiasis (006)	0	-	-	-	0	0	0	-	-
Other protozoal intestinal diseases (007)	1	4	1	1	1	1	-	-	-
Intestinal infections due to other organisms (008)	6	20	6	6	6	4	3	5	3
Ill-defined intestinal infections (009)	408	2,011	387	366	284	198	233	311	445
Primary tuberculous infection (010)	0	-	-	-	0	-	-	-	-
Pulmonary tuberculosis (011)	0	-	-	0	0	1	1	1	-
Other respiratory tuberculosis (012)	0	-	-	-	0	0	-	-	-
Tuberculosis of bones and joints (015)	0	-	-	-	0	-	-	-	-
Tuberculosis of genitourinary system (016)	0	-	-	-	-	0	-	1	-
Tuberculosis of other organs (017)	0	-	0	0	0	-	-	0	-
Anthrax (022)	0	-	-	-	-	0	-	-	-
Brucellosis (023)	0	-	-	-	-	0	-	-	-
Other zoonotic bacterial diseases (027)	0	-	1	-	0	-	-	-	-
Leprosy (030)	0	-	-	0	-	-	-	-	-
Diseases due to other mycobacteria (031)	0	-	0	-	0	-	1	-	-
Diphtheria (032)	0	-	0	-	-	-	-	-	-
Whooping cough (033)	1	11	3	0	0	-	-	-	-
Streptococcal sore throat and scarlatina (034)	9	31	22	10	6	2	1	2	1
Erysipelas (035)	3	3	1	1	2	5	7	4	4
Meningococcal infection (036)	0	2	1	0	0	0	-	0	-
Tetanus (037)	0	-	0	0	0	1	0	1	1
Septicaemia (038)	1	1	0	0	0	1	2	7	10
Actinomycotic infections (039)	1	-	0	-	1	1	-	-	-
Other bacterial diseases (040)	0	-	-	0	0	0	-	-	-
Bacterial infection in conditions classified elsewhere and of unspecified site (041)	2	7	2	2	1	2	1	1	-
Slow virus infection of central nervous system (046)	0	-	-	0	0	-	-	-	-
Meningitis due to enterovirus (047)	0	0	0	1	0	0	-	-	-
Other non-arthropod-borne viral diseases of central nervous system (049)	1	1	1	0	1	1	0	-	-
Cowpox and paravaccinia (051)	0	0	0	-	0	0	-	-	-
Chickenpox (052)	68	459	148	52	29	4	1	3	-
Herpes zoster (053)	45	10	27	24	28	61	108	118	130
Herpes simplex (054)	79	80	77	109	98	58	52	34	22
Measles (055)	4	41	4	1	0	0	-	-	-
Rubella (056)	7	56	15	4	1	0	0	0	-
Other viral exanthemata (057)	24	209	43	8	6	2	1	2	-
Mosquito-borne viral encephalitis (062)	0	-	-	-	0	-	-	-	-
Viral hepatitis (070)	3	1	6	4	3	2	1	1	1
Rabies (071)	0	-	-	-	0	-	-	-	-
Mumps (072)	4	22	9	2	1	1	1	1	1
Ornithosis (073)	0	-	-	-	0	0	-	-	-
Specific diseases due to Coxsackie virus (074)	10	84	9	5	5	3	1	0	3
Infectious mononucleosis (075)	9	2	14	38	5	1	1	-	-
Trachoma (076)	0	-	-	-	-	0	-	-	-
Other diseases of conjunctiva due to viruses and Chlamydiae (077)	0	-	0	-	0	-	-	0	-
Other diseases due to viruses and Chlamydiae (078)	191	201	599	266	127	69	49	36	24
Viral infection in conditions classified elsewhere and of unspecified site (079)	67	337	118	48	42	26	20	20	27

By age-group and sex

Total		0-4		5-15		16-24		25-44		45-64		65-74		75-84		85 and over	
Male	Female	Male	Female	Male	Female	Male	Female	Male	Female	Male	Female	Male	Female	Male	Female	Male	Female
-	0	-	1	-	-	-	-	-	-	-	-	-	-	-	-	-	-
-	0	-	-	-	-	-	1	-	-	-	0	-	-	-	-	-	-
3	2	4	6	1	1	2	2	3	3	3	3	1	2	3	1	6	-
1	2	5	6	3	3	-	0	1	2	0	0	1	0	-	-	-	-
2	2	1	1	1	1	2	2	3	3	2	1	1	3	-	2	6	-
0	0	-	-	-	-	-	-	-	0	0	1	-	0	-	-	-	-
1	1	4	4	2	1	0	2	1	1	1	1	-	-	-	-	-	-
6	6	18	22	9	3	5	7	5	6	4	5	4	3	6	4	-	4
370	446	2062	1958	385	388	277	455	228	341	153	243	174	280	240	354	357	475
-	0	-	-	-	-	-	-	-	0	-	-	-	-	-	-	-	-
1	0	-	-	-	-	-	0	0	0	1	1	2	-	2	-	-	-
-	0	-	-	-	-	-	-	-	0	-	0	-	-	-	-	-	-
0	-	-	-	-	-	-	-	0	-	-	-	-	-	-	-	-	-
0	-	-	-	-	-	-	-	-	-	0	-	-	-	2	-	-	-
0	0	-	-	-	0	-	0	0	0	-	-	-	-	-	1	-	-
-	0	-	-	-	-	-	-	-	-	-	0	-	-	-	-	-	-
0	-	-	-	-	-	-	-	-	-	0	-	-	-	-	-	-	-
0	0	-	-	1	1	-	-	0	-	-	-	-	-	-	-	-	-
-	0	-	-	-	-	-	0	-	-	-	-	-	-	-	-	-	-
0	0	-	-	0	-	-	-	-	0	-	-	1	0	-	-	-	-
0	-	-	-	0	-	-	-	-	-	-	-	-	-	-	-	-	-
1	2	9	13	3	3	-	0	0	1	-	-	-	-	-	-	-	-
7	10	29	34	19	26	8	11	4	8	1	3	-	2	1	2	-	2
3	3	4	3	-	2	2	1	1	3	5	5	6	8	8	2	-	6
0	0	2	2	1	0	0	0	0	0	0	0	-	-	-	1	-	-
0	0	-	-	0	-	0	-	0	0	0	1	-	0	1	1	-	2
1	1	1	2	0	-	1	-	0	0	1	1	2	1	14	3	-	14
0	1	-	-	0	1	-	-	0	1	1	1	-	-	-	-	-	-
0	0	-	-	-	-	-	0	0	0	-	0	-	-	-	-	-	-
2	2	8	6	2	2	1	2	0	3	2	2	2	-	-	1	-	-
0	0	-	-	-	-	0	-	0	0	-	-	-	-	-	-	-	-
0	0	1	-	0	0	1	1	0	1	-	0	-	-	-	-	-	-
0	1	1	1	2	1	0	-	-	1	-	1	1	-	-	-	-	-
0	0	-	1	0	-	-	-	0	-	0	-	-	-	-	-	-	-
70	67	455	463	149	146	48	55	28	30	4	4	-	2	2	4	-	-
39	52	9	11	26	27	23	25	26	30	51	71	90	122	113	120	143	126
48	108	77	84	60	95	58	160	48	149	31	86	46	56	26	39	30	20
4	3	41	41	4	4	1	1	0	0	0	0	-	-	-	-	-	-
6	7	55	57	13	16	1	7	1	1	0	-	-	0	1	-	-	-
23	24	207	211	42	44	3	12	4	8	1	2	1	1	1	2	-	-
-	0	-	-	-	-	-	-	-	0	-	-	-	-	-	-	-	-
4	2	2	1	8	4	6	2	4	2	3	2	1	1	1	1	-	2
-	0	-	-	-	-	-	-	-	0	-	-	-	-	-	-	-	-
4	4	29	16	8	10	2	2	1	1	0	1	-	1	-	1	-	2
-	0	-	-	-	-	-	-	-	0	-	0	-	-	-	-	-	-
11	9	102	65	10	8	4	7	4	5	2	3	-	1	-	1	6	2
8	10	4	1	13	15	31	46	5	5	0	1	-	1	-	-	-	-
0	-	-	-	-	-	-	-	-	-	0	-	-	-	-	-	-	-
0	0	-	-	-	1	-	-	0	-	-	-	-	-	-	1	-	-
182	200	196	206	568	631	232	299	110	145	66	73	55	45	34	38	48	16
59	75	349	324	109	127	26	70	28	56	20	33	17	23	15	23	12	32

New and first ever episodes

Table 22 - *continued*

Disease Group	Persons, by age group								
	Total	0-4	5-15	16-24	25-44	45-64	65-74	75-84	85 and over
Other rickettsioses (083)	0	-	0	-	-	-	-	-	-
Malaria (084)	0	1	0	0	1	1	0	-	1
Relapsing fever (087)	0	-	-	-	0	0	0	-	-
Congenital syphilis (090)	0	0	-	-	-	0	-	-	-
Neurosyphilis (094)	0	-	-	-	-	0	-	-	-
Other and unspecified syphilis (097)	0	-	-	0	0	-	-	-	-
Gonococcal infections (098)	0	0	-	2	1	-	0	-	1
Other venereal diseases (099)	5	1	1	13	7	2	2	1	-
Leptospirosis (100)	0	-	-	0	0	0	-	-	-
Vincent's angina (101)	0	1	1	-	0	1	0	0	-
Yaws (102)	0	-	-	-	-	-	-	0	-
Dermatophytosis (110)	141	107	179	160	151	130	121	75	59
Dermatomycosis, other and unspecified (111)	16	6	15	31	21	9	8	6	1
Candidiasis (112)	347	565	79	561	537	188	143	143	135
Other mycoses (117)	0	1	0	0	0	0	0	-	-
Echinococcosis (122)	0	-	-	0	0	0	-	-	-
Other cestode infection (123)	0	0	0	0	0	-	-	-	-
Filarial infection and dracontiasis (125)	0	1	0	0	0	0	-	-	-
Other intestinal helminthiases (127)	42	169	139	25	23	5	1	1	4
Other and unspecified helminthiases (128)	1	3	2	1	0	-	-	-	-
Toxoplasmosis (130)	0	-	-	-	0	-	0	-	-
Trichomoniasis (131)	3	-	0	4	6	3	1	-	-
Pediculosis and phthirus infestation (132)	33	85	118	27	21	3	1	3	6
Acariasis (133)	34	51	60	59	28	17	7	17	41
Sarcoidosis (135)	1	-	-	0	1	1	-	1	-
Other and unspecified infectious and parasitic diseases (136)	17	98	28	9	9	7	4	7	-
Late effects of acute poliomyelitis (138)	0	-	-	-	0	-	-	-	-
Malignant neoplasm of lip (140)	0	-	-	-	-	-	-	0	-
Malignant neoplasm of tongue (141)	0	-	-	-	-	0	1	-	-
Malignant neoplasm of major salivary glands (142)	0	-	-	-	-	0	1	-	-
Malignant neoplasm of gum (143)	0	-	-	-	0	0	0	-	1
Malignant neoplasm of other and unspecified parts of mouth (145)	0	-	-	-	-	0	0	-	-
Malignant neoplasm of oropharynx (146)	0	-	-	-	-	0	-	0	-
Malignant neoplasm of other and ill-defined sites within the lip,oral cavity and pharynx (149)	0	-	-	-	-	0	1	-	-
Malignant neoplasm of oesophagus (150)	1	-	-	-	0	1	4	5	9
Malignant neoplasm of stomach (151)	1	-	-	-	-	1	4	7	10
Malignant neoplasm of colon (153)	2	-	-	0	0	2	9	17	13
Malignant neoplasm of rectum, rectosigmoid junction and anus (154)	1	-	-	-	0	2	3	9	10
Malignant neoplasm of liver and intrahepatic bile ducts (155)	0	-	-	-	-	0	-	-	1
Malignant neoplasm of gallbladder and extrahepatic bile ducts (156)	0	-	-	-	-	0	-	1	-
Malignant neoplasm of pancreas (157)	0	-	-	-	-	0	2	2	4
Malignant neoplasm of other and ill-defined sites within the digestive organs and peritoneum (159)	0	-	-	-	-	0	-	-	-
Malignant neoplasm of larynx (161)	0	-	-	-	0	1	2	2	-
Malignant neoplasm of trachea, bronchus and lung (162)	4	-	-	-	0	5	13	20	21
Malignant neoplasm of pleura (163)	0	-	-	-	-	-	0	-	-
Malignant neoplasm of thymus, heart and mediastinum (164)	0	-	-	-	-	-	0	-	-

By age-group and sex

Total		0-4		5-15		16-24		25-44		45-64		65-74		75-84		85 and over	
Male	Female	Male	Female	Male	Female	Male	Female	Male	Female	Male	Female	Male	Female	Male	Female	Male	Female
0	-	-	-	0	-	-	-	-	-	-	-	-	-	-	-	-	-
0	1	2	-	0	-	-	0	0	1	0	1	1	-	-	-	6	-
0	0	-	-	-	-	-	-	-	0	-	0	1	-	-	-	-	-
0	0	-	1	-	-	-	-	-	-	0	-	-	-	-	-	-	-
0	-	-	-	-	-	-	-	-	-	0	-	-	-	-	-	-	-
0	-	-	-	-	-	0	-	0	-	-	-	-	-	-	-	-	-
0	0	1	-	-	-	2	1	1	1	-	-	-	-	0	-	-	2
7	2	2	-	1	1	21	6	10	3	4	0	2	3	1	1	-	-
0	0	-	-	-	-	0	-	-	-	0	-	0	-	-	-	-	-
0	1	1	1	1	0	-	-	-	1	0	1	-	0	1	-	-	-
0	-	-	-	-	-	-	-	-	-	-	-	-	-	1	-	-	-
166	117	118	96	191	165	175	145	188	115	148	111	153	95	89	66	71	55
15	17	8	4	13	18	24	38	20	23	10	8	10	6	3	8	-	2
97	586	461	674	33	127	78	1,041	78	998	59	319	88	188	119	158	101	146
0	0	1	1	-	1	0	0	0	0	-	0	-	0	-	-	-	-
-	0	-	-	-	-	-	0	-	0	-	0	-	-	-	-	-	-
0	0	-	1	1	-	-	0	-	0	-	-	-	-	-	-	-	-
0	0	1	-	0	0	-	0	-	0	0	-	-	-	-	-	-	-
33	51	142	197	107	173	17	32	14	33	4	5	1	1	1	1	-	6
1	1	2	4	2	3	1	0	0	0	-	-	-	-	-	-	-	-
0	0	-	-	-	-	-	-	0	-	-	-	-	0	-	-	-	-
1	6	-	-	-	1	1	7	1	11	0	6	-	1	-	-	-	-
22	43	67	105	71	167	21	33	12	29	2	3	-	2	2	3	-	8
29	38	52	50	53	67	48	70	23	33	13	21	8	7	14	19	24	47
1	1	-	-	-	-	0	-	-	1	1	1	-	-	-	1	-	-
17	16	105	92	29	26	7	10	8	9	5	9	3	4	3	9	-	-
-	0	-	-	-	-	-	-	-	0	-	-	-	-	-	-	-	-
0	-	-	-	-	-	-	-	-	-	-	-	-	-	1	-	-	-
0	-	-	-	-	-	-	-	-	-	0	-	2	-	-	-	-	-
0	0	-	-	-	-	-	-	-	-	0	-	1	0	-	-	-	-
-	0	-	-	-	-	-	-	-	0	-	0	-	0	-	-	-	2
0	0	-	-	-	-	-	-	-	-	0	-	-	0	-	-	-	-
0	0	-	-	-	-	-	-	-	-	0	-	-	-	-	1	-	-
0	0	-	-	-	-	-	-	-	-	0	0	1	-	-	-	-	-
1	1	-	-	-	-	-	-	0	-	1	-	5	4	11	1	18	6
2	1	-	-	-	-	-	-	-	-	2	0	8	2	9	5	24	6
2	2	-	-	-	-	-	0	0	-	2	2	10	7	22	14	12	14
1	1	-	-	-	-	-	-	0	0	2	1	3	3	17	5	6	12
-	0	-	-	-	-	-	-	-	-	-	0	-	-	-	-	-	2
0	0	-	-	-	-	-	-	-	-	0	0	-	-	2	1	-	-
0	0	-	-	-	-	-	-	-	-	0	0	2	2	1	2	6	4
0	-	-	-	-	-	-	-	-	-	0	-	-	-	-	-	-	-
1	0	-	-	-	-	-	-	0	0	1	0	2	1	5	-	-	-
5	3	-	-	-	-	-	-	0	-	7	4	19	8	31	14	53	10
-	0	-	-	-	-	-	-	-	-	-	-	-	0	-	-	-	-
0	-	-	-	-	-	-	-	-	-	-	-	1	-	-	-	-	-

Table 22 - *continued*

Disease Group	Persons, by age group								
	Total	0-4	5-15	16-24	25-44	45-64	65-74	75-84	85 and over
Malignant neoplasm of bone and articular cartilage (170)	0	0	0	-	0	0	1	0	-
Malignant neoplasm of connective and other soft tissue (171)	0	-	-	0	-	-	0	-	-
Malignant melanoma of skin (172)	2	-	0	1	2	2	3	2	4
Other malignant neoplasm of skin (173)	6	-	-	0	1	6	20	39	41
Malignant neoplasm of female breast (174)	5	-	-	-	2	11	15	18	28
Malignant neoplasm of male breast (175)	0	-	-	-	-	-	1	0	-
Malignant neoplasm of uterus, part unspecified (179)	0	-	-	-	-	1	1	1	3
Malignant neoplasm of cervix uteri (180)	0	-	-	-	0	1	1	1	1
Malignant neoplasm of body of uterus (182)	0	-	-	-	-	1	3	1	-
Malignant neoplasm of ovary and other uterine adnexa (183)	1	1	1	1	0	3	2	2	4
Malignant neoplasm of other and unspecified female genital organs(184)	0	-	-	-	0	0	1	0	-
Malignant neoplasm of prostate (185)	2	-	-	-	-	2	9	17	9
Malignant neoplasm of testis (186)	1	-	-	-	1	2	1	0	-
Malignant neoplasm of penis and other male genital organs (187)	0	-	-	-	-	0	0	-	-
Malignant neoplasm of bladder (188)	1	-	-	-	-	1	4	12	9
Malignant neoplasm of kidney and other and unspecified urinary organs (189)	0	-	-	-	0	1	2	2	-
Malignant neoplasm of eye (190)	0	0	-	-	0	-	-	-	-
Malignant neoplasm of brain (191)	1	-	0	0	0	1	1	2	-
Malignant neoplasm of other and unspecified parts of nervous system (192)	0	-	-	-	-	0	0	-	-
Malignant neoplasm of thyroid gland (193)	0	-	-	-	0	0	0	-	-
Malignant neoplasm of other and ill-defined sites (195)	6	-	-	0	1	9	24	32	38
Secondary and unspecified malignant neoplasm of lymph nodes (196)	0	-	-	-	0	1	1	0	1
Secondary malignant neoplasm of respiratory and digestive systems (197)	2	-	0	-	0	-	6	9	7
Secondary malignant neoplasm of other specified sites (198)	2	-	-	-	0	3	8	10	9
Malignant neoplasm without specification of site (199)	1	-	-	-	0	1	3	7	1
Lymphosarcoma and reticulosarcoma (200)	0	-	-	-	0	-	-	-	1
Hodgkin's disease (201)	0	-	0	0	0	0	1	0	-
Other malignant neoplasm of lymphoid and histiocytic tissue (202)	0	0	0	1	-	0	1	-	-
Multiple myeloma and immunoproliferative neoplasms (203)	0	-	-	-	-	1	1	2	-
Lymphoid leukaemia (204)	0	1	0	0	0	0	2	2	1
Myeloid leukaemia (205)	0	-	-	-	0	0	1	1	-
Other specified leukaemia (207)	0	1	-	0	0	-	1	0	-
Leukaemia of unspecified cell type (208)	1	-	-	1	0	0	2	3	1
Benign neoplasm of lip, oral cavity and pharynx (210)	1	0	0	2	1	2	2	2	-
Benign neoplasm of other parts of digestive system (211)	1	1	0	-	0	1	1	2	3
Benign neoplasm of respiratory and intrathoracic organs (212)	0	-	-	-	0	0	0	-	-
Benign neoplasm of bone and articular cartilage (213)	1	1	1	2	1	1	1	-	-
Lipoma (214)	19	3	4	13	25	29	21	15	7
Other benign neoplasm of connective and other soft tissue (215)	3	1	1	3	5	3	2	1	-
Benign neoplasm of skin (216)	69	18	50	72	89	79	64	41	18
Benign neoplasm of breast (217)	6	0	0	6	11	5	1	0	-
Uterine leiomyoma (218)	4	-	-	0	8	9	-	0	-
Other benign neoplasm of uterus (219)	0	-	-	-	0	0	0	-	-
Benign neoplasm of ovary (220)	0	-	-	0	1	0	1	1	-
Benign neoplasm of other female genital organs (221)	0	0	-	0	1	0	-	-	-

By age-group and sex

Total Male	Total Female	0-4 Male	0-4 Female	5-15 Male	5-15 Female	16-24 Male	16-24 Female	25-44 Male	25-44 Female	45-64 Male	45-64 Female	65-74 Male	65-74 Female	75-84 Male	75-84 Female	85 and over Male	85 and over Female
0	0	-	1	0	-	-	-	0	-	-	0	2	0	1	-	-	-
0	0	-	-	-	-	0	-	-	-	-	-	-	0	-	-	-	-
1	2	-	-	0	-	1	1	1	2	2	3	2	3	3	1	-	6
5	6	-	-	-	-	0	-	1	1	6	6	20	20	46	35	36	43
-	11	-	-	-	-	-	-	-	4	-	22	-	27	-	29	-	37
0	-	-	-	-	-	-	-	-	-	-	-	1	-	1	-	-	-
-	1	-	-	-	-	-	-	-	-	-	1	-	1	-	1	-	4
-	1	-	-	-	-	-	-	-	1	-	2	-	1	-	2	-	2
-	1	-	-	-	-	-	-	-	-	-	2	-	5	-	1	-	-
-	3	-	2	-	2	-	1	-	1	-	6	-	3	-	3	-	6
-	0	-	-	-	-	-	-	-	0	-	0	-	1	-	1	-	-
4	-	-	-	-	-	-	-	-	-	4	-	19	-	46	-	36	-
2	-	-	-	-	-	-	-	3	-	4	-	1	-	1	-	-	-
0	-	-	-	-	-	-	-	-	-	0	-	1	-	-	-	-	-
2	1	-	-	-	-	-	-	-	-	2	0	7	1	17	10	18	6
0	1	-	-	-	-	-	-	0	-	0	1	1	3	2	1	-	-
0	0	-	1	-	-	-	-	0	0	-	-	-	-	-	-	-	-
1	1	-	-	0	-	1	-	0	0	1	1	1	2	2	1	-	-
0	0	-	-	-	-	-	-	-	-	0	0	-	0	-	-	-	-
-	0	-	-	-	-	-	-	-	0	-	1	-	0	-	-	-	-
6	6	-	-	-	-	0	-	1	0	11	7	26	23	38	28	42	37
0	0	-	-	-	-	-	-	0	-	0	1	1	2	-	1	-	2
2	1	-	-	-	0	-	-	0	1	1	2	8	5	16	4	18	4
2	2	-	-	-	-	-	-	0	0	2	4	7	8	16	6	18	6
1	1	-	-	-	-	-	-	0	0	1	1	4	2	7	8	-	2
0	0	-	-	-	-	-	-	0	-	-	-	-	-	-	-	-	2
0	0	-	-	0	-	0	-	0	0	0	-	2	0	1	-	-	-
0	0	-	1	-	0	1	0	-	-	0	1	2	1	-	-	-	-
0	0	-	-	-	-	-	-	-	-	1	0	1	1	2	2	-	-
1	0	1	1	0	0	0	-	-	0	0	0	2	1	3	1	6	-
0	0	-	-	-	-	-	-	0	1	-	0	2	0	1	1	-	-
0	0	1	1	-	-	-	0	0	-	-	-	1	-	-	1	-	-
1	0	-	-	-	-	0	1	0	0	0	0	2	1	6	1	-	2
1	1	1	-	1	-	2	2	1	1	2	2	2	2	2	2	-	-
0	1	-	1	-	0	-	-	0	1	1	2	1	1	1	2	-	4
0	0	-	-	-	-	-	-	0	-	0	1	1	-	-	-	-	-
1	1	1	1	2	0	2	1	1	1	0	2	1	0	-	-	-	-
19	19	3	3	4	3	13	12	28	22	27	31	14	26	9	18	-	10
2	4	1	1	1	1	2	4	3	7	4	3	1	3	-	1	-	-
50	86	18	18	46	53	42	102	53	125	64	94	65	64	37	43	12	20
0	11	1	-	-	1	0	12	-	23	0	9	-	2	-	1	-	-
-	8	-	-	-	-	-	0	-	15	-	18	-	-	-	1	-	-
-	0	-	-	-	-	-	-	-	0	-	1	-	0	-	-	-	-
-	1	-	-	-	-	1	-	2	-	1	-	1	-	1	-	1	-
-	1	-	1	-	-	-	0	-	2	-	1	-	-	-	-	-	-

Table 22 - *continued*

Disease Group	Persons, by age group								
	Total	0-4	5-15	16-24	25-44	45-64	65-74	75-84	85 and over
Benign neoplasm of male genital organs (222)	0	-	-	0	1	0	2	-	-
Benign neoplasm of kidney and other urinary organs (223)	0	-	-	-	-	0	1	2	-
Benign neoplasm of eye (224)	0	-	-	-	0	1	1	-	-
Benign neoplasm of brain and other parts of nervous system (225)	0	-	0	0	0	1	1	-	-
Benign neoplasm of thyroid gland (226)	1	-	-	-	1	1	0	0	1
Benign neoplasm of other endocrine glands and related structures (227)	0	-	-	-	0	0	-	-	-
Haemangioma and lymphangioma, any site (228)	3	7	2	2	3	4	3	3	3
Benign neoplasm of other and unspecified sites (229)	2	1	1	2	2	2	2	1	1
Carcinoma in situ of digestive organs (230)	1	-	-	-	0	1	3	5	9
Carcinoma in situ of respiratory system (231)	0	-	-	-	-	0	2	2	-
Carcinoma in situ of skin (232)	0	-	-	-	-	0	0	2	-
Carcinoma in situ of breast and genitourinary system (233)	1	-	-	-	1	2	3	3	10
Carcinoma in situ of other and unspecified sites (234)	0	-	-	-	-	0	1	1	-
Neoplasm of uncertain behaviour of digestive and respiratory systems (235)	1	0	-	0	0	1	1	2	1
Neoplasm of uncertain behaviour of genitourinary organs (236)	1	-	-	1	0	1	1	0	-
Neoplasm of uncertain behaviour of endocrine glands and nervous system (237)	1	1	1	1	1	1	1	1	-
Neoplasm of uncertain behaviour of other and unspecified sites and tissues (238)	2	-	0	0	1	2	4	5	12
Neoplasm of unspecified nature (239)	22	8	18	12	24	26	33	35	16
Simple and unspecified goitre (240)	3	1	1	4	4	4	3	1	3
Nontoxic nodular goitre (241)	1	-	-	0	2	3	0	2	3
Thyrotoxicosis with or without goitre (242)	4	-	-	2	5	6	7	6	7
Congenital hypothyroidism (243)	0	-	-	-	0	0	-	-	-
Acquired hypothyroidism (244)	13	-	1	2	8	25	34	39	28
Thyroiditis (245)	1	-	0	0	1	1	1	-	-
Other disorders of thyroid (246)	1	-	-	0	1	2	2	2	-
Diabetes mellitus (250)	30	1	3	6	12	51	101	110	70
Other disorders of pancreatic internal secretion (251)	5	1	1	3	4	6	9	16	6
Disorders of parathyroid gland (252)	0	-	-	-	0	1	1	1	1
Disorders of the pituitary gland and its hypothalamic control (253)	0	-	0	-	0	0	-	-	-
Disorders of adrenal glands (255)	0	1	0	0	0	-	1	1	-
Ovarian dysfunction (256)	3	-	0	4	7	2	-	-	-
Testicular dysfunction (257)	0	-		1	0	0	-	-	-
Other endocrine disorders (259)	0	0	2	-	0	0	0	-	-
Nutritional marasmus (261)	0	0	-	-	-	-	-	-	-
Vitamin A deficiency (264)	0	0	0	-	-	-	-	-	-
Thiamine and niacin deficiency states (265)	0	-	-	-	-	0	-	-	-
Deficiency of B-complex components (266)	1	0	0	0	0	1	1	4	3
Ascorbic acid deficiency (267)	0	-	-	-	0	-	-	-	1
Vitamin D deficiency (268)	0	-	0	-	0	-	-	-	1
Other nutritional deficiencies (269)	0	0	1	-	0	-	2	0	1
Disorders of amino-acid transport and metabolism (270)	0	-	0	-	0	0	0	-	-
Disorders of carbohydrate transport and metabolism (271)	2	29	0	0	0	0	-	1	1
Disorders of lipoid metabolism (272)	26	0	1	4	21	72	44	6	-
Disorders of plasma protein metabolism (273)	0	-	-	-	0	0	0	-	3
Gout (274)	31	-	0	1	20	54	92	92	95

By age-group and sex

Total		0-4		5-15		16-24		25-44		45-64		65-74		75-84		85 and over	
Male	Female	Male	Female	Male	Female	Male	Female	Male	Female	Male	Female	Male	Female	Male	Female	Male	Female
1	-	-	-	-	-	1	-	1	-	1	-	4	-	-	-	-	-
0	0	-	-	-	-	-	-	-	-	1	0	1	1	3	1	-	-
0	0	-	-	-	-	-	-	0	0	1	0	1	0	-	-	-	-
0	1	-	-	-	0	-	0	0	0	-	1	1	1	-	-	-	-
0	1	-	-	-	-	-	-	0	1	0	2	-	0	-	1	-	2
0	0	-	-	-	-	-	-	-	-	0	0	-	-	-	-	-	-
2	4	5	8	1	3	1	3	2	4	3	5	3	2	-	4	12	-
2	1	2	-	1	1	2	2	2	1	2	2	-	3	1	1	-	2
1	1	-	-	-	-	-	-	0	-	1	1	4	1	6	4	18	6
0	0	-	-	-	-	-	-	-	-	1	-	2	1	3	1	-	-
0	0	-	-	-	-	-	-	-	-	-	0	-	0	1	3	-	-
0	2	-	-	-	-	-	-	-	2	1	3	1	5	1	5	6	12
0	0	-	-	-	-	-	-	-	-	-	0	1	-	1	1	-	-
1	0	-	1	-	-	0	0	-	0	1	1	2	1	5	-	-	2
1	0	-	-	-	-	1	1	0	0	1	1	2	0	1	-	-	-
1	1	1	1	1	0	1	0	1	1	1	1	1	0	2	-	-	-
1	2	-	-	1	-	0	-	1	1	1	3	4	3	5	5	12	12
17	26	6	10	17	19	9	16	14	34	21	30	34	31	41	31	18	16
1	6	1	1	0	1	-	7	1	7	1	8	1	5	-	2	-	4
0	3	-	-	-	-	-	0	0	4	-	5	-	0	-	3	6	2
1	7	-	-	-	-	1	2	1	9	2	10	2	11	1	8	12	6
-	0	-	-	-	-	-	-	-	0	-	0	-	-	-	-	-	-
4	22	-	-	-	1	0	3	2	14	6	45	13	51	17	51	12	33
0	1	-	-	-	0	-	0	0	2	-	2	-	1	-	-	-	-
0	2	-	-	-	-	-	0	1	2	1	3	-	3	1	2	-	-
32	28	-	1	2	3	7	4	15	8	58	43	109	95	120	103	65	71
4	5	1	1	0	1	4	2	3	4	6	6	8	10	9	21	12	4
0	1	-	-	-	-	-	-	0	0	-	1	-	2	-	1	-	2
0	0	-	-	1	0	-	-	0	0	-	0	-	-	-	-	-	-
0	0	-	1	-	0	0	-	0	0	-	-	1	0	-	2	-	-
-	6	-	-	-	0	-	8	-	15	-	4	-	-	-	-	-	-
0	-	-	-	1	-	1	-	1	-	0	-	-	-	-	-	-	-
0	1	-	1	1	3	-	-	0	0	-	0	1	-	-	-	-	-
0	-	1	-	-	-	-	-	-	-	-	-	-	-	-	-	-	-
-	0	-	1	-	0	-	-	-	-	-	-	-	-	-	-	-	-
-	0	-	-	-	-	-	-	-	-	-	-	0	-	-	-	-	-
0	1	1	-	-	0	-	1	-	0	0	2	-	1	5	4	6	2
-	0	-	-	-	-	-	-	-	-	0	-	-	-	-	-	-	2
0	0	-	-	-	0	-	-	0	0	-	-	-	-	-	-	-	-
0	1	-	1	1	2	-	-	-	0	-	-	2	1	-	1	-	2
0	0	-	-	0	-	-	-	0	-	0	0	-	-	0	-	-	-
0	0	-	-	-	-	-	-	-	0	0	-	1	-	-	-	-	-
2	2	32	25	0	-	-	0	-	0	0	0	-	-	-	-	1	-
27	26	1	-	1	2	3	6	28	14	67	78	34	52	5	7	-	-
0	0	-	-	-	-	-	-	-	0	0	-	1	-	-	-	12	-
50	14	-	-	1	-	1	2	36	4	91	17	150	45	143	62	172	69

New and first ever episodes

Table 22 - *continued*

Disease Group	Persons, by age group								
	Total	0-4	5-15	16-24	25-44	45-64	65-74	75-84	85 and over
Disorders of mineral metabolism (275)	1	1	0	-	0	1	4	3	-
Disorders of fluid, electrolyte, and acid-base balance (276)	11	6	1	6	10	16	18	25	49
Other and unspecified disorders of metabolism (277)	2	4	2	3	1	1	2	1	1
Obesity and other hyperalimentation (278)	43	3	12	42	59	65	42	18	3
Disorders involving the immune mechanism (279)	0	1	-	-	0	0	0	0	-
Iron deficiency anaemias (280)	39	16	9	28	42	39	55	113	154
Other deficiency anaemias (281)	5	0	-	1	2	5	15	29	34
Hereditary haemolytic anaemias (282)	1	1	1	1	1	0	0	0	-
Acquired haemolytic anaemias (283)	0	0	-	0	0	0	0	-	1
Aplastic anaemia (284)	0	-	-	-	0	-	0	-	-
Other and unspecified anaemias (285)	10	6	2	8	8	9	20	25	36
Coagulation defects (286)	0	1	1	-	0	0	1	-	-
Purpura and other haemorrhagic conditions (287)	4	3	5	3	2	3	10	11	12
Diseases of white blood cells (288)	0	0	0	0	0	1	1	-	-
Other diseases of blood and blood-forming organs (289)	8	23	35	4	2	2	1	2	-
Senile and presenile organic psychotic conditions (290)	8	0	-	-	-	2	12	76	192
Alcoholic psychoses (291)	1	-	-	1	2	2	2	-	4
Drug psychoses (292)	1	-	-	2	1	1	3	1	4
Transient organic psychotic conditions (293)	8	-	0	1	1	4	18	66	154
Other organic psychotic conditions (chronic) (294)	1	-	-	0	0	0	1	7	19
Schizophrenic psychoses (295)	3	-	-	2	3	4	3	2	3
Affective psychoses (296)	37	-	1	27	43	55	52	64	89
Paranoid states (297)	2	-	-	3	2	3	3	7	10
Other nonorganic psychoses (298)	3	-	-	2	4	2	2	9	6
Psychoses with origin specific to childhood (299)	0	-	0	-	0	-	-	-	-
Neurotic disorders (300)	271	13	44	282	353	351	312	310	265
Personality disorders (301)	6	-	1	10	7	7	4	13	13
Sexual deviations and disorders (302)	12	-	-	10	13	24	16	3	1
Alcohol dependence syndrome (303)	6	-	-	3	11	10	5	3	1
Drug dependence (304)	7	-	1	15	8	7	7	6	7
Nondependent abuse of drugs (305)	11	-	2	13	16	15	7	3	4
Physiological malfunction arising from mental factors (306)	9	3	7	12	11	10	7	8	4
Special symptoms or syndromes not elsewhere classified (307)	74	92	49	75	73	82	69	75	117
Acute reaction to stress (308)	24	1	3	27	40	30	13	7	3
Adjustment reaction (309)	27	-	2	16	28	39	52	60	47
Specific nonpsychotic mental disorders following organic brain damage (310)	4	1	2	4	2	4	5	16	7
Depressive disorder, not elsewhere classified (311)	75	0	5	67	100	100	84	109	123
Disturbance of conduct not elsewhere classified (312)	11	35	34	9	4	1	2	12	31
Disturbance of emotions specific to childhood and adolescence (313)	1	4	5	2	0	0	-	-	-
Hyperkinetic syndrome of childhood (314)	1	10	2	-	-	-	-	-	-
Specific delays in development (315)	4	38	7	1	0	0	0	0	-
Mild mental retardation (317)	0	-	-	0	0	-	-	-	-
Other specified mental retardation (318)	0	-	-	1	0	0	-	-	-
Unspecified mental retardation (319)	0	0	-	0	0	0	-	-	-
Bacterial meningitis (320)	0	2	0	0	0	0	-	-	-
Meningitis of unspecified cause (322)	1	3	1	1	1	1	0	-	-
Encephalitis, myelitis and encephalomyelitis (323)	1	-	0	-	1	1	-	-	-
Intracranial and intraspinal abscess (324)	0	-	0	0	0	0	-	-	-
Phlebitis and thrombophlebitis of intracranial venous sinuses (325)	0	-	-	-	0	0	0	1	-

210

By age-group and sex

Total		0-4		5-15		16-24		25-44		45-64		65-74		75-84		85 and over	
Male	Female	Male	Female	Male	Female	Male	Female	Male	Female	Male	Female	Male	Female	Male	Female	Male	Female
1	1	1	-	0	-	-	-	0	1	1	1	5	3	-	4	-	-
4	18	7	4	1	1	0	12	1	20	4	28	15	21	19	28	48	49
2	2	3	4	2	2	3	2	1	2	1	1	1	2	-	1	-	2
19	67	3	3	9	15	11	72	22	95	32	100	23	57	9	23	-	4
0	0	-	1	-	-	-	-	-	0	0	0	0	1	-	-	1	-
14	63	15	16	8	9	2	55	4	80	14	64	50	59	77	135	101	171
3	7	1	-	-	-	-	2	2	3	2	8	13	17	26	31	48	30
1	1	-	1	1	1	1	1	1	1	0	0	-	0	-	1	-	-
0	0	1	-	-	-	1	-	-	-	0	0	-	-	-	-	-	2
-	0	-	-	-	-	-	-	-	0	-	-	-	0	-	-	-	-
4	15	6	5	1	4	1	14	1	16	4	14	16	23	14	31	18	41
0	0	1	-	1	0	-	-	0	0	0	0	-	1	-	-	-	-
4	5	5	2	5	5	1	4	1	3	3	4	9	10	11	10	30	6
0	1	-	1	-	1	-	1	0	0	1	1	1	0	-	-	-	-
7	8	20	26	31	38	3	4	2	1	2	1	1	1	2	1	-	-
5	11	-	1	-	-	-	-	-	-	3	2	8	16	62	84	238	177
2	1	-	-	-	-	0	1	2	1	3	1	2	1	-	-	6	4
1	2	-	-	-	-	2	1	1	1	0	2	1	4	1	1	-	6
6	10	-	-	1	-	0	1	1	2	5	2	17	18	64	68	166	150
0	1	-	-	-	-	-	0	0	0	0	1	-	1	5	8	24	18
3	2	-	-	-	-	4	1	5	2	4	3	2	4	-	3	12	-
21	53	-	-	1	1	18	36	24	62	33	78	23	75	39	79	59	99
2	2	-	-	-	-	4	1	3	1	2	4	2	3	2	10	12	10
2	3	-	-	-	-	1	4	2	5	2	2	1	4	13	8	-	8
0	0	-	-	0	-	-	-	0	0	-	-	-	-	-	-	-	-
154	383	13	13	33	56	152	410	188	520	213	492	185	416	187	384	184	292
5	8	-	-	1	-	11	9	5	9	3	11	3	6	8	16	12	14
17	7	-	-	-	-	9	10	12	14	43	5	36	-	9	-	-	2
9	4	-	-	-	-	5	0	16	5	14	6	5	5	2	4	-	2
8	6	-	-	1	-	23	6	10	6	5	9	1	12	5	6	6	8
14	8	-	-	2	2	17	8	19	13	18	12	10	4	9	-	12	2
6	12	2	4	4	11	7	16	7	15	7	12	8	7	7	8	-	6
52	94	96	88	50	48	40	109	42	105	55	109	62	75	61	83	83	128
15	32	1	-	2	4	15	39	25	54	21	40	6	18	2	10	6	2
12	41	-	-	2	2	7	24	12	43	16	63	25	73	37	73	42	49
4	4	1	-	2	2	4	4	2	2	4	5	7	4	16	16	6	8
40	109	1	-	3	7	32	103	45	156	62	140	62	101	65	135	113	126
14	7	45	24	44	22	12	5	5	3	2	1	2	2	14	10	53	24
1	2	2	6	4	5	1	3	-	0	-	0	-	-	-	-	-	-
2	0	15	5	5	-	-	-	-	-	-	-	-	-	-	-	-	-
5	3	46	29	11	4	1	1	1	-	-	1	1	-	-	1	-	-
0	-	-	-	-	-	0	-	0	-	-	-	-	-	-	-	-	-
0	0	-	-	-	-	1	0	-	0	0	0	-	-	-	-	-	-
0	0	1	-	-	-	0	0	0	-	0	-	-	-	-	-	-	-
0	0	1	2	-	0	-	0	0	0	-	0	-	-	-	-	-	-
1	1	3	3	1	0	1	-	0	1	0	1	-	0	-	-	-	-
1	0	-	-	0	0	-	-	2	1	1	0	-	-	-	-	-	-
0	0	-	-	-	0	0	-	0	0	0	0	-	-	-	-	-	-
0	0	-	-	-	-	-	-	0	0	-	0	-	0	2	1	-	-

Table 22 - *continued*

Disease Group	Persons, by age group								
	Total	0-4	5-15	16-24	25-44	45-64	65-74	75-84	85 and over
Cerebral degenerations usually manifest in childhood (330)	0	1	0	-	0	0	-	-	-
Other cerebral degenerations (331)	1	-	-	-	0	1	5	11	18
Parkinson's disease (332)	5	-	-	0	0	3	20	45	53
Other extrapyramidal disease and abnormal movement disorders (333)	9	2	5	7	8	13	21	11	13
Spinocerebellar disease (334)	0	-	0	-	0	0	1	0	-
Anterior horn cell disease (335)	0	-	-	-	0	0	1	1	-
Other diseases of spinal cord (336)	0	-	-	-	0	0	1	1	-
Disorders of autonomic nervous system (337)	0	-	-	-	0	1	0	0	-
Multiple sclerosis (340)	2	-	-	1	4	4	1	-	-
Other demyelinating diseases of central nervous system (341)	0	-	-	0	0	0	-	-	-
Hemiplegia (342)	2	0	0	0	0	2	3	11	38
Infantile cerebral palsy (343)	0	2	0	0	0	0	0	-	-
Other paralytic syndromes (344)	1	-	0	0	0	1	2	1	3
Epilepsy (345)	12	12	12	17	10	9	16	17	13
Migraine (346)	94	3	87	128	130	93	43	28	12
Cataplexy and narcolepsy (347)	0	-	-	0	0	0	-	-	-
Other conditions of brain (348)	0	-	-	0	1	1	1	1	-
Other and unspecified disorders of the nervous system (349)	1	-	-	0	1	1	1	0	-
Trigeminal nerve disorders (350)	7	1	1	2	6	12	16	16	9
Facial nerve disorders (351)	3	0	1	2	4	5	6	5	3
Disorders of other cranial nerves (352)	0	-	-	-	0	0	0	1	-
Nerve root and plexus disorders (353)	2	-	0	1	2	4	2	3	1
Mononeuritis of upper limb and mononeuritis multiplex (354)	17	-	0	6	23	29	21	21	15
Mononeuritis of lower limb (355)	2	-	0	1	2	5	4	5	1
Hereditary and idiopathic peripheral neuropathy (356)	0	-	-	-	0	1	1	2	1
Inflammatory and toxic neuropathy (357)	2	-	-	0	1	3	4	3	-
Myoneural disorders (358)	0	-	-	0	-	0	1	1	-
Muscular dystrophies and other myopathies (359)	0	-	0	-	1	1	1	0	-
Disorders of the globe (360)	0	-	-	-	1	0	-	-	4
Retinal detachments and defects (361)	1	-	0	1	1	3	4	3	-
Other retinal disorders (362)	8	-	1	0	2	8	25	46	59
Chorioretinal inflammations and scars and other disorders of choroid (363)	0	-	0	-	0	1	1	1	1
Disorders of iris and ciliary body (364)	4	1	1	4	5	6	5	6	4
Glaucoma (365)	10	-	-	-	2	17	33	44	34
Cataract (366)	22	1	1	1	1	12	86	173	209
Disorders of refraction and accommodation (367)	3	6	4	2	2	3	3	3	-
Visual disturbances (368)	18	5	15	8	13	22	42	46	46
Blindness and low vision (369)	5	2	2	1	1	3	11	32	67
Keratitis (370)	5	-	1	4	5	8	8	9	9
Corneal opacity and other disorders of cornea (371)	2	0	0	1	2	4	2	3	1
Disorders of conjunctiva (372)	447	2,094	407	237	268	318	440	458	589
Inflammation of eyelids (373)	80	79	89	71	72	79	101	98	70
Other disorders of eyelids (374)	11	8	4	5	8	15	18	37	52
Disorders of lacrimal system (375)	21	12	4	3	9	28	72	75	75
Disorders of the orbit (376)	2	4	2	1	2	2	2	2	4
Disorders of optic nerve and visual pathways (377)	1	1	0	0	1	1	1	1	-
Strabismus and other disorders of binocular eye movements (378)	6	57	10	2	1	1	2	1	-
Other disorders of eye (379)	17	10	7	9	14	25	40	33	19
Disorders of external ear (380)	424	222	238	272	392	521	709	812	808
Nonsuppurative otitis media and Eustachian tube disorders (381)	393	2,426	853	179	167	114	84	51	36
Suppurative and unspecified otitis media (382)	185	1,269	395	69	64	45	39	27	18

By age-group and sex

| Total | | 0-4 | | 5-15 | | 16-24 | | 25-44 | | 45-64 | | 65-74 | | 75-84 | | 85 and over | |
Male	Female	Male	Female	Male	Female	Male	Female	Male	Female	Male	Female	Male	Female	Male	Female	Male	Female
0	0	1	1	0	-	-	-	-	0	0	-	-	-	-	-	-	-
1	2	-	-	-	-	-	-	0	-	1	1	6	4	11	11	6	22
5	6	-	-	-	-	0	-	1	0	4	2	19	21	61	36	83	43
7	12	3	1	5	6	6	9	5	11	9	17	14	27	11	11	-	18
0	0	-	-	0	-	-	-	-	0	0	0	1	0	1	-	-	-
0	0	-	-	-	-	-	-	0	-	0	0	-	2	1	1	-	-
0	0	-	-	-	-	-	-	0	1	0	0	1	1	2	1	-	-
0	0	-	-	-	-	-	-	0	0	-	1	1	-	-	1	-	-
1	3	-	-	-	-	1	2	2	5	2	5	1	1	-	-	-	-
0	0	-	-	-	-	0	-	0	0	-	0	-	-	-	-	-	-
2	2	-	1	-	0	0	0	0	0	2	2	3	3	14	10	36	39
0	0	2	1	1	-	-	0	0	-	0	-	1	-	-	-	-	-
1	1	-	-	0	-	1	-	0	0	1	1	2	1	1	1	-	4
12	12	10	15	13	12	19	15	9	11	10	8	16	16	18	16	12	14
47	138	3	3	77	99	56	200	53	208	41	146	29	55	18	34	6	14
0	0	-	-	-	-	0	-	-	0	-	0	-	-	-	-	-	-
0	0	-	-	-	-	-	0	1	1	0	1	1	0	1	1	-	-
1	1	-	-	-	-	0	0	0	2	2	1	1	1	1	1	-	-
5	9	1	1	1	0	1	3	4	9	8	15	12	19	15	16	12	8
3	3	1	-	1	2	1	2	3	4	5	4	7	5	9	3	-	4
0	0	-	-	-	-	-	-	-	0	-	0	1	-	1	1	-	-
2	2	-	-	-	0	1	1	2	3	3	4	2	2	5	2	-	2
9	25	-	-	-	0	2	10	10	37	17	42	19	23	17	23	18	14
2	3	-	-	0	0	1	1	2	2	3	6	3	4	3	6	6	-
1	0	-	-	-	-	-	-	0	0	1	0	1	1	3	1	6	-
2	2	-	-	-	-	0	0	2	1	2	4	6	2	3	3	-	-
0	0	-	-	-	-	-	0	-	-	0	0	1	1	1	1	-	-
0	0	-	-	0	-	-	-	0	1	1	0	1	0	-	1	-	-
0	0	-	-	-	-	-	-	0	1	0	0	-	-	-	-	6	4
1	1	-	-	0	-	0	1	1	1	3	2	3	5	2	3	-	-
7	9	-	-	0	1	1	-	2	2	9	8	22	28	50	43	65	57
1	0	-	-	-	0	-	-	0	0	1	1	2	-	1	1	6	-
4	5	-	1	1	1	3	4	5	5	5	7	2	8	7	5	6	4
9	11	-	-	-	-	-	-	2	2	17	17	31	34	41	46	48	30
16	27	1	1	0	1	1	0	1	1	11	12	68	101	159	181	220	205
3	3	5	6	5	4	1	2	2	3	3	3	1	4	6	1	-	-
17	19	6	4	15	15	10	5	11	15	22	21	38	46	52	42	18	55
4	6	2	3	1	3	1	1	1	2	2	4	13	9	27	34	53	71
5	5	-	-	1	2	6	2	6	4	6	10	10	6	8	10	30	2
2	2	1	-	0	1	1	1	2	2	4	3	4	1	3	3	-	2
382	511	2,103	2,085	379	437	167	307	189	347	226	411	358	507	392	497	452	634
62	98	74	85	76	103	51	91	51	94	58	100	84	114	84	107	53	75
9	13	9	7	3	5	3	6	6	10	11	19	19	17	47	31	77	43
12	30	8	17	4	3	1	4	4	14	15	42	46	92	48	90	59	81
1	2	5	2	1	3	1	1	1	3	0	3	3	2	-	3	-	6
1	1	1	1	0	-	0	0	1	1	1	2	1	1	-	1	-	-
7	6	60	54	11	9	2	3	1	2	0	1	2	2	2	1	-	-
14	21	10	10	8	6	8	9	11	17	18	33	34	45	26	38	30	16
432	416	230	212	197	280	249	295	385	399	555	487	883	568	1,024	685	981	751
375	410	2,477	2,372	815	892	124	234	118	216	83	145	79	88	39	58	6	45
188	181	1,334	1,200	393	397	56	81	53	75	35	55	31	46	35	23	-	24

New and first ever episodes

Table 22 - *continued*

Disease Group	Persons, by age group								
	Total	0-4	5-15	16-24	25-44	45-64	65-74	75-84	85 and over
Mastoiditis and related conditions (383)	1	1	1	1	1	1	1	2	-
Other disorders of tympanic membrane (384)	7	15	11	5	6	5	5	3	3
Other disorders of middle ear and mastoid (385)	1	0	0	-	1	1	2	2	1
Vertiginous syndromes and other disorders of vestibular system (386)	65	2	8	29	58	104	136	149	135
Otosclerosis (387)	0	-	-	0	0	0	1	-	-
Other disorders of ear (388)	107	280	198	64	70	79	94	87	108
Deafness (389)	33	44	34	10	16	33	62	99	117
Rheumatic fever without mention of heart involvement (390)	0	-	0	0	0	-	-	-	-
Rheumatic fever with heart involvement (391)	0	-	-	-	-	0	-	-	-
Rheumatic chorea (392)	0	-	-	-	0	-	-	-	-
Diseases of mitral valve (394)	0	-	-	-	0	1	1	2	-
Diseases of aortic valve (395)	0	-	-	-	-	1	0	0	1
Diseases of mitral and aortic valves (396)	0	-	-	-	0	1	0	-	3
Diseases of other endocardial structures (397)	0	-	-	-	-	0	-	-	-
Other rheumatic heart disease (398)	0	-	-	-	-	0	0	0	-
Essential hypertension (401)	95	0	0	4	32	192	336	289	95
Hypertensive heart disease (402)	2	-	-	0	1	4	4	5	-
Hypertensive renal disease (403)	0	-	-	-	0	0	1	-	-
Secondary hypertension (405)	0	-	-	1	0	1	1	0	-
Acute myocardial infarction (410)	23	-	-	0	2	34	88	116	114
Other acute and subacute forms of ischaemic heart disease (411)	1	-	-	-	0	1	2	3	1
Old myocardial infarction (412)	1	-	-	-	0	1	3	2	3
Angina pectoris (413)	52	0	-	-	6	87	198	242	213
Other forms of chronic ischaemic heart disease (414)	9	-	0	-	1	15	32	39	37
Acute pulmonary heart disease (415)	4	-	-	1	2	4	12	23	18
Chronic pulmonary heart disease (416)	0	-	0	0	0	0	2	3	1
Other diseases of pulmonary circulation (417)	0	-	-	-	0	-	-	0	-
Acute pericarditis (420)	1	-	0	1	0	1	1	1	1
Acute and subacute endocarditis (421)	0	-	-	-	0	0	1	0	1
Acute myocarditis (422)	0	-	-	0	-	-	-	-	-
Other diseases of pericardium (423)	0	1	-	-	0	0	1	0	-
Other diseases of endocardium (424)	2	1	1	0	1	3	7	9	15
Cardiomyopathy (425)	1	-	0	-	0	1	2	0	-
Conduction disorders (426)	2	1	-	1	0	2	4	9	13
Cardiac dysrhythmias (427)	23	1	0	3	7	27	75	127	148
Heart failure (428)	51	1	0	0	1	24	166	422	780
Ill-defined descriptions and complications of heart disease (429)	1	-	0	1	0	1	1	3	4
Subarachnoid haemorrhage (430)	1	-	-	1	1	2	2	-	-
Intracerebral haemorrhage (431)	1	-	-	1	-	2	3	3	13
Other and unspecified intracranial haemorrhage (432)	0	-	0	-	-	1	1	1	1
Occlusion and stenosis of precerebral arteries (433)	1	-	-	-	0	2	5	7	7
Occlusion of cerebral arteries (434)	2	-	-	-	-	1	5	11	21
Transient cerebral ischaemia (435)	25	-	-	0	1	18	81	195	297
Acute but ill-defined cerebrovascular disease (436)	18	-	-	-	1	11	58	134	268
Other and ill-defined cerebrovascular disease (437)	3	-	-	-	0	2	10	27	43
Late effects of cerebrovascular disease (438)	0	-	-	-	-	0	1	1	1
Atherosclerosis (440)	1	-	-	-	-	1	3	8	13
Aortic aneurysm (441)	2	-	-	-	0	2	8	13	16
Other aneurysm (442)	0	-	-	-	0	0	1	1	3
Other peripheral vascular disease (443)	24	1	2	6	9	33	90	103	75

By age-group and sex

Total		0-4		5-15		16-24		25-44		45-64		65-74		75-84		85 and over	
Male	Female	Male	Female	Male	Female	Male	Female	Male	Female	Male	Female	Male	Female	Male	Female	Male	Female
1	1	1	1	1	1	1	1	1	1	0	1	1	1	-	3	-	-
7	7	14	17	11	11	6	5	5	7	5	5	8	3	1	5	6	2
1	1	1	-	0	0	-	-	1	1	1	1	2	1	1	2	-	2
43	87	2	1	7	9	17	41	31	85	71	137	110	157	126	163	149	130
0	0	-	-	-	-	-	0	-	1	0	0	-	1	-	-	-	-
87	126	272	288	146	253	44	85	45	96	71	87	95	93	72	96	101	110
33	32	52	36	35	33	7	13	15	17	39	27	71	55	105	95	131	112
0	0	-	-	-	0	0	-	-	0	-	-	-	-	-	-	-	-
0	-	-	-	-	-	-	-	-	-	0	-	-	-	-	-	-	-
0	-	-	-	-	-	-	-	0	-	-	-	-	-	-	-	-	-
0	0	-	-	-	-	-	-	0	0	0	1	1	1	5	1	-	-
0	0	-	-	-	-	-	-	-	-	1	0	1	-	-	1	-	2
0	0	-	-	-	-	-	-	0	-	0	1	-	0	-	-	-	4
0	-	-	-	-	-	-	-	-	-	0	-	-	-	-	-	-	-
0	0	-	-	-	-	-	-	-	-	0	1	1	-	1	-	-	-
83	106	1	-	1	-	2	5	33	32	187	198	293	372	227	327	71	102
2	2	-	-	-	-	-	1	1	1	4	5	6	3	-	8	-	-
0	0	-	-	-	-	-	-	-	1	0	-	1	0	-	-	-	-
0	1	-	-	-	-	1	0	1	1	1	1	1	0	-	1	-	-
29	16	-	-	-	-	0	-	3	1	53	15	126	58	153	94	143	104
1	0	-	-	-	-	-	-	0	0	2	0	1	3	7	1	6	-
1	0	-	-	-	-	-	-	0	-	1	1	5	3	3	1	6	2
55	49	-	1	-	-	-	-	9	4	108	66	225	176	273	224	202	217
11	7	-	-	0	-	-	-	2	1	21	9	43	24	56	29	36	37
3	5	-	-	-	-	-	2	0	3	4	5	13	10	24	22	36	12
1	0	-	-	0	-	0	-	-	0	1	0	4	1	5	1	6	-
0	-	-	-	-	-	-	-	0	-	-	-	-	-	1	-	-	-
1	0	-	-	0	0	1	0	1	0	1	1	2	-	1	1	6	-
0	0	-	-	-	-	-	-	1	-	0	0	2	0	-	1	6	-
0	-	-	-	-	-	0	-	-	-	-	-	-	-	-	-	-	-
0	0	1	1	-	-	-	-	0	-	0	-	1	0	1	-	-	-
2	2	1	1	1	1	0	-	1	1	3	3	8	5	14	7	24	12
1	0	-	-	0	-	-	-	1	-	2	1	2	2	-	1	-	-
2	1	2	-	-	-	0	1	1	0	2	2	6	2	14	6	18	12
21	26	1	1	1	-	3	4	6	9	29	25	79	71	133	124	95	165
45	58	1	1	0	0	-	1	1	1	25	24	200	138	471	393	826	764
1	1	-	-	-	0	1	1	0	0	1	1	1	1	3	3	-	6
1	1	-	-	-	-	1	1	1	0	1	3	3	1	-	-	-	-
1	1	-	-	-	-	1	0	-	-	2	2	4	3	3	3	18	12
0	0	-	-	0	-	-	-	-	-	1	0	2	-	2	1	-	2
1	2	-	-	-	-	-	-	0	-	1	2	3	7	5	9	6	8
2	1	-	-	-	-	-	-	-	-	1	1	8	3	16	8	30	18
23	27	-	-	-	-	-	1	1	2	18	18	100	66	240	168	333	286
16	20	-	-	-	-	-	-	0	1	15	8	73	46	137	132	244	276
3	4	-	-	-	-	-	-	0	0	3	1	9	10	31	25	30	47
0	0	-	-	-	-	-	-	-	-	1	-	-	1	1	1	-	2
1	1	-	-	-	-	-	-	-	-	1	1	3	3	10	6	12	14
3	1	-	-	-	-	-	-	0	0	3	1	15	2	25	5	24	14
0	0	-	-	-	-	-	-	0	-	0	0	1	0	3	-	6	2
25	24	1	1	0	4	2	11	5	13	43	23	115	70	121	92	113	63

Table 22 - *continued*

Disease Group	Persons, by age group								
	Total	0-4	5-15	16-24	25-44	45-64	65-74	75-84	85 and over
Arterial embolism and thrombosis (444)	1	-	-	-	0	1	2	5	6
Polyarteritis nodosa and allied conditions (446)	2	-	-	-	0	2	6	9	10
Other disorders of arteries and arterioles (447)	0	-	-	0	-	0	0	1	-
Diseases of capillaries (448)	5	3	6	6	5	4	3	4	1
Phlebitis and thrombophlebitis (451)	22	-	1	5	12	36	59	83	47
Other venous embolism and thrombosis (453)	3	-	0	0	1	5	12	14	10
Varicose veins of lower extremities (454)	63	0	1	18	49	104	153	183	148
Haemorrhoids (455)	92	4	4	69	134	117	125	98	87
Varicose veins of other sites (456)	2	-	0	2	2	1	2	2	-
Noninfective disorders of lymphatic channels (457)	2	1	1	2	2	3	2	1	4
Hypotension (458)	10	-	2	5	4	9	29	49	101
Other disorders of circulatory system (459)	3	2	0	1	2	5	8	8	12
Acute nasopharyngitis (common cold) (460)	364	2,520	447	203	158	139	168	167	216
Acute sinusitis (461)	274	19	126	283	401	335	217	128	86
Acute pharyngitis (462)	436	506	690	679	442	268	200	164	121
Acute tonsillitis (463)	467	1,238	1,157	743	335	90	38	28	15
Acute laryngitis and tracheitis (464)	143	449	121	106	122	137	120	98	80
Acute upper respiratory infections of multiple or unspecified site (465)	906	4,403	1,165	639	518	514	584	675	743
Acute bronchitis and bronchiolitis (466)	834	1,973	472	460	539	874	1,383	1,645	1,975
Deflected nasal septum (470)	4	-	2	8	4	3	3	1	1
Nasal polyps (471)	6	1	3	3	6	11	14	6	1
Chronic pharyngitis and nasopharyngitis (472)	82	137	75	56	68	87	120	92	59
Chronic sinusitis (473)	18	0	6	17	25	25	21	12	4
Chronic disease of tonsils and adenoids (474)	5	17	13	9	2	1	1	1	-
Peritonsillar abscess (475)	3	1	2	7	4	1	1	-	-
Chronic laryngitis and laryngotracheitis (476)	2	0	2	1	2	4	5	3	3
Allergic rhinitis (477)	245	147	459	428	258	122	91	66	25
Other diseases of upper respiratory tract (478)	8	9	7	6	8	8	11	6	6
Viral pneumonia (480)	1	3	1	0	1	1	1	3	9
Pneumococcal pneumonia (481)	5	8	5	1	3	5	11	19	25
Other bacterial pneumonia (482)	2	2	1	1	1	2	5	7	12
Pneumonia due to other specified organism (483)	0	-	0	1	0	0	0	0	-
Bronchopneumonia, organism unspecified (485)	10	7	3	1	2	5	20	61	218
Pneumonia, organism unspecified (486)	8	13	5	4	4	7	16	29	44
Influenza (487)	202	192	169	228	222	205	165	172	166
Bronchitis, not specified as acute or chronic (490)	44	95	17	16	25	44	86	120	194
Chronic bronchitis (491)	35	4	2	5	6	51	150	155	98
Emphysema (492)	4	-	-	-	1	6	16	12	7
Asthma (493)	297	883	545	275	190	182	223	180	109
Bronchiectasis (494)	3	1	0	0	1	5	7	7	6
Extrinsic allergic alveolitis (495)	0	-	0	-	0	0	1	-	3
Chronic airways obsruction, not elsewhere classified (496)	24	0	0	-	2	35	107	121	90
Coalworkers' pneumoconiosis (500)	0	-	-	-	-	-	-	1	-
Asbestosis (501)	0	-	-	-	-	0	1	0	-
Pneumoconiosis due to other inorganic dust (503)	0	-	0	-	-	-	-	-	-
Respiratory conditions due to chemical fumes and vapours (506)	0	-	-	-	0	0	0	-	-
Pneumonitis due to solids and liquids (507)	0	-	-	-	0	-	1	1	1
Respiratory conditions due to other and unspecified external agents (508)	0	-	-	-	-	0	-	-	-

By age-group and sex

Total		0-4		5-15		16-24		25-44		45-64		65-74		75-84		85 and over	
Male	Female	Male	Female	Male	Female	Male	Female	Male	Female	Male	Female	Male	Female	Male	Female	Male	Female
1	1	-	-	-	-	-	-	-	0	1	1	3	1	8	3	6	6
1	2	-	-	-	-	-	-	0	0	1	2	3	8	8	10	6	12
0	0	-	-	-	-	0	-	-	-	0	-	-	0	-	1	-	-
3	6	4	3	5	6	3	9	2	8	2	5	2	3	1	6	-	2
14	29	-	-	0	1	3	7	6	17	24	49	50	66	66	92	12	59
3	4	-	-	0	-	1	-	1	1	3	7	12	13	10	16	-	14
40	85	-	1	1	1	8	27	24	75	70	138	123	177	166	193	119	158
81	102	5	3	2	6	50	88	108	159	116	118	127	123	109	91	95	85
2	1	-	-	1	-	4	-	2	2	2	1	3	1	5	1	-	-
2	2	1	1	1	2	2	2	3	2	2	3	2	1	1	1	-	6
9	11	-	-	2	1	4	5	2	6	10	8	34	25	60	42	95	102
2	4	1	3	1	-	0	1	1	2	3	6	6	10	7	8	12	12
334	393	2,518	2,522	414	481	136	269	104	211	109	170	149	183	163	169	166	232
169	375	18	19	110	143	180	384	229	575	187	485	151	270	100	146	53	97
340	528	501	511	559	828	470	887	311	573	206	330	169	225	150	172	101	128
394	538	1,333	1,139	942	1,383	535	950	237	435	62	120	35	40	27	29	12	16
107	178	530	364	117	125	53	159	60	184	74	200	87	147	79	109	59	87
796	1,010	4,463	4,340	1,092	1,241	449	829	346	691	377	653	502	650	624	705	874	699
748	916	2,097	1,843	494	449	376	542	398	682	722	1,028	1,413	1,359	1,886	1,501	2,288	1,872
5	2	-	-	3	2	12	5	5	3	4	2	3	2	2	-	-	2
9	4	-	1	5	2	4	2	8	3	16	5	22	7	9	3	6	-
73	90	133	141	79	70	50	62	52	85	72	103	118	121	97	88	89	49
13	23	-	1	7	5	12	23	18	31	18	32	12	29	6	16	6	4
4	6	19	15	11	15	2	15	1	3	1	2	-	1	1	1	-	-
3	2	1	1	2	2	9	5	4	4	1	1	2	1	-	-	-	-
2	3	-	1	1	3	0	2	2	3	3	4	6	4	2	3	-	4
229	259	176	117	508	407	363	493	204	311	102	143	82	99	74	60	42	20
7	8	10	7	8	7	6	5	7	9	6	10	9	12	6	5	18	2
1	1	5	2	1	1	0	-	1	1	1	0	1	1	5	2	6	10
6	5	11	5	6	4	1	0	2	3	5	5	12	10	26	14	42	20
2	2	2	3	2	0	1	2	1	1	2	1	7	3	10	5	24	8
0	0	-	-	0	-	-	1	0	0	0	0	-	0	-	1	-	-
10	11	8	6	4	2	1	1	3	1	6	4	22	18	76	53	256	205
9	7	15	11	6	3	3	4	4	4	8	6	20	12	39	23	65	37
178	224	207	176	160	179	194	261	193	251	167	243	143	183	150	185	184	160
38	49	102	88	19	15	17	15	19	31	35	54	85	86	115	123	202	191
42	29	4	4	2	3	5	5	6	7	55	47	218	95	252	98	214	59
5	2	-	-	-	-	-	-	1	1	9	4	28	7	26	3	24	2
300	295	1,017	742	626	460	249	301	157	224	150	215	197	244	158	194	125	104
2	3	1	1	-	0	1	-	1	2	4	6	3	11	10	5	6	6
0	0	-	-	0	-	-	-	0	0	-	1	1	1	-	-	-	4
29	20	1	-	-	0	-	-	2	3	39	32	158	65	172	90	178	61
0	-	-	-	-	-	-	-	-	-	-	-	-	-	2	-	-	-
0	-	-	-	-	-	-	-	-	-	1	-	1	-	1	-	-	-
0	-	-	-	0	-	-	-	-	-	-	-	-	-	-	-	-	-
0	-	-	-	-	-	-	-	0	-	0	-	1	-	-	-	-	-
0	0	-	-	-	-	-	-	-	-	-	0	-	-	1	2	1	6
-	0	-	-	-	-	-	-	-	-	-	-	0	-	-	-	-	-

Table 22 - *continued*

Disease Group	Persons, by age group								
	Total	0-4	5-15	16-24	25-44	45-64	65-74	75-84	85 and over
Empyema (510)	0	-	-	0	0	0	1	1	-
Pleurisy (511)	18	0	3	12	18	24	33	43	49
Pneumothorax (512)	2	-	0	2	2	1	2	2	4
Abscess of lung and mediastinum (513)	0	-	-	-	0	-	-	-	-
Pulmonary congestion and hypostasis (514)	1	-	-	0	-	1	2	8	16
Postinflammatory pulmonary fibrosis (515)	0	-	-	-	-	-	-	-	1
Other alveolar and parietoalveolar pneumopathy (516)	1	0	-	-	0	1	2	6	3
Other diseases of lung (518)	0	0	-	-	-	0	1	-	-
Other diseases of respiratory system (519)	8	31	6	6	6	7	10	6	4
Disorders of tooth development and eruption (520)	5	64	0	0	0	0	-	-	-
Diseases of hard tissues of teeth (521)	12	122	3	5	5	4	4	2	1
Diseases of pulp and periapical tissues (522)	34	8	23	36	48	41	21	11	7
Gingival and periodontal diseases (523)	8	15	5	9	9	8	6	5	6
Dentofacial anomalies, including malocclusion (524)	13	1	6	21	17	15	7	6	4
Other diseases and conditions of the teeth and supporting structures (525)	2	-	0	4	2	1	2	2	6
Diseases of the jaws (526)	0	0	0	1	0	0	1	-	-
Diseases of the salivary glands (527)	8	4	6	5	9	12	7	13	10
Diseases of the oral soft tissues, excluding lesions specific for gingiva and tongue (528)	62	122	72	66	51	49	68	63	58
Diseases and other conditions of the tongue (529)	9	10	6	5	8	11	13	20	13
Diseases of oesophagus (530)	81	21	4	38	78	132	157	153	139
Gastric ulcer (531)	3	-	-	1	3	5	7	13	10
Duodenal ulcer (532)	20	-	-	7	24	36	33	26	22
Peptic ulcer, site unspecified (533)	9	-	0	6	10	14	12	18	13
Gastritis and duodenitis (535)	66	46	36	70	72	74	72	91	86
Disorders of function of stomach (536)	128	3	12	84	129	186	253	254	209
Other disorders of stomach and duodenum (537)	0	2	0	0	-	1	1	0	-
Acute appendicitis (540)	3	0	8	6	4	2	1	1	-
Appendicitis, unqualified (541)	5	0	11	11	5	2	1	0	-
Other appendicitis (542)	0	0	0	1	1	0	0	-	-
Other diseases of appendix (543)	0	-	0	-	0	-	-	-	-
Inguinal hernia (550)	24	27	5	6	11	34	58	77	75
Other hernia of abdominal cavity with obstruction, without mention of gangrene (552)	0	0	-	-	0	0	1	2	3
Other hernia of abdominal cavity without mention of obstruction or gangrene (553)	23	33	2	3	14	34	54	64	44
Regional enteritis (555)	3	0	1	2	4	4	3	4	-
Idiopathic proctocolitis (556)	5	1	0	2	6	8	5	9	4
Vascular insufficiency of intestine (557)	0	-	-	-	-	0	1	1	3
Other noninfective gastroenteritis and colitis (558)	15	38	10	13	13	14	16	18	18
Intestinal obstruction without mention of hernia (560)	5	3	0	1	2	7	13	23	53
Diverticula of intestine (562)	16	-	0	0	3	25	56	82	92
Functional digestive disorders, not elsewhere classified (564)	172	236	71	165	159	152	223	347	568
Anal fissure and fistula (565)	24	49	11	34	31	19	9	12	10
Abscess of anal and rectal regions (566)	6	2	2	6	9	9	5	4	-
Peritonitis (567)	0	-	0	-	0	0	1	-	1
Other disorders of peritoneum (568)	1	0	0	0	1	1	1	1	-
Other disorders of intestine (569)	31	24	7	20	28	35	55	74	118

By age-group and sex

| Total | | 0-4 | | 5-15 | | 16-24 | | 25-44 | | 45-64 | | 65-74 | | 75-84 | | 85 and over | |
Male	Female	Male	Female	Male	Female	Male	Female	Male	Female	Male	Female	Male	Female	Male	Female	Male	Female
0	0	-	-	-	-	-	0	0	0	1	-	1	-	1	1	-	-
14	22	-	1	3	3	8	16	12	23	19	29	30	36	54	37	59	45
2	1	-	-	0	-	4	1	3	1	2	1	3	1	3	1	6	4
0	-	-	-	-	-	-	-	0	-	-	-	-	-	-	-	-	-
1	1	-	-	-	-	-	0	-	-	1	1	1	2	11	6	18	16
0	-	-	-	-	-	-	-	-	-	-	-	-	-	-	-	6	-
1	1	-	1	-	-	-	-	0	0	1	1	2	2	9	4	6	2
0	0	-	1	-	-	-	-	-	-	1	0	1	0	-	-	-	-
7	9	33	29	5	8	5	7	5	7	5	8	8	11	7	5	6	4
5	4	63	65	0	-	-	1	0	0	0	-	-	-	-	-	-	-
13	11	139	105	2	4	2	8	4	5	4	4	4	4	5	-	-	2
32	36	10	6	26	20	31	40	39	57	38	44	25	17	13	10	12	6
7	9	16	13	4	5	7	11	6	12	7	9	6	6	2	6	-	8
8	18	-	1	5	8	12	29	10	25	8	21	2	11	8	5	12	2
1	2	-	-	-	1	1	6	2	3	1	1	2	2	3	1	-	8
0	0	1	-	-	0	1	1	0	1	1	0	1	0	-	-	-	-
6	10	4	4	4	7	5	5	7	10	7	17	6	7	6	17	12	10
49	75	114	131	63	81	42	90	39	62	34	65	59	75	48	72	42	63
7	11	9	11	5	6	5	5	6	10	8	14	7	18	15	23	12	14
69	93	22	19	4	4	33	43	67	89	113	152	142	169	139	162	149	136
3	3	-	-	-	-	1	0	3	2	5	4	8	6	14	13	-	14
27	13	-	-	-	-	12	2	34	13	47	25	45	23	37	19	30	20
10	7	-	-	-	1	7	5	12	8	17	11	15	9	24	15	6	16
62	71	46	46	40	32	64	75	66	77	67	81	69	74	89	92	77	89
119	136	2	4	12	12	83	84	120	137	171	200	262	246	255	252	250	195
1	0	2	3	0	-	0	-	-	-	1	0	1	-	-	1	-	-
3	4	1	-	8	8	3	9	3	5	2	2	1	-	-	1	-	-
4	5	1	-	11	11	10	12	4	6	1	3	1	1	-	1	-	-
1	0	-	1	1	0	1	0	1	1	0	-	-	0	-	-	-	-
0	-	-	-	0	-	-	-	0	-	-	-	-	-	-	-	-	-
43	5	46	8	9	2	11	1	21	2	62	5	118	9	182	14	190	37
0	0	1	-	-	-	-	-	0	0	-	0	-	1	1	3	-	4
21	24	39	27	4	1	4	1	13	15	33	36	52	55	49	73	30	49
2	4	1	-	-	2	1	3	3	4	3	5	1	5	-	6	-	-
4	5	-	1	0	-	2	2	5	7	7	9	4	6	7	10	12	2
0	0	-	-	-	-	-	-	-	-	0	-	1	1	2	1	-	4
14	16	39	36	11	9	11	15	10	15	14	15	16	16	15	20	12	20
5	6	4	2	0	-	0	2	2	2	6	9	13	12	26	21	65	49
9	23	-	-	-	0	-	0	2	3	14	36	41	68	55	99	77	97
106	235	233	238	53	90	55	273	72	247	91	214	188	252	356	341	618	552
20	29	53	45	11	11	16	51	20	42	19	19	10	7	14	11	18	8
9	4	4	1	2	1	8	4	13	6	12	5	10	0	6	3	-	-
0	0	-	-	-	0	-	-	0	-	1	0	-	-	1	-	-	2
0	1	1	-	0	0	-	1	-	1	0	1	1	1	-	2	-	-
27	35	27	21	9	5	14	27	25	31	34	35	47	61	65	79	107	122

New and first ever episodes

Table 22 - *continued*

Disease Group	Persons, by age group								
	Total	0-4	5-15	16-24	25-44	45-64	65-74	75-84	85 and over
Acute and subacute necrosis of liver (570)	0	-	0	1	0	0	-	-	-
Chronic liver disease and cirrhosis (571)	2	-	-	0	2	4	3	2	-
Liver abscess and sequelae of chronic liver disease (572)	0	-	-	-	0	1	1	0	-
Other disorders of liver (573)	0	-	-	-	0	1	1	0	-
Cholelithiasis (574)	8	-	0	3	7	15	15	13	15
Other disorders of gallbladder (575)	9	-	-	3	8	15	18	18	19
Other disorders of biliary tract (576)	2	-	-	0	1	4	7	12	19
Diseases of pancreas (577)	2	-	0	1	2	3	3	6	4
Gastrointestinal haemorrhage (578)	11	4	1	5	7	11	26	51	92
Intestinal malabsorption (579)	1	4	1	1	1	1	2	1	1
Acute glomerulonephritis (580)	0	1	0	1	0	0	0	-	-
Nephrotic syndrome (581)	0	2	1	0	0	0	0	1	-
Chronic glomerulonephritis (582)	0	-	-	0	0	0	0	-	-
Nephritis and nephropathy, not specified as acute or chronic (583)	0	-	0	0	0	-	0	-	-
Acute renal failure (584)	1	-	-	0	0	1	4	5	6
Chronic renal failure (585)	2	-	-	-	0	2	4	8	34
Renal failure, unspecified (586)	1	1	-	-	0	1	2	5	10
Infections of kidney (590)	14	0	5	26	19	12	8	10	9
Hydronephrosis (591)	1	2	0	0	1	1	1	-	3
Calculus of kidney and ureter (592)	5	-	1	3	6	8	6	3	3
Other disorders of kidney and ureter (593)	1	2	1	1	1	1	1	1	-
Calculus of lower urinary tract (594)	1	-	0	0	0	1	3	0	-
Cystitis (595)	120	23	32	148	135	132	166	187	188
Other disorders of bladder (596)	3	-	0	1	3	5	8	8	7
Urethritis, not sexually transmitted, and urethral syndrome (597)	2	1	1	2	2	3	1	3	1
Urethral stricture (598)	1	-	1	-	0	1	2	3	6
Other disorders of urethra and urinary tract (599)	305	217	147	303	283	277	468	666	951
Hyperplasia of prostate (600)	9	-	-	-	0	15	43	45	18
Inflammatory diseases of prostate (601)	4	-	-	1	4	6	8	12	1
Other disorders of prostate (602)	0	-	-	-	-	0	-	2	-
Hydrocele (603)	5	23	3	2	2	4	7	7	13
Orchitis and epididymitis (604)	15	1	2	13	25	16	16	8	3
Redundant prepuce and phimosis (605)	12	68	28	7	4	3	3	4	7
Infertility, male (606)	2	-	-	1	6	4	0	-	-
Disorders of penis (607)	32	171	62	15	15	13	14	14	7
Other disorders of male genital organs (608)	12	4	8	12	16	14	14	6	-
Benign mammary dysplasias (610)	15	0	3	14	28	19	2	2	-
Other disorders of breast (611)	77	13	37	66	129	86	42	29	12
Inflammatory disease of ovary, fallopian tube, pelvic cellular tissue and peritoneum (614)	30	-	1	76	61	6	0	0	-
Inflammatory diseases of uterus, except cervix (615)	4	-	-	8	8	1	-	-	-
Inflammatory disease of cervix, vagina and vulva (616)	68	48	31	101	103	51	36	39	50
Endometriosis (617)	4	-	-	4	8	2	0	-	-
Genital prolapse (618)	15	-	0	1	8	27	45	53	34
Fistulae involving female genital tract (619)	0	-	-	-	0	0	1	1	3
Noninflammatory disorders of ovary, fallopian tube and broad ligament (620)	4	-	0	5	7	4	1	1	-
Disorders of uterus, not elsewhere classified (621)	2	0	-	2	4	3	1	-	-
Noninflammatory disorders of cervix (622)	10	-	0	11	16	15	4	3	-
Noninflammatory disorders of vagina (623)	29	9	9	48	50	18	12	9	31
Noninflammatory disorders of vulva and perineum (624)	2	1	0	1	3	2	2	3	6

By age-group and sex

Total		0-4		5-15		16-24		25-44		45-64		65-74		75-84		85 and over	
Male	Female	Male	Female	Male	Female	Male	Female	Male	Female	Male	Female	Male	Female	Male	Female	Male	Female
0	0	-	-	0	-	1	0	0	-	0	-	-	-	-	-	-	-
3	1	-	-	-	-	0	-	3	1	5	3	3	2	3	1	-	-
0	0	-	-	-	-	-	-	0	-	1	0	1	0	-	1	-	-
0	0	-	-	-	-	-	-	0	-	1	0	1	1	-	1	-	-
4	12	-	-	0	-	0	6	2	11	6	24	12	18	14	12	12	16
4	13	-	-	-	-	0	6	2	14	9	21	12	22	17	18	24	18
3	2	-	-	-	-	-	0	1	1	3	4	10	5	18	8	30	16
2	1	-	-	0	-	0	1	2	1	4	2	3	2	8	5	-	6
13	10	4	4	2	1	7	3	9	5	14	8	35	18	62	44	125	81
1	2	4	5	1	0	0	2	1	2	1	2	1	3	2	1	-	2
0	0	1	1	1	-	1	0	0	0	0	0	-	0	-	-	-	-
1	0	3	-	1	-	-	0	0	-	0	-	1	-	1	1	-	-
0	0	-	-	-	-	0	-	0	-	0	0	1	-	-	-	-	-
-	0	-	-	-	0	-	1	-	0	-	-	-	0	-	-	-	-
1	1	-	-	-	-	1	-	0	0	1	0	5	3	7	3	12	4
2	1	-	-	-	-	-	-	0	0	2	1	6	2	13	5	48	30
1	1	1	-	-	-	-	-	-	0	1	0	2	2	7	4	36	2
5	22	-	1	2	8	3	50	6	31	6	18	8	8	6	12	-	12
1	1	2	1	0	-	-	0	1	1	1	0	2	1	-	-	6	2
6	3	-	-	1	0	3	3	7	4	11	5	9	3	6	2	-	4
1	1	2	1	-	1	1	0	0	1	1	1	1	1	2	-	-	-
1	0	-	-	0	-	0	-	0	0	1	0	5	2	1	-	-	-
14	222	5	41	6	59	5	290	9	262	21	246	34	274	45	272	71	227
3	4	-	-	-	1	1	1	2	3	3	8	10	7	8	8	12	6
2	2	2	-	1	1	1	3	2	2	4	2	1	1	7	-	-	2
1	0	-	-	1	-	-	-	1	-	2	-	3	-	8	1	18	2
129	473	123	316	65	234	50	554	68	498	131	426	340	571	602	705	826	993
19	-	-	-	-	-	-	-	1	-	29	-	96	-	121	-	71	-
8	-	-	-	-	-	2	-	7	-	12	-	17	-	31	-	6	-
0	-	-	-	-	-	-	-	-	-	0	-	-	-	5	-	-	-
9	-	45	-	6	-	3	-	3	-	8	-	15	-	18	-	53	-
30	-	2	-	5	-	26	-	49	-	32	-	36	-	21	-	12	-
24	-	134	-	54	-	15	-	7	-	7	-	7	-	11	-	30	-
4	-	-	-	-	-	1	-	12	-	1	-	1	-	-	-	-	-
65	-	333	-	121	-	30	-	31	-	25	-	32	-	37	-	30	-
25	-	7	-	17	-	25	-	32	-	28	-	30	-	16	-	-	-
1	29	-	1	2	3	1	27	0	56	1	37	-	3	-	3	-	-
12	140	8	18	38	35	16	116	3	255	6	168	7	70	10	40	12	12
-	58	-	-	-	1	-	151	-	123	-	12	-	0	-	1	-	-
-	7	-	-	-	-	-	15	-	16	-	2	-	-	-	-	-	-
0	134	-	99	-	64	-	202	0	206	-	102	-	65	-	62	-	67
-	7	-	-	-	-	-	8	-	16	-	5	-	0	-	-	-	-
-	30	-	-	-	0	-	1	-	16	-	55	-	82	-	85	-	45
-	1	-	-	-	-	-	-	-	0	-	1	-	1	-	1	-	4
-	7	-	-	-	0	-	10	-	13	-	8	-	1	-	1	-	-
-	4	-	1	-	-	-	3	-	7	-	6	-	1	-	-	-	-
-	19	-	-	-	0	-	21	-	33	-	29	-	7	-	4	-	-
-	57	-	18	-	18	-	96	-	99	-	36	-	22	-	14	-	41
-	4	-	3	-	1	-	2	-	7	-	4	-	3	-	5	-	8

Table 22 - *continued*

Disease Group	Persons, by age group								
	Total	0-4	5-15	16-24	25-44	45-64	65-74	75-84	85 and over
Pain and other symptoms associated with female genital organs (625)	108	-	53	190	208	49	12	10	10
Disorders of menstruation and other abnormal bleeding from female genital tract (626)	207	1	52	434	385	121	1	2	-
Menopausal and postmenopausal disorders (627)	98	0	-	1	57	336	74	47	65
Infertility, female (628)	9	-	-	11	24	0	-	-	-
Other disorders of female genital organs (629)	0	-	0	0	-	0	-	-	-
Hydatidiform mole (630)	0	-	-	0	0	-	-	-	-
Other abnormal product of conception (631)	1	0	0	0	2	0	-	-	-
Missed abortion (632)	2	-	0	5	5	-	-	-	-
Ectopic pregnancy (633)	3	-	0	6	7	-	-	-	-
Spontaneous abortion (634)	13	-	0	32	29	1	-	-	-
Legally induced abortion (635)	4	-	1	16	7	0	-	-	-
Unspecified abortion (637)	0	-	-	1	0	-	-	-	-
Failed attempted abortion (638)	0	-	-	0	-	-	-	-	-
Complications following abortion and ectopic and molar pregnancies (639)	0	-	-	1	0	-	-	-	-
Haemorrhage in early pregnancy (640)	20	-	1	52	44	0	-	-	-
Antepartum haemorrhage, abruptio placentae, and placenta praevia (641)	2	-	-	4	5	-	-	-	-
Hypertension complicating pregnancy, childbirth and the puerperium (642)	2	-	-	5	5	0	-	-	-
Excessive vomiting in pregnancy (643)	7	-	0	22	14	0	-	-	-
Early or threatened labour (644)	2	-	-	6	3	-	-	-	-
Prolonged pregnancy (645)	0	-	-	1	0	-	-	-	-
Other complications of pregnancy, not elsewhere classified (646)	11	-	1	31	21	0	-	-	1
Infective and parasitic conditions in the mother classifiable elsewhere but complicating pregnancy, childbirth and the puerperium (647)	0	-	-	0	0	-	-	-	-
Other current conditions in the mother classifiable elsewhere but complicating pregnancy, childbirth and the puerperium (648)	4	-	0	10	10	-	-	-	-
Delivery in a completely normal case (650)	25	-	1	55	57	-	-	-	-
Multiple gestation (651)	1	-	-	2	2	-	-	-	-
Malposition and malpresentation of fetus (652)	1	-	-	2	3	-	-	-	-
Disproportion (653)	0	-	-	0	0	-	-	-	-
Abnormality of organs and soft tissues of pelvis (654)	0	-	-	-	-	0	-	-	-
Known or suspected fetal abnormality affecting management of mother (655)	0	-	-	1	0	-	-	-	-
Other fetal and placental problems affecting management of mother (656)	1	1	-	4	3	-	-	-	-
Polyhydramnios (657)	0	-	-	0	1	-	-	-	-
Other problems associated with amniotic cavity and membranes (658)	0	-	-	1	0	-	-	-	-
Other indications for care or intervention related to labour and delivery and not elsewhere classified (659)	0	-	-	0	-	-	-	-	-
Obstructed labour (660)	0	-	-	0					
Abnormality of forces of labour (661)	0	-	-	1	0	-	-	-	-
Long labour (662)	0	-	-	0	0	-	-	-	-
Umbilical cord complications (663)	0	4	-	0	0	-	-	-	-
Trauma to perineum and vulva during delivery (664)	1	0	-	2	2	-	-	-	-
Other obstetrical trauma (665)	0	-	-	1	0	0	-	-	-
Postpartum haemorrhage (666)	2	-	-	4	6	-	-	-	-

By age-group and sex

Total		0-4		5-15		16-24		25-44		45-64		65-74		75-84		85 and over	
Male	Female	Male	Female	Male	Female	Male	Female	Male	Female	Male	Female	Male	Female	Male	Female	Male	Female
-	211	-	-	-	109	-	379	-	418	-	98	-	21	-	16	-	14
-	405	-	2	-	106	-	865	-	773	-	244	-	2	-	3	-	-
-	192	-	1	-	-	-	1	-	115	-	678	-	134	-	75	-	87
-	18	-	-	-	-	-	22	-	49	-	0	-	-	-	-	-	-
-	0	-	-	-	0	-	0	-	-	-	0	-	-	-	-	-	-
-	0	-	-	-	-	-	1	-	1	-	-	-	-	-	-	-	-
-	1	-	1	-	0	-	0	-	3	-	0	-	-	-	-	-	-
-	4	-	-	-	0	-	10	-	10	-	-	-	-	-	-	-	-
-	6	-	-	-	0	-	12	-	13	-	-	-	-	-	-	-	-
-	26	-	-	-	0	-	64	-	58	-	1	-	-	-	-	-	-
-	9	-	-	-	2	-	33	-	14	-	0	-	-	-	-	-	-
-	0	-	-	-	-	-	2	-	1	-	-	-	-	-	-	-	-
-	0	-	-	-	-	-	1	-	-	-	-	-	-	-	-	-	-
-	1	-	-	-	-	-	2	-	1	-	-	-	-	-	-	-	-
-	40	-	-	-	2	-	104	-	89	-	0	-	-	-	-	-	-
-	4	-	-	-	-	-	7	-	9	-	-	-	-	-	-	-	-
-	4	-	-	-	-	-	10	-	10	-	0	-	-	-	-	-	-
-	14	-	-	-	0	-	44	-	29	-	0	-	-	-	-	-	-
-	3	-	-	-	-	-	12	-	5	-	-	-	-	-	-	-	-
-	0	-	-	-	-	-	1	-	0	-	-	-	-	-	-	-	-
-	21	-	-	-	1	-	62	-	43	-	0	-	-	-	-	-	2
-	0	-	-	-	-	-	0	-	0	-	-	-	-	-	-	-	-
-	8	-	-	-	0	-	19	-	20	-	-	-	-	-	-	-	-
-	48	-	3	-	1	-	109	-	115	-	-	-	-	-	-	-	-
-	1	-	-	-	-	-	3	-	4	-	-	-	-	-	-	-	-
-	2	-	-	-	-	-	4	-	6	-	-	-	-	-	-	-	-
-	0	-	-	-	-	-	1	-	0	-	-	-	-	-	-	-	-
-	0	-	-	-	-	-	-	-	-	-	0	-	-	-	-	-	-
-	0	-	-	-	-	-	2	-	1	-	-	-	-	-	-	-	-
-	3	-	1	-	-	-	8	-	6	-	-	-	-	-	-	-	-
-	0	-	-	-	-	-	1	-	1	-	-	-	-	-	-	-	-
-	0	-	-	-	-	-	2	-	1	-	-	-	-	-	-	-	-
-	0	-	-	-	-	-	1	-	-	-	-	-	-	-	-	-	-
-	0	-	-	-	-	-	0	-	0	-	-	-	-	-	-	-	-
-	0	-	-	-	-	-	2	-	1	-	-	-	-	-	-	-	-
-	0	-	-	-	-	-	0	-	1	-	-	-	-	-	-	-	-
0	1	1	7	-	-	-	1	-	0	-	-	-	-	-	-	-	-
-	2	-	1	-	-	-	4	-	5	-	-	-	-	-	-	-	-
-	0	-	-	-	-	-	1	-	1	-	0	-	-	-	-	-	-
-	5	-	-	-	-	-	8	-	12	-	-	-	-	-	-	-	-

Table 22 - *continued*

Disease Group	Persons, by age group								
	Total	0-4	5-15	16-24	25-44	45-64	65-74	75-84	85 and over
Retained placenta or membranes, without haemorrhage (667)	1	-	-	2	3	0	-	-	-
Other complications of labour and delivery, not elsewhere classified (669)	7	1	0	13	17	0	-	-	-
Major puerperal infection (670)	1	-	-	2	2	-	-	-	-
Venous complications in pregnancy and the puerperium (671)	4	-	-	6	8	0	1	0	-
Pyrexia of unknown origin during the puerperium (672)	0	-	0	-	0	-	-	-	-
Other and unspecified complications of the puerperium, not elsewhere classified (674)	1	-	-	2	3	-	-	-	-
Infections of the breast and nipple associated with childbirth (675)	9	-	-	11	25	0	-	-	-
Other disorders of the breast associated with childbirth, and disorders of lactation (676)	4	0	0	7	9	2	1	0	-
Carbuncle and furuncle (680)	62	32	45	84	84	56	41	31	22
Cellulitis and abscess of finger and toe (681)	61	114	93	47	45	53	60	63	80
Other cellulitis and abscess (682)	103	54	55	75	95	114	159	223	355
Acute lymphadenitis (683)	18	39	34	26	18	7	3	3	6
Impetigo (684)	67	292	171	65	28	17	21	21	21
Pilonidal cyst (685)	5	2	1	16	7	2	2	1	-
Other local infections of skin and subcutaneous tissue (686)	42	67	46	37	39	35	38	53	75
Erythematosquamous dermatosis (690)	67	147	56	63	61	54	76	75	62
Atopic dermatitis and related conditions (691)	266	1,624	240	201	149	135	154	127	135
Contact dermatitis and other eczema (692)	176	333	155	225	166	141	155	146	118
Dermatitis due to substances taken internally (693)	1	2	1	1	1	2	2	3	1
Bullous dermatoses (694)	2	1	1	1	1	1	4	4	7
Erythematous conditions (695)	57	50	18	31	54	76	98	96	123
Psoriasis and similar disorders (696)	48	18	49	65	55	46	47	30	18
Lichen (697)	3	1	1	3	3	6	4	6	1
Pruritus and related conditions (698)	67	42	34	44	61	83	110	121	146
Corns and callosities (700)	15	2	7	11	11	16	34	42	38
Other hypertrophic and atrophic conditions of skin (701)	8	4	10	9	7	7	9	15	9
Other dermatoses (702)	35	2	6	7	16	57	107	119	83
Diseases of nail (703)	58	33	102	109	39	41	45	51	43
Diseases of hair and hair follicles (704)	37	30	26	54	52	28	20	13	6
Disorders of sweat glands (705)	21	24	18	29	27	16	10	3	7
Diseases of sebaceous glands (706)	162	33	184	411	173	93	70	59	43
Chronic ulcer of skin (707)	15	1	1	2	2	12	43	93	228
Urticaria (708)	67	130	93	67	61	50	54	40	37
Other disorders of skin and subcutaneous tissue (709)	17	24	16	15	19	17	16	14	7
Diffuse diseases of connective tissue (710)	1	-	0	1	1	2	2	2	-
Arthropathy associated with infections (711)	1	1	0	1	1	1	2	0	7
Crystal arthropathies (712)	0	-	-	-	-	0	-	-	-
Rheumatoid arthritis and other inflammatory polyarthropathies (714)	13	0	1	3	11	24	29	23	25
Osteoarthrosis and allied disorders (715)	173	0	1	6	49	325	560	676	645
Other and unspecified arthropathies (716)	17	1	2	9	18	30	25	21	16
Internal derangement of knee (717)	25	-	35	46	29	21	10	6	1
Other derangement of joint (718)	2	1	1	3	3	1	3	1	1
Other and unspecified disorder of joint (719)	201	40	111	151	201	281	276	312	286

By age-group and sex

Total		0-4		5-15		16-24		25-44		45-64		65-74		75-84		85 and over	
Male	Female	Male	Female	Male	Female	Male	Female	Male	Female	Male	Female	Male	Female	Male	Female	Male	Female
-	2	-	-	-	-	-	4	-	5	-	0	-	-	-	-	-	-
-	13	-	1	-	0	-	26	-	34	-	0	-	-	-	-	-	-
-	1	-	-	-	-	-	4	-	3	-	-	-	-	-	-	-	-
-	7	-	-	-	-	-	12	-	17	-	0	-	1	-	1	-	-
-	0	-	-	-	0	-	-	-	1	-	-	-	-	-	-	-	-
-	2	-	-	-	-	-	4	-	6	-	-	-	-	-	-	-	-
-	18	-	-	-	-	-	21	-	49	-	0	-	-	-	-	-	-
-	8	-	1	-	0	-	13	-	19	-	4	-	2	-	1	-	-
58	66	33	31	46	44	73	94	76	91	49	63	43	39	26	34	18	24
59	62	123	104	95	91	52	41	42	48	43	63	57	63	62	64	101	73
91	115	58	50	57	52	70	81	87	103	107	120	140	174	169	255	208	404
15	21	48	29	32	35	18	34	12	25	4	11	2	4	2	3	6	6
69	65	303	281	180	161	55	74	25	31	16	17	23	19	24	18	42	14
6	4	1	3	1	0	19	13	9	4	2	1	3	-	-	1	-	-
36	47	81	52	41	50	30	43	30	47	30	40	30	45	48	56	71	77
63	71	156	138	45	67	52	74	55	68	53	55	81	71	93	65	36	71
231	299	1,502	1,752	211	271	122	280	105	193	113	157	167	144	139	120	166	124
136	214	326	340	130	182	140	310	106	227	112	171	148	161	159	138	119	118
1	2	3	1	1	1	1	0	-	1	1	3	1	2	-	5	-	2
1	2	1	1	2	1	1	1	1	2	0	2	3	4	2	5	6	8
42	72	44	57	16	21	21	41	41	67	57	96	69	121	68	114	59	144
44	53	22	13	42	56	48	82	48	61	47	46	48	46	24	33	18	18
3	4	2	1	1	2	2	4	2	4	6	5	5	3	5	6	-	2
46	87	26	59	22	46	24	63	39	84	64	103	84	131	102	132	155	144
11	19	3	1	2	11	7	14	9	14	11	22	30	37	41	43	36	39
6	10	5	3	8	11	6	12	4	10	6	9	10	9	19	13	6	10
32	38	4	1	7	4	6	7	11	22	53	62	113	101	137	108	101	77
67	49	40	26	110	94	145	72	47	32	37	46	47	44	63	44	65	35
30	43	28	31	22	30	42	65	43	60	22	34	13	26	8	16	6	6
15	26	16	32	16	21	15	44	18	36	14	19	8	11	2	3	6	8
145	179	36	29	164	204	397	424	126	220	87	100	73	67	74	50	59	37
12	18	1	1	2	0	1	2	2	2	12	11	41	45	82	100	220	231
47	85	120	140	82	105	38	97	35	86	29	71	43	63	26	49	24	41
15	20	28	20	16	16	12	18	14	24	13	21	15	18	7	18	12	6
1	2	-	-	-	0	1	1	0	1	1	3	2	3	1	3	-	-
1	1	2	1	1	-	1	1	1	1	0	1	1	3	1	-	6	8
-	0	-	-	-	-	-	-	-	-	-	0	-	-	-	-	-	-
8	18	1	-	0	1	2	4	7	15	15	33	20	37	14	29	6	32
130	215	1	-	1	0	7	6	40	58	267	384	452	648	538	759	517	688
13	21	1	1	2	3	5	12	14	23	24	36	23	28	15	25	12	18
28	22	-	-	25	45	46	45	38	21	25	17	13	7	7	5	6	-
3	2	2	-	1	1	3	3	4	2	2	1	3	3	-	1	-	2
167	233	45	34	107	115	142	160	171	231	220	344	235	309	239	355	256	296

Table 22 - *continued*

Disease Group	Persons, by age group								
	Total	0-4	5-15	16-24	25-44	45-64	65-74	75-84	85 and over
Ankylosing spondylitis and other inflammatory spondylopathies (720)	7	-	0	4	10	12	6	10	3
Spondylosis and allied disorders (721)	81	-	0	8	56	178	187	168	123
Intervertebral disc disorders (722)	26	-	1	10	34	46	31	21	12
Other disorders of cervical region (723)	81	18	47	59	114	102	72	57	61
Other and unspecified disorders of back (724)	316	6	53	233	392	463	410	425	374
Polymyalgia rheumatica (725)	4	-	-	-	0	5	16	32	15
Peripheral enthesopathies and allied syndromes (726)	180	1	40	67	187	362	243	206	130
Other disorders of synovium, tendon and bursa (727)	73	9	29	65	83	106	96	75	64
Disorders of muscle, ligament and fascia (728)	35	4	15	21	29	57	66	51	44
Other disorders of soft tissues (729)	164	34	67	92	145	232	320	338	302
Osteomyelitis, periostitis and other infections involving bone (730)	1	1	1	1	1	1	2	3	1
Osteitis deformans and osteopathies associated with other disorders classified elsewhere (731)	1	-	-	-	-	1	2	6	6
Osteochondropathies (732)	7	1	41	4	1	1	0	-	-
Other disorders of bone and cartilage (733)	21	1	7	19	19	27	34	52	52
Flat foot (734)	3	10	7	2	1	3	3	3	1
Acquired deformities of toe (735)	8	10	8	4	5	12	13	14	6
Other acquired deformities of limbs (736)	3	5	3	2	2	3	4	2	4
Curvature of spine (737)	2	0	3	2	2	2	3	3	3
Other acquired deformity (738)	1	1	1	1	1	1	2	2	1
Spina bifida (741)	0	1	-	-	-	0	-	-	1
Other congenital anamolies of nervous system (742)	0	1	-	0	-	-	-	-	-
Congenital anomalies of eye (743)	2	14	1	1	1	1	1	6	4
Congenital anomalies of ear, face and neck (744)	2	6	4	2	1	1	-	1	-
Bulbus cordis anomalies and anomalies of cardiac septal closure (745)	1	9	1	0	-	0	-	-	-
Other congenital anomalies of heart (746)	0	2	0	1	0	0	-	1	-
Other congenital anomalies of ciculatory system (747)	0	1	0	1	0	0	0	0	-
Congenital anomalies of respiratory system (748)	0	1	-	0	-	-	0	-	-
Cleft palate and cleft lip (749)	0	2	-	-	0	-	0	-	-
Other congenital anomalies of upper alimentary tract (750)	3	17	1	0	1	2	5	4	6
Other congenital anomalies of digestive system (751)	1	2	0	-	0	1	1	2	4
Congenital anomalies of genital organs (752)	5	38	14	2	1	0	0	0	-
Congenital anomalies of urinary system (753)	1	4	-	1	0	1	-	-	-
Certain congenital musculoskeletal deformities (754)	4	30	6	2	1	1	1	-	-
Other congenital anomalies of limbs (755)	2	7	2	1	1	1	1	1	3
Other congenital musculoskeletal anomalies (756)	2	6	1	1	2	3	2	-	-
Congenital anomalies of the integument (757)	13	26	7	8	14	16	11	7	3
Chromosomal anomalies (758)	0	2	-	0	0	-	-	-	-
Other and unspecified congenital anomalies (759)	1	3	2	1	1	1	0	-	-
Fetus or newborn affected by maternal complications of pregnancy (761)	0	-	-	0	0	-	-	-	-
Fetus or newborn affected by complications of placenta, cord and membranes (762)	0	5	-	-	0	-	-	-	-

By age-group and sex

Total		0-4		5-15		16-24		25-44		45-64		65-74		75-84		85 and over	
Male	Female	Male	Female	Male	Female	Male	Female	Male	Female	Male	Female	Male	Female	Male	Female	Male	Female
5	10	-	-	0	0	3	5	6	15	8	17	6	6	10	10	6	2
64	98	-	-	-	0	7	9	38	74	149	208	166	205	156	176	83	136
25	26	-	-	1	2	10	11	35	34	44	49	29	34	26	18	6	14
64	98	16	19	48	45	44	74	80	148	81	124	67	76	53	60	77	55
272	358	10	2	39	68	181	286	345	438	409	517	354	456	377	454	428	357
2	6	-	-	-	-	-	-	0	1	2	8	9	22	32	32	18	14
178	182	2	1	36	44	65	70	189	185	351	372	256	233	213	201	172	116
57	89	12	6	24	35	41	89	65	100	82	130	83	106	70	78	36	73
37	32	6	3	18	12	23	20	28	29	61	54	79	56	64	42	59	39
132	196	39	28	68	65	74	110	109	181	179	287	287	348	330	343	297	303
1	1	1	1	1	1	1	0	1	0	2	1	3	1	-	4	-	2
1	1	-	-	-	-	-	-	-	-	2	1	2	2	6	6	12	4
9	5	1	1	52	29	3	4	1	1	1	1	1	-	-	-	-	-
12	30	1	1	7	7	15	22	13	25	14	41	15	49	13	75	18	63
3	3	11	8	7	8	2	3	1	1	2	3	2	3	6	1	-	2
5	12	11	10	6	10	2	6	1	8	6	18	7	18	10	16	-	8
3	3	5	5	2	3	2	2	2	1	3	4	5	3	5	1	6	4
2	2	1	-	4	2	2	2	2	2	2	2	1	4	1	4	-	4
1	1	1	1	1	1	2	-	1	0	1	1	1	2	2	1	6	-
0	0	1	1	-	-	-	-	-	-	-	0	-	-	-	-	-	2
0	0	2	1	-	-	-	0	-	-	-	-	-	-	-	-	-	-
2	2	15	13	-	1	-	1	1	1	0	2	2	1	6	5	-	6
2	2	6	6	3	5	1	3	1	1	1	0	-	-	1	1	-	-
1	1	8	10	1	1	0	-	-	-	0	-	-	-	-	-	-	-
0	0	2	1	0	0	1	1	0	0	0	0	-	-	2	-	-	-
0	0	1	1	-	0	1	0	0	0	-	0	1	-	-	1	-	-
0	0	1	1	-	-	0	-	-	-	-	-	-	0	-	-	-	-
0	0	1	2	-	-	-	-	0	-	-	-	-	0	-	-	-	-
3	3	24	10	2	0	0	0	1	1	2	3	5	6	1	6	6	6
0	1	2	2	0	1	-	-	0	0	-	1	1	0	2	1	6	4
10	1	74	1	27	1	2	2	1	0	0	0	-	0	-	1	-	-
1	1	5	2	-	-	0	1	0	1	1	1	-	-	-	-	-	-
4	4	31	29	6	6	1	2	1	2	1	1	2	-	-	-	-	-
1	2	7	8	2	2	1	2	0	1	1	2	1	1	1	1	-	4
2	2	9	3	1	2	1	1	2	2	3	2	-	4	-	-	-	-
11	15	23	30	5	9	5	10	11	17	14	18	13	10	7	8	6	2
0	0	1	3	-	-	1	-	0	0	-	-	-	-	-	-	-	-
1	1	4	3	1	2	0	1	1	1	1	1	-	0	-	-	-	-
-	0	-	-	-	-	-	0	-	0	-	-	-	-	-	-	-	-
1	0	9	-	-	-	-	-	-	0	-	-	-	-	-	-	-	-

Table 22 - *continued*

Disease Group	Persons, by age group								
	Total	0-4	5-15	16-24	25-44	45-64	65-74	75-84	85 and over
Fetus or newborn affected by other complications of labour and delivery (763)	0	-	-	-	0	-	-	-	-
Slow fetal growth and fetal malnutrition (764)	0	0	-	0	-	-	-	-	-
Disorders relating to short gestation and unspecified low birthweight (765)	0	7	-	-	-	-	-	-	-
Disorders relating to long gestation and high birthweight (766)	0	-	-	-	0	-	-	-	-
Birth trauma (767)	0	1	-	0	-	-	-	-	-
Intrauterine hypoxia and birth asphyxia (768)	0	1	-	-	0	-	-	-	-
Respiratory distress syndrome (769)	0	2	-	-	-	-	-	-	-
Other respiratory conditions of fetus and newborn (770)	0	6	-	-	0	-	-	0	-
Infections specific to the perinatal period (771)	9	123	0	1	0	0	-	0	-
Fetal and neonatal haemorrhage (772)	0	-	-	0	0	-	-	1	-
Haemolytic disease of fetus or newborn, due to isoimmunization (773)	0	0	-	-	-	-	-	0	-
Other perinatal jaundice (774)	1	9	-	-	-	-	-	-	-
Endocrine and metabolic disturbances specific to the fetus and newborn (775)	0	1	-	-	-	-	-	-	-
Conditions involving the integument and temperature regulation of fetus and newborn (778)	0	1	-	-	0	-	-	-	-
Other and ill-defined conditions originating in the perinatal period (779)	1	14	-	1	0	-	-	-	-
Fracture of vault of skull (800)	0	1	0	-	0	0	-	-	-
Fracture of base of skull (801)	0	-	-	0	0	0	-	-	-
Fracture of face bones (802)	5	1	6	13	6	3	2	3	4
Other and unqualified skull fractures (803)	1	1	1	1	1	0	-	0	4
Multiple fractures involving skull or face with other bones (804)	0	0	0	-	0	-	-	-	-
Fracture of vertebral column without mention of spinal cord lesion (805)	3	-	0	2	3	3	3	10	22
Fracture of vertebral column with spinal cord lesion (806)	0	-	-	-	0	-	-	0	1
Fracture of rib(s), sternum, larynx and trachea (807)	10	1	1	5	10	15	19	24	36
Fracture of pelvis (808)	1	0	0	1	1	0	2	6	12
Ill-defined fractures of trunk (809)	0	-	-	-	-	0	-	-	-
Fracture of clavicle (810)	4	7	7	5	3	2	3	2	7
Fracture of scapula (811)	0	-	-	1	0	0	1	0	-
Fracture of humerus (812)	4	3	5	2	1	3	11	12	25
Fracture of radius and ulna (813)	16	13	29	13	8	12	21	35	43
Fracture of carpal bone(s) (814)	4	-	3	7	5	3	3	3	1
Fracture of metacarpal bone(s) (815)	6	0	9	15	6	3	2	6	1
Fracture of one or more phalanges of hand (816)	6	1	13	8	6	4	4	2	-
Ill-defined fractures of upper limb (818)	0	-	-	0	0	0	1	1	3
Multiple fractures involving both upper limbs, and upper limb with rib(s) and sternum (819)	0	-	-	-	0	1	1	1	-
Fracture of neck of femur (820)	5	-	-	-	0	2	13	36	136
Fracture of other and unspecified parts of femur (821)	2	1	1	1	1	1	3	9	37
Fracture of patella (822)	1	0	2	2	1	1	1	3	3
Fracture of tibia and fibula (823)	5	5	5	8	5	4	4	2	9
Fracture of ankle (824)	5	0	2	9	5	6	8	7	3
Fracture of one or more tarsal and metatarsal bones (825)	5	2	7	5	6	6	5	3	1
Fracture of one or more phalanges of foot (826)	5	1	5	7	5	5	3	2	3

By age-group and sex

Total		0-4		5-15		16-24		25-44		45-64		65-74		75-84		85 and over	
Male	Female	Male	Female	Male	Female	Male	Female	Male	Female	Male	Female	Male	Female	Male	Female	Male	Female
-	0	-	-	-	-	-	-	-	0	-	-	-	-	-	-	-	-
0	0	1	-	-	-	-	1	-	-	-	-	-	-	-	-	-	-
0	1	5	10	-	-	-	-	-	-	-	-	-	-	-	-	-	-
-	0	-	-	-	-	-	-	-	0	-	-	-	-	-	-	-	-
-	0	-	1	-	-	-	0	-	-	-	-	-	-	-	-	-	-
0	0	1	-	-	-	-	-	-	0	-	-	-	-	-	-	-	-
0	0	2	1	-	-	-	-	-	-	-	-	-	-	-	-	-	-
1	0	7	4	-	-	-	-	0	-	-	-	-	-	-	1	-	-
8	10	106	140	0	0	-	1	0	1	-	1	-	-	-	-	1	-
0	0	-	-	-	-	-	0	-	0	-	-	-	-	-	1	1	-
-	0	-	1	-	-	-	-	-	-	-	-	-	-	-	1	-	-
1	0	12	5	-	-	-	-	-	-	-	-	-	-	-	-	-	-
0	-	1	-	-	-	-	-	-	-	-	-	-	-	-	-	-	-
0	0	1	1	-	-	-	-	0	-	-	-	-	-	-	-	-	-
1	1	15	13	-	-	-	1	-	1	-	-	-	-	-	-	-	-
0	0	1	2	0	0	-	-	1	0	0	-	-	-	-	-	-	-
0	-	-	-	-	-	0	-	0	-	0	-	-	-	-	-	-	-
7	4	1	1	7	5	21	5	8	3	2	3	-	4	1	5	6	4
1	0	1	-	1	0	1	0	1	0	0	-	-	-	-	1	-	6
0	0	-	1	-	0	-	-	0	-	-	-	-	-	-	-	-	-
2	4	-	-	0	-	2	1	2	3	2	4	1	5	3	14	6	28
0	0	-	-	-	-	-	-	0	-	-	-	-	-	-	-	1	2
12	9	1	1	2	1	7	4	14	5	16	13	20	18	23	25	24	39
1	2	1	-	0	0	1	1	1	0	0	0	1	3	1	10	6	14
-	0	-	-	-	-	-	-	-	-	0	-	-	-	-	-	-	-
5	3	6	8	10	4	7	2	4	1	1	2	2	3	2	1	12	6
0	0	-	-	-	-	0	1	0	0	0	-	-	1	-	1	-	-
2	6	2	4	5	5	2	1	1	1	1	5	3	18	5	16	12	30
14	18	13	13	33	25	18	8	10	7	7	18	6	33	8	51	18	51
5	3	-	-	4	3	9	5	6	3	2	4	3	2	2	4	6	-
10	3	-	1	14	3	27	2	10	2	4	2	1	3	5	6	-	2
8	4	1	1	14	12	12	5	10	3	5	3	2	6	2	2	-	-
0	0	-	-	-	-	1	-	1	0	0	0	0	-	1	-	6	2
0	0	-	-	-	-	-	-	1	0	1	0	1	0	-	1	-	-
2	9	-	-	-	-	-	-	0	0	1	3	4	19	15	49	77	156
1	3	1	1	1	0	3	-	1	0	1	1	1	4	5	12	12	45
1	1	-	1	3	0	2	1	1	1	1	1	1	2	-	5	-	4
6	4	6	4	6	3	12	3	8	2	3	5	3	5	3	-	3	12
6	5	-	1	4	1	14	4	7	3	6	6	2	13	1	10	6	2
6	5	4	1	10	4	6	3	6	6	5	8	3	8	2	4	-	2
5	5	1	1	6	4	9	6	6	4	4	7	2	3	-	3	-	4

Table 22 - *continued*

Disease Group	Persons, by age group								
	Total	0-4	5-15	16-24	25-44	45-64	65-74	75-84	85 and over
Other, multiple and ill-defined fractures of lower limb (827)	0	-	-	0	0	0	0	0	-
Multiple fractures involving both lower limbs, lower with upper limb, and lower limb(s) with rib(s) and sternum (828)	0	-	-	-	-	0	-	-	-
Fracture of unspecified bones (829)	2	1	1	2	2	1	2	3	4
Dislocation of jaw (830)	0	-	-	1	0	0	0	0	-
Dislocation of shoulder (831)	3	1	1	7	3	2	3	6	10
Dislocation of elbow (832)	1	8	1	1	0	0	0	-	1
Dislocation of wrist (833)	0	-	1	1	0	0	-	0	1
Dislocation of finger (834)	2	1	2	2	1	3	1	2	1
Dislocation of hip (835)	0	1	0	1	0	0	2	1	1
Dislocation of knee (836)	2	-	3	4	3	1	2	1	-
Dislocation of ankle (837)	1	-	1	0	1	0	1	0	1
Dislocation of foot (838)	0	-	1	0	0	0	1	0	-
Other, multiple and ill-defined dislocations (839)	2	0	1	1	2	2	1	3	-
Sprains and strains of shoulder and upper arm (840)	46	8	15	44	56	62	52	46	41
Sprains and strains of elbow and forearm (841)	13	16	15	11	13	15	6	5	3
Sprains and strains of wrist and hand (842)	40	12	73	56	38	31	26	28	33
Sprains and strains of hip and thigh (843)	32	8	31	32	32	39	31	41	37
Sprains and strains of knee and leg (844)	74	12	76	108	84	77	55	42	33
Sprains and strains of ankle and foot (845)	85	28	121	117	82	74	80	60	47
Sprains and strains of sacroiliac region (846)	40	-	5	30	59	61	38	29	27
Sprains and strains of other and unspecified parts of back (847)	156	5	53	210	229	177	94	96	84
Other and ill-defined sprains and strains (848)	60	4	34	64	74	72	60	66	73
Concussion (850)	12	38	26	15	6	4	3	9	12
Cerebral laceration and contusion (851)	0	2	1	0	0	0	-	1	-
Subarachnoid, subdural and extradural haemorrhage, following injury (852)	0	0	-	0	0	0	-	1	-
Intracranial injury of other and unspecified nature (854)	10	41	21	9	4	3	4	4	7
Traumatic pneumothorax and haemothorax (860)	0	-	0	0	0	0	-	0	-
Injury to heart and lung (861)	0	0	-	-	-	-	-	0	-
Injury to other and unspecified intrathoracic organs (862)	0	-	-	0	0	0	0	-	-
Injury to gastrointestinal tract (863)	0	0	1	0	0	0	1	-	-
Injury to spleen (865)	0	-	-	0	0	-	-	-	-
Injury to kidney (866)	0	-	0	0	0	-	-	-	-
Injury to pelvic organs (867)	0	-	-	0	0	0	0	-	-
Internal injury to unspecified or ill-defined organs (869)	0	-	-	0	0	1	0	1	-
Open wound of ocular adnexa (870)	2	4	3	2	2	2	1	1	-
Open wound of eyeball (871)	3	2	3	2	4	3	2	0	-
Open wound of ear (872)	2	4	6	3	1	1	1	0	1
Other open wound of head (873)	38	160	66	31	17	16	21	42	121
Open wound of neck (874)	0	1	0	1	0	0	-	-	-
Open wound of chest (wall) (875)	0	-	0	1	-	-	-	-	1
Open wound of back (876)	0	0	1	0	0	0	-	-	-
Open wound of buttock (877)	0	-	1	0	0	0	0	-	3
Open wound of genital organs (external), including traumatic amputation (878)	2	4	5	3	1	1	1	2	1
Open wound of other and unspecified sites, except limbs (879)	2	4	4	3	2	2	1	6	6

By age-group and sex

Total		0-4		5-15		16-24		25-44		45-64		65-74		75-84		85 and over	
Male	Female	Male	Female	Male	Female	Male	Female	Male	Female	Male	Female	Male	Female	Male	Female	Male	Female
0	0	-	-	-	-	1	-	0	0	0	-	-	0	1	-	-	-
-	0	-	-	-	-	-	-	-	-	-	0	-	-	-	-	-	-
2	2	-	3	2	1	2	1	2	1	1	1	1	3	2	3	-	6
0	0	-	-	-	-	-	1	0	1	0	0	1	-	-	1	-	-
4	3	-	1	1	2	10	3	4	2	2	2	2	5	2	9	12	10
1	1	4	12	1	-	1	1	0	0	0	-	-	0	-	-	-	2
0	1	-	-	0	1	-	1	0	0	-	1	-	-	-	1	-	2
2	2	1	1	3	2	2	2	2	1	3	2	1	1	3	1	-	2
1	0	1	1	0	-	0	1	-	0	1	-	3	-	1	1	-	2
3	2	-	-	2	3	4	3	4	3	2	1	1	2	1	1	-	-
0	1	-	-	1	2	0	-	1	1	-	1	1	1	-	1	6	-
0	0	-	-	0	1	0	-	0	0	-	0	1	1	-	1	-	-
2	2	1	-	2	1	2	1	3	2	3	2	1	1	1	3	-	-
46	46	6	10	14	16	47	41	57	55	63	60	45	57	53	42	24	47
14	11	12	19	13	16	14	9	16	11	16	14	8	5	3	5	-	4
37	44	12	11	72	74	60	52	35	40	21	43	17	33	19	34	36	32
37	27	10	6	40	21	42	22	38	27	40	37	34	28	49	36	36	37
85	64	12	11	78	73	132	83	103	66	81	74	62	49	30	50	-	43
79	90	37	19	114	129	133	100	82	82	55	93	47	107	39	73	24	55
35	46	-	-	4	5	25	34	51	67	53	70	34	41	26	30	12	32
157	155	6	4	53	53	210	210	232	226	174	181	80	106	93	98	113	75
60	61	3	4	38	31	74	54	80	68	62	83	44	73	61	69	53	79
13	11	40	36	37	15	15	15	5	7	3	5	1	5	9	9	12	12
0	0	2	2	1	0	-	0	0	0	0	1	-	-	1	1	-	-
0	0	1	-	-	-	0	-	0	-	0	0	-	-	1	1	-	-
10	9	38	43	26	16	11	7	4	4	3	4	3	5	3	4	6	8
0	0	-	-	0	-	0	0	-	0	0	-	-	-	-	-	1	-
-	0	-	1	-	-	-	-	-	-	-	-	-	-	-	-	1	-
0	0	-	-	-	-	-	0	0	0	0	-	1	-	-	-	-	-
0	0	1	-	1	1	-	0	0	-	0	0	1	1	-	-	-	-
0	-	-	-	-	-	0	-	0	-	-	-	-	-	-	-	-	-
0	0	-	-	1	-	0	0	0	-	-	-	-	-	-	-	-	-
0	0	-	-	-	-	-	0	0	0	0	-	1	-	-	-	-	-
0	0	-	-	-	-	0	-	0	0	1	1	1	-	2	-	-	-
3	1	4	4	3	2	3	-	4	1	3	1	1	1	3	-	-	-
4	2	1	3	4	2	4	1	6	2	3	2	2	1	-	1	-	-
2	2	6	2	5	6	2	3	2	1	0	1	2	1	1	-	-	2
49	28	204	114	92	38	47	15	24	11	18	14	20	21	38	44	119	122
0	0	2	-	0	0	1	0	0	0	0	0	0	-	-	-	-	-
0	0	-	-	1	0	1	-	-	-	-	-	-	-	-	-	-	2
0	0	-	1	1	-	0	-	-	0	0	-	-	-	-	-	-	-
1	0	-	-	2	1	0	-	0	0	0	-	1	-	-	-	6	2
2	2	2	5	5	4	4	2	2	1	0	1	1	1	3	1	6	-
3	2	6	3	5	2	4	1	2	2	1	2	1	0	2	8	-	8

Table 22 - *continued*

Disease Group	Persons, by age group								
	Total	0-4	5-15	16-24	25-44	45-64	65-74	75-84	85 and over
Open wound of shoulder and upper arm (880)	2	1	2	3	2	2	2	3	3
Open wound of elbow, forearm and wrist (881)	9	2	12	11	6	5	5	22	43
Open wound of hand except finger(s) alone (882)	11	8	11	19	11	10	8	9	13
Open wound of finger(s) (883)	31	29	25	40	32	33	28	18	22
Multiple and unspecified open wounds of upper limb (884)	1	-	0	1	0	0	2	2	3
Traumatic amputation of thumb (complete) (partial) (885)	0	-	-	-	0	-	-	-	-
Traumatic amputation of other finger(s) (complete) (partial) (886)	0	-	0	0	1	1	1	-	-
Traumatic amputation of arm and hand (complete) (partial) (887)	0	-	-	-	-	0	-	0	-
Open wound of hip and thigh (890)	1	1	3	2	1	1	1	1	1
Open wound of knee, leg (except thigh) and ankle (891)	19	7	29	13	8	13	34	77	73
Open wound of foot except toe(s) alone (892)	6	7	11	8	5	4	5	5	3
Open wound of toe(s) (893)	3	8	4	2	2	3	4	9	4
Multiple and unspecified open wound of lower limb (894)	2	-	2	2	1	2	3	6	9
Traumatic amputation of toe(s) (complete) (partial) (895)	0	-	-	-	-	0	0	-	-
Traumatic amputation of leg(s) (complete) (partial) (897)	0	-	-	-	-	-	-	0	-
Injury to blood vessels of head and neck (900)	0	-	0	-	-	-	-	-	-
Injury to blood vessels of abdomen and pelvis (902)	0	-	0	0	0	-	-	0	-
Injury to blood vessels of upper extremity (903)	0	-	-	-	-	0	0	-	-
Injury to blood vessels of lower extremity and unspecified sites (904)	0	-	-	0	0	1	1	0	-
Late effects of musculoskeletal and connective tissue injuries (905)	0	-	-	0	0	0	1	-	1
Late effects of injuries to skin and subcutaneous tissues (906)	0	-	0	-	0	0	1	0	1
Late effects of injuries to the nervous system (907)	0	1	0	0	0	0	-	0	1
Late effects of other and unspecified external causes (909)	1	0	1	1	0	0	1	1	1
Superficial injury of face, neck and scalp except eye (910)	20	73	36	16	9	9	15	30	58
Superficial injury of trunk (911)	13	8	19	14	11	11	15	24	36
Superficial injury of shoulder and upper arm (912)	9	4	12	11	8	6	8	15	22
Superficial injury of elbow, forearm and wrist (913)	3	1	4	2	2	2	4	6	6
Superficial injury of hand(s) except finger(s) alone (914)	20	30	30	24	15	17	14	15	28
Superficial injury of finger(s) (915)	4	7	4	3	3	5	5	6	3
Superficial injury of hip, thigh, leg and ankle (916)	31	17	36	28	22	27	43	75	86
Superficial injury of foot and toe(s) (917)	22	23	38	24	17	16	21	17	22
Superficial injury of eye and adnexa (918)	10	11	11	6	12	10	5	6	-
Superficial injury of other, multiple and unspecified sites (919)	23	34	33	22	9	18	17	27	33
Contusion of face, scalp, and neck except eye(s) (920)	19	69	33	18	9	7	12	25	41
Contusion of eye and adnexa (921)	7	10	12	10	5	3	6	10	19
Contusion of trunk (922)	23	8	18	19	21	22	28	47	107
Contusion of upper limb (923)	27	22	47	34	21	18	23	42	50
Contusion of lower limb and of other and unspecified sites (924)	49	24	61	58	40	41	52	83	117

By age-group and sex

Total		0-4		5-15		16-24		25-44		45-64		65-74		75-84		85 and over	
Male	Female	Male	Female	Male	Female	Male	Female	Male	Female	Male	Female	Male	Female	Male	Female	Male	Female
2	2	1	1	3	1	4	2	3	2	2	2	1	2	2	3	-	4
11	7	3	1	17	8	18	5	9	3	5	5	3	7	24	21	53	39
16	7	9	8	15	7	30	9	13	8	13	7	15	3	13	6	24	10
39	23	30	27	31	19	58	21	39	25	39	27	38	20	19	17	42	16
1	1	-	-	1	0	2	1	0	1	0	0	2	2	1	2	6	2
0	-	-	-	-	-	-	-	0	-	-	-	-	-	-	-	-	-
1	0	-	-	0	0	0	-	1	0	1	0	1	1	-	-	-	-
0	-	-	-	-	-	-	-	-	-	0	-	-	-	1	-	-	-
2	1	1	1	4	2	4	0	1	0	1	0	1	0	1	1	-	2
15	23	7	6	36	21	18	8	8	8	8	17	13	52	21	110	30	87
6	6	8	6	14	8	9	6	4	6	2	5	5	6	3	5	6	2
3	4	9	6	4	5	2	1	2	2	2	4	6	3	8	10	6	4
1	2	-	-	2	2	1	2	1	1	2	2	1	5	2	9	-	12
0	0	-	-	-	-	-	-	-	-	0	0	-	0	-	-	-	-
-	0	-	-	-	-	-	-	-	-	-	-	-	-	-	1	-	-
0	-	-	-	0	-	-	-	-	-	-	-	-	-	-	-	-	-
0	-	-	-	0	-	0	-	0	-	-	-	-	-	1	-	-	-
-	0	-	-	-	-	-	-	-	-	-	-	0	-	0	-	-	-
0	1	-	-	-	-	-	-	0	-	0	-	2	1	0	-	1	-
0	0	-	-	-	-	0	-	-	0	0	0	1	1	-	-	-	2
0	0	-	-	0	1	-	-	1	0	0	0	-	1	-	1	-	2
0	0	1	1	1	-	1	-	1	0	0	0	-	-	-	1	-	2
1	0	1	-	2	0	1	1	0	0	1	0	2	0	-	2	-	2
20	20	74	71	43	28	17	14	8	9	7	12	9	20	30	30	42	63
13	14	7	10	21	17	14	13	11	10	9	13	10	18	26	23	48	32
8	9	2	7	14	10	12	10	8	7	5	7	5	10	10	18	6	28
3	2	1	1	5	3	3	2	2	1	2	2	4	4	7	5	12	4
23	16	30	29	35	24	30	18	19	12	17	16	16	12	21	12	48	22
4	4	7	6	3	4	3	3	3	3	5	4	6	4	8	4	12	-
23	38	20	15	36	36	32	24	16	27	18	37	19	62	35	98	59	95
20	23	23	22	37	39	25	23	16	19	13	19	20	22	11	20	12	26
11	8	12	10	14	8	9	4	13	11	10	9	8	3	6	6	-	-
19	26	36	32	35	32	17	27	14	23	13	24	13	20	16	34	18	37
18	19	74	63	42	24	19	18	7	10	4	9	4	18	9	34	30	45
6	8	9	11	14	10	9	10	5	4	2	4	2	9	7	12	12	22
21	25	9	8	19	16	21	17	22	20	21	24	17	37	32	56	113	104
28	27	25	18	50	44	37	31	22	19	17	19	18	27	33	48	65	45
42	54	22	27	73	48	63	52	35	45	29	54	32	68	50	103	71	132

Table 22 - *continued*

Disease Group	Persons, by age group								
	Total	0-4	5-15	16-24	25-44	45-64	65-74	75-84	85 and over
Crushing injury of face, scalp and neck (925)	0	-	0	0	0	-	-	-	-
Crushing injury of trunk (926)	0	1	1	-	0	0	-	0	-
Crushing injury of upper limb (927)	4	11	6	6	3	2	1	2	1
Crushing injury of lower limb (928)	2	3	2	3	2	2	1	0	-
Crushing injury of multiple and unspecified sites (929)	0	1	0	1	0	1	-	-	-
Foreign body on external eye (930)	12	8	8	14	16	12	9	5	7
Foreign body in ear (931)	4	12	10	1	2	2	3	3	1
Foreign body in nose (932)	1	15	2	-	-	-	-	-	-
Foreign body in pharynx and larynx (933)	1	1	0	1	1	1	1	2	-
Foreign body in trachea, bronchus and lung (934)	0	-	-	-	0	0	-	-	-
Foreign body in mouth, oesophagus and stomach (935)	1	3	1	1	0	1	0	-	3
Foreign body in intestine and colon (936)	0	-	0	0	-	-	-	-	-
Foreign body in anus and rectum (937)	0	-	-	-	0	-	-	-	-
Foreign body in digestive system, unspecified (938)	0	2	0	0	0	0	-	-	-
Foreign body in genitourinary tract (939)	2	0	0	3	5	1	-	-	-
Burn confined to eye and adnexa (940)	0	1	1	1	0	1	0	-	-
Burn of face, head and neck (941)	2	5	2	4	2	1	1	0	1
Burn of trunk (942)	2	7	2	1	1	1	3	3	4
Burn of upper limb, except wrist and hand (943)	4	8	2	4	4	3	3	4	3
Burn of wrist(s) and hand(s) (944)	7	21	6	8	6	5	5	7	7
Burn of lower limb(s) (945)	5	12	5	6	4	4	5	9	18
Burns of multiple specified sites (946)	0	-	0	0	0	0	-	-	-
Burn of internal organs (947)	0	-	0	1	0	1	0	-	1
Burns classified according to extent of body surface involved (948)	1	2	0	1	1	1	1	-	-
Burn, unspecified (949)	2	8	1	3	2	1	1	2	6
Injury to other cranial nerve(s) (951)	0	-	-	-	0	0	0	0	-
Spinal cord lesion without evidence of spinal bone injury (952)	0	-	-	-	-	0	0	0	-
Injury to nerve roots and spinal plexus (953)	0	-	0	0	0	1	0	1	-
Injury to other nerve(s) of trunk excluding shoulder and pelvic girdles (954)	0	-	-	0	-	-	-	-	-
Injury to peripheral nerve(s) of shoulder girdle and upper limb (955)	2	-	1	1	3	2	2	1	-
Injury to peripheral nerve(s) of pelvic girdle and lower limb (956)	1	-	-	0	1	1	1	2	-
Injury to other and unspecified nerves (957)	2	9	2	3	1	1	1	1	-
Certain early complications of trauma (958)	3	1	3	3	3	3	3	3	13
Injury, other and unspecified (959)	41	29	52	57	38	31	32	45	75
Poisoning by antibiotics (960)	0	-	-	-	0	0	-	1	-
Poisoning by other anti-infectives (961)	0	-	-	-	-	0	1	0	3
Poisoning by hormones and synthetic substitutes (962)	0	1	-	-	0	-	-	-	-
Poisoning by primarily systemic agents (963)	0	-	-	0	0	-	-	-	-
Poisoning by agents primarily affecting blood constituents (964)	0	0	-	-	-	-	-	-	-
Poisoning by analgesics, antipyretics and antirheumatics (965)	0	0	0	1	0	-	1	-	-
Poisoning by anticonvulsants and anti-Parkinsonism drugs (966)	0	-	-	-	-	0	-	-	-
Poisoning by sedatives and hypnotics (967)	0	-	-	-	-	0	-	-	-
Poisoning by psychotropic agents (969)	0	-	-	1	-	0	-	-	-
Poisoning by agents primarily affecting the cardiovascular system (972)	0	-	-	-	0	0	0	3	4
Poisoning by water, mineral and uric acid metabolism drugs (974)	0	-	-	-	-	-	-	-	1
Poisoning by other and unspecified drugs and medicaments (977)	1	2	0	1	1	0	1	0	-
Poisoning by bacterial vaccines (978)	0	0	0	0	0	-	-	-	-
Poisoning by other vaccines and biological substances (979)	0	1	-	-	0	0	-	-	-

By age-group and sex

Total		0-4		5-15		16-24		25-44		45-64		65-74		75-84		85 and over	
Male	Female	Male	Female	Male	Female	Male	Female	Male	Female	Male	Female	Male	Female	Male	Female	Male	Female
0	0	-	-	0	-	0	-	-	0	-	-	-	-	-	-	-	-
1	0	2	-	1	0	-	-	1	0	0	-	-	-	1	-	-	-
5	2	17	5	7	6	8	3	4	1	3	2	1	1	2	1	6	-
2	1	4	3	2	3	4	3	2	1	3	1	1	0	-	1	-	-
1	0	1	-	-	0	1	0	1	0	1	1	-	-	-	-	-	-
18	6	10	5	10	7	24	5	24	7	18	5	13	6	7	3	18	4
4	4	12	13	10	10	1	1	2	3	2	2	3	3	6	1	6	-
1	2	11	20	2	2	-	-	-	-	-	-	-	-	-	-	-	-
1	1	-	2	1	0	1	2	1	2	1	1	1	1	-	3	-	-
0	0	-	-	-	-	-	-	-	-	0	0	-	-	-	-	-	-
1	1	5	1	1	1	0	1	0	1	1	0	1	-	-	-	-	4
0	0	-	-	0	0	0	-	-	-	-	-	-	-	-	-	-	-
0	-	-	-	-	-	-	-	0	-	-	-	-	-	-	-	-	-
0	0	3	2	0	1	-	1	0	0	0	0	-	-	-	-	-	-
0	4	1	-	0	1	-	6	-	10	0	3	-	-	-	-	-	-
1	0	-	1	1	1	1	0	0	1	1	0	1	-	-	-	-	-
2	2	7	3	1	3	4	3	2	2	1	1	2	1	-	1	-	2
2	2	9	4	2	3	1	1	1	2	1	2	1	5	2	3	6	4
3	4	7	9	2	1	3	5	3	5	2	4	2	5	2	5	6	2
7	8	23	18	8	5	7	8	6	7	3	8	3	8	6	8	6	8
5	6	9	16	6	4	7	5	3	4	2	5	3	7	9	8	6	22
0	0	-	-	-	0	0	0	0	0	-	0	-	-	-	-	-	-
0	0	-	-	-	0	1	0	0	0	0	0	1	1	-	-	-	2
1	1	2	3	0	1	-	2	1	1	0	1	1	1	-	-	-	-
2	3	8	8	1	1	2	4	1	3	1	1	2	1	2	1	6	6
0	0	-	-	-	-	-	-	1	0	0	0	-	0	-	1	-	-
0	0	-	-	-	-	-	-	-	-	0	0	-	0	1	-	-	-
0	1	-	-	-	0	-	1	0	1	1	1	-	0	-	1	-	-
-	0	-	-	-	-	-	1	-	-	-	-	-	-	-	-	-	-
2	1	-	-	1	1	1	1	3	2	3	1	3	1	2	1	-	-
1	1	-	-	-	-	1	-	1	1	1	1	1	0	1	2	-	-
2	1	12	6	2	2	4	2	2	1	1	1	1	0	1	1	-	-
3	2	1	1	3	2	4	1	3	2	3	2	3	4	5	3	24	10
44	37	30	28	59	44	76	38	44	32	29	34	24	39	26	56	59	81
-	0	-	-	-	-	-	-	0	-	0	-	-	-	-	-	2	-
0	0	-	-	-	-	-	-	-	-	0	0	1	0	-	1	6	2
0	0	1	1	-	-	-	-	0	-	-	-	-	-	-	-	-	-
0	0	-	-	-	-	-	1	0	-	-	-	-	-	-	-	-	-
-	0	-	1	-	-	-	-	-	-	-	-	-	-	-	-	-	-
0	0	-	1	-	0	1	1	0	0	-	-	1	1	-	-	-	-
-	0	-	-	-	-	-	-	-	-	-	0	-	-	-	-	-	-
-	0	-	-	-	-	-	-	-	-	-	0	-	-	-	-	-	-
0	0	-	-	-	-	1	0	-	-	-	1	-	-	-	-	-	-
0	1	-	-	-	-	-	-	0	0	0	0	-	0	1	4	-	6
0	-	-	-	-	-	-	-	-	-	-	-	-	-	-	-	6	-
1	1	2	3	0	-	0	1	0	1	-	1	2	1	-	1	-	-
-	0	-	1	-	1	-	0	-	0	-	-	-	-	-	-	-	-
0	0	1	-	-	-	-	-	-	-	0	-	0	-	-	-	-	-

New and first ever episodes

Table 22 - *continued*

Disease Group	Persons, by age group								
	Total	0-4	5-15	16-24	25-44	45-64	65-74	75-84	85 and over
Toxic effect of alcohol (980)	1	-	0	1	0	1	-	-	-
Toxic effect of petroleum products (981)	0	-	-	0	-	-	-	-	-
Toxic effect of solvents other than petroleum-based (982)	0	-	1	1	0	0	-	-	-
Toxic effect of corrosive aromatics, acids and caustic alkalis (983)	0	1	-	-	0	-	-	-	-
Toxic effect of lead and its compounds (including fumes) (984)	0	-	-	0	0	-	-	-	-
Toxic effect of other metals (985)	0	-	0	0	0	-	-	-	-
Toxic effect of carbon monoxide (986)	0	0	-	0	0	0	0	-	-
Toxic effect of other gases, fumes or vapours (987)	0	-	0	1	0	0	0	0	1
Toxic effect of noxious substances eaten as food (988)	1	1	1	1	2	1	1	1	3
Toxic effect of other substances, chiefly nonmedicinal as to source (989)	2	2	3	4	2	2	4	3	1
Effects of radiation, unspecified (990)	0	-	-	-	0	1	1	0	-
Effects of reduced temperature (991)	8	4	9	6	5	7	15	17	24
Effects of heat and light (992)	1	3	1	1	2	1	2	2	1
Effects of air pressure (993)	1	-	1	1	1	1	0	-	-
Effects of other external causes (994)	4	9	5	2	3	4	5	6	1
Certain adverse effects not elsewhere classified (995)	287	445	284	283	240	241	275	466	737
Complications peculiar to certain specified procedures (996)	3	1	0	1	2	2	5	20	50
Complications affecting specified body systems, not elsewhere classified (997)	0	-	0	-	0	1	0	0	1
Other complications of procedures, not elsewhere classified (998)	37	13	14	27	48	44	49	50	27
Complications of medical care, not elsewhere classified (999)	1	7	1	1	1	1	1	1	3
Contact with or exposure to communicable diseases (V01)	15	37	30	14	19	5	2	0	1
Carrier or suspected carrier of infectious diseases (V02)	1	-	1	1	1	1	-	-	1
Need for prophylactic vaccination and inoculation against bacterial diseases (V03)	413	186	220	320	480	574	489	342	207
Need for prophylactic vaccination and inoculation against certain viral diseases (V04)	645	271	346	196	291	704	1,958	2,429	2,339
Need for other prophylactic vaccination and inoculation against single diseases (V05)	15	3	4	25	23	16	3	2	-
Need for prophylactic vaccination and inoculation against combinations of diseases (V06)	386	4,753	214	46	48	34	16	7	1
Need for isolation and other prophylactic measures (V07)	47	7	22	56	62	71	30	6	-
Health supervision of infant or child (V20)	131	1,883	9	1	1	-	0	-	-
Normal pregnancy (V22)	94	-	3	223	212	1	-	-	-
Supervision of high-risk pregnancy (V23)	2	-	-	4	4	-	-	-	-
Postpartum care and examination (V24)	113	8	2	239	265	1	0	0	-
Contraceptive management (V25)	502	2	68	1,688	871	47	1	-	-
Procreative management (V26)	8	1	0	24	17	0	0	-	-
Attention to artificial openings (V55)	0	-	-	-	-	0	-	-	-
Housing, household and economic circumstances (V60)	8	6	1	15	9	6	8	15	10
Other family circumstances (V61)	72	12	9	55	94	89	95	124	78
Other psychosocial circumstances (V62)	10	-	3	18	15	13	2	5	4
Other persons seeking consultation without complaint or sickness (V65)	38	31	24	51	41	43	33	32	27
Encounters for administrative purposes (V68)	383	15	12	425	556	650	120	116	109

By age-group and sex

Total		0-4		5-15		16-24		25-44		45-64		65-74		75-84		85 and over	
Male	Female	Male	Female	Male	Female	Male	Female	Male	Female	Male	Female	Male	Female	Male	Female	Male	Female
1	0	-	-	1	0	1	0	0	0	2	-	-	-	-	-	-	-
0	-	-	-	-	-	0	-	-	-	-	-	-	-	-	-	-	-
0	0	-	-	1	0	1	1	0	-	0	-	-	-	-	-	-	-
0	0	1	-	-	-	-	-	0	0	-	-	-	-	-	-	-	-
0	-	-	-	-	-	0	-	0	-	-	-	-	-	-	-	-	-
-	0	-	-	-	0	-	1	-	0	-	-	-	-	-	-	-	-
0	0	1	-	-	-	-	0	0	0	0	0	-	0	-	-	-	-
1	0	-	-	1	-	2	1	0	0	0	0	-	0	1	-	6	-
1	1	1	1	1	1	1	1	1	2	1	1	1	0	1	1	12	-
2	3	4	1	4	3	2	5	1	3	1	2	2	5	1	4	-	2
0	0	-	-	-	-	-	-	0	-	0	1	1	1	1	-	-	-
4	11	4	4	4	14	1	12	1	10	4	10	15	15	17	17	42	18
1	2	2	3	2	1	1	1	1	2	1	1	2	1	1	2	-	2
1	1	-	-	2	1	1	1	1	0	1	0	1	-	-	-	-	-
3	5	9	8	5	5	1	2	2	3	2	6	3	7	6	6	-	2
230	342	464	426	275	294	229	336	179	302	172	310	219	320	335	544	541	802
4	3	-	1	-	0	1	2	0	4	2	2	9	1	40	8	196	2
0	0	-	-	-	0	-	-	0	0	2	0	-	0	-	1	-	2
32	42	21	4	15	12	17	37	32	64	40	48	56	43	68	40	12	32
1	1	9	6	0	1	-	1	1	2	1	0	-	1	1	1	6	2
15	16	35	40	27	32	11	16	16	21	6	5	3	1	-	1	-	2
1	1	-	-	2	0	1	2	1	1	1	1	-	-	-	-	-	2
367	458	190	182	228	211	262	378	402	558	491	660	489	489	366	328	256	191
529	757	276	266	147	556	148	243	237	346	612	798	1,927	1,983	2,602	2,327	2,353	2,335
12	18	3	4	3	4	14	36	20	26	12	21	2	3	2	1	-	-
397	375	4,791	4,712	207	221	37	56	35	61	27	42	12	20	5	8	-	2
44	50	5	10	23	21	41	71	55	68	71	71	27	33	8	5	-	-
134	128	1,854	1,914	7	11	1	1	1	2	-	-	1	-	-	-	-	-
0	184	-	-	-	7	-	444	0	425	0	2	-	-	-	-	-	-
-	4	-	-	-	-	-	9	-	9	-	-	-	-	-	-	-	-
1	221	8	9	-	3	-	477	0	531	1	1	-	0	-	1	-	-
19	967	1	3	1	139	6	3,359	53	1,695	6	89	1	1	-	-	-	-
2	14	1	-	-	1	2	45	6	28	-	0	-	0	-	-	-	-
-	0	-	-	-	-	-	-	-	-	-	0	-	-	-	-	-	-
4	12	7	5	2	0	3	27	4	14	4	8	7	8	5	22	12	10
36	107	11	13	7	11	11	98	43	146	45	134	57	127	104	135	119	65
11	10	-	-	3	2	15	21	16	14	15	11	-	3	5	5	18	-
30	46	38	24	20	27	36	66	27	54	34	52	29	37	25	36	24	28
419	348	12	18	13	12	410	440	569	543	742	556	187	65	171	84	155	95

New and first ever episodes

237

Table 22 - *continued*

Disease Group	Persons, by age group								
	Total	0-4	5-15	16-24	25-44	45-64	65-74	75-84	85 and over
General medical examination (V70)	381	54	155	331	334	355	224	1,865	1,716
Special investigations and examinations (V72)	59	2	6	146	98	39	9	9	4
Special screening examination for viral diseases (V73)	31	1	9	89	55	4	2	0	1
Special screening examination for bacterial and spirochaetal diseases (V74)	1	2	0	2	1	0	0	0	-
Special screening examination for other infectious diseases (V75)	1	1	1	2	1	0	0	0	-
Special screening for malignant neoplasms (V76)	367	-	3	483	577	557	106	12	7
Special screening for endocrine, nutritional, metabolic and immunity disorders (V77)	117	2	8	55	126	237	176	104	52
Special screening for disorders of blood and blood-forming organs (V78)	10	2	2	14	13	10	10	18	19
Special screening for mental disorders and developmental handicaps (V79)	8	91	1	1	1	2	2	0	3
Special screening for neurological, eye and ear diseases (V80)	10	9	4	2	3	9	42	39	34
Special screening for cardiovascular, respiratory and genitourinary diseases (V81)	206	35	54	119	196	337	363	341	175
Special screening for other conditions (V82)	12	15	6	11	13	13	12	12	3

By age-group and sex

Total		0-4		5-15		16-24		25-44		45-64		65-74		75-84		85 and over	
Male	Female	Male	Female	Male	Female	Male	Female	Male	Female	Male	Female	Male	Female	Male	Female	Male	Female
299	460	60	48	155	155	229	432	242	427	303	409	219	227	1,873	1,860	1,771	1,698
2	114	1	4	2	10	1	289	1	195	3	75	-	17	7	10	-	6
7	53	1	1	7	10	15	162	10	101	5	4	3	-	1	-	-	2
1	1	1	2	-	1	3	1	1	1	0	0	1	-	1	-	-	-
1	1	1	-	2	1	1	2	1	2	0	0	1	-	1	-	-	-
1	718	-	-	-	6	1	963	1	1,158	1	1,124	2	190	-	20	-	10
106	128	2	3	8	8	42	69	112	140	215	259	167	183	115	98	77	43
5	15	2	2	1	3	5	22	6	21	7	13	8	12	11	21	6	24
8	7	87	96	2	0	1	0	2	1	1	2	2	2	-	1	6	2
9	11	5	13	5	2	2	1	2	3	8	10	41	43	42	37	48	30
182	228	35	34	57	51	80	158	160	232	315	360	370	357	341	341	178	173
7	16	10	20	5	6	3	18	7	20	9	18	10	12	13	12	6	2

New and first ever episodes

Table 23: Consultations with doctor - rates per 10,000 person years at risk:
ICD chapter and category of severity by age and sex

Disease group	Persons, by age group								
	Total	0-4	5-15	16-24	25-44	45-64	65-74	75-84	85 and over
All diseases and conditions (I-XVIII)	34,785	49,691	21,513	30,237	31,024	36,898	45,532	53,331	55,873
Serious	5,451	2,751	1,848	1,841	2,846	7,596	13,666	17,865	19,423
Intermediate	14,370	21,752	10,037	11,674	12,708	15,322	19,020	20,341	19,226
Minor	14,963	25,188	9,628	16,721	15,470	13,980	12,846	15,125	17,224
All illnesses (I-XVII)	30,021	43,316	20,667	22,642	24,593	32,856	43,161	50,005	52,438
I Infectious and parasitic diseases (001-139)	2,006	5,640	2,573	2,297	1,835	1,096	1,150	1,191	1,335
Serious	12	16	7	7	11	14	12	23	28
Intermediate	1,635	4,955	2,002	1,887	1,494	832	914	1,002	1,138
Minor	359	668	564	404	330	250	224	166	169
II Neoplasms (140-239)	492	75	110	166	315	676	1,312	1,675	1,373
Serious	287	13	6	12	68	415	1,051	1,433	1,173
Intermediate	206	62	104	154	246	261	261	242	200
Minor	-	-	-	-	-	-	-	-	-
III Endocrine, nutritional and metabolic diseases and immunity disorders (240-279)	710	89	62	181	462	1,296	1,885	1,679	1,231
Serious	419	16	18	76	203	714	1,331	1,397	991
Intermediate	290	73	44	106	259	582	554	281	240
Minor	-	-	-	-	-	-	-	-	-
IV Diseases of blood and blood-forming organs (280-289)	151	76	82	71	101	143	298	584	737
Serious	12	10	21	6	8	10	25	23	22
Intermediate	138	66	60	64	93	133	272	561	715
Minor	-	-	-	-	-	-	-	-	-
V Mental disorders (290-319)	1,761	276	258	1,246	2,162	2,474	2,221	2,620	3,260
Serious	350	1	5	212	419	427	422	898	1,654
Intermediate	1,180	174	203	856	1,492	1,745	1,442	1,354	1,190
Minor	231	101	49	179	251	302	357	368	416
VI Diseases of the nervous system and sense organs (320-389)	2,848	8,135	3,002	1,533	1,976	2,498	3,434	4,004	4,248
Serious	378	53	69	150	256	485	889	1,411	1,486
Intermediate	1,499	5,472	2,217	790	956	1,102	1,291	1,271	1,264
Minor	971	2,610	715	592	764	911	1,254	1,322	1,499
VII Diseases of the circulatory system (390-459)	2,397	30	30	181	643	3,956	8,465	10,039	9,706
Serious	977	12	8	28	108	1,344	3,485	5,370	7,010
Intermediate	1,399	13	12	140	523	2,594	4,936	4,583	2,566
Minor	21	4	11	13	11	18	44	86	130
VIII Diseases of the respiratory system (460-519)	6,200	16,394	7,237	5,355	4,441	4,840	6,695	6,974	7,081
Serious	1,314	2,231	1,543	809	700	1,245	2,508	2,549	2,289
Intermediate	1,933	4,285	2,092	1,715	1,370	1,615	2,288	2,703	3,097
Minor	2,953	9,879	3,602	2,831	2,371	1,980	1,899	1,722	1,696
IX Diseases of the digestive system (520-579)	1,493	1,104	397	946	1,302	1,957	2,726	3,137	3,305
Serious	414	84	41	167	356	673	865	920	880
Intermediate	527	647	222	389	451	621	851	992	940
Minor	552	373	134	390	496	663	1,010	1,225	1,486
X Diseases of the genitourinary system (580-629)	2,050	793	653	2,189	2,613	2,592	1,712	2,007	2,339
Serious	53	12	10	52	51	71	82	96	146
Intermediate	1,356	573	448	1,551	1,785	1,302	1,408	1,781	1,997
Minor	640	209	195	586	777	1,220	222	129	195
XI Complications of pregnancy, childbirth and the puerperium (630-676)	183	7	5	421	412	6	2	1	3
Serious	25	-	1	56	58	1	-	-	1
Intermediate	153	7	4	357	343	4	1	0	1
Minor	5	0	0	8	12	2	1	0	-
XII Diseases of the skin and subcutaneous tissue (680-709)	2,289	4,417	2,083	2,754	1,920	1,848	2,377	2,566	2,928
Serious	-	-	-	-	-	-	-	-	-
Intermediate	1,678	3,677	1,437	2,103	1,371	1,288	1,714	1,849	2,153
Minor	612	740	646	651	548	560	664	717	775

By age-group and sex

	Total		0-4		5-15		16-24		25-44		45-64		65-74		75-84		85 and over	
	Male	Female	Male	Female	Male	Female	Male	Female	Male	Female	Male	Female	Male	Female	Male	Female	Male	Female
	27,194	42,071	51,027	48,288	20,142	22,954	17,198	43,186	19,290	42,846	30,622	43,291	43,138	47,478	51,708	54,301	57,761	55,247
	5,148	5,743	3,180	2,301	2,111	1,572	1,692	1,989	2,465	3,231	7,469	7,726	14,592	12,913	19,243	17,041	22,213	18,498
	11,282	17,334	22,082	21,405	9,200	10,917	7,510	15,810	8,147	17,303	12,396	18,303	17,044	20,626	18,495	21,445	18,719	19,394
	10,765	18,994	25,765	24,582	8,831	10,466	7,996	25,387	8,678	22,313	10,758	17,262	11,502	13,939	13,971	15,815	16,829	17,355
	24,583	35,240	44,649	41,917	19,522	21,871	15,775	29,462	16,970	32,273	26,871	38,952	40,753	45,119	48,422	50,950	54,118	51,880
	1,602	2,393	5,563	5,721	2,367	2,791	1,448	3,139	1,146	2,529	843	1,354	1,020	1,256	1,067	1,265	1,284	1,352
	14	10	18	15	8	6	9	4	11	12	18	11	14	11	45	10	18	32
	1,227	2,026	4,867	5,048	1,853	2,159	1,078	2,689	798	2,195	565	1,104	724	1,068	842	1,098	1,135	1,139
	361	357	678	659	506	626	361	446	338	321	260	239	281	177	181	157	131	181
	426	556	69	81	108	112	117	214	200	431	514	841	1,493	1,165	2,233	1,342	2,436	1,021
	275	297	15	11	5	8	14	10	49	89	325	507	1,230	905	2,026	1,079	2,246	818
	150	259	54	70	104	104	103	204	151	342	189	334	262	260	207	263	190	203
	-	-	-	-	-	-	-	-	-	-	-	-	-	-	-	-	-	-
	587	827	83	95	52	73	99	263	335	590	1,141	1,455	1,768	1,980	1,675	1,681	1,414	1,170
	335	501	13	19	14	21	68	84	137	268	604	827	1,199	1,438	1,316	1,446	1,076	963
	252	326	70	76	37	52	31	179	197	321	537	628	569	542	360	235	339	207
	-	-	-	-	-	-	-	-	-	-	-	-	-	-	-	-	-	-
	81	219	77	76	76	88	12	129	17	185	71	216	257	330	434	673	755	731
	12	13	15	6	22	21	4	9	4	11	10	11	23	27	34	16	42	16
	69	205	62	70	54	67	8	120	13	174	62	205	234	303	400	657	713	715
	-	-	-	-	-	-	-	-	-	-	-	-	-	-	-	-	-	-
	1,241	2,260	315	235	261	255	893	1,597	1,500	2,830	1,786	3,175	1,512	2,797	1,849	3,081	2,680	3,452
	289	409	1	1	6	4	230	194	399	440	332	524	289	531	718	1,006	1,492	1,708
	810	1,534	206	141	217	189	565	1,145	952	2,036	1,265	2,235	998	1,803	879	1,638	909	1,283
	143	316	108	93	38	62	99	258	148	354	190	416	226	463	252	437	279	461
	2,504	3,179	8,344	7,916	2,796	3,218	1,141	1,922	1,474	2,482	2,085	2,918	3,310	3,535	4,017	3,996	4,279	4,238
	327	428	57	49	67	72	132	168	202	310	464	507	846	924	1,467	1,377	1,587	1,452
	1,289	1,700	5,643	5,293	2,087	2,354	524	1,054	621	1,294	806	1,403	1,157	1,401	1,191	1,319	1,248	1,269
	889	1,051	2,645	2,574	641	792	484	700	651	877	815	1,008	1,307	1,211	1,359	1,300	1,444	1,517
	2,273	2,516	34	25	28	32	125	236	580	705	4,250	3,656	9,001	8,030	10,265	9,904	10,358	9,490
	1,077	881	16	8	7	9	19	36	119	98	1,792	887	4,548	2,620	6,403	4,753	8,183	6,622
	1,179	1,611	13	12	11	13	98	182	456	591	2,440	2,750	4,403	5,370	3,761	5,074	2,068	2,731
	17	24	4	4	11	11	8	18	6	17	18	19	49	41	101	77	107	138
	5,538	6,835	17,288	15,455	7,023	7,462	4,069	6,632	3,184	5,707	3,910	5,787	6,919	6,513	8,058	6,326	9,258	6,360
	1,343	1,287	2,550	1,896	1,783	1,290	707	909	558	843	1,172	1,319	2,967	2,136	3,374	2,056	3,738	1,809
	1,714	2,142	4,627	3,926	1,859	2,337	1,346	2,080	1,040	1,702	1,338	1,897	2,333	2,252	3,071	2,483	3,637	2,918
	2,480	3,406	10,112	9,634	3,381	3,835	2,015	3,642	1,586	3,161	1,401	2,571	1,620	2,125	1,612	1,787	1,884	1,633
	1,319	1,660	1,173	1,031	385	410	710	1,180	1,084	1,522	1,774	2,143	2,768	2,692	3,255	3,066	3,708	3,172
	436	392	114	53	44	37	171	163	377	334	709	636	990	764	1,146	785	1,135	796
	465	587	682	610	225	219	318	460	385	517	554	689	806	887	854	1,075	939	940
	418	680	377	369	116	154	221	558	322	671	511	818	972	1,041	1,255	1,207	1,634	1,436
	589	3,451	869	713	412	908	270	4,096	386	4,856	620	4,601	1,249	2,089	1,767	2,150	1,991	2,455
	46	60	18	6	9	12	18	86	37	65	76	65	93	73	113	86	196	130
	470	2,207	469	681	263	643	218	2,874	316	3,265	518	2,101	1,104	1,655	1,616	1,880	1,753	2,079
	74	1,184	382	26	140	253	33	1,135	33	1,527	27	2,435	52	360	38	184	42	246
	-	359	-	15	-	11	-	839	-	828	-	13	-	4	-	1	-	4
	-	49	-	-	-	2	-	112	-	116	-	1	-	-	-	-	-	2
	-	299	-	15	-	9	-	711	-	688	-	7	-	2	-	1	-	2
	-	11	-	1	-	1	-	16	-	24	-	4	-	2	-	1	-	-
	2,016	2,552	4,367	4,469	1,898	2,278	2,322	3,183	1,512	2,330	1,620	2,080	2,332	2,414	2,598	2,547	3,037	2,892
	-	-	-	-	-	-	-	-	-	-	-	-	-	-	-	-	-	-
	1,471	1,876	3,613	3,744	1,262	1,620	1,719	2,484	1,066	1,679	1,162	1,416	1,722	1,706	1,887	1,827	2,068	2,181
	545	676	754	725	636	657	603	699	446	651	458	664	610	707	711	720	969	711

Table 23 - *continued*

Disease group		Persons, by age group								
		Total	0-4	5-15	16-24	25-44	45-64	65-74	75-84	85 and over
XIII	Diseases of then musculoskeletal system and connective tissue (710-739)	3,070	187	633	1,299	2,589	5,242	5,842	6,743	5,896
	Serious	1,067	7	21	133	504	2,083	2,836	3,463	3,193
	Intermediate	1,629	115	478	934	1,742	2,626	2,320	2,534	2,023
	Minor	374	65	134	232	343	533	687	746	681
XIV	Congenital anomalies (740-759)	69	275	69	44	46	56	64	60	59
	Serious	41	168	45	24	23	31	44	41	49
	Intermediate	28	107	24	20	24	25	20	19	10
	Minor	-	-	-	-	-	-	-	-	-
XV	Certain conditions originating in the perinatal period (760-779)	16	224	0	2	1	0	-	2	-
	Serious	4	59	0	0	1	0	-	2	-
	Intermediate	12	166	-	2	1	-	-	-	-
	Minor	-	-	-	-	-	-	-	-	-
XVI	Symptoms, signs and ill-defined conditions (780-799)	2,340	4,175	1,863	1,834	1,769	2,217	3,194	4,208	5,327
	Serious	7	1	0	-	1	4	24	48	98
	Intermediate	287	919	312	183	176	200	306	507	721
	Minor	2,046	3,255	1,551	1,651	1,592	2,013	2,864	3,654	4,508
XVII	Injury and poisoning (800-999)	1,946	1,418	1,609	2,124	2,006	1,959	1,784	2,515	3,609
	Serious	90	68	53	109	80	79	92	190	401
	Intermediate	421	441	377	426	381	394	442	662	974
	Minor	1,435	909	1,179	1,589	1,545	1,486	1,250	1,663	2,234
XVIII	Supplementary Classification of factors influencing health status and contact with Health Services (V01-V82)	4,764	6,375	846	7,595	6,431	4,042	2,371	3,327	3,436
	Serious	-	-	-	-	-	-	-	-	-
	Intermediate	-	-	-	-	-	-	-	-	-
	Minor	4,764	6,375	846	7,595	6,431	4,042	2,371	3,327	3,436

By age-group and sex

Total		0-4		5-15		16-24		25-44		45-64		65-74		75-84		85 and over	
Male	Female	Male	Female	Male	Female	Male	Female	Male	Female	Male	Female	Male	Female	Male	Female	Male	Female
2,572	3,548	223	149	586	682	1,100	1,497	2,276	2,904	4,647	5,847	4,848	6,650	5,284	7,615	4,647	6,310
841	1,283	7	6	16	26	134	133	440	568	1,854	2,315	2,268	3,297	2,418	4,087	2,139	3,542
1,438	1,814	137	92	442	516	797	1,070	1,575	1,910	2,379	2,877	1,981	2,595	2,202	2,732	1,830	2,086
294	452	79	51	128	140	170	294	261	426	414	655	598	759	664	795	677	682
70	69	323	226	86	51	35	53	41	51	47	65	55	71	48	68	53	61
46	36	220	114	64	25	24	25	23	22	27	34	34	52	30	48	48	49
24	33	103	112	22	27	11	28	18	29	19	31	21	19	18	20	6	12
-	-	-	-	-	-	-	-	-	-	-	-	-	-	-	-	-	-
15	17	213	236	-	0	-	4	0	3	-	1	-	-	2	2	-	-
5	4	67	49	-	0	-	0	0	1	-	1	-	-	2	2	-	-
10	13	146	187	-	-	-	3	-	2	-	-	-	-	-	-	-	-
-	-	-	-	-	-	-	-	-	-	-	-	-	-	-	-	-	-
1,829	2,830	4,209	4,141	1,716	2,018	1,082	2,581	1,149	2,394	1,732	2,710	2,780	3,530	3,969	4,351	5,253	5,351
7	7	-	1	1	-	-	-	-	1	5	-	32	17	62	39	125	89
268	305	888	952	309	314	148	218	138	215	178	223	348	273	668	410	879	668
1,554	2,518	3,321	3,187	1,406	1,704	934	2,363	1,009	2,178	1,550	2,484	2,401	3,240	3,239	3,902	4,249	4,594
1,922	1,969	1,499	1,333	1,729	1,482	2,352	1,897	2,086	1,926	1,830	2,090	1,441	2,062	1,901	2,882	2,965	3,822
96	84	69	67	64	41	162	57	107	53	82	76	59	118	89	250	190	471
446	397	503	376	455	295	546	306	421	342	384	404	381	491	539	735	1,004	963
1,380	1,488	927	889	1,210	1,147	1,645	1,533	1,558	1,531	1,364	1,610	1,000	1,453	1,272	1,897	1,771	2,388
2,612	6,830	6,379	6,371	620	1,083	1,424	13,724	2,320	10,573	3,751	4,339	2,385	2,359	3,286	3,351	3,643	3,367
-	-	-	-	-	-	-	-	-	-	-	-	-	-	-	-	-	-
2,612	6,830	6,379	6,371	620	1,083	1,424	13,724	2,320	10,573	3,751	4,339	2,385	2,359	3,286	3,351	3,643	3,367

Table 24 Consultations with doctor - rates per 10,000 person years at risk:
disease related groups by age and sex

Disease group	Persons, by age group								
	Total	0-4	5-15	16-24	25-44	45-64	65-74	75-84	85 and over
Intestinal infectious diseases (001-009)	518	2,593	447	444	360	261	311	423	593
Tuberculosis (010-018)	3	-	1	1	2	5	6	9	1
Zoonotic bacterial diseases (020-027)	0	0	1	-	0	1	-	-	-
Other bacterial diseases (030-041)	24	70	36	20	15	18	18	22	25
Poliomyelitis and other non-arthropod-borne viral diseases of central nervous system (045-049)	2	2	2	3	2	1	1	-	-
Viral diseases accompanied by exanthem (050-057)	287	937	342	235	203	178	304	304	331
Other diseases due to viruses and Chlamydiae (070-079)	400	754	1,039	551	284	150	105	92	65
Rickettsioses and other arthropod- borne diseases (080-088)	1	1	0	0	1	1	1	-	4
Syphilis and other venereal diseases (090-099)	7	2	1	18	10	5	6	2	4
Other spirochaetal diseases (100-104)	1	1	1	0	0	1	1	1	-
Mycoses (110-118)	617	844	337	884	853	421	372	296	241
Helminthiases (120-129)	45	180	148	26	26	6	2	1	4
Other infectious and parasitic diseases (130-136)	101	256	220	115	77	47	23	39	64
Late effects of infectious and parasitic diseases (137-139)	1	0	0	-	0	1	-	1	-
Malignant neoplasm of lip, oral cavity and pharynx (140-149)	4	-	-	-	1	6	14	17	4
Malignant neoplasm of digestive organs and peritoneum (150-159)	54	-	0	0	5	63	212	367	249
Malignant neoplasm of respiratory and intrathoracic organs (160-165)	32	-	-	1	2	54	139	144	105
Malignant neoplasm of bone, connective tissue, skin and breast (170-175)	56	1	1	3	17	110	152	226	231
Malignant neoplasm of genitourinary organs (179-189)	57	2	2	2	16	74	183	335	302
Malignant neoplasm of other and unspecified sites (190-199)	48	3	0	1	14	61	210	212	176
Malignant neoplasm of lymphatic and haematopoietic tissue (200-208)	13	7	1	3	5	16	46	51	18
Benign neoplasms (210-229)	159	49	80	132	212	206	156	94	81
Carcinoma in situ (230-234)	17	-	-	1	4	21	77	75	87
Neoplasms of uncertain behaviour (235-238)	8	2	1	3	5	12	20	25	27
Neoplasms of unspecified nature (239)	45	12	24	20	35	54	103	129	93
Disorders of thyroid gland (240-246)	128	2	6	26	92	225	343	306	352
Diseases of other endocrine glands (250-259)	296	6	19	62	133	493	968	1,054	589
Nutritional deficiencies (260-269)	4	3	4	1	3	3	12	16	31
Other metabolic disorders and immunity disorders (270-279)	280	78	34	93	234	576	561	303	259
Diseases of blood and blood-forming organs (280-289)	151	76	82	71	101	143	298	584	737
Organic psychotic conditions (290-294)	62	0	1	6	17	22	95	516	1,259
Other psychoses (295-299)	228	0	4	114	259	388	328	382	399
Neurotic disorders, personality disorders and other nonpsychotic mental disorders (300-316)	1,466	274	253	1,117	1,882	2,059	1,796	1,722	1,599
Mental retardation (317-319)	4	1	1	9	4	5	2	-	1
Inflammatory diseases of the central nervous system (320-326)	4	7	2	2	5	6	2	4	-
Hereditary and degenerative diseases of the central nervous system (330-337)	76	5	7	10	18	80	270	443	466
Other disorders of the central nervous system (340-349)	296	42	183	318	384	371	228	182	175
Disorders of the peripheral nervous system (350-359)	77	1	7	25	77	137	135	151	77
Disorders of the eye and adnexa (360-379)	866	2,558	614	421	514	765	1,381	1,781	2,032
Diseases of the ear and mastoid process (380-389)	1,531	5,523	2,188	757	978	1,138	1,418	1,443	1,499
Acute rheumatic fever (390-392)	0	-	0	0	0	0	0	-	-
Chronic rheumatic heart disease (393-398)	10	0	0	-	1	25	31	24	15
Hypertensive disease (401-405)	1,034	1	1	19	253	2,075	4,009	3,344	1,388
Ischaemic heart disease (410-414)	428	0	0	1	44	812	1,654	1,758	1,352
Diseases of pulmonary circulation (415-417)	14	-	0	2	4	22	50	59	59
Other forms of heart disease (420-429)	346	13	4	11	25	246	1,151	2,545	4,357
Cerebrovascular disease (430-438)	130	-	0	3	6	130	445	898	1,341
Diseases of arteries, arterioles and capillaries (440-448)	103	5	12	18	26	138	373	505	417
Diseases of veins and lymphatics, and other diseases of circulatory system (451-459)	331	10	12	127	283	508	753	906	777

By age-group and sex

Total		0-4		5-15		16-24		25-44		45-64		65-74		75-84		85 and over	
Male	Female	Male	Female	Male	Female	Male	Female	Male	Female	Male	Female	Male	Female	Male	Female	Male	Female
473	560	2,648	2,535	456	438	336	552	297	424	205	317	236	373	349	467	576	599
4	2	-	-	0	1	1	1	2	2	8	3	7	5	23	1	-	2
1	0	1	-	1	1	-	-	0	-	1	0	-	-	-	-	-	-
20	27	61	80	29	42	15	24	9	20	16	20	17	19	39	12	-	33
1	2	2	1	2	1	4	1	1	4	0	2	1	-	-	-	-	-
240	331	924	952	321	364	162	307	143	264	133	223	262	339	258	332	362	321
377	421	796	710	984	1,096	462	640	243	326	133	168	105	104	74	103	65	65
1	1	2	-	1	-	-	0	1	1	1	1	2	-	-	-	18	-
11	4	2	1	2	1	27	9	15	5	9	2	3	8	3	1	-	6
0	1	1	1	1	0	0	-	-	1	0	1	-	1	2	-	-	-
355	869	724	970	291	384	333	1,431	362	1,348	291	554	368	376	292	299	232	244
36	55	150	211	114	183	17	34	15	36	5	6	1	3	1	1	-	6
82	119	251	262	163	279	91	140	57	98	37	56	17	28	25	47	30	75
1	0	1	-	0	-	-	-	0	1	2	1	-	-	-	-	1	-
4	3	-	-	-	-	-	-	0	2	9	3	18	11	23	13	-	6
65	44	-	-	-	0	-	1	5	4	72	53	278	159	595	230	499	165
42	22	-	-	-	-	1	-	3	0	67	41	199	91	254	78	267	51
14	97	-	1	2	1	4	2	5	30	17	204	48	236	94	305	65	286
72	43	-	4	-	3	2	1	14	18	68	81	274	109	655	144	933	93
46	50	5	1	0	0	2	-	12	17	51	73	235	190	267	179	345	120
14	11	9	5	1	1	3	3	5	5	17	15	71	27	61	46	42	10
114	202	45	53	76	84	84	180	130	295	152	260	151	160	77	104	48	93
13	21	-	-	-	-	0	1	1	6	11	32	88	67	68	80	95	85
9	7	2	1	2	0	4	3	4	5	12	11	29	14	33	20	30	26
35	55	9	16	27	21	17	24	22	47	38	70	102	103	106	142	113	87
31	222	2	3	1	10	6	46	18	166	46	407	117	527	103	428	238	390
306	288	2	10	15	23	65	60	131	136	561	424	1,074	883	1,189	973	796	520
3	6	2	4	5	3	1	1	1	4	2	4	5	17	24	11	12	37
247	312	77	78	31	37	28	157	185	283	532	620	572	553	360	269	368	223
81	219	77	76	76	88	12	129	17	185	71	216	257	330	434	673	755	731
43	81	-	1	1	-	6	6	16	18	24	20	89	99	428	568	1,188	1,283
162	292	1	-	4	3	103	125	184	334	283	496	204	429	291	437	309	429
1,031	1,884	313	234	255	250	774	1,458	1,294	2,475	1,472	2,657	1,219	2,265	1,130	2,076	1,183	1,738
5	3	1	-	1	2	10	9	6	3	6	3	-	4	-	-	-	2
4	4	9	5	2	2	2	1	6	4	5	8	2	1	7	3	-	-
72	80	6	3	7	7	9	10	14	22	84	76	278	264	577	363	458	469
202	386	44	40	168	199	192	443	221	549	259	485	195	255	188	179	196	167
56	96	1	1	8	7	12	38	46	107	104	171	130	139	148	153	77	77
719	1,006	2,576	2,538	578	652	321	520	378	651	588	946	1,160	1,561	1,580	1,901	1,991	2,045
1,451	1,607	5,708	5,328	2,033	2,351	604	910	809	1,148	1,046	1,232	1,546	1,315	1,517	1,398	1,557	1,480
0	0	-	-	-	0	0	-	0	0	0	-	-	0	-	-	-	-
7	12	-	1	0	-	-	-	1	1	14	36	25	36	33	18	18	14
884	1,178	1	1	2	1	12	26	251	255	1,978	2,175	3,545	4,385	2,605	3,785	1,016	1,511
534	326	-	1	0	-	1	0	63	24	1,157	461	2,223	1,191	2,169	1,513	1,688	1,241
14	14	-	-	1	-	0	3	2	7	25	18	67	37	66	54	83	51
319	373	19	6	5	3	10	12	28	22	287	204	1,389	958	2,774	2,409	4,706	4,242
133	128	-	-	1	-	3	4	5	7	163	95	577	337	1,066	798	1,587	1,259
114	92	5	6	9	15	11	26	17	35	180	95	495	274	671	406	565	368
267	392	9	10	11	13	89	166	213	355	446	572	680	812	881	921	695	804

Consultations with doctor

Table 24 - *continued*

Disease group	Persons, by age group								
	Total	0-4	5-15	16-24	25-44	45-64	65-74	75-84	85 and over
Acute respiratory infections (460-466)	4,083	13,485	4,710	3,535	2,928	2,901	3,485	3,827	4,375
Other diseases of upper respiratory tract (470-478)	537	399	786	746	543	404	434	301	197
Pneumonia and influenza (480-487)	293	287	218	271	282	299	306	445	763
Chronic obstructive pulmonary disease and allied conditions (490-496)	1,233	2,177	1,511	774	646	1,170	2,355	2,251	1,629
Pneumoconioses and other lung diseases due to external agents (500-508)	2	-	0	-	0	3	8	7	1
Other diseases of respiratory system (510-519)	52	46	11	29	41	64	108	143	115
Diseases of oral cavity, salivary glands and jaws (520-529)	185	392	140	173	175	179	178	165	144
Diseases of oesophagus, stomach and duodenum (530-537)	584	95	64	299	530	916	1,236	1,182	981
Appendicitis (540-543)	12	1	23	26	14	6	2	1	-
Hernia of abdominal cavity (550-553)	104	91	11	19	49	157	292	351	286
Noninfective enteritis and colitis (555-558)	67	49	16	46	78	93	86	82	73
Other diseases of intestines and peritoneum (560-569)	460	461	140	358	396	472	760	1,140	1,562
Other diseases of digestive system (570-579)	80	16	4	25	59	133	172	216	260
Nephritis, nephrotic syndrome and nephrosis (580-589)	19	8	2	6	9	26	47	60	112
Other diseases of urinary system (590-599)	617	356	254	619	577	622	974	1,311	1,672
Diseases of male genital organs (600-608)	143	330	131	73	112	135	225	201	104
Disorders of breast (610-611)	132	16	44	112	228	155	64	43	15
Inflammatory disease of female pelvic organs (614-616)	152	69	42	276	254	88	62	70	59
Other disorders of female genital tract (617-629)	987	13	181	1,103	1,432	1,565	340	321	377
Pregnancy with abortive outcome (630-639)	35	0	2	84	78	2	-	-	-
Complications mainly related to pregnancy (640-648)	76	-	2	200	164	1	-	-	1
Normal delivery, and other indications for care in pregnancy, labour and delivery (650-659)	32	2	1	73	73	0	-	-	-
Complications occurring mainly in the course of labour and delivery (660-669)	14	5	0	28	33	1	-	-	-
Complications of the puerperium (670-676)	26	0	1	36	65	3	2	1	1
Infections of skin and subcutaneous tissue (680-686)	471	710	521	442	400	406	493	638	885
Other inflammatory conditions of skin and subcutaneous tissue (690-698)	1,112	3,360	831	1,000	887	925	1,199	1,113	1,135
Other diseases of skin and subcutaneous tissue (700-709)	706	346	731	1,312	633	517	684	815	908
Arthropathies and related disorders (710-719)	1,134	56	220	372	609	1,916	2,823	3,580	3,442
Dorsopathies (720-724)	1,060	29	121	522	1,229	1,875	1,414	1,374	1,138
Rheumatism, excluding the back (725-729)	782	61	189	352	697	1,346	1,419	1,542	1,040
Osteopathies, chondropathies and acquired musculoskeletal deformities (730-739)	94	41	103	54	53	104	185	248	277
Congenital anomalies (740-759)	69	275	69	44	46	56	64	60	59
Certain conditions originating in the perinatal period (760-779)	16	224	0	2	1	0	-	2	-
Symptoms, signs and ill-defined conditions (780-789)	2,136	3,782	1,721	1,700	1,618	2,005	2,931	3,881	4,532
Nonspecific abnormal findings (790-796)	163	377	133	118	129	185	196	152	115
Ill-defined and unknown causes of morbidity and mortality (797-799)	41	16	10	15	22	27	66	175	679
Fracture of skull (800-804)	10	4	8	23	12	5	5	5	10
Fracture of spine and trunk (805-809)	27	1	2	15	25	39	36	72	133
Fracture of upper limb (810-819)	67	29	78	85	58	60	75	96	142
Fracture of lower limb (820-829)	63	14	27	65	61	64	74	145	331
Dislocation (830-839)	19	12	13	32	19	15	18	21	27
Sprains and strains of joints and adjacent muscles (840-848)	774	98	463	906	992	933	603	567	500
Intracranial injury, excluding those with skull fracture (850-854)	26	79	50	34	15	11	10	17	30
Internal injury of chest, abdomen and pelvis (860-869)	2	0	1	3	2	2	2	2	-
Open wound of head, neck and trunk (870-879)	45	142	70	39	26	25	25	56	172
Open wound of upper limb (880-887)	47	30	36	70	48	44	33	62	89
Open wound of lower limb (890-897)	32	17	41	25	16	29	46	108	126

By age-group and sex

Total		0-4		5-15		16-24		25-44		45-64		65-74		75-84		85 and over	
Male	Female	Male	Female	Male	Female	Male	Female	Male	Female	Male	Female	Male	Female	Male	Female	Male	Female
3,462	4,679	13,997	12,948	4,194	5,252	2,505	4,558	1,958	3,906	2,161	3,654	3,275	3,655	4,039	3,700	4,950	4,185
497	576	438	358	861	708	634	858	435	651	341	468	426	440	339	278	339	150
265	320	308	265	212	224	230	311	249	316	260	339	295	314	472	430	951	701
1,261	1,205	2,491	1,847	1,744	1,266	677	870	509	785	1,085	1,256	2,797	1,995	2,991	1,809	2,882	1,214
3	0	-	-	0	0	-	-	1	0	6	0	16	2	17	1	6	-
48	55	55	37	10	12	24	34	33	49	59	69	110	106	200	109	131	110
152	217	405	378	130	150	119	226	131	220	135	223	156	196	133	184	131	148
580	589	98	91	69	57	310	288	540	520	902	930	1,331	1,159	1,255	1,138	1,099	942
12	13	1	1	23	23	25	28	12	16	6	5	2	2	-	1	-	-
133	76	128	52	17	4	33	5	66	33	211	102	380	220	495	265	469	225
60	74	50	48	17	14	31	60	65	91	87	100	104	70	63	94	83	69
313	601	477	445	123	158	175	538	226	568	317	631	621	873	1,047	1,196	1,616	1,545
68	91	13	18	6	3	16	34	44	73	117	151	173	172	263	188	309	244
20	17	15	1	4	1	8	3	9	9	30	21	54	41	76	51	178	91
261	958	201	519	110	405	90	1,144	148	1,010	312	939	680	1,213	1,136	1,415	1,379	1,769
292	-	645	-	255	-	147	-	223	-	268	-	502	-	537	-	416	-
16	244	9	25	43	44	24	199	6	453	10	303	13	106	18	58	18	14
0	297	-	141	-	85	-	551	0	509	-	178	-	113	-	112	-	79
-	1,935	-	27	-	371	-	2,199	-	2,875	-	3,160	-	616	-	513	-	502
-	69	-	1	-	4	-	167	-	156	-	3	-	-	-	-	-	-
-	149	-	-	-	4	-	399	-	328	-	2	-	-	-	-	-	2
-	63	-	4	-	1	-	146	-	147	-	0	-	-	-	-	-	-
-	28	-	10	-	0	-	56	-	66	-	1	-	-	-	-	-	-
-	51	-	1	-	2	-	72	-	131	-	7	-	4	-	1	-	2
446	495	786	630	532	509	406	477	370	430	368	445	465	516	595	664	749	930
941	1,276	3,227	3,500	675	996	644	1,355	663	1,112	812	1,040	1,185	1,211	1,176	1,075	1,183	1,119
629	781	354	339	691	773	1,272	1,351	480	788	440	595	682	687	827	808	1,105	843
870	1,387	68	43	184	258	345	398	518	702	1,615	2,223	2,215	3,318	2,492	4,230	2,401	3,787
954	1,162	33	26	102	140	422	621	1,104	1,354	1,775	1,977	1,263	1,538	1,171	1,495	1,165	1,129
683	878	78	43	179	199	283	421	616	779	1,195	1,501	1,263	1,545	1,539	1,544	951	1,070
65	122	44	38	121	84	50	57	38	69	63	146	106	250	82	346	131	325
70	69	323	226	86	51	35	53	41	51	47	65	55	71	48	68	53	61
15	17	213	236	-	0	-	4	0	3	-	1	-	-	2	2	-	-
1,664	2,588	3,812	3,751	1,585	1,864	1,005	2,392	1,048	2,193	1,549	2,469	2,555	3,237	3,643	4,023	4,380	4,583
134	192	383	372	119	147	68	168	84	173	160	211	167	220	133	163	149	104
31	50	14	17	12	7	9	22	16	28	24	31	59	72	192	165	725	664
14	6	4	4	10	7	37	9	18	6	6	3	5	5	1	8	6	12
28	25	1	1	3	1	20	11	34	16	42	35	31	40	61	79	71	154
73	62	27	30	93	63	136	34	82	34	45	75	31	111	32	135	65	167
66	61	16	12	35	19	101	29	84	37	65	64	36	106	48	203	143	394
22	16	8	16	12	14	41	23	25	13	19	11	17	18	17	23	18	30
792	755	102	94	465	461	979	834	1,054	929	913	954	505	682	488	614	458	514
28	23	77	82	66	33	36	31	15	14	10	12	7	12	18	16	30	30
2	2	-	1	2	1	3	3	3	2	3	2	3	1	2	2	-	-
56	35	177	105	94	46	57	20	36	16	25	26	24	25	47	62	166	173
62	33	32	29	45	26	108	33	67	29	54	34	44	25	62	62	119	79
28	36	18	16	51	31	34	17	18	14	27	31	24	63	41	148	36	156

Table 24 - *continued*

Disease group	Persons, by age group								
	Total	0-4	5-15	16-24	25-44	45-64	65-74	75-84	85 and over
Injury to blood vessels (900-904)	1	-	0	1	0	1	1	1	-
Late effects of injuries, poisonings, toxic effects and other external causes (905-909)	3	2	2	3	3	4	6	3	7
Superficial injury (910-919)	159	197	207	154	124	134	156	261	346
Contusion with intact skin surface (920-924)	141	129	169	151	110	111	155	252	451
Crushing injury (925-929)	8	14	8	11	8	9	1	2	-
Effects of foreign body entering through orifice (930-939)	22	43	22	19	25	17	13	9	12
Burns (940-949)	28	63	19	28	23	21	30	45	56
Injury to nerves and spinal cord (950-957)	8	9	2	8	10	9	8	8	1
Certain traumatic complications and unspecified injuries (958-959)	54	26	54	70	56	48	49	59	107
Poisoning by drugs, medicaments and biological substances (960-979)	3	4	1	3	2	2	3	7	12
Toxic effects of substances chiefly nonmedicinal as to source (980-989)	6	4	6	10	6	5	4	5	6
Other and unspecified effects of external causes (990-995)	337	470	308	325	287	293	341	593	910
Complications of surgical and medical care not elsewhere classified (996-999)	66	30	19	44	77	77	90	119	141
Persons with potential health hazards related to communicable diseases (V01-V07)	807	4,000	461	298	384	609	1,089	1,417	1,681
Persons encountering health services in circumstances related to reproduction and development (V20-V28)	1,954	2,095	138	5,390	3,523	99	3	1	1
Persons encountering health services for specific procedures and aftercare (V50-V59)	0	-	-	-	0	0	-	1	1
Persons encountering health services in other circumstances (V60-V68)	1,169	76	56	1,057	1,606	2,204	463	383	315
Persons without reported diagnosis encountered during examination and investigation of individuals and populations (V70-V82)	834	204	191	850	919	1,129	817	1,525	1,437

By age-group and sex

Total		0-4		5-15		16-24		25-44		45-64		65-74		75-84		85 and over	
Male	Female	Male	Female	Male	Female	Male	Female	Male	Female	Male	Female	Male	Female	Male	Female	Male	Female
0	1	-	-	1	-	0	1	0	0	0	2	1	1	1	1	-	-
4	3	2	1	3	1	4	2	4	1	6	3	5	7	3	3	-	10
149	169	198	196	223	190	165	144	122	126	110	157	124	182	189	304	261	374
129	151	132	124	196	141	161	141	110	110	93	130	97	201	149	313	357	483
12	5	19	8	8	8	16	6	13	4	14	3	1	2	2	2	-	-
26	18	43	43	22	22	25	14	29	22	23	12	18	9	13	6	18	10
26	29	65	61	21	16	32	25	21	25	18	24	21	38	54	39	42	61
11	6	13	6	2	3	11	5	15	6	10	8	11	6	10	6	-	2
60	48	24	27	63	44	90	50	69	43	50	46	36	60	39	70	101	108
2	3	4	5	0	1	2	4	2	2	1	3	3	3	3	10	6	14
6	6	7	2	7	4	9	11	4	7	5	4	3	5	5	5	18	2
266	405	486	453	287	331	256	394	212	362	213	374	279	391	449	679	707	977
59	72	43	16	19	19	30	57	49	106	77	77	114	71	166	91	345	73
737	875	4,051	3,946	372	554	243	352	327	441	522	698	1,037	1,130	1,394	1,431	1,723	1,667
176	3,660	2,052	2,139	11	271	13	10,730	74	6,998	9	191	2	3	1	1	-	2
0	0	-	-	-	-	-	-	-	0	-	0	-	-	1	1	6	-
1,247	1,094	80	72	47	66	938	1,174	1,586	1,625	2,513	1,890	624	332	401	373	464	266
452	1,201	195	213	189	193	229	1,467	333	1,509	707	1,559	722	894	1,490	1,545	1,450	1,432

**Table 25 Consultations with doctor - rates per 10,000 person years at risk:
first 3 ICD digits by age and sex**

Disease group	Persons, by age group								
	Total	0-4	5-15	16-24	25-44	45-64	65-74	75-84	85 and over
Cholera (001)	0	0	-	-	-	-	-	-	-
Typhoid and paratyphoid fevers (002)	0	-	-	0	-	-	-	-	-
Other salmonella infections (003)	6	12	2	4	8	7	4	2	7
Shigellosis (004)	2	8	6	0	2	1	2	-	-
Other food poisoning (bacterial) (005)	2	1	1	2	3	2	3	1	1
Amoebiasis (006)	0	-	-	0	0	1	0	-	-
Other protozoal intestinal diseases (007)	1	5	2	1	2	1	-	-	-
Intestinal infections due to other organisms (008)	9	26	7	9	8	6	7	5	4
Ill-defined intestinal infections (009)	497	2,541	428	428	337	242	296	415	580
Primary tuberculous infection (010)	0	-	-	-	0	-	0	-	-
Pulmonary tuberculosis (011)	2	-	0	0	1	4	6	7	1
Other respiratory tuberculosis (012)	0	-	-	-	0	0	-	-	-
Tuberculosis of meninges and central nervous system (013)	0	-	-	0	0	0	-	-	-
Tuberculosis of bones and joints (015)	0	-	-	0	0	0	-	-	-
Tuberculosis of genitourinary system (016)	0	-	-	-	-	1	-	2	-
Tuberculosis of other organs (017)	0	-	0	0	1	0	-	0	-
Miliary tuberculosis (018)	0	-	-	-	-	-	-	0	-
Anthrax (022)	0	-	-	-	-	0	-	-	-
Brucellosis (023)	0	-	-	-	-	1	-	-	-
Other zoonotic bacterial diseases (027)	0	0	1	-	0	-	-	-	-
Leprosy (030)	0	-	-	0	-	-	-	-	-
Diseases due to other mycobacteria (031)	0	-	0	-	0	-	1	-	-
Diphtheria (032)	0	-	0	-	-	-	-	-	-
Whooping cough (033)	2	16	5	0	0	-	-	-	-
Streptococcal sore throat and scarlatina (034)	11	38	25	13	7	3	2	2	1
Erysipelas (035)	5	4	1	2	3	9	13	9	6
Meningococcal infection (036)	1	2	1	0	1	0	-	-	-
Tetanus (037)	0	-	-	0	0	0	-	0	-
Septicaemia (038)	1	2	0	0	0	2	2	9	18
Actinomycotic infections (039)	1	-	0	0	1	2	-	-	-
Other bacterial diseases (040)	0	-	-	0	0	0	-	-	-
Bacterial infection in conditions classified elsewhere and of unspecified site (041)	3	9	3	3	2	3	1	2	-
Acute poliomyelitis (045)	0	-	-	-	0	0	-	-	-
Slow virus infection of central nervous system (046)	0	-	-	0	0	-	-	-	-
Meningitis due to enterovirus (047)	1	1	0	2	1	0	-	-	-
Other non-arthropod-borne viral diseases of central nervous system (049)	1	1	1	1	1	1	1	-	-
Cowpox and paravaccinia (051)	0	0	0	-	1	0	-	-	-
Chickenpox (052)	78	504	159	67	38	4	2	3	-
Herpes zoster (053)	81	13	32	31	42	102	240	259	308
Herpes simplex (054)	91	92	86	124	114	69	61	39	24
Measles (055)	4	43	4	1	0	0	-	-	-
Rubella (056)	6	56	13	3	1	0	1	0	-
Other viral exanthemata (057)	26	229	47	9	7	2	1	2	-
Viral hepatitis (070)	8	2	10	11	11	5	3	4	1
Rabies (071)	0	-	-	-	0	-	-	-	-
Mumps (072)	4	26	11	3	2	1	1	1	1
Ornithosis (073)	0	-	-	-	0	0	-	-	-
Specific diseases due to Coxsackie virus (074)	11	89	10	6	6	4	1	0	3
Infectious mononucleosis (075)	17	4	23	77	10	1	2	-	-
Other diseases of conjunctiva due to viruses and Chlamydiae (077)	0	0	0	0	0	-	-	0	-
Other diseases due to viruses and Chlamydiae (078)	281	254	852	393	204	107	74	66	30
Viral infection in conditions classified elsewhere and of unspecified site (079)	79	380	133	62	51	33	25	21	30

By age-group and sex

Total		0-4		5-15		16-24		25-44		45-64		65-74		75-84		85 and over	
Male	Female	Male	Female	Male	Female	Male	Female	Male	Female	Male	Female	Male	Female	Male	Female	Male	Female
-	0	-	1	-	-	-	-	-	-	-	-	-	-	-	-	-	-
-	0	-	-	-	-	-	1	-	-	-	-	-	-	-	-	-	-
6	6	12	12	1	3	4	3	9	7	8	7	1	6	3	1	18	4
2	3	8	8	6	7	-	1	1	4	0	1	1	3	-	-	-	-
2	2	1	1	1	1	2	2	4	3	2	2	1	5	-	2	6	-
0	0	-	-	-	-	0	0	-	0	0	1	-	0	-	-	-	-
1	2	5	4	3	1	1	2	1	3	1	1	-	-	-	-	-	-
9	8	24	29	11	4	8	9	8	8	5	7	8	6	6	5	6	4
453	539	2,598	2,481	435	422	321	534	275	399	187	299	225	353	340	460	547	591
0	0	-	-	-	-	-	-	-	0	-	-	1	-	-	-	-	-
3	1	-	-	0	-	-	0	1	1	6	2	6	5	17	1	-	2
-	0	-	-	-	-	-	-	-	0	-	0	-	-	-	-	-	-
0	0	-	-	-	-	1	-	-	0	0	-	-	-	-	-	-	-
0	0	-	-	-	-	-	0	0	-	0	0	-	-	-	-	-	-
0	-	-	-	-	-	-	-	-	-	1	-	-	-	5	-	-	-
0	0	-	-	-	1	0	0	1	0	-	0	-	-	-	1	-	-
0	-	-	-	-	-	-	-	-	-	-	-	-	-	1	-	-	-
-	0	-	-	-	-	-	-	-	-	-	0	-	-	-	-	-	-
0	-	-	-	-	-	-	-	-	-	1	-	-	-	-	-	-	-
0	0	1	-	1	1	-	-	0	-	-	-	-	-	-	-	-	-
-	0	-	-	-	-	-	1	-	-	-	-	-	-	-	-	-	-
0	0	-	-	0	-	-	-	0	-	-	-	1	0	-	-	-	-
0	-	-	-	0	-	-	-	-	-	-	-	-	-	-	-	-	-
1	2	11	20	4	6	-	0	0	1	-	-	-	-	-	-	-	-
9	13	34	43	20	30	9	17	5	10	2	4	1	2	1	2	-	2
4	5	4	4	-	2	2	1	1	4	8	9	10	14	19	2	-	8
1	0	2	2	2	0	0	0	1	0	0	0	-	-	-	-	-	-
0	-	-	-	-	-	0	-	0	-	0	-	-	-	1	-	-	-
2	1	1	2	0	-	1	-	0	0	2	1	2	2	17	4	-	24
0	1	-	-	0	1	-	0	0	2	2	2	-	-	-	-	-	-
0	0	-	-	-	-	-	0	0	0	0	0	-	-	-	-	-	-
2	3	9	10	3	3	2	4	0	3	2	4	2	0	-	3	-	-
0	0	-	-	-	-	-	-	0	0	-	0	-	-	-	-	-	-
0	0	-	-	-	-	0	-	0	0	-	-	-	-	-	-	-	-
1	1	1	-	0	0	3	1	0	1	-	0	-	-	-	-	-	-
1	1	1	1	2	1	1	0	0	2	0	1	1	-	-	-	-	-
1	0	-	1	0	1	-	-	1	-	0	-	-	-	-	-	-	-
80	77	500	508	158	161	60	73	38	38	5	4	-	3	2	4	-	-
66	95	11	15	31	34	28	34	39	44	87	118	205	267	216	284	327	301
57	123	89	96	68	105	67	181	58	171	39	99	56	66	35	42	36	20
4	4	43	43	5	4	1	1	1	0	0	0	-	-	-	-	-	-
7	6	56	57	13	12	1	4	1	2	0	-	-	1	1	-	-	-
26	27	225	233	46	49	4	14	5	9	2	2	1	1	2	2	-	-
10	6	2	1	12	8	12	9	14	8	6	3	2	4	2	5	-	2
-	0	-	-	-	-	-	-	-	0	-	-	-	-	-	-	-	-
5	4	33	18	10	12	2	3	2	2	1	1	-	1	-	1	-	2
-	0	-	-	-	-	-	-	-	0	-	0	-	-	-	-	-	-
12	10	107	70	11	9	5	8	5	6	2	5	-	1	-	1	6	2
16	18	6	1	24	22	68	85	10	11	1	2	-	3	-	-	-	-
0	0	-	1	-	1	-	0	0	-	-	-	-	-	-	1	-	-
266	295	252	255	804	902	339	446	179	229	100	114	82	68	56	71	42	26
69	88	395	365	123	143	35	88	33	70	23	42	21	28	16	24	18	33

Table 25 - *continued*

Disease group	Persons, by age group								
	Total	0-4	5-15	16-24	25-44	45-64	65-74	75-84	85 and over
Other rickettsioses (083)	0	-	0	-	0	-	-	-	-
Malaria (084)	1	1	0	0	1	1	1	-	4
Relapsing fever (087)	0	-	-	-	0	-	0	-	-
Congenital syphilis (090)	0	0	-	-	-	0	-	-	-
Neurosyphilis (094)	0	-	-	-	-	1	-	-	3
Other and unspecified syphilis (097)	0	-	-	0	-	-	-	-	-
Gonococcal infections (098)	1	0	-	2	1	-	0	0	1
Other venereal diseases (099)	7	1	1	15	9	5	6	2	-
Leptospirosis (100)	0	-	-	0	0	0	-	-	-
Vincent's angina (101)	0	1	1	-	0	1	1	0	-
Yaws (102)	0	-	-	-	-	-	-	0	-
Dermatophytosis (110)	184	136	225	196	196	178	176	109	74
Dermatomycosis, other and unspecified (111)	22	9	18	45	28	14	11	7	1
Candidiasis (112)	411	699	93	642	629	228	185	180	166
Other mycoses (117)	1	1	0	1	0	2	0	0	-
Echinococcosis (122)	0	-	-	0	0	0	-	-	-
Other cestode infection (123)	0	0	0	0	0	-	-	-	-
Filarial infection and dracontiasis (125)	0	1	0	0	0	0	-	-	-
Other intestinal helminthiases (127)	44	175	145	25	25	5	2	1	4
Other and unspecified helminthiases (128)	1	3	2	1	0	-	-	-	-
Toxoplasmosis (130)	0	-	-	-	0	-	1	-	-
Trichomoniasis (131)	4	-	0	4	7	3	1	-	-
Pediculosis and phthirus infestation (132)	32	81	116	27	21	3	1	3	6
Acariasis (133)	42	63	72	74	34	22	11	27	58
Sarcoidosis (135)	3	-	-	0	4	6	4	1	-
Other and unspecified infectious and parasitic diseases (136)	20	113	32	11	11	12	5	8	-
Late effects of acute poliomyelitis (138)	0	0	-	-	0	1	-	1	-
Late effects of other infectious and parasitic diseases (139)	0	-	0	-	-	0	-	-	-
Malignant neoplasm of lip (140)	0	-	-	-	-	-	-	0	-
Malignant neoplasm of tongue (141)	2	-	-	-	-	3	7	6	-
Malignant neoplasm of major salivary glands (142)	1	-	-	-	-	1	2	5	3
Malignant neoplasm of gum (143)	0	-	-	-	1	0	1	5	1
Malignant neoplasm of floor of mouth (144)	0	-	-	-	0	0	-	-	-
Malignant neoplasm of other and unspecified parts of mouth (145)	0	-	-	-	0	0	1	-	-
Malignant neoplasm of oropharynx (146)	0	-	-	-	-	1	0	0	-
Malignant neoplasm of nasopharynx (147)	0	-	-	-	-	0	1	-	-
Malignant neoplasm of other and ill-defined sites within the lip,oral cavity and pharynx (149)	0	-	-	-	-	0	3	-	-
Malignant neoplasm of oesophagus (150)	10	-	-	-	1	8	45	69	37
Malignant neoplasm of stomach (151)	10	-	-	-	-	10	36	91	52
Malignant neoplasm of small intestine, including duodenum (152)	0	-	-	-	-	-	1	-	-
Malignant neoplasm of colon (153)	18	-	0	0	1	28	67	107	61
Malignant neoplasm of rectum, rectosigmoid junction and anus (154)	11	-	-	-	1	13	41	72	67
Malignant neoplasm of liver and intrahepatic bile ducts (155)	1	-	-	-	1	2	0	1	1
Malignant neoplasm of gallbladder and extrahepatic bile ducts (156)	0	-	-	-	-	1	-	3	-
Malignant neoplasm of pancreas (157)	4	-	-	-	-	2	21	24	31
Malignant neoplasm of other and ill-defined sites within the digestive organs and peritoneum (159)	0	-	-	-	-	0	1	-	-

By age-group and sex

Total		0-4		5-15		16-24		25-44		45-64		65-74		75-84		85 and over	
Male	Female	Male	Female	Male	Female	Male	Female	Male	Female	Male	Female	Male	Female	Male	Female	Male	Female
0	-	-	-	0	-	-	-	0	-	-	-	-	-	-	-	-	-
1	1	2	-	0	-	-	0	1	1	1	1	1	-	-	-	18	-
0	0	-	-	-	-	-	-	-	0	-	-	1	-	-	-	-	-
0	0	-	1	-	-	-	-	-	-	0	-	-	-	-	-	-	-
0	0	-	-	-	-	-	-	-	-	1	-	-	-	-	-	-	4
0	-	-	-	-	-	0	-	-	-	-	-	-	-	-	-	-	-
1	1	1	-	-	-	3	2	1	1	-	-	-	0	1	-	-	2
10	3	2	-	2	1	24	7	14	4	8	2	3	8	2	1	-	-
0	0	-	-	-	-	0	-	-	0	-	0	-	-	-	-	-	-
0	1	1	1	1	0	-	-	-	1	0	1	-	1	1	-	-	-
0	-	-	-	-	-	-	-	-	-	-	-	-	-	1	-	-	-
215	155	143	128	237	213	214	178	238	153	201	155	236	127	140	90	83	71
20	23	9	8	15	21	33	58	25	31	16	11	16	8	5	8	-	2
120	690	572	832	39	149	86	1,195	98	1,164	73	385	117	240	148	200	149	171
0	1	1	1	-	1	1	0	0	0	1	2	-	0	-	1	-	-
-	0	-	-	-	-	-	0	-	0	-	0	-	-	-	-	-	-
0	0	-	1	1	-	-	0	-	0	-	-	-	-	-	-	-	-
0	0	1	-	0	0	-	0	-	0	0	-	-	-	-	-	-	-
35	54	146	205	111	179	17	33	15	35	5	6	1	3	1	1	-	6
1	1	2	4	2	3	1	0	0	0	-	-	-	-	-	-	-	-
0	0	-	-	-	-	-	-	0	0	-	-	-	1	-	-	-	-
1	7	-	-	-	1	1	7	1	14	0	7	-	2	-	-	-	-
22	43	64	98	68	167	21	32	12	29	3	4	-	2	2	3	-	8
36	47	67	59	63	81	58	89	29	39	17	27	9	12	18	31	30	67
3	3	-	-	-	-	0	-	5	3	4	8	3	6	-	2	-	-
21	20	120	105	32	31	10	11	9	13	13	11	5	4	5	10	-	-
1	0	1	-	-	-	-	-	0	1	2	0	-	-	-	1	-	-
0	0	-	-	0	-	-	-	-	-	-	0	-	-	-	-	-	-
0	-	-	-	-	-	-	-	-	-	-	-	-	-	1	-	-	-
2	1	-	-	-	-	-	-	-	-	6	0	8	6	-	10	-	-
1	1	-	-	-	-	-	-	-	-	1	1	2	2	9	2	-	4
1	0	-	-	-	-	-	-	-	1	-	0	1	0	13	-	-	2
0	0	-	-	-	-	-	-	0	-	-	0	-	-	-	-	-	-
0	0	-	-	-	-	-	-	-	1	0	-	-	1	-	-	-	-
0	0	-	-	-	-	-	-	-	-	1	0	1	-	-	1	-	-
-	0	-	-	-	-	-	-	-	-	-	1	-	1	-	-	-	-
1	0	-	-	-	-	-	-	-	-	0	0	7	-	-	-	-	-
14	6	-	-	-	-	-	-	3	-	11	4	57	35	148	23	65	28
17	4	-	-	-	-	-	-	-	-	17	3	69	10	175	40	172	12
0	-	-	-	-	-	-	-	-	-	-	-	2	-	-	-	-	-
16	20	-	-	-	0	-	1	1	2	25	31	83	53	84	122	53	63
15	7	-	-	-	-	-	-	1	1	15	10	58	26	160	18	119	49
0	1	-	-	-	-	-	-	-	2	1	2	1	-	2	-	-	2
0	0	-	-	-	-	-	-	-	-	1	1	-	-	5	1	-	-
3	5	-	-	-	-	-	-	-	-	3	2	8	32	22	25	89	12
0	0	-	-	-	-	-	-	-	-	0	-	-	2	-	-	-	-

Table 25 - *continued*

Disease group	Persons, by age group								
	Total	0-4	5-15	16-24	25-44	45-64	65-74	75-84	85 and over
Malignant neoplasm of nasal cavities, middle ear and accessory sinuses (160)	0	-	-	-	-	-	-	2	-
Malignant neoplasm of larynx (161)	2	-	-	-	0	7	6	3	-
Malignant neoplasm of trachea, bronchus and lung (162)	30	-	-	1	1	47	133	140	105
Malignant neoplasm of pleura (163)	0	-	-	-	-	-	0	-	-
Malignant neoplasm of thymus, heart and mediastinum (164)	0	-	-	-	-	-	1	-	-
Malignant neoplasm of bone and articular cartilage (170)	1	1	1	-	1	0	2	3	-
Malignant neoplasm of connective and other soft tissue (171)	0	-	0	1	-	0	1	1	-
Malignant melanoma of skin (172)	4	-	0	2	3	10	6	8	18
Other malignant neoplasm of skin (173)	10	-	-	0	1	12	36	69	68
Malignant neoplasm of female breast (174)	40	-	-	-	12	87	103	144	145
Malignant neoplasm of male breast (175)	0	-	-	-	-	-	3	1	-
Malignant neoplasm of uterus, part unspecified (179)	1	-	-	-	-	1	4	3	6
Malignant neoplasm of cervix uteri (180)	6	-	-	-	8	6	15	25	4
Malignant neoplasm of body of uterus (182)	2	-	-	-	0	4	11	10	1
Malignant neoplasm of ovary and other uterine adnexa (183)	7	2	2	1	1	24	10	10	15
Malignant neoplasm of other and unspecified female genital organs(184)	1	-	-	-	0	0	2	7	-
Malignant neoplasm of prostate (185)	21	-	-	-	-	17	79	174	167
Malignant neoplasm of testis (186)	2	-	-	1	3	2	-	0	-
Malignant neoplasm of penis and other male genital organs (187)	0	-	-	-	-	0	2	0	-
Malignant neoplasm of bladder (188)	11	-	-	-	0	13	42	74	107
Malignant neoplasm of kidney and other and unspecified urinary organs (189)	6	-	-	-	4	7	19	32	1
Malignant neoplasm of eye (190)	0	0	-	-	0	-	1	-	-
Malignant neoplasm of brain (191)	5	-	0	1	5	6	16	8	-
Malignant neoplasm of other and unspecified parts of nervous system (192)	0	-	-	-	-	1	0	-	-
Malignant neoplasm of thyroid gland (193)	1	-	-	-	1	3	3	3	-
Malignant neoplasm of other endocrine glands and related structures (194)	0	-	-	-	-	-	-	3	-
Malignant neoplasm of other and ill-defined sites (195)	11	-	-	0	1	16	39	69	62
Secondary and unspecified malignant neoplasm of lymph nodes (196)	1	-	-	-	0	2	4	1	1
Secondary malignant neoplasm of respiratory and digestive systems (197)	10	2	0	-	2	9	43	61	30
Secondary malignant neoplasm of other specified sites (198)	13	-	-	-	2	20	69	33	64
Malignant neoplasm without specification of site (199)	7	-	-	-	2	6	34	34	19
Lymphosarcoma and reticulosarcoma (200)	0	-	-	-	1	1	1	0	1
Hodgkin's disease (201)	1	-	0	1	1	2	2	2	-
Other malignant neoplasm of lymphoid and histiocytic tissue (202)	1	0	0	1	0	2	4	2	-
Multiple myeloma and immunoproliferative neoplasms (203)	2	-	-	-	0	3	7	17	3
Lymphoid leukaemia (204)	3	6	1	1	0	3	12	15	7
Myeloid leukaemia (205)	2	-	-	0	1	2	10	4	-
Monocytic leukaemia (206)	0	-	-	-	-	0	-	0	1
Other specified leukaemia (207)	0	1	-	0	0	-	2	0	1
Leukaemia of unspecified cell type (208)	2	-	-	1	1	3	9	10	3
Benign neoplasm of lip, oral cavity and pharynx (210)	2	0	1	2	2	2	2	3	-
Benign neoplasm of other parts of digestive system (211)	2	2	0	0	1	3	4	5	4
Benign neoplasm of respiratory and intrathoracic organs (212)	0	-	-	-	0	1	1	0	-

By age-group and sex

Total		0-4		5-15		16-24		25-44		45-64		65-74		75-84		85 and over	
Male	Female	Male	Female	Male	Female	Male	Female	Male	Female	Male	Female	Male	Female	Male	Female	Male	Female
-	0	-	-	-	-	-	-	-	-	-	-	-	-	-	3	-	-
3	1	-	-	-	-	-	-	0	0	11	3	7	5	7	-	-	-
39	21	-	-	-	-	1	-	3	0	56	38	191	85	247	75	267	51
-	0	-	-	-	-	-	-	-	-	-	-	-	0	-	-	-	-
0	-	-	-	-	-	-	-	-	-	-	-	1	-	-	-	-	-
1	1	-	1	1	1	-	-	1	0	0	0	2	3	8	-	-	-
0	0	-	-	-	0	3	-	-	-	-	0	-	2	-	1	-	-
3	6	-	-	1	-	1	2	3	3	6	14	6	7	10	7	-	24
9	12	-	-	-	-	0	-	1	2	11	13	35	37	73	66	65	69
-	78	-	-	-	-	-	-	-	25	-	176	-	186	-	231	-	193
1	-	-	-	-	-	-	-	-	-	-	-	-	6	-	2	-	-
-	1	-	-	-	-	-	-	-	-	-	2	-	7	-	5	-	8
-	12	-	-	-	-	-	-	-	15	-	11	-	27	-	40	-	6
-	5	-	-	-	-	-	-	-	0	-	8	-	20	-	16	-	2
-	14	-	4	-	3	-	1	-	2	-	49	-	18	-	16	-	20
-	1	-	-	-	-	-	-	-	0	-	1	-	3	-	11	-	-
43	-	-	-	-	-	-	-	-	-	34	-	176	-	465	-	671	-
3	-	-	-	-	-	2	-	6	-	4	-	-	-	1	-	-	-
0	-	-	-	-	-	-	-	-	-	0	-	3	-	1	-	-	-
18	5	-	-	-	-	-	-	0	-	21	4	82	10	149	29	256	57
6	5	-	-	-	-	-	-	7	-	8	6	12	24	39	27	6	-
0	0	-	1	-	-	-	-	0	1	-	-	1	-	-	-	-	-
5	4	-	-	0	-	2	-	6	3	7	4	18	15	5	10	-	-
0	0	-	-	-	-	-	-	-	-	1	0	-	0	-	-	-	-
1	2	-	-	-	-	-	-	0	1	2	3	2	4	-	5	-	-
0	-	-	-	-	-	-	-	-	-	-	-	-	-	-	7	-	-
12	11	-	-	-	-	0	-	1	1	18	13	46	34	93	55	71	59
0	1	-	-	-	-	-	-	1	-	1	3	1	7	1	1	-	2
12	8	5	-	-	0	-	-	1	4	10	9	68	23	89	44	77	14
9	17	-	-	-	-	-	-	0	4	7	33	53	81	55	21	155	33
6	7	-	-	-	-	-	-	2	2	5	7	45	25	17	44	42	12
1	0	-	-	-	-	-	-	1	-	1	1	1	-	1	-	-	2
1	1	-	-	0	-	0	1	1	1	2	1	3	1	1	2	-	-
1	1	-	1	0	0	1	1	-	1	2	2	7	1	-	3	-	-
2	2	-	-	-	-	-	-	-	0	3	4	12	2	16	18	12	-
4	3	7	4	1	1	1	-	1	0	4	3	18	7	16	15	24	2
2	2	-	-	-	-	-	0	0	2	3	1	16	6	8	1	-	-
0	0	-	-	-	-	-	-	-	-	0	-	-	-	-	1	-	2
1	0	1	1	-	-	-	0	0	-	-	-	4	-	-	1	6	-
3	2	-	-	-	-	1	1	2	1	3	4	9	9	18	5	-	4
2	1	1	-	1	-	2	2	2	2	3	2	2	2	2	3	-	-
2	2	-	3	-	0	-	1	1	1	4	2	3	4	6	4	-	6
0	0	-	-	-	-	-	-	1	-	0	2	1	-	-	1	-	-

Table 25 - *continued*

Disease group	Persons, by age group								
	Total	0-4	5-15	16-24	25-44	45-64	65-74	75-84	85 and over
Benign neoplasm of bone and articular cartilage (213)	2	1	1	2	2	2	2	-	-
Lipoma (214)	24	4	4	14	32	40	28	18	10
Other benign neoplasm of connective and other soft tissue (215)	4	2	1	4	7	4	2	2	-
Benign neoplasm of skin (216)	92	23	66	93	117	108	93	49	37
Benign neoplasm of breast (217)	8	0	0	9	17	8	2	0	-
Uterine leiomyoma (218)	9	-	-	0	17	19	0	0	1
Other benign neoplasm of uterus (219)	0	-	-	-	0	0	0	-	-
Benign neoplasm of ovary (220)	1	-	-	1	2	1	1	1	-
Benign neoplasm of other female genital organs (221)	0	1	-	0	1	0	0	0	-
Benign neoplasm of male genital organs (222)	1	-	-	0	1	1	2	1	-
Benign neoplasm of kidney and other urinary organs (223)	1	-	-	0	0	1	3	7	-
Benign neoplasm of eye (224)	0	-	-	0	0	1	1	-	-
Benign neoplasm of brain and other parts of nervous system (225)	2	-	0	0	3	3	7	1	-
Benign neoplasm of thyroid gland (226)	1	-	0	0	1	2	0	1	1
Benign neoplasm of other endocrine glands and related structures (227)	0	-	-	0	0	1	-	-	-
Haemangioma and lymphangioma, any site (228)	5	14	4	4	5	5	5	3	6
Benign neoplasm of other and unspecified sites (229)	2	1	1	2	3	2	3	1	21
Carcinoma in situ of digestive organs (230)	7	-	-	0	1	9	22	42	49
Carcinoma in situ of respiratory system (231)	3	-	-	-	-	2	24	9	1
Carcinoma in situ of skin (232)	0	-	-	-	-	0	0	4	-
Carcinoma in situ of breast and genitourinary system (233)	7	-	-	0	3	10	29	18	37
Carcinoma in situ of other and unspecified sites (234)	0	-	-	-	-	0	1	3	-
Neoplasm of uncertain behaviour of digestive and respiratory systems (235)	1	0	-	1	0	2	5	4	1
Neoplasm of uncertain behaviour of genitourinary organs (236)	1	-	-	1	1	1	2	3	3
Neoplasm of uncertain behaviour of endocrine glands and nervous system (237)	2	1	1	2	2	2	2	2	-
Neoplasm of uncertain behaviour of other and unspecified sites and tissues (238)	4	-	0	0	2	6	12	15	22
Neoplasm of unspecified nature (239)	45	12	24	20	35	54	103	129	93
Simple and unspecified goitre (240)	6	-	1	6	8	8	7	3	9
Nontoxic nodular goitre (241)	3	-	-	0	4	5	2	3	12
Thyrotoxicosis with or without goitre (242)	19	-	-	5	23	27	52	27	21
Congenital hypothyroidism (243)	1	2	1	1	1	1	0	-	-
Acquired hypothyroidism (244)	95	1	3	12	51	175	271	271	308
Thyroiditis (245)	2	-	0	0	3	4	6	1	-
Other disorders of thyroid (246)	2	-	-	1	2	4	5	2	3
Diabetes mellitus (250)	274	2	11	45	100	470	945	1,019	567
Other disorders of pancreatic internal secretion (251)	6	2	1	4	5	8	13	26	7
Disorders of parathyroid gland (252)	1	-	-	1	1	2	5	4	9
Disorders of the pituitary gland and its hypothalamic control (253)	3	-	1	0	5	4	1	2	4
Disorders of adrenal glands (255)	2	2	0	0	2	1	3	3	1
Ovarian dysfunction (256)	8	-	0	10	18	7	-	-	-
Testicular dysfunction (257)	1	-	0	1	1	1	-	-	-
Polyglandular dysfunction and related disorders (258)	0	-	-	-	0	-	-	-	-
Other endocrine disorders (259)	1	0	5	1	0	1	1	-	-

By age-group and sex

Total		0-4		5-15		16-24		25-44		45-64		65-74		75-84		85 and over	
Male	Female	Male	Female	Male	Female	Male	Female	Male	Female	Male	Female	Male	Female	Male	Female	Male	Female
2	2	1	1	2	1	2	2	2	2	1	4	4	0	-	-	-	-
24	24	3	4	5	3	15	13	35	29	37	43	21	33	11	22	6	12
3	5	2	3	1	1	2	6	6	8	5	4	1	3	-	3	-	-
69	114	24	22	62	71	59	127	72	163	87	129	99	89	46	51	18	43
0	16	1	-	-	1	0	18	-	34	0	15	-	3	-	1	-	-
-	18	-	-	-	-	-	0	-	34	-	39	-	0	-	1	-	2
-	1	-	-	-	-	-	-	-	1	-	1	-	0	-	-	-	-
-	2	-	-	-	-	-	1	-	4	-	2	-	1	-	1	-	-
-	1	-	2	-	-	-	0	-	2	-	1	-	0	-	1	-	-
1	-	-	-	-	-	1	-	2	-	2	-	5	-	3	-	-	-
1	1	-	-	-	-	-	0	0	0	1	1	5	2	6	8	-	-
1	0	-	-	-	-	0	-	1	0	1	1	1	1	-	-	-	-
2	3	-	-	-	1	-	1	2	3	3	3	2	11	1	1	-	-
0	2	-	-	-	0	-	1	0	2	0	4	-	0	-	1	-	2
0	0	-	-	-	-	-	1	-	1	2	-	-	-	-	-	-	-
4	6	11	17	3	6	1	6	3	7	4	7	6	4	-	5	24	-
2	2	2	-	1	1	2	2	3	2	2	2	2	4	1	1	-	28
5	8	-	-	-	-	0	-	1	0	4	13	32	15	37	44	59	45
4	2	-	-	-	-	-	-	-	-	4	-	30	19	19	2	6	-
0	0	-	-	-	-	-	-	-	-	0	0	-	0	1	5	-	-
3	11	-	-	-	-	-	1	0	6	2	18	24	33	6	25	30	39
0	0	-	-	-	-	-	-	-	-	-	0	2	0	5	3	-	-
2	1	-	1	-	-	0	1	-	0	3	1	9	1	6	3	-	2
1	1	-	-	-	-	1	1	1	0	1	1	3	0	9	-	12	-
2	1	2	1	2	0	2	1	2	2	3	2	3	1	5	-	-	-
4	4	-	-	1	-	0	-	2	2	6	6	13	11	14	16	18	24
35	55	9	16	27	21	17	24	22	47	38	70	102	103	106	142	113	87
1	11	-	-	0	2	-	11	1	15	1	15	5	9	1	5	-	12
1	5	-	-	-	-	-	0	0	8	0	10	3	1	2	3	36	4
7	32	-	-	-	-	2	8	5	41	9	46	29	71	8	38	24	20
1	1	2	1	1	1	1	1	1	1	-	2	-	0	-	-	-	-
21	166	-	2	-	7	2	22	9	93	33	320	76	429	92	378	178	351
1	4	-	-	-	1	-	1	1	5	1	8	5	7	-	1	-	-
1	4	-	-	-	-	0	2	1	4	2	7	-	9	-	3	-	4
292	256	1	3	12	10	55	35	113	86	544	394	1,053	858	1,164	932	778	496
6	7	2	1	0	1	4	4	5	5	8	8	12	13	21	29	18	4
0	2	-	-	-	-	2	-	1	1	-	4	1	9	-	6	-	12
4	2	-	-	1	2	1	-	7	3	5	3	-	1	3	1	-	6
1	2	-	5	-	1	1	-	1	3	0	1	5	2	-	4	-	2
-	17	-	-	-	1	-	20	-	37	-	14	-	-	-	-	-	-
2	-	-	-	1	-	1	-	3	-	3	-	-	-	-	-	-	-
-	0	-	-	-	-	-	-	-	0	-	-	-	-	-	-	-	-
1	1	-	1	2	8	1	0	0	1	1	0	3	-	-	-	-	-

Table 25 - *continued*

Disease group	Persons, by age group								
	Total	0-4	5-15	16-24	25-44	45-64	65-74	75-84	85 and over
Nutritional marasmus (261)	0	0	-	-	-	-	2	0	3
Vitamin A deficiency (264)	0	1	0	-	-	-	1	-	-
Thiamine and niacin deficiency states (265)	0	-	-	-	0	0	1	0	-
Deficiency of B-complex components (266)	2	0	0	0	1	3	5	13	24
Ascorbic acid deficiency (267)	0	-	-	-	0	-	1	-	1
Vitamin D deficiency (268)	0	1	0	0	1	-	0	-	-
Other nutritional deficiencies (269)	1	1	3	-	1	0	2	2	3
Disorders of amino-acid transport and metabolism (270)	0	1	1	1	0	0	1	-	-
Disorders of carbohydrate transport and metabolism (271)	4	49	0	0	0	0	-	1	1
Disorders of lipoid metabolism (272)	75	0	2	7	41	219	167	18	-
Disorders of plasma protein metabolism (273)	0	-	-	-	0	0	1	1	4
Gout (274)	68	-	0	1	39	130	210	181	158
Disorders of mineral metabolism (275)	3	1	0	1	1	5	10	10	7
Disorders of fluid, electrolyte, and acid-base balance (276)	20	7	1	7	19	29	39	42	78
Other and unspecified disorders of metabolism (277)	5	14	8	5	4	2	4	2	1
Obesity and other hyperalimentation (278)	105	5	20	72	130	188	129	41	7
Disorders involving the immune mechanism (279)	1	1	-	-	0	1	0	6	-
Iron deficiency anaemias (280)	84	30	16	48	69	85	148	316	432
Other deficiency anaemias (281)	23	2	-	2	6	25	70	146	178
Hereditary haemolytic anaemias (282)	1	1	3	1	2	1	1	1	-
Acquired haemolytic anaemias (283)	1	1	0	0	0	1	4	1	1
Aplastic anaemia (284)	0	-	-	-	0	0	2	1	6
Other and unspecified anaemias (285)	21	8	4	10	15	19	48	83	101
Coagulation defects (286)	1	2	2	-	1	1	2	-	-
Purpura and other haemorrhagic conditions (287)	8	7	16	4	4	7	15	20	15
Diseases of white blood cells (288)	1	0	0	1	1	1	2	0	-
Other diseases of blood and blood-forming organs (289)	11	26	41	4	3	4	5	15	4
Senile and presenile organic psychotic conditions (290)	37	0	-	-	0	6	59	370	888
Alcoholic psychoses (291)	3	-	-	1	4	4	3	-	4
Drug psychoses (292)	4	-	-	4	8	4	4	1	4
Transient organic psychotic conditions (293)	15	-	1	1	3	6	28	113	291
Other organic psychotic conditions (chronic) (294)	4	-	-	0	2	2	1	31	71
Schizophrenic psychoses (295)	39	-	0	20	48	80	39	27	15
Affective psychoses (296)	167	-	3	79	184	282	264	304	277
Paranoid states (297)	12	-	-	9	11	14	16	36	96
Other nonorganic psychoses (298)	9	-	-	5	15	12	8	16	12
Psychoses with origin specific to childhood (299)	0	0	1	1	1	-	-	-	-
Neurotic disorders (300)	707	18	64	544	917	1,040	909	827	713
Personality disorders (301)	32	1	1	25	36	51	36	50	49
Sexual deviations and disorders (302)	22	-	-	13	25	46	30	6	1
Alcohol dependence syndrome (303)	32	-	-	8	55	60	13	14	1
Drug dependence (304)	94	-	1	108	192	69	64	28	25
Nondependent abuse of drugs (305)	22	-	2	20	35	34	13	7	6
Physiological malfunction arising from mental factors (306)	13	4	10	17	15	13	12	12	13
Special symptoms or syndromes not elsewhere classified (307)	128	124	84	111	113	144	181	188	305
Acute reaction to stress (308)	37	1	3	37	64	50	17	9	3
Adjustment reaction (309)	65	-	2	26	63	97	149	160	96
Specific nonpsychotic mental disorders following organic brain damage (310)	6	1	2	6	4	6	13	27	16
Depressive disorder, not elsewhere classified (311)	280	0	9	184	352	446	357	379	326

By age-group and sex

Total		0-4		5-15		16-24		25-44		45-64		65-74		75-84		85 and over	
Male	Female	Male	Female	Male	Female	Male	Female	Male	Female	Male	Female	Male	Female	Male	Female	Male	Female
0	0	1	-	-	-	-	-	-	-	-	-	-	4	1	-	-	4
-	0	-	1	-	0	-	-	-	-	-	-	-	2	-	-	-	-
0	0	-	-	-	-	-	-	0	-	-	0	1	1	-	1	-	-
1	3	1	-	-	0	-	1	-	2	2	3	2	8	23	8	12	28
0	0	-	-	-	-	-	-	-	0	-	-	1	-	-	-	-	2
0	0	-	2	-	0	1	-	1	1	-	-	-	0	-	-	-	-
1	1	1	1	5	2	-	-	-	1	-	0	2	2	-	3	-	4
1	0	2	1	2	-	0	1	0	0	0	0	-	1	-	-	-	-
4	3	53	45	1	-	-	0	0	1	0	0	-	-	-	2	-	2
74	75	1	-	2	3	6	7	59	23	209	230	118	207	16	20	-	-
0	0	-	-	-	-	-	-	-	0	0	-	1	-	-	1	18	-
110	29	-	-	1	-	0	2	73	5	221	39	340	105	289	117	273	120
2	4	1	-	0	0	0	1	0	1	3	8	7	13	3	14	-	10
6	33	9	6	1	1	0	14	1	37	7	51	20	55	31	49	77	79
5	4	7	21	11	5	5	4	5	2	2	1	5	3	1	3	-	2
45	162	5	4	13	28	15	128	47	213	89	289	80	169	19	53	-	10
0	1	1	1	-	-	-	-	-	1	1	2	1	-	-	10	-	-
34	131	30	31	17	15	4	92	6	134	33	138	131	162	194	390	428	433
16	30	1	3	-	-	0	4	3	9	17	33	58	80	137	150	244	156
1	2	-	2	4	2	1	1	1	2	1	1	-	1	1	1	-	-
1	1	1	-	0	-	1	-	-	0	1	0	6	3	2	-	-	2
0	1	-	-	-	-	-	-	-	1	0	0	1	2	1	1	-	8
8	32	9	7	2	5	1	19	2	28	7	32	36	58	58	98	36	122
1	1	3	1	4	0	-	-	1	0	0	1	1	3	-	-	-	-
8	9	10	3	14	18	1	7	2	6	6	7	15	16	30	14	42	6
1	1	-	1	-	1	1	1	0	1	1	1	1	2	-	1	-	-
10	12	22	30	35	47	3	5	2	3	6	3	8	3	10	18	6	4
23	51	-	1	-	-	-	-	-	0	8	5	52	64	294	415	856	898
4	2	-	-	-	-	1	1	6	2	6	2	3	3	-	-	6	4
3	5	-	-	-	-	5	2	6	10	1	6	3	5	1	1	-	6
11	18	-	-	1	-	0	2	2	4	9	3	31	26	113	114	279	296
2	5	-	-	-	-	-	0	2	1	0	3	-	2	19	38	48	79
44	34	-	-	0	-	30	11	62	33	77	83	45	34	7	38	18	14
101	231	-	-	3	3	57	00	95	272	187	379	148	359	239	342	273	278
11	14	-	-	-	-	13	6	17	5	8	21	9	23	24	43	18	122
6	13	-	-	-	-	3	7	8	22	10	14	2	13	21	14	-	16
1	0	1	-	1	0	1	0	1	0	-	-	-	-	-	-	-	-
424	979	18	18	48	81	325	761	524	1,313	656	1,431	577	1,178	499	1,023	440	804
30	33	-	1	2	1	34	17	35	37	48	55	31	39	26	64	42	51
33	12	-	-	-	-	14	12	27	24	78	13	64	2	15	-	-	2
51	14	-	-	-	-	12	3	90	20	90	29	13	13	19	11	-	2
110	79	-	-	1	2	146	70	241	142	58	80	23	96	24	30	18	28
28	16	-	-	2	2	27	14	42	28	42	26	20	6	13	3	12	4
9	17	4	4	4	15	9	24	10	20	10	17	13	11	10	13	-	18
89	166	125	124	90	78	60	163	64	162	101	187	137	216	139	217	190	343
26	48	1	-	2	5	24	51	45	83	37	63	8	25	3	12	6	2
30	99	-	-	2	3	9	42	30	97	43	152	71	211	100	196	83	100
6	6	1	-	2	3	6	5	5	3	6	5	15	11	21	31	6	20
160	395	1	-	7	12	84	283	170	536	300	595	240	451	239	462	315	329

Table 25 - *continued*

Disease group	Persons, by age group								
	Total	0-4	5-15	16-24	25-44	45-64	65-74	75-84	85 and over
Disturbance of conduct not elsewhere classified (312)	18	47	51	14	10	3	4	16	44
Disturbance of emotions specific to childhood and adolescence (313)	2	4	8	3	0	-	-	-	-
Hyperkinetic syndrome of childhood (314)	1	15	4	-	-	-	-	-	-
Specific delays in development (315)	6	60	11	2	0	1	0	0	-
Mild mental retardation (317)	1	-	0	2	1	0	0	-	-
Other specified mental retardation (318)	1	-	1	4	1	1	1	-	1
Unspecified mental retardation (319)	2	1	0	3	1	3	1	-	-
Bacterial meningitis (320)	0	2	0	0	0	0	-	0	-
Meningitis of unspecified cause (322)	2	5	1	1	2	2	0	-	-
Encephalitis, myelitis and encephalomyelitis (323)	2	-	0	1	3	4	1	3	-
Intracranial and intraspinal abscess (324)	0	-	0	0	0	0	-	-	-
Phlebitis and thrombophlebitis of intracranial venous sinuses (325)	0	-	-	-	0	0	0	1	-
Cerebral degenerations usually manifest in childhood (330)	0	2	0	0	0	0	-	2	-
Other cerebral degenerations (331)	10	1	0	0	0	4	24	96	139
Parkinson's disease (332)	41	-	-	0	1	37	172	295	299
Other extrapyramidal disease and abnormal movement disorders (333)	18	2	6	9	14	27	48	29	27
Spinocerebellar disease (334)	2	-	0	-	1	4	4	6	-
Anterior horn cell disease (335)	2	-	-	-	1	4	8	8	1
Other diseases of spinal cord (336)	2	-	-	-	1	2	10	6	-
Disorders of autonomic nervous system (337)	1	-	-	-	0	2	4	0	-
Multiple sclerosis (340)	24	-	-	2	35	51	24	6	-
Other demyelinating diseases of central nervous system (341)	0	-	-	0	1	0	1	-	-
Hemiplegia (342)	6	0	0	1	2	8	16	34	70
Infantile cerebral palsy (343)	2	7	2	3	2	1	0	2	-
Other paralytic syndromes (344)	3	0	0	2	2	4	5	6	13
Epilepsy (345)	81	31	48	99	94	89	88	84	75
Migraine (346)	172	3	132	209	241	205	88	48	15
Cataplexy and narcolepsy (347)	0	-	-	0	0	0	1	-	-
Other conditions of brain (348)	4	0	1	1	6	9	3	2	1
Other and unspecified disorders of the nervous system (349)	2	-	0	1	2	3	2	1	-
Trigeminal nerve disorders (350)	17	1	1	3	13	29	47	54	21
Facial nerve disorders (351)	9	0	3	4	9	15	17	15	12
Disorders of other cranial nerves (352)	0	-	-	-	0	0	0	1	-
Nerve root and plexus disorders (353)	4	-	0	2	4	8	3	5	1
Mononeuritis of upper limb and mononeuritis multiplex (354)	32	-	0	11	41	60	38	45	34
Mononeuritis of lower limb (355)	4	-	0	2	3	8	5	7	1
Hereditary and idiopathic peripheral neuropathy (356)	1	-	-	-	1	2	3	5	4
Inflammatory and toxic neuropathy (357)	4	-	-	1	3	10	9	9	1
Myoneural disorders (358)	2	-	-	2	0	2	9	8	-
Muscular dystrophies and other myopathies (359)	2	0	2	0	2	5	4	1	1
Disorders of the globe (360)	0	0	-	0	1	0	-	0	4
Retinal detachments and defects (361)	3	-	0	1	2	7	7	6	-
Other retinal disorders (362)	16	0	1	1	3	18	47	104	123
Chorioretinal inflammations and scars and other disorders of choroid (363)	1	-	0	1	1	2	1	1	3
Disorders of iris and ciliary body (364)	7	1	1	6	8	12	8	15	7
Glaucoma (365)	31	-	0	-	4	42	116	183	169
Cataract (366)	46	1	1	2	2	28	169	371	448
Disorders of refraction and accommodation (367)	4	7	5	3	3	4	4	4	1
Visual disturbances (368)	25	7	18	10	16	32	57	69	74
Blindness and low vision (369)	9	3	2	2	3	7	22	50	108
Keratitis (370)	8	-	1	5	7	14	14	13	10

By age-group and sex

Total		0-4		5-15		16-24		25-44		45-64		65-74		75-84		85 and over	
Male	Female	Male	Female	Male	Female	Male	Female	Male	Female	Male	Female	Male	Female	Male	Female	Male	Female
23	12	64	28	70	32	21	7	11	9	3	3	4	4	22	13	71	35
1	2	2	6	6	10	1	4	-	0	-	-	-	-	-	-	-	-
2	1	22	6	5	2	-	-	-	-	-	-	-	-	-	-	-	-
8	4	74	46	16	6	2	2	1	-	1	1	1	-	-	1	-	-
1	1	-	-	-	0	1	2	2	1	0	0	-	0	-	-	-	-
1	1	-	-	0	1	5	4	2	1	1	1	-	2	-	-	-	2
2	1	1	-	0	-	4	3	2	1	5	1	-	1	-	-	-	-
0	1	2	3	-	1	-	0	0	0	0	0	-	-	-	1	-	-
2	1	7	3	1	0	2	-	1	2	1	2	-	0	-	-	-	-
2	2	-	-	1	0	0	1	4	2	3	4	2	-	5	1	-	-
0	0	-	-	-	1	0	-	0	0	0	-	-	-	-	-	-	-
0	0	-	-	-	-	-	-	0	0	-	0	-	0	2	1	-	-
1	0	2	2	1	-	1	-	-	0	0	-	-	-	3	1	-	-
7	12	1	-	0	-	0	-	0	0	5	4	22	26	100	94	95	154
42	40	-	-	-	-	0	-	1	1	45	29	181	165	421	220	362	278
14	22	3	1	5	7	8	10	10	18	20	35	40	55	27	30	-	35
2	1	-	-	0	-	-	-	1	1	6	1	7	2	5	6	-	-
2	2	-	-	-	-	-	-	2	0	5	3	8	9	10	6	-	2
2	1	-	-	-	-	-	-	1	1	3	1	13	8	10	4	-	-
1	1	-	-	-	-	-	-	0	0	0	3	8	-	-	1	-	-
17	30	-	-	-	-	1	3	20	50	46	56	10	35	11	2	-	-
0	0	-	-	-	-	0	-	1	1	-	0	2	-	-	-	-	-
6	7	-	1	0	0	0	2	1	3	11	5	22	12	33	35	71	69
2	2	10	4	2	2	2	4	2	3	1	2	1	-	1	2	-	-
4	2	-	1	0	-	5	-	4	1	4	4	8	2	11	2	6	16
81	82	29	33	47	48	95	103	89	99	99	78	84	92	85	83	107	65
86	255	4	3	118	148	88	329	100	382	89	324	64	107	41	51	6	18
0	0	-	-	-	-	0	-	0	0	0	0	-	1	-	-	-	-
2	6	1	-	0	2	-	2	3	9	5	13	3	4	1	3	6	-
2	2	-	-	0	-	0	1	2	2	4	3	2	1	3	-	-	-
12	23	1	1	2	0	2	3	8	17	20	37	37	55	35	66	18	22
9	9	1	-	3	4	2	6	9	8	16	14	16	18	24	10	-	16
0	0	-	-	-	-	-	-	-	0	-	0	1	-	1	1	-	-
3	4	-	-	-	1	1	3	3	5	8	8	3	3	6	5	-	2
17	47	-	-	-	0	3	19	17	65	32	89	37	38	41	47	36	33
4	4	-	-	0	0	3	1	3	4	7	8	3	7	7	7	6	-
1	1	-	-	-	-	-	-	1	1	3	1	1	4	8	3	18	-
5	3	-	-	-	-	1	1	4	2	12	7	15	4	7	10	-	2
2	2	-	-	-	-	-	5	-	1	1	3	12	7	18	2	-	-
2	2	-	1	2	1	-	0	1	4	6	3	6	3	-	2	-	2
0	1		-	-	-	0	0	0	1	0	0	-	-	-	1	6	4
3	3	-	-	0	-	1	1	2	2	7	7	8	6	5	8	-	2
13	18	-	1	0	1	1	-	3	4	20	15	41	52	89	112	137	118
1	1	-	-	-	1	-	1	1	0	2	2	3	-	2	1	12	-
6	8	1	1	1	1	5	8	8	8	8	16	3	11	22	10	18	4
27	35	-	-	-	0	-	-	5	3	43	41	114	119	161	196	208	156
34	57	1	1	0	1	2	1	4	1	30	26	136	195	318	402	475	439
4	4	7	6	6	4	3	3	3	3	5	4	2	5	8	2	-	2
25	25	8	6	19	16	13	7	14	18	35	29	55	59	79	62	59	79
7	11	2	4	1	3	3	2	3	4	7	7	22	23	53	48	95	112
8	8	-	-	1	2	8	2	7	7	11	18	15	12	11	14	36	2

Table 25 - *continued*

Disease group	Persons, by age group								
	Total	0-4	5-15	16-24	25-44	45-64	65-74	75-84	85 and over
Corneal opacity and other disorders of cornea (371)	3	0	0	3	3	5	3	8	4
Disorders of conjunctiva (372)	521	2,314	444	278	321	387	558	573	709
Inflammation of eyelids (373)	100	94	104	85	90	100	140	135	101
Other disorders of eyelids (374)	16	10	6	6	10	19	32	61	83
Disorders of lacrimal system (375)	36	21	4	4	13	45	133	137	144
Disorders of the orbit (376)	3	4	3	1	3	3	5	3	18
Disorders of optic nerve and visual pathways (377)	1	1	0	0	2	2	2	1	-
Strabismus and other disorders of binocular eye movements (378)	10	81	16	4	3	2	3	3	-
Other disorders of eye (379)	24	12	8	9	19	35	59	43	25
Disorders of external ear (380)	467	287	287	315	455	553	742	762	809
Nonsuppurative otitis media and Eustachian tube disorders (381)	507	3,155	1,076	218	218	152	115	71	55
Suppurative and unspecified otitis media (382)	252	1,680	523	88	94	74	68	45	28
Mastoiditis and related conditions (383)	2	2	1	3	1	3	2	3	-
Other disorders of tympanic membrane (384)	13	23	21	9	11	11	9	12	7
Other disorders of middle ear and mastoid (385)	1	0	0	1	2	1	3	2	1
Vertiginous syndromes and other disorders of vestibular system (386)	107	2	10	38	86	181	243	250	212
Otosclerosis (387)	1	-	0	0	2	1	1	-	-
Other disorders of ear (388)	134	321	223	71	86	114	144	143	181
Deafness (389)	47	52	45	14	23	49	91	155	206
Rheumatic fever without mention of heart involvement (390)	0	-	0	0	0	-	0	-	-
Rheumatic fever with heart involvement (391)	0	-	-	-	-	0	-	-	-
Rheumatic chorea (392)	0	-	-	-	0	-	-	-	-
Diseases of mitral valve (394)	6	-	0	-	1	16	22	15	7
Diseases of aortic valve (395)	2	0	-	-	0	3	5	6	4
Diseases of mitral and aortic valves (396)	0	-	-	-	0	1	2	-	1
Diseases of other endocardial structures (397)	0	-	-	-	-	0	-	-	-
Other rheumatic heart disease (398)	1	-	-	-	-	5	2	3	1
Essential hypertension (401)	1,012	1	1	16	238	2,032	3,950	3,280	1,361
Hypertensive heart disease (402)	14	-	0	1	3	31	46	51	19
Hypertensive renal disease (403)	4	-	0	-	7	5	6	1	-
Hypertensive heart and renal disease (404)	0	-	-	-	-	1	0	-	-
Secondary hypertension (405)	4	0	0	2	4	8	7	12	7
Acute myocardial infarction (410)	53	-	-	0	8	99	193	226	206
Other acute and subacute forms of ischaemic heart disease (411)	2	-	-	-	0	3	4	7	6
Old myocardial infarction (412)	11	-	-	-	1	23	53	35	15
Angina pectoris (413)	264	0	-	0	25	505	1,021	1,096	812
Other forms of chronic ischaemic heart disease (414)	97	-	0	0	10	182	383	395	314
Acute pulmonary heart disease (415)	11	-	-	1	4	17	37	49	56
Chronic pulmonary heart disease (416)	3	-	0	0	0	5	13	9	3
Other diseases of pulmonary circulation (417)	0	-	0		0	-	-	1	-
Acute pericarditis (420)	2	-	1	1	1	4	2	2	1
Acute and subacute endocarditis (421)	1	-	-	-	1	1	2	1	6
Acute myocarditis (422)	0	-	-	1	-	-	-	-	-
Other diseases of pericardium (423)	0	1	-	-	0	0	1	0	-
Other diseases of endocardium (424)	12	6	1	1	3	18	45	39	52
Cardiomyopathy (425)	4	-	0	0	1	9	14	10	-
Conduction disorders (426)	3	2	1	1	1	3	10	21	27
Cardiac dysrhythmias (427)	92	2	1	5	16	101	340	573	616
Heart failure (428)	231	2	0	1	2	107	736	1,894	3,650

By age-group and sex

Total		0-4		5-15		16-24		25-44		45-64		65-74		75-84		85 and over	
Male	Female	Male	Female	Male	Female	Male	Female	Male	Female	Male	Female	Male	Female	Male	Female	Male	Female
4	3	1	-	0	1	3	2	3	4	6	5	6	1	9	8	-	6
444	595	2,336	2,291	422	466	203	353	226	416	274	503	463	636	494	621	570	755
78	122	91	98	91	119	59	111	65	116	76	125	115	160	108	152	65	112
13	19	10	11	4	8	4	7	7	13	13	24	30	33	84	47	131	67
20	51	19	24	5	3	3	5	6	20	22	69	87	170	96	162	101	158
2	4	5	2	2	4	1	1	2	4	1	5	4	6	-	5	36	12
1	2	2	1	1	-	0	0	1	2	1	3	2	2	-	2	-	-
10	10	81	82	17	16	3	4	3	3	1	3	4	2	5	1	-	-
19	28	12	12	9	6	8	10	15	23	26	44	48	69	37	47	42	20
461	473	303	270	243	334	286	343	432	478	563	542	901	613	890	686	891	782
486	527	3,232	3,075	1,030	1,125	152	284	158	279	110	194	110	119	54	81	18	67
255	249	1,774	1,582	514	532	70	106	79	109	55	93	56	78	69	31	6	35
2	2	2	3	1	2	4	1	1	1	2	4	1	2	-	4	-	-
12	14	22	23	21	21	8	10	9	13	9	13	11	8	13	12	6	8
2	1	1	-	0	0	1	-	2	1	1	1	3	2	2	2	-	2
76	136	2	1	10	11	23	53	51	122	140	222	194	282	220	268	250	199
1	1	-	-	1	-	-	0	1	2	1	1	-	2	-	-	-	-
109	158	312	330	165	285	48	95	55	118	103	124	155	136	113	160	131	197
49	46	60	44	49	41	11	17	20	26	60	38	115	72	157	153	256	189
0	0	-	-	-	0	0	-	-	0	-	-	-	0	-	-	-	-
0	-	-	-	-	-	-	-	0	-	0	-	-	-	-	-	-	-
0	-	-	-	-	-	-	-	0	-	-	-	-	-	-	-	-	-
4	9	-	-	0	-	-	-	1	1	8	24	16	28	18	12	18	4
2	1	-	1	-	-	-	-	1	-	4	3	6	4	13	2	-	6
0	1	-	-	-	-	-	-	0	-	1	1	2	3	-	-	-	2
0	-	-	-	-	-	-	-	-	-	0	-	-	-	-	-	-	-
1	2	-	-	-	-	-	-	-	-	2	7	2	1	2	4	-	2
862	1,156	1	1	1	1	11	21	238	238	1,927	2,138	3,479	4,333	2,548	3,717	981	1,487
14	14	-	-	0	-	-	2	4	3	32	29	52	41	50	51	6	24
4	4	-	-	0	0	-	-	4	9	9	1	5	6	1	1	-	-
0	0	-	-	-	-	-	-	-	-	1	-	-	0	-	-	-	-
4	4	-	1	-	0	1	3	4	4	9	7	9	5	6	16	30	-
75	33	-	-	-	-	0	-	14	2	163	35	278	124	309	176	273	183
2	1	-	-	-	-	-	-	0	0	6	1	3	5	13	3	18	2
18	6	-	-	-	-	-	-	2	0	36	10	84	27	68	15	36	8
306	224	-	1	-	-	0	0	31	19	670	337	1,281	809	1,247	1,006	927	774
133	62	-	-	0	-	0	-	16	4	283	79	576	226	532	313	434	274
10	12	-	-	-	-	-	3	2	7	20	14	44	31	48	49	71	51
4	1	-	-	0	-	0	-	-	0	6	3	23	5	16	5	12	-
0	0	-	-	0	-	-	-	0	0	-	-	-	-	2	-	-	-
3	1	-	-	0	1	2	1	2	0	5	2	5	-	3	1	6	-
1	0	-	-	-	-	-	-	1	-	2	0	3	1	1	1	24	-
0	-	-	-	-	-	1	-	-	-	-	-	-	-	-	-	-	-
1	0	1	1	-	-	-	-	1	-	0	-	1	0	1	-	-	-
13	11	10	3	1	1	1	2	3	2	22	15	50	41	46	35	65	47
5	3	-	-	0	0	-	1	2	1	14	4	12	16	9	11	-	-
5	2	3	-	2	-	1	1	1	0	4	2	18	3	3	14	30	26
82	102	3	2	2	-	4	6	14	17	116	87	361	323	547	588	529	644
208	252	2	1	0	0	-	1	2	1	122	92	937	573	2,127	1,755	4,047	3,519

Consultations with doctor

Table 25 - *continued*

Disease group	Persons, by age group								
	Total	0-4	5-15	16-24	25-44	45-64	65-74	75-84	85 and over
Ill-defined descriptions and complications of heart disease (429)	1	-	0	1	0	2	1	4	6
Subarachnoid haemorrhage (430)	3	-	-	1	1	9	7	-	-
Intracerebral haemorrhage (431)	3	-	-	1	0	4	12	8	25
Other and unspecified intracranial haemorrhage (432)	0	-	0	0	-	1	1	1	4
Occlusion and stenosis of precerebral arteries (433)	2	-	-	-	0	3	11	14	12
Occlusion of cerebral arteries (434)	5	-	-	0	1	5	20	38	37
Transient cerebral ischaemia (435)	47	-	-	1	2	41	163	353	476
Acute but ill-defined cerebrovascular disease (436)	56	-	-	0	1	51	193	398	633
Other and ill-defined cerebrovascular disease (437)	12	-	-	-	1	14	35	82	139
Late effects of cerebrovascular disease (438)	1	-	-	-	0	1	2	4	13
Atherosclerosis (440)	4	-	-	-	0	4	12	30	38
Aortic aneurysm (441)	6	-	-	-	0	8	26	37	34
Other aneurysm (442)	1	-	-	-	0	1	1	7	3
Other peripheral vascular disease (443)	71	1	3	9	16	109	260	338	249
Arterial embolism and thrombosis (444)	2	-	-	-	1	2	8	8	10
Polyarteritis nodosa and allied conditions (446)	12	-	-	1	2	8	58	78	81
Other disorders of arteries and arterioles (447)	0	-	-	1	-	0	2	2	-
Diseases of capillaries (448)	7	4	9	8	7	5	5	6	1
Phlebitis and thrombophlebitis (451)	41	-	1	8	22	74	107	149	87
Other venous embolism and thrombosis (453)	7	-	0	1	3	12	20	21	34
Varicose veins of lower extremities (454)	133	1	1	25	76	223	371	463	365
Haemorrhoids (455)	125	5	5	82	169	169	190	169	130
Varicose veins of other sites (456)	3	-	1	2	3	3	6	6	1
Noninfective disorders of lymphatic channels (457)	3	1	2	2	3	6	3	3	7
Hypotension (458)	14	-	2	5	5	13	39	80	129
Other disorders of circulatory system (459)	6	2	0	2	3	8	17	15	22
Acute nasopharyngitis (common cold) (460)	410	2,960	477	214	170	156	190	185	250
Acute sinusitis (461)	318	20	141	329	464	393	260	149	96
Acute pharyngitis (462)	486	549	759	753	498	306	226	179	145
Acute tonsillitis (463)	539	1,428	1,312	878	389	104	43	36	18
Acute laryngitis and tracheitis (464)	162	514	131	119	137	158	140	113	95
Acute upper respiratory infections of multiple or unspecified site (465)	1,075	5,451	1,329	710	599	613	704	827	932
Acute bronchitis and bronchiolitis (466)	1,091	2,563	562	533	672	1,171	1,922	2,338	2,839
Deflected nasal septum (470)	6	-	4	13	8	6	5	2	1
Nasal polyps (471)	11	1	4	6	9	21	23	12	9
Chronic pharyngitis and nasopharyngitis (472)	123	176	109	82	106	134	197	145	112
Chronic sinusitis (473)	34	0	10	32	44	48	42	26	13
Chronic disease of tonsils and adenoids (474)	10	26	26	16	5	2	1	1	-
Peritonsillar abscess (475)	4	1	2	11	7	2	2	-	-
Chronic laryngitis and laryngotracheitis (476)	5	1	2	2	4	9	9	9	3
Allergic rhinitis (477)	333	182	622	577	349	170	138	97	52
Other diseases of upper respiratory tract (478)	10	12	8	7	11	11	16	9	6
Viral pneumonia (480)	2	4	2	0	2	1	3	6	21
Pneumococcal pneumonia (481)	11	11	10	1	7	13	23	36	46
Other bacterial pneumonia (482)	4	5	1	2	2	4	8	12	13
Pneumonia due to other specified organism (483)	1	-	0	1	1	1	1	0	-

By age-group and sex

| Total | | 0-4 | | 5-15 | | 16-24 | | 25-44 | | 45-64 | | 65-74 | | 75-84 | | 85 and over | |
Male	Female	Male	Female	Male	Female	Male	Female	Male	Female	Male	Female	Male	Female	Male	Female	Male	Female
1	1	-	-	-	0	1	1	1	0	2	2	2	1	6	3	6	6
2	4	-	-	-	-	1	1	1	1	3	15	8	5	-	-	-	-
3	2	-	-	-	-	1	1	0	-	6	3	19	5	5	10	30	24
1	0	-	-	1	-	-	0	-	-	1	0	2	-	2	1	-	6
2	3	-	-	-	-	-	-	0	-	3	3	10	12	10	16	6	14
8	3	-	-	-	-	-	0	1	-	9	2	26	15	78	14	48	33
48	47	-	-	-	-	0	1	1	3	47	34	212	124	437	303	612	431
57	55	-	-	-	-	0	-	1	2	71	31	258	140	433	377	731	601
13	12	-	-	-	-	-	-	1	1	22	6	38	32	95	75	155	134
1	1	-	-	-	-	-	-	0	-	2	0	1	3	6	3	6	16
5	3	-	-	-	-	-	-	0	0	7	2	22	4	46	20	71	28
10	3	-	-	-	-	-	-	0	0	12	3	50	7	80	11	30	35
1	1	-	-	-	-	-	-	0	-	0	1	1	2	8	6	6	2
85	58	1	1	0	5	3	14	10	22	151	67	387	157	440	277	386	203
1	2	-	-	-	-	-	-	0	2	1	2	10	6	10	7	12	10
8	17	-	-	-	-	1	-	3	1	5	12	23	87	84	74	59	89
0	1	-	-	-	-	2	0	-	-	0	0	-	4	1	3	-	-
4	9	4	4	8	9	4	12	4	10	3	8	3	7	2	8	-	2
30	52	-	-	0	2	4	12	16	27	55	92	93	119	127	162	18	110
6	7	-	-	0	-	1	-	3	3	12	12	18	21	21	21	-	45
95	169	-	3	1	1	14	37	42	111	177	270	296	431	432	482	368	364
114	136	7	4	3	7	58	106	141	198	172	167	204	178	180	162	190	110
4	2	-	-	2	-	5	-	4	3	5	2	10	2	11	3	-	2
3	4	1	1	1	2	2	2	3	3	5	7	2	3	1	3	-	10
13	15	-	-	2	1	4	6	2	7	14	11	46	34	98	69	107	136
3	8	1	3	1	-	0	3	2	4	6	11	10	23	10	18	12	26
378	441	2,954	2,966	440	516	143	284	113	226	121	192	174	202	172	192	220	260
198	434	19	20	122	160	209	449	269	660	221	568	184	321	118	167	71	104
379	589	540	559	612	912	522	983	353	644	235	378	193	253	161	189	107	158
455	621	1,550	1,301	1,067	1,570	639	1,115	273	507	68	140	40	45	35	37	24	16
121	202	605	418	130	131	59	177	67	207	85	232	104	170	93	126	83	99
949	1,196	5,572	5,324	1,237	1,426	500	919	391	808	452	777	606	784	769	861	1,099	877
983	1,195	2,757	2,360	586	538	434	631	493	853	978	1,368	1,974	1,880	2,690	2,128	3,346	2,672
9	4	-	-	5	2	20	7	10	5	9	3	7	3	6	-	-	2
15	7	1	1	5	3	7	4	12	7	31	10	33	16	19	7	18	6
113	134	172	181	115	102	70	93	83	129	112	156	211	186	172	129	196	85
25	43	-	1	11	9	19	45	32	56	37	60	26	55	13	34	36	6
8	11	27	26	24	29	5	27	4	6	2	3	-	2	1	1	-	-
5	4	1	1	2	2	14	8	7	6	1	3	2	1	-	-	-	-
4	6	1	1	1	3	2	3	3	5	6	13	12	7	9	8	-	4
309	355	222	140	689	551	488	665	274	425	136	205	121	152	113	88	71	45
9	11	14	9	9	8	8	6	9	13	9	13	13	18	6	12	18	2
2	2	5	3	2	3	0	-	2	1	2	1	3	2	8	5	24	20
13	10	14	8	13	6	2	0	7	6	16	10	20	25	46	29	77	35
4	3	3	8	2	0	2	3	1	2	6	1	12	4	17	10	24	10
1	1	-	-	0	-	1	1	2	1	0	1	-	2	-	1	-	-

Consultations with doctor

Table 25 - *continued*

Disease group	Persons, by age group								
	Total	0-4	5-15	16-24	25-44	45-64	65-74	75-84	85 and over
Bronchopneumonia, organism unspecified (485)	20	11	4	1	4	11	35	119	399
Pneumonia, organism unspecified (486)	18	19	9	7	10	20	40	57	89
Influenza (487)	237	236	192	258	257	250	197	215	195
Bronchitis, not specified as acute or chronic (490)	63	125	20	20	34	64	135	184	318
Chronic bronchitis (491)	103	5	3	6	10	149	468	485	290
Emphysema (492)	18	-	-	-	3	30	73	69	78
Asthma (493)	913	2,045	1,486	746	587	734	1,050	844	463
Bronchiectasis (494)	12	1	0	1	6	26	31	36	21
Extrinsic allergic alveolitis (495)	1	-	0	-	0	1	2	3	4
Chronic airways obsruction, not elsewhere classified (496)	124	1	1	-	6	166	595	630	454
Coalworkers' pneumoconiosis (500)	0	-	-	-	-	-	1	2	-
Asbestosis (501)	1	-	-	-	0	2	3	2	-
Pneumoconiosis due to other silica or silicates (502)	0	-	-	-	-	0	0	-	-
Pneumoconiosis due to other inorganic dust (503)	0	-	0	-	-	-	-	-	-
Pneumoconiosis, unspecified (505)	0	-	-	-	-	-	0	-	-
Respiratory conditions due to chemical fumes and vapours (506)	0	-	-	-	0	1	2	-	-
Pneumonitis due to solids and liquids (507)	0	-	-	-	0	-	1	3	1
Respiratory conditions due to ther and unspecified external agents (508)	0	-	-	-	-	1	-	-	-
Empyema (510)	1	-	-	1	0	1	1	1	4
Pleurisy (511)	30	1	3	15	27	43	60	79	65
Pneumothorax (512)	3	-	0	5	4	2	4	2	4
Abscess of lung and mediastinum (513)	0	-	-	-	0	-	-	-	-
Pulmonary congestion and hypostasis (514)	2	-	-	0	0	1	3	12	22
Postinflammatory pulmonary fibrosis (515)	0	-	-	-	-	-	-	-	4
Other alveolar and parietoalveolar pneumopathy (516)	6	3	0	-	1	6	25	38	7
Other diseases of lung (518)	0	0	-	-	-	1	1	-	-
Other diseases of respiratory system (519)	11	42	7	8	8	9	13	11	7
Disorders of tooth development and eruption (520)	5	73	0	0	0	0	-	-	-
Diseases of hard tissues of teeth (521)	14	130	4	6	6	5	5	3	1
Diseases of pulp and periapical tissues (522)	38	8	25	39	54	48	23	13	7
Gingival and periodontal diseases (523)	9	18	5	11	10	9	9	6	7
Dentofacial anomalies, including malocclusion (524)	16	1	8	24	22	18	12	11	6
Other diseases and conditions of the teeth and supporting structures (525)	2	-	1	3	2	1	2	2	12
Diseases of the jaws (526)	1	0	0	1	0	1	2	-	-
Diseases of the salivary glands (527)	12	4	8	7	13	17	11	19	12
Diseases of the oral soft tissues, excluding lesions specific for gingiva and tongue (528)	75	144	84	75	57	63	93	79	74
Diseases and other conditions of the tongue (529)	13	12	6	6	10	16	22	32	24
Diseases of oesophagus (530)	169	36	6	55	138	276	418	381	293
Gastric ulcer (531)	11	-	-	2	5	18	28	41	55
Duodenal ulcer (532)	59	-	0	17	60	112	115	78	65
Peptic ulcer, site unspecified (533)	20	-	1	10	21	35	29	46	31
Gastritis and duodenitis (535)	101	51	41	90	103	129	139	154	144
Disorders of function of stomach (536)	224	4	15	124	203	344	506	482	392
Other disorders of stomach and duodenum (537)	1	3	0	0	-	1	1	1	1
Acute appendicitis (540)	5	0	9	9	5	3	1	1	-
Appendicitis, unqualified (541)	7	0	13	17	7	3	1	-	-
Other appendicitis (542)	1	0	1	1	1	0	0	-	-
Other diseases of appendix (543)	0	-	0	-	0	-	-	-	-

By age-group and sex

| Total | | 0-4 | | 5-15 | | 16-24 | | 25-44 | | 45-64 | | 65-74 | | 75-84 | | 85 and over | |
Male	Female	Male	Female	Male	Female	Male	Female	Male	Female	Male	Female	Male	Female	Male	Female	Male	Female
17	22	13	9	4	3	1	1	5	3	11	12	41	30	142	106	446	384
20	17	21	17	12	7	8	6	9	10	23	17	45	35	74	47	149	69
208	266	251	220	179	205	216	300	222	293	202	298	173	217	184	233	232	183
54	72	136	114	23	17	19	22	25	43	53	76	135	136	173	191	315	319
125	81	5	4	2	4	6	6	9	11	165	132	666	307	777	311	701	154
25	11	-	-	-	-	-	-	2	4	41	19	110	43	132	31	285	10
892	933	2,347	1,727	1,719	1,242	651	841	465	710	613	858	953	1,129	875	826	541	437
9	15	1	1	0	0	1	1	3	9	15	37	27	34	56	24	30	18
0	1	-	-	0	-	-	-	0	1	1	1	1	3	1	4	-	6
157	92	1	-	-	2	-	-	4	8	197	134	905	344	977	422	1,010	270
0	-	-	-	-	-	-	-	-	-	-	-	3	-	5	-	-	-
2	-	-	-	-	-	-	-	0	-	3	-	8	-	5	-	-	-
0	-	-	-	-	-	-	-	-	-	0	-	1	-	-	-	-	-
0	0	-	-	0	0	-	-	-	-	-	-	-	-	-	-	-	-
0	-	-	-	-	-	-	-	-	-	-	-	1	-	-	-	-	-
1	-	-	-	-	-	-	-	0	-	1	-	4	-	-	-	-	-
0	0	-	-	-	-	-	-	-	0	-	-	-	2	8	1	6	-
0	0	-	-	-	-	-	-	-	-	1	0	-	-	-	-	-	-
1	0	-	-	-	-	-	1	0	0	2	0	2	0	2	1	-	6
24	35	-	2	3	3	9	21	19	35	36	51	57	63	103	64	77	61
4	2	-	-	0	-	7	2	5	3	3	1	8	1	5	1	-	6
0	0	-	-	-	-	-	-	0	0	-	-	-	-	-	-	-	-
1	2	-	-	-	-	-	1	-	0	1	2	2	3	19	8	18	24
0	-	-	-	-	-	-	-	-	-	-	-	-	-	-	-	18	-
7	5	5	1	-	1	-	-	1	0	8	5	28	22	60	25	12	6
0	0	-	1	-	-	-	-	-	-	1	0	1	0	-	-	-	-
11	11	50	34	7	8	7	9	7	9	8	10	11	15	11	10	6	8
5	5	72	74	0	-	-	1	0	0	0	-	-	-	-	-	-	-
14	13	150	109	2	5	2	10	5	7	5	5	5	6	7	1	-	2
35	42	10	6	28	22	33	46	44	65	44	52	29	18	15	12	12	6
8	11	18	19	5	6	8	14	7	13	8	11	9	9	3	7	-	10
10	23	-	2	6	9	14	35	13	31	10	27	4	18	11	11	18	2
1	3	-	-	1	1	1	5	2	3	1	2	2	2	3	1	-	16
1	1	1	-	-	0	1	1	0	1	1	1	2	1	-	-	-	-
9	15	5	4	8	8	6	7	10	16	11	23	10	12	10	25	12	12
59	90	136	154	76	92	48	102	43	72	44	82	83	101	60	91	65	77
9	16	15	10	5	6	7	5	7	13	11	21	12	30	23	37	24	24
148	189	42	31	7	6	49	61	129	147	237	316	390	441	360	393	315	286
12	10	-	-	-	-	4	1	7	4	23	13	26	30	44	39	36	61
81	37	-	-	0	-	30	4	88	33	144	80	169	71	120	53	113	49
26	15	-	-	0	1	14	7	27	16	46	23	36	24	68	33	18	35
98	104	50	52	46	36	86	94	99	107	126	133	145	134	150	156	137	146
215	233	4	5	16	14	127	121	191	215	325	364	565	459	513	463	475	364
1	0	3	3	0	-	0	-	-	-	1	1	1	-	1	1	6	-
4	5	1	-	8	9	7	11	4	7	3	2	1	0	-	1	-	-
7	7	1	-	13	13	17	16	6	8	3	3	1	1	-	-	-	-
1	1	-	1	1	1	1	1	1	1	0	-	-	0	-	-	-	-
0	0	-	-	1	-	-	-	0	0	-	-	-	-	-	-	-	-

Table 25 - *continued*

Disease group	Persons, by age group								
	Total	0-4	5-15	16-24	25-44	45-64	65-74	75-84	85 and over
Inguinal hernia (550)	46	45	7	14	22	72	107	151	138
Other hernia of abdominal cavity, with gangrene (551)	0	-	-	-	-	-	1	-	-
Other hernia of abdominal cavity with obstruction, without mention of gangrene (552)	1	0	-	-	0	0	2	3	7
Other hernia of abdominal cavity without mention of obstruction or gangrene (553)	57	45	4	5	28	85	181	197	141
Regional enteritis (555)	20	1	3	20	29	24	18	20	13
Idiopathic proctocolitis (556)	26	1	0	9	30	47	42	38	34
Vascular insufficiency of intestine (557)	0	-	-	-	-	0	2	2	3
Other noninfective gastroenteritis and colitis (558)	21	47	12	16	18	21	24	23	22
Intestinal obstruction without mention of hernia (560)	8	3	0	1	3	12	18	37	73
Diverticula of intestine (562)	40	-	0	0	6	54	149	226	219
Functional digestive disorders, not elsewhere classified (564)	318	360	113	260	285	308	484	729	1,080
Anal fissure and fistula (565)	33	65	14	43	43	28	14	18	12
Abscess of anal and rectal regions (566)	15	4	2	28	19	18	7	6	-
Peritonitis (567)	1	-	0	-	1	1	1	-	1
Other disorders of peritoneum (568)	1	0	0	0	2	1	1	2	1
Other disorders of intestine (569)	44	29	9	25	37	51	87	122	176
Acute and subacute necrosis of liver (570)	0	1	0	0	0	0	0	-	-
Chronic liver disease and cirrhosis (571)	10	-	-	1	6	23	23	17	-
Liver abscess and sequelae of chronic liver disease (572)	1	-	-	-	0	1	3	0	-
Other disorders of liver (573)	0	-	-	-	0	1	1	1	-
Cholelithiasis (574)	19	-	0	7	16	35	37	39	21
Other disorders of gallbladder (575)	17	-	-	7	15	31	38	33	30
Other disorders of biliary tract (576)	5	1	0	1	2	7	14	23	53
Diseases of pancreas (577)	6	-	0	1	5	14	10	14	9
Gastrointestinal haemorrhage (578)	16	5	2	6	8	15	38	82	144
Intestinal malabsorption (579)	5	9	2	3	5	5	8	6	4
Acute glomerulonephritis (580)	1	1	1	1	1	0	1	-	-
Nephrotic syndrome (581)	3	6	2	1	1	6	3	9	-
Chronic glomerulonephritis (582)	1	-	-	2	2	1	2	0	-
Nephritis and nephropathy, not specified as acute or chronic (583)	1	-	0	1	1	1	0	-	-
Acute renal failure (584)	2	-	-	0	0	2	7	9	12
Chronic renal failure (585)	9	-	-	1	4	12	27	33	83
Renal failure, unspecified (586)	2	1	-	-	1	4	6	8	18
Renal sclerosis, unspecified (587)	0	0	-	-	-	-	-	-	-
Disorders resulting from impaired renal function (588)	0	-	-	0	-	-	0	-	-
Infections of kidney (590)	21	0	6	39	27	20	14	22	12
Hydronephrosis (591)	1	3	0	1	1	1	3	0	9
Calculus of kidney and ureter (592)	11	0	1	7	13	21	12	12	7
Other disorders of kidney and ureter (593)	2	8	2	2	1	3	3	5	-
Calculus of lower urinary tract (594)	1	-	0	0	1	2	6	1	6
Cystitis (595)	147	29	35	173	158	168	220	256	240
Other disorders of bladder (596)	10	-	1	2	6	16	29	29	24
Urethritis, not sexually transmitted, and urethral syndrome (597)	3	1	1	3	4	5	1	3	6
Urethral stricture (598)	2	-	1	-	1	3	6	12	7
Other disorders of urethra and urinary tract (599)	418	314	206	392	366	383	680	972	1,361
Hyperplasia of prostate (600)	22	-	-	-	0	33	103	113	46
Inflammatory diseases of prostate (601)	8	-	-	1	7	15	18	20	3
Other disorders of prostate (602)	0	-	-	-	-	1	1	4	-
Hydrocele (603)	9	33	5	3	5	7	14	17	27
Orchitis and epididymitis (604)	26	1	4	21	41	31	33	14	4
Redundant prepuce and phimosis (605)	16	92	38	9	5	5	4	6	7
Infertility, male (606)	4	-	-	2	12	1	0	-	-

By age-group and sex

Total		0-4		5-15		16-24		25-44		45-64		65-74		75-84		85 and over	
Male	Female	Male	Female	Male	Female	Male	Female	Male	Female	Male	Female	Male	Female	Male	Female	Male	Female
85	9	77	11	13	2	26	3	38	5	132	11	220	16	357	27	404	49
-	0	-	-	-	-	-	-	-	-	-	-	-	1	-	-	-	-
0	1	1	-	-	-	-	-	-	0	0	0	1	3	1	3	-	10
49	66	50	40	5	2	7	2	27	28	79	91	159	200	136	234	65	165
16	24	1	1	3	3	15	25	24	35	16	33	17	18	14	24	24	10
26	27	-	1	1	-	3	15	26	35	51	44	60	28	29	43	42	32
0	0	-	-	-	-	-	-	-	-	0	-	2	2	3	1	-	4
19	22	49	45	13	11	13	20	15	22	20	23	25	22	17	26	18	24
7	9	4	2	0	0	0	2	3	3	9	15	19	17	52	29	113	59
22	57	-	-	-	0	-	1	6	6	28	81	103	186	139	278	137	246
195	435	365	355	94	133	89	430	125	446	178	439	395	557	729	729	1,153	1,056
27	39	67	63	14	15	20	65	30	57	28	27	16	11	21	16	18	10
23	7	8	1	4	1	49	8	28	11	24	12	14	0	9	5	-	-
0	1	-	-	-	0	-	-	1	1	0	1	1	2	-	-	-	2
0	2	1	-	0	1	-	1	0	3	0	2	1	1	-	3	-	2
38	50	33	24	11	7	17	33	34	41	49	54	72	99	97	136	196	169
1	0	-	2	0	-	1	-	1	-	1	-	1	-	-	-	-	-
11	9	-	-	-	-	2	-	10	3	21	25	22	24	29	10	-	-
1	0	-	-	-	-	-	-	0	0	1	1	5	1	-	1	-	-
0	0	-	-	-	-	-	-	0	-	2	1	-	1	-	2	-	-
10	27	-	-	0	-	0	13	4	28	21	50	33	41	33	43	12	24
9	24	-	-	-	-	3	11	4	25	18	44	26	47	41	29	36	28
6	5	2	-	-	0	-	1	2	3	8	7	19	10	40	13	53	53
9	4	-	-	0	-	1	1	8	2	21	6	9	11	25	7	-	12
19	14	5	5	2	1	9	3	11	5	20	10	55	24	95	74	208	122
3	7	6	11	3	1	1	5	3	7	3	7	4	12	-	10	-	6
1	1	1	1	1	0	1	0	1	2	0	0	-	1	-	-	-	-
5	2	12	-	3	1	-	2	1	1	11	1	3	2	10	8	-	-
1	1	-	-	-	-	4	0	0	3	2	1	5	-	1	-	-	-
1	0	-	-	-	0	-	1	1	1	2	0	-	0	-	-	-	-
2	2	-	-	-	-	1	-	0	0	2	2	6	8	10	9	6	14
9	9	-	-	-	-	2	-	5	3	11	12	31	24	42	28	119	71
2	2	1	-	-	-	-	-	1	0	2	5	8	4	11	6	53	6
-	0	-	1	-	-	-	-	-	-	-	-	-	-	-	-	-	-
0	0	-	-	-	-	1	-	-	-	-	-	-	0	-	-	-	-
7	33	-	1	3	10	4	74	9	44	10	29	10	17	15	26	-	16
1	2	3	3	1	-	-	1	1	2	1	1	3	3	-	1	18	6
15	8	-	1	2	0	6	7	17	9	30	13	16	8	17	8	-	10
3	2	10	6	2	3	2	1	1	1	3	2	1	4	10	1	-	-
2	1	-	-	0	-	0	0	1	1	3	0	9	4	2	-	-	8
21	269	6	54	7	65	8	336	12	304	34	305	52	357	61	373	107	284
8	11	-	-	-	2	1	3	4	8	10	22	36	24	42	21	24	24
4	3	2	-	1	1	3	4	4	4	7	4	1	1	8	-	-	8
4	0	-	-	2	-	-	-	2	0	6	1	13	0	30	1	24	2
197	630	180	455	93	324	66	717	97	637	209	561	540	794	950	985	1,206	1,413
44	-	-	-	-	-	-	-	1	-	65	-	229	-	302	-	184	-
16	-	-	-	-	-	3	-	14	-	31	-	40	-	53	-	12	-
1	-	-	-	-	-	-	-	-	-	2	-	1	-	10	-	-	-
18	-	65	-	9	-	6	-	10	-	14	-	32	-	46	-	107	-
53	-	2	-	8	-	42	-	82	-	62	-	75	-	38	-	18	-
33	-	180	-	74	-	18	-	11	-	10	-	9	-	15	-	30	-
8	-	-	-	-	-	4	-	24	-	2	-	1	-	-	-	-	-

Consultations with doctor

Table 25 - *continued*

Disease group	Persons, by age group								
	Total	0-4	5-15	16-24	25-44	45-64	65-74	75-84	85 and over
Disorders of penis (607)	40	199	74	20	19	18	30	16	15
Other disorders of male genital organs (608)	18	4	11	17	23	23	22	12	1
Benign mammary dysplasias (610)	25	1	3	20	46	32	3	2	-
Other disorders of breast (611)	108	16	41	92	182	123	61	42	15
Inflammatory disease of ovary, fallopian tube, pelvic cellular tissue and peritoneum (614)	50	0	1	133	101	11	0	1	-
Inflammatory diseases of uterus, except cervix (615)	6	-	-	12	13	1	-	1	-
Inflammatory disease of cervix, vagina and vulva (616)	95	68	41	131	140	76	62	69	59
Endometriosis (617)	12	-	-	14	30	5	0	-	-
Genital prolapse (618)	36	-	0	1	13	55	114	174	163
Fistulae involving female genital tract (619)	0	-	-	-	0	1	2	1	3
Noninflammatory disorders of ovary, fallopian tube and broad ligament (620)	7	-	0	10	13	7	1	5	1
Disorders of uterus, not elsewhere classified (621)	3	1	-	2	5	5	1	0	-
Noninflammatory disorders of cervix (622)	13	-	0	13	22	18	6	3	-
Noninflammatory disorders of vagina (623)	40	11	12	72	66	27	14	15	37
Noninflammatory disorders of vulva and perineum (624)	3	1	1	2	4	3	5	5	9
Pain and other symptoms associated with female genital organs (625)	201	-	85	322	400	101	28	26	28
Disorders of menstruation and other abnormal bleeding from female genital tract (626)	345	0	82	643	650	243	2	1	-
Menopausal and postmenopausal disorders (627)	298	-	-	1	146	1,099	166	90	136
Infertility, female (628)	29	-	-	25	83	1	-	-	-
Other disorders of female genital organs (629)	0	-	0	0	-	0	-	-	-
Hydatidiform mole (630)	0	-	-	1	1	0	-	-	-
Other abnormal product of conception (631)	1	0	0	1	2	0	-	-	-
Missed abortion (632)	3	-	0	6	7	-	-	-	-
Ectopic pregnancy (633)	4	-	0	9	11	-	-	-	-
Spontaneous abortion (634)	20	-	0	45	46	1	-	-	-
Legally induced abortion (635)	5	-	1	20	9	0	-	-	-
Unspecified abortion (637)	0	-	-	2	0	-	-	-	-
Failed attempted abortion (638)	0	-	-	0	-	-	-	-	-
Complications following abortion and ectopic and molar pregnancies (639)	1	-	-	1	1	-	-	-	-
Haemorrhage in early pregnancy (640)	34	-	1	87	73	0	-	-	-
Antepartum haemorrhage, abruptio placentae, and placenta praevia (641)	2	-	-	5	5	-	-	-	-
Hypertension complicating pregnancy, childbirth and the puerperium (642)	4	-	-	9	8	0	-	-	-
Excessive vomiting in pregnancy (643)	15	-	0	42	32	0	-	-	-
Early or threatened labour (644)	2	-	-	7	3	-	-	-	-
Prolonged pregnancy (645)	0	-	-	1	0	-	-	-	-
Other complications of pregnancy, not elsewhere classified (646)	13	-	1	38	27	0	-	-	1
Infective and parasitic conditions in the mother classifiable elsewhere but complicating pregnancy, childbirth and the puerperium (647)	0	-	-	0	0	-	-	-	-
Other current conditions in the mother classifiable elsewhere but complicating pregnancy, childbirth and the puerperium (648)	6	-	0	12	14	-	-	-	-
Delivery in a completely normal case (650)	26	1	1	56	60	-	-	-	-
Multiple gestation (651)	2	-	-	4	4	-	-	-	-

By age-group and sex

Total		0-4		5-15		16-24		25-44		45-64		65-74		75-84		85 and over	
Male	Female	Male	Female	Male	Female	Male	Female	Male	Female	Male	Female	Male	Female	Male	Female	Male	Female
81	-	389	-	143	-	40	-	38	-	37	-	66	-	42	-	59	-
37	-	9	-	21	-	34	-	45	-	46	-	50	-	31	-	6	-
0	48	-	2	2	4	0	39	0	93	0	65	-	6	-	3	-	-
15	196	9	23	41	40	24	160	5	360	9	238	13	100	18	55	18	14
-	99	1	-	2	-	266	-	202	-	22	-	0	-	1	-	-	-
-	11	-	-	-	-	-	23	-	26	-	2	-	-	-	1	-	-
0	187	-	140	-	84	-	261	0	280	-	153	-	112	-	109	-	79
-	24	-	-	-	-	-	28	-	61	-	9	-	0	-	-	-	-
-	71	-	-	-	0	-	1	-	27	-	110	-	207	-	278	-	217
-	1	-	-	-	-	-	-	-	0	-	1	-	3	-	2	-	4
-	14	-	-	-	1	-	19	-	25	-	15	-	2	-	8	-	2
-	6	-	1	-	-	-	5	-	10	-	10	-	1	-	1	-	-
-	26	-	-	-	0	-	26	-	45	-	37	-	11	-	5	-	-
-	78	-	22	-	25	-	143	-	132	-	54	-	26	-	25	-	49
-	6	-	3	-	2	-	3	-	8	-	5	-	9	-	8	-	12
-	394	-	-	-	173	-	642	-	802	-	205	-	51	-	42	-	37
-	676	-	1	-	169	-	1,281	-	1,304	-	491	-	4	-	1	-	-
-	583	-	-	-	-	-	1	-	293	-	2,219	-	302	-	144	-	181
-	57	-	-	-	-	-	49	-	168	-	2	-	-	-	-	-	-
-	0	-	-	-	0	-	0	-	-	-	0	-	-	-	-	-	-
-	1	-	-	-	-	-	2	-	1	-	0	-	-	-	-	-	-
-	2	-	1	-	1	-	1	-	4	-	0	-	-	-	-	-	-
-	6	-	-	-	1	-	12	-	15	-	-	-	-	-	-	-	-
-	9	-	-	-	0	-	17	-	22	-	-	-	-	-	-	-	-
-	39	-	-	-	1	-	89	-	92	-	2	-	-	-	-	-	-
-	11	-	-	-	2	-	40	-	17	-	0	-	-	-	-	-	-
-	1	-	-	-	-	-	3	-	1	-	-	-	-	-	-	-	-
-	0	-	-	-	-	-	0	-	-	-	-	-	-	-	-	-	-
-	1	-	-	-	-	-	2	-	3	-	-	-	-	-	-	-	-
-	66	-	-	-	2	-	173	-	148	-	1	-	-	-	-	-	-
-	5	-	-	-	-	-	11	-	11	-	-	-	-	-	-	-	-
-	7	-	-	-	-	-	17	-	17	-	0	-	-	-	-	-	-
-	30	-	-	-	0	-	83	-	65	-	0	-	-	-	-	-	-
-	4	-	-	-	-	-	14	-	6	-	-	-	-	-	-	-	-
-	0	-	-	-	-	-	1	-	0	-	-	-	-	-	-	-	-
-	26	-	-	-	1	-	75	-	53	-	1	-	-	-	-	-	2
-	0	-	-	-	-	-	1	-	1	-	-	-	-	-	-	-	-
-	11	-	-	-	0	-	23	-	28	-	-	-	-	-	-	-	-
-	50	-	3	-	1	-	112	-	120	-	-	-	-	-	-	-	-
-	3	-	-	-	-	-	8	-	8	-	-	-	-	-	-	-	-

Consultations
with doctor

Table 25 - *continued*

Disease group	Persons, by age group								
	Total	0-4	5-15	16-24	25-44	45-64	65-74	75-84	85 and over
Malposition and malpresentation of fetus (652)	2	-	-	3	4	-	-	-	-
Disproportion (653)	0	-	-	1	0	-	-	-	-
Abnormality of organs and soft tissues of pelvis (654)	0	-	-	-	0	0	-	-	-
Known or suspected fetal abnormality affecting management of mother (655)	0	-	-	1	0	-	-	-	-
Other fetal and placental problems affecting management of mother (656)	2	1	-	6	4	-	-	-	-
Polyhydramnios (657)	0	-	-	0	1	-	-	-	-
Other problems associated with amniotic cavity and membranes (658)	0	-	-	1	0	-	-	-	-
Other indications for care or intervention related to labour and delivery and not elsewhere classified (659)	0	-	-	1	0	-	-	-	-
Obstructed labour (660)	0	-	-	0	0	-	-	-	-
Abnormality of forces of labour (661)	0	-	-	1	0	-	-	-	-
Long labour (662)	0	-	-	0	0	-	-	-	-
Umbilical cord complications (663)	0	4	-	0	0	-	-	-	-
Trauma to perineum and vulva during delivery (664)	1	-	-	3	3	-	-	-	-
Other obstetrical trauma (665)	0	-	-	1	0	0	-	-	-
Postpartum haemorrhage (666)	3	-	-	7	8	-	-	-	-
Retained placenta or membranes, without haemorrhage (667)	1	-	-	3	3	0	-	-	-
Other complications of labour and delivery, not elsewhere classified (669)	7	1	0	14	18	0	-	-	-
Major puerperal infection (670)	1	-	-	2	2	-	-	-	1
Venous complications in pregnancy and the puerperium (671)	4	-	0	8	11	0	1	0	-
Pyrexia of unknown origin during the puerperium (672)	0	-	0	-	0	-	-	-	-
Other and unspecified complications of the puerperium, not elsewhere classified (674)	2	-	-	3	5	-	-	-	-
Infections of the breast and nipple associated with childbirth (675)	13	-	-	15	35	1	-	-	-
Other disorders of the breast associated with childbirth, and disorders of lactation (676)	5	0	0	8	12	2	1	0	-
Carbuncle and furuncle (680)	75	36	54	99	100	72	51	38	24
Cellulitis and abscess of finger and toe (681)	74	128	105	56	53	71	79	83	104
Other cellulitis and abscess (682)	158	69	70	101	133	181	271	417	613
Acute lymphadenitis (683)	22	49	41	32	21	10	5	4	9
Impetigo (684)	78	346	192	74	33	20	25	25	22
Pilonidal cyst (685)	10	3	1	37	14	4	2	1	-
Other local infections of skin and subcutaneous tissue (686)	54	78	58	43	46	49	61	70	114
Erythematosquamous dermatosis (690)	99	213	75	89	90	83	129	117	80
Atopic dermatitis and related conditions (691)	429	2,458	384	346	245	222	291	262	237
Contact dermatitis and other eczema (692)	266	542	221	321	238	218	268	248	228
Dermatitis due to substances taken internally (693)	1	2	1	1	1	2	3	4	1
Bullous dermatoses (694)	4	1	2	1	3	2	13	10	43
Erythematous conditions (695)	89	64	24	52	86	124	154	144	167
Psoriasis and similar disorders (696)	113	25	81	127	130	130	134	99	55
Lichen (697)	7	1	1	4	6	11	14	13	3
Pruritus and related conditions (698)	104	54	42	60	88	132	193	216	321
Corns and callosities (700)	18	3	8	13	13	19	42	56	50
Other hypertrophic and atrophic conditions of skin (701)	12	7	12	11	11	12	17	27	21
Other dermatoses (702)	52	3	7	9	22	81	171	201	148
Diseases of nail (703)	91	37	169	184	62	65	59	71	64

By age-group and sex

Total		0-4		5-15		16-24		25-44		45-64		65-74		75-84		85 and over	
Male	Female	Male	Female	Male	Female	Male	Female	Male	Female	Male	Female	Male	Female	Male	Female	Male	Female
-	3	-	-	-	-	-	7	-	7	-	-	-	-	-	-	-	-
-	0	-	-	-	-	-	1	-	0	-	-	-	-	-	-	-	-
-	0	-	-	-	-	-	-	-	0	-	0	-	-	-	-	-	-
-	1	-	-	-	-	-	3	-	1	-	-	-	-	-	-	-	-
-	4	-	1	-	-	-	11	-	8	-	-	-	-	-	-	-	-
-	1	-	-	-	-	-	1	-	2	-	-	-	-	-	-	-	-
-	0	-	-	-	-	-	2	-	1	-	-	-	-	-	-	-	-
-	0	-	-	-	-	-	2	-	0	-	-	-	-	-	-	-	-
-	0	-	-	-	-	-	0	-	0	-	-	-	-	-	-	-	-
-	0	-	-	-	-	-	2	-	1	-	-	-	-	-	-	-	-
-	0	-	-	-	-	-	1	-	1	-	-	-	-	-	-	-	-
-	1	-	9	-	-	-	1	-	0	-	-	-	-	-	-	-	-
-	2	-	-	-	-	-	5	-	6	-	-	-	-	-	-	-	-
-	1	-	-	-	-	-	1	-	1	-	1	-	-	-	-	-	-
-	6	-	-	-	-	-	13	-	16	-	-	-	-	-	-	-	-
-	3	-	-	-	-	-	5	-	6	-	0	-	-	-	-	-	-
-	14	-	1	-	0	-	28	-	35	-	0	-	-	-	-	-	-
-	2	-	-	-	-	-	5	-	5	-	-	-	-	-	-	-	2
-	9	-	-	-	0	-	16	-	21	-	1	-	2	-	1	-	-
-	0	-	-	-	0	-	-	-	1	-	-	-	-	-	-	-	-
-	4	-	-	-	-	-	5	-	10	-	-	-	-	-	-	-	-
-	25	-	-	-	-	-	30	-	71	-	2	-	-	-	-	-	-
-	11	-	1	-	1	-	16	-	24	-	4	-	2	-	1	-	-
70	80	39	33	56	52	83	115	91	109	64	80	52	50	37	39	18	26
73	75	139	116	108	102	65	48	50	55	60	81	73	83	85	81	160	85
140	176	71	68	72	68	92	109	125	142	170	193	252	286	371	445	410	680
20	25	68	29	40	43	23	41	14	27	5	15	5	5	5	3	6	10
82	74	374	316	203	181	64	84	30	36	18	21	27	23	33	20	48	14
14	6	2	4	2	1	45	29	21	7	6	2	5	-	1	1	-	-
48	59	92	64	52	63	35	51	38	54	45	53	51	69	64	74	107	116
97	101	230	196	59	92	71	107	86	95	84	81	160	103	142	103	59	87
377	478	2,330	2,591	323	448	201	491	175	316	199	247	317	270	334	219	279	223
211	318	537	547	176	267	204	437	161	316	180	257	256	278	269	235	208	234
1	2	3	2	1	1	1	1	-	1	1	3	1	4	1	5	-	2
3	5	1	1	3	1	1	1	1	4	2	3	13	14	9	11	59	37
67	110	60	68	21	26	34	70	62	110	100	148	124	178	115	161	83	195
104	122	29	20	62	101	94	160	117	142	134	125	139	131	92	103	125	32
6	7	2	1	1	2	3	5	5	7	13	10	16	12	10	14	-	4
73	133	35	74	28	57	36	84	57	120	99	166	158	222	204	223	368	305
13	23	3	3	3	14	7	18	9	18	15	23	37	46	53	58	59	47
9	15	10	4	9	14	8	15	7	15	9	16	16	18	25	27	18	22
48	56	5	1	8	5	7	10	15	29	76	86	187	158	230	184	196	132
110	74	47	26	190	146	256	113	76	47	59	71	58	59	87	62	107	49

Table 25 - *continued*

Disease group	Persons, by age group								
	Total	0-4	5-15	16-24	25-44	45-64	65-74	75-84	85 and over
Diseases of hair and hair follicles (704)	51	41	34	75	72	41	31	18	7
Disorders of sweat glands (705)	28	28	23	35	37	25	14	6	7
Diseases of sebaceous glands (706)	302	41	346	873	306	144	116	102	58
Chronic ulcer of skin (707)	37	1	1	3	4	33	121	239	466
Urticaria (708)	88	158	110	84	79	72	87	76	68
Other disorders of skin and subcutaneous tissue (709)	25	27	21	25	27	26	26	19	19
Diffuse diseases of connective tissue (710)	9	-	0	3	9	19	15	9	7
Arthropathy associated with infections (711)	2	1	0	1	3	2	5	3	9
Crystal arthropathies (712)	0	-	-	-	-	0	-	-	-
Rheumatoid arthritis and other inflammatory polyarthropathies (714)	107	1	3	10	57	225	313	268	107
Osteoarthrosis and allied disorders (715)	583	1	1	15	103	1,056	1,893	2,637	2,699
Other and unspecified arthropathies (716)	35	1	4	15	35	62	55	68	55
Internal derangement of knee (717)	47	-	53	85	58	42	17	9	1
Other derangement of joint (718)	4	1	2	6	6	2	5	3	1
Other and unspecified disorder of joint (719)	347	51	156	236	340	509	520	583	562
Ankylosing spondylitis and other inflammatory spondylopathies (720)	18	-	1	9	26	32	11	17	4
Spondylosis and allied disorders (721)	205	-	1	14	123	499	440	388	278
Intervertebral disc disorders (722)	79	-	2	30	107	151	78	56	28
Other disorders of cervical region (723)	120	20	50	78	169	168	112	82	71
Other and unspecified disorders of back (724)	639	10	67	390	804	1,025	772	831	756
Polymyalgia rheumatica (725)	43	-	-	-	3	33	187	360	139
Peripheral enthesopathies and allied syndromes (726)	319	2	52	102	312	679	446	390	218
Other disorders of synovium, tendon and bursa (727)	113	13	38	99	127	166	146	120	120
Disorders of muscle, ligament and fascia (728)	56	7	19	26	42	101	117	84	86
Other disorders of soft tissues (729)	252	39	81	125	213	368	522	588	478
Osteomyelitis, periostitis and other infections involving bone (730)	3	2	1	1	2	3	10	7	3
Osteitis deformans and osteopathies associated with other disorders classified elsewhere (731)	4	-	0	-	-	3	16	30	37
Osteochondropathies (732)	12	1	65	10	3	1	0	0	-
Other disorders of bone and cartilage (733)	46	2	8	24	29	57	111	163	206
Flat foot (734)	5	12	9	3	2	4	5	6	4
Acquired deformities of toe (735)	13	14	9	7	9	22	20	29	10
Other acquired deformities of limbs (736)	5	7	4	4	3	7	8	4	7
Curvature of spine (737)	5	1	5	3	4	4	12	6	7
Other acquired deformity (738)	2	2	1	3	1	1	4	3	1
Spina bifida (741)	1	1	0	2	0	0	-	-	1
Other congenital anamolies of nervous system (742)	1	4	-	1	0	0	1	-	-
Congenital anomalies of eye (743)	3	21	1	1	1	2	2	7	10
Congenital anomalies of ear, face and neck (744)	2	6	5	3	2	1	-	1	1
Bulbus cordis anomalies and anomalies of cardiac septal closure (745)	4	26	6	2	1	1	1	1	-
Other congenital anomalies of heart (746)	2	5	2	3	1	1	1	2	-
Other congenital anomalies of circulatory system (747)	1	4	1	2	1	1	2	1	-
Congenital anomalies of respiratory system (748)	0	1	-	0	-	0	1	-	-
Cleft palate and cleft lip (749)	0	3	0	0	0	-	1	-	-
Other congenital anomalies of upper alimentary tract (750)	7	22	1	1	2	7	26	22	25
Other congenital anomalies of digestive system (751)	1	3	1	0	0	1	1	2	7

By age-group and sex

Total		0-4		5-15		16-24		25-44		45-64		65-74		75-84		85 and over	
Male	Female	Male	Female	Male	Female	Male	Female	Male	Female	Male	Female	Male	Female	Male	Female	Male	Female
42	61	41	40	29	39	54	95	59	86	30	52	23	37	11	23	12	6
20	35	18	38	21	25	18	53	25	49	23	26	10	18	3	8	6	8
274	329	47	34	310	384	855	891	217	395	139	148	127	108	145	76	77	51
32	43	1	1	2	0	2	4	4	5	29	37	141	104	232	243	570	431
61	114	148	169	99	122	45	122	48	110	41	102	61	109	30	103	30	81
20	30	32	22	19	23	19	30	20	34	19	33	21	30	9	25	30	16
4	14	-	-	-	1	0	6	2	16	11	26	8	20	2	14	-	10
2	2	2	1	1	-	1	1	3	2	1	3	2	8	2	4	6	10
-	0	-	-	-	-	-	-	-	-	-	0	-	-	-	-	-	-
60	152	1	1	1	6	3	16	26	87	154	297	181	420	109	363	18	136
432	728	1	1	1	2	18	12	86	121	936	1,177	1,509	2,206	1,863	3,100	1,878	2,971
28	42	1	1	3	4	12	17	27	43	52	72	51	57	46	81	36	61
53	40	-	-	35	72	86	84	76	39	50	33	23	12	10	8	6	-
5	3	2	1	1	3	7	6	7	4	3	2	6	5	1	4	-	2
287	405	61	40	142	170	218	255	291	389	406	613	436	589	458	657	458	597
19	17	-	-	2	1	9	9	28	24	33	30	11	11	16	18	12	2
174	234	-	-	-	1	13	15	86	160	467	532	404	470	326	425	160	317
82	76	-	-	1	3	32	28	119	95	150	153	71	84	42	64	18	32
96	143	19	20	50	51	57	98	122	216	143	193	101	122	71	89	77	69
583	693	14	5	50	85	310	470	749	859	982	1,069	676	851	716	900	897	709
24	61	-	-	-	-	-	-	1	5	14	51	79	275	370	354	95	154
314	324	4	-	46	57	94	110	314	311	657	702	462	433	423	371	238	211
83	140	17	10	29	47	60	138	99	155	121	211	114	173	97	134	71	136
59	52	11	3	21	16	27	25	40	43	109	94	147	93	109	70	89	85
202	300	46	31	83	79	102	149	162	265	294	443	461	571	540	616	458	485
3	3	2	3	2	1	2	1	2	1	4	2	12	9	-	11	-	4
4	4	-	-	-	0	-	-	-	-	5	1	20	12	21	36	89	20
16	8	2	1	86	44	12	7	3	3	1	2	1	-	-	1	-	-
18	72	1	2	8	8	18	29	20	39	22	93	35	174	21	248	24	266
5	4	14	10	9	9	2	4	2	2	5	3	4	5	11	2	-	6
7	19	15	13	7	11	4	9	3	14	12	32	9	28	16	36	-	14
5	5	9	6	4	4	4	3	4	3	8	7	7	9	8	2	6	8
4	5	1	1	5	5	3	3	3	5	5	4	16	8	2	9	6	8
2	1	2	1	2	1	5	0	1	1	2	1	2	6	3	2	6	-
0	1	1	1	-	1	1	3	1	0	0	0	-	-	-	-	-	2
1	1	6	1	-	-	-	2	0	0	0	-	-	2	-	-	-	-
3	4	20	22	1	2	0	1	1	1	0	4	3	2	6	8	-	14
2	3	6	6	4	7	2	4	1	3	1	1	-	-	2	1	-	2
3	4	18	34	8	3	3	2	0	2	1	2	1	0	-	2	-	-
2	1	6	3	4	1	1	4	1	1	2	1	1	1	3	1	-	-
1	1	5	4	-	3	3	1	1	1	0	1	1	3	-	1	-	-
0	0	1	1	-	-	0	-	-	-	0	0	-	1	-	-	-	-
0	0	2	4	0	0	1	-	0	-	-	-	-	1	-	-	-	-
7	8	31	13	2	0	0	1	2	2	6	8	23	28	15	26	36	22
1	1	4	3	1	1	-	0	0	0	-	2	1	1	2	2	6	8

Table 25- *continued*

Disease group	Persons, by age group								
	Total	0-4	5-15	16-24	25-44	45-64	65-74	75-84	85 and over
Congenital anomalies of genital organs (752)	8	57	20	4	1	1	1	0	-
Congenital anomalies of urinary system (753)	2	6	0	1	3	3	-	-	-
Certain congenital musculoskeletal deformities (754)	7	46	10	5	5	2	2	3	-
Other congenital anomalies of limbs (755)	3	14	4	3	1	2	1	3	6
Other congenital musculoskeletal anomalies (756)	5	7	2	4	5	8	8	3	1
Congenital anomalies of the integument (757)	18	39	10	11	19	22	17	15	6
Chromosomal anomalies (758)	2	6	2	1	2	1	-	-	-
Other and unspecified congenital anomalies (759)	2	4	3	2	1	2	1	-	-
Fetus or newborn affected by maternal complications of pregnancy (761)	0	-	-	0	0	-	-	-	-
Fetus or newborn affected by complications of placenta, cord and membranes (762)	1	7	-	-	0	-	-	-	-
Fetus or newborn affected by other complications of labour and delivery (763)	0	-	-	-	0	-	-	-	-
Slow fetal growth and fetal malnutrition (764)	0	0	-	0	0	-	-	-	-
Disorders relating to short gestation and unspecified low birthweight (765)	1	12	-	-	-	-	-	-	-
Disorders relating to long gestation and high birthweight (766)	0	-	-	-	0	-	-	-	-
Birth trauma (767)	0	1	-	-	-	-	-	-	-
Intrauterine hypoxia and birth asphyxia (768)	0	3	-	-	0	-	-	-	-
Respiratory distress syndrome (769)	0	2	-	-	-	-	-	-	-
Other respiratory conditions of fetus and newborn (770)	1	8	-	-	0	-	-	0	-
Infections specific to the perinatal period (771)	11	156	0	0	0	0	-	0	-
Fetal and neonatal haemorrhage (772)	0	0	-	0	0	-	-	1	-
Haemolytic disease of fetus or newborn, due to isoimmunization (773)	0	0	-	-	-	-	-	-	-
Other perinatal jaundice (774)	1	12	-	-	-	-	-	0	-
Endocrine and metabolic disturbances specific to the fetus and newborn (775)	0	1	-	-	-	-	-	-	-
Conditions involving the integument and temperature regulation of fetus and newborn (778)	0	1	-	-	0	-	-	-	-
Other and ill-defined conditions originating in the perinatal period (779)	2	22	-	1	0	-	-	-	-
General symptoms (780)	397	445	155	264	298	444	681	1,039	1,268
Symptoms involving nervous and musculoskeletal systems (781)	20	27	10	13	12	23	46	53	37
Symptoms involving skin and other integumentary tissue (782)	260	574	211	189	182	228	337	497	726
Symptoms concerning nutrition, metabolism and development (783)	55	185	35	58	33	35	74	99	124
Symptoms involving head and neck (784)	226	107	263	270	211	220	232	280	263
Symptoms involving cardiovascular system (785)	82	149	64	67	68	75	124	121	121
Symptoms involving respiratory system and other chest symptoms (786)	479	1,509	414	233	294	460	659	721	743
Symptoms involving digestive system (787)	127	309	77	101	85	101	196	277	358
Symptoms involving urinary system (788)	115	123	105	63	72	108	188	352	386
Other symptoms involving abdomen and pelvis (789)	374	354	388	442	363	311	395	442	505
Nonspecific findings on examination of blood (790)	83	364	122	68	52	47	45	47	52
Nonspecific findings on examination of urine (791)	10	2	3	8	10	15	17	21	21

By age-group and sex

Total		0-4		5-15		16-24		25-44		45-64		65-74		75-84		85 and over	
Male	Female	Male	Female	Male	Female	Male	Female	Male	Female	Male	Female	Male	Female	Male	Female	Male	Female
15	1	108	4	39	1	3	4	2	0	1	0	1	0	-	1	-	-
2	2	10	3	0	1	0	2	3	3	3	3	-	-	-	-	-	-
7	8	43	49	10	11	5	4	5	5	1	4	2	1	2	3	-	-
3	3	15	12	4	3	1	4	1	1	2	3	1	2	1	3	-	8
5	6	11	4	2	3	4	3	5	6	8	8	5	9	-	5	6	-
15	21	31	47	8	13	7	15	15	23	18	25	16	18	16	14	6	6
1	2	2	10	1	2	2	1	1	2	1	2	-	-	-	-	-	-
2	2	4	4	3	2	1	3	1	1	2	1	1	0	-	-	-	-
-	0	-	-	-	-	-	0	-	0	-	-	-	-	-	-	-	-
1	0	14	1	-	-	-	-	-	0	-	-	-	-	-	-	-	-
-	0	-	-	-	-	-	-	-	0	-	-	-	-	-	-	-	-
0	0	1	-	-	-	-	1	-	0	-	-	-	-	-	-	-	-
1	1	9	15	-	-	-	-	-	-	-	-	-	-	-	-	-	-
-	0	-	-	-	-	-	-	-	0	-	-	-	-	-	-	-	-
0	0	1	2	-	-	-	-	-	-	-	-	-	-	-	-	-	-
0	0	5	-	-	-	-	-	-	0	-	-	-	-	-	-	-	-
0	0	2	1	-	-	-	-	-	-	-	-	-	-	-	-	-	-
1	0	10	6	-	-	-	-	-	0	-	-	-	-	1	-	-	-
10	12	131	181	-	0	-	1	0	1	-	1	-	-	-	1	-	-
0	0	-	1	-	-	-	0	-	0	-	-	-	-	1	1	-	-
-	0	-	1	-	-	-	-	-	-	-	-	-	-	-	-	-	-
1	1	15	8	-	-	-	-	-	-	-	-	-	-	-	1	-	-
0	-	1	-	-	-	-	-	-	-	-	-	-	-	-	-	-	-
0	0	1	1	-	-	-	-	-	0	-	-	-	-	-	-	-	-
2	2	24	20	-	-	-	2	-	1	-	-	-	-	-	-	-	-
281	509	431	460	140	171	162	366	181	416	324	566	510	819	883	1,133	1,224	1,283
17	24	21	33	11	8	11	14	10	14	20	26	34	56	49	55	30	39
188	328	575	572	191	232	106	271	116	248	155	303	250	407	323	601	565	780
42	68	183	187	33	37	33	82	14	52	27	43	69	78	96	101	113	128
174	276	118	96	257	269	166	374	139	283	166	276	211	248	251	298	256	266
64	100	175	121	71	57	57	77	44	93	46	104	92	151	80	145	18	156
442	515	1,534	1,484	385	444	185	282	254	335	413	508	643	671	720	722	909	688
91	162	316	302	77	78	40	161	40	131	67	135	167	219	266	284	327	368
113	116	97	151	99	111	53	73	62	83	104	111	244	143	526	248	600	315
251	491	362	346	322	457	192	691	188	539	227	397	334	445	450	438	339	560
76	91	374	353	114	131	56	81	39	66	37	56	36	53	42	50	53	51
10	11	1	3	4	3	5	11	6	13	18	11	22	14	23	19	30	18

Consultations
with doctor

Table 25- *continued*

Disease group	Persons, by age group								
	Total	0-4	5-15	16-24	25-44	45-64	65-74	75-84	85 and over
Nonspecific abnormal findings in other body substances (792)	15	10	6	25	23	13	7	5	3
Nonspecific abnormal findings on radiological and other examinatiion of body structure (793)	2	1	0	0	0	4	4	2	-
Nonspecific abnormal results of function studies (794)	3	1	1	1	2	6	10	7	4
Nonspecific abnormal histological and immunological findings (795)	4	0	0	7	9	2	1	1	1
Other nonspecific abnormal findings (796)	45	-	-	9	32	99	113	69	34
Senility without mention of psychosis (797)	11	-	-	-	0	0	6	66	497
Sudden death, cause unknown (798)	6	0	0	-	1	4	21	44	98
Other ill-defined and unknown causes of morbidity and mortality (799)	23	15	9	15	22	23	39	65	84
Fracture of vault of skull (800)	0	2	0	-	0	0	-	-	-
Fracture of base of skull (801)	0	-	-	0	0	0	0	-	-
Fracture of face bones (802)	8	1	7	20	10	3	3	5	6
Other and unqualified skull fractures (803)	1	1	1	2	1	1	1	0	4
Multiple fractures involving skull or face with other bones (804)	0	0	0	0	0	-	1	-	-
Fracture of vertebral column without mention of spinal cord lesion (805)	6	-	0	4	7	7	7	23	41
Fracture of vertebral column with spinal cord lesion (806)	0	-	-	1	0	0	-	0	1
Fracture of rib(s), sternum, larynx and trachea (807)	17	1	2	9	15	29	26	37	50
Fracture of pelvis (808)	3	0	0	2	2	2	4	12	40
Ill-defined fractures of trunk (809)	0	-	-	-	-	0	-	-	-
Fracture of clavicle (810)	5	8	9	9	4	3	4	2	12
Fracture of scapula (811)	0	-	-	1	0	0	1	0	-
Fracture of humerus (812)	8	4	7	5	3	8	21	21	37
Fracture of radius and ulna (813)	26	14	32	20	17	28	34	55	84
Fracture of carpal bone(s) (814)	8	0	4	11	11	7	6	4	3
Fracture of metacarpal bone(s) (815)	10	0	10	26	10	5	3	7	1
Fracture of one or more phalanges of hand (816)	9	1	16	12	11	7	4	3	1
Multiple fractures of hand bones (817)	0	-	-	0	-	-	-	-	-
Ill-defined fractures of upper limb (818)	0	-	-	1	0	0	1	2	3
Multiple fractures involving both upper limbs, and upper limb with rib(s) and sternum (819)	1	-	-	-	1	1	2	1	-
Fracture of neck of femur (820)	10	-	-	0	1	4	22	77	225
Fracture of other and unspecified parts of femur (821)	5	1	2	3	4	4	9	19	61
Fracture of patella (822)	3	0	2	4	3	3	5	7	1
Fracture of tibia and fibula (823)	13	7	6	22	15	13	4	6	25
Fracture of ankle (824)	13	0	3	17	13	18	16	23	6
Fracture of one or more tarsal and metatarsal bones (825)	10	3	8	6	12	13	10	5	1
Fracture of one or more phalanges of foot (826)	6	1	6	9	7	8	4	3	3
Other, multiple and ill-defined fractures of lower limb (827)	0	-	-	0	1	1	0	0	-
Multiple fractures involving both lower limbs, lower with upper limb, and lower limb(s) with rib(s) and sternum (828)	0	-	-	-	0	0	-	-	-
Fracture of unspecified bones (829)	3	1	2	3	3	2	4	5	9
Dislocation of jaw (830)	0	-	-	1	0	0	0	0	-
Dislocation of shoulder (831)	5	1	1	13	5	4	5	11	19
Dislocation of elbow (832)	1	9	1	2	0	1	0	-	1
Dislocation of wrist (833)	0	-	1	1	0	0	-	0	1
Dislocation of finger (834)	2	1	2	2	2	3	2	3	1
Dislocation of hip (835)	1	1	0	1	0	0	4	1	1

By age-group and sex

Total		0-4		5-15		16-24		25-44		45-64		65-74		75-84		85 and over	
Male	Female	Male	Female	Male	Female	Male	Female	Male	Female	Male	Female	Male	Female	Male	Female	Male	Female
2	29	4	16	1	10	1	49	2	45	3	24	1	11	-	8	-	4
1	2	1	1	0	0	0	0	0	1	2	6	4	4	2	2	-	-
3	3	1	-	0	1	0	1	4	1	5	7	8	11	7	8	-	6
0	8	1	-	-	1	0	13	0	17	-	5	1	1	-	2	6	-
42	48	-	-	-	-	6	12	34	30	96	102	95	127	58	75	59	26
7	15	-	-	-	-	-	-	-	0	0	0	3	9	77	60	541	483
6	7	-	1	1	-	-	-	0	1	4	4	27	16	60	35	125	89
18	29	14	17	11	7	9	22	16	27	19	27	29	47	56	70	59	93
0	0	1	2	0	0	-	-	0	0	0	-	-	-	-	-	-	-
0	-	-	-	-	-	0	-	0	-	1	-	1	-	-	-	-	-
11	5	1	1	8	6	33	8	15	5	3	3	-	5	1	7	6	6
2	1	1	-	2	0	4	1	2	1	2	-	3	-	-	1	-	6
0	0	-	1	-	0	0	-	0	-	-	-	1	-	-	-	-	-
5	7	-	-	0	-	4	4	8	6	8	7	3	9	15	27	12	51
1	0	-	-	-	-	2	-	1	-	0	0	-	-	-	1	-	2
20	14	1	1	2	1	11	6	23	8	32	26	27	25	44	33	36	55
2	3	1	-	0	0	2	1	3	2	3	1	1	6	2	18	24	45
-	0	-	-	-	-	-	-	-	-	-	1	-	-	-	-	-	-
7	4	7	10	12	5	15	2	7	2	2	4	3	5	2	2	12	12
0	0	-	-	-	-	1	1	1	0	0	-	-	1	-	1	-	-
5	11	3	5	8	7	6	3	3	3	3	14	7	33	5	31	12	45
22	30	15	13	35	29	30	10	23	12	17	39	8	55	14	80	30	102
9	6	1	-	5	2	16	6	13	9	6	8	8	4	2	5	6	2
16	4	-	1	17	4	47	5	18	3	6	4	2	4	6	8	-	2
12	6	1	1	17	15	18	6	16	5	10	4	2	6	1	4	-	2
0	-	-	-	-	-	0	-	-	-	-	-	-	-	-	-	-	-
1	0	-	-	-	-	1	-	1	0	0	0	-	1	2	2	6	2
1	0	-	-	-	-	-	-	1	0	2	1	2	1	-	1	-	-
4	16	-	-	-	-	0	-	2	0	3	5	6	34	27	107	107	264
4	6	1	1	2	1	6	-	5	3	4	4	3	13	6	27	18	75
4	3	-	1	3	0	7	2	3	4	4	2	9	2	-	11	-	2
18	7	9	5	6	6	38	6	25	5	16	11	3	5	-	10	-	33
14	11	-	1	5	1	25	9	19	7	18	18	3	26	9	31	12	4
11	8	5	1	11	5	8	4	16	9	12	13	5	14	2	7	-	2
7	6	1	1	6	5	12	5	9	6	6	9	2	6	-	4	-	4
1	0	-	-	-	-	1	-	1	0	1	-	-	0	1	-	-	-
0	0	-	-	-	-	-	-	0	1	-	0	-	-	-	-	-	-
3	3	-	3	2	2	4	2	4	3	2	3	3	4	2	7	6	10
0	1	-	-	-	-	-	2	0	1	0	0	1	-	-	1	-	-
7	4	-	1	1	2	19	7	7	3	5	3	3	7	7	13	12	22
1	2	4	13	2	-	3	2	0	1	1	0	-	0	-	-	-	2
0	1	-	-	0	1	0	1	0	0	-	1	-	-	-	1	-	2
3	2	2	1	3	2	3	2	4	1	3	2	3	2	6	1	-	2
1	0	1	1	0	-	1	1	-	0	1	-	8	0	1	1	-	2

Table 25 - *continued*

Disease group	Persons, by age group								
	Total	0-4	5-15	16-24	25-44	45-64	65-74	75-84	85 and over
Dislocation of knee (836)	5	-	4	10	6	3	2	2	-
Dislocation of ankle (837)	1	-	1	-	1	0	1	0	1
Dislocation of foot (838)	0	-	1	0	0	0	1	0	-
Other, multiple and ill-defined dislocations (839)	2	0	1	1	3	3	3	3	-
Sprains and strains of shoulder and upper arm (840)	65	8	17	58	79	96	76	69	58
Sprains and strains of elbow and forearm (841)	16	17	16	13	18	20	7	6	3
Sprains and strains of wrist and hand (842)	50	11	74	69	52	43	37	37	41
Sprains and strains of hip and thigh (843)	43	9	36	41	42	53	49	58	49
Sprains and strains of knee and leg (844)	107	14	92	144	129	121	75	65	38
Sprains and strains of ankle and foot (845)	111	30	129	147	115	109	106	79	59
Sprains and strains of sacroiliac region (846)	65	-	5	47	96	103	56	36	36
Sprains and strains of other and unspecified parts of back (847)	243	5	58	315	371	293	124	138	130
Other and ill-defined sprains and strains (848)	74	4	36	73	91	95	73	78	86
Concussion (850)	14	36	27	20	7	6	4	11	22
Cerebral laceration and contusion (851)	1	2	1	0	0	1	-	1	-
Subarachnoid, subdural and extradural haemorrhage, following injury (852)	0	1	-	1	0	0	-	1	-
Intracranial injury of other and unspecified nature (854)	11	41	22	13	7	4	5	4	7
Traumatic pneumothorax and haemothorax (860)	0	-	0	1	0	0	-	1	-
Injury to heart and lung (861)	0	0	-	-	-	-	-	0	-
Injury to other and unspecified intrathoracic organs (862)	0	-	-	1	0	0	0	-	-
Injury to gastrointestinal tract (863)	0	-	1	0	0	0	1	-	-
Injury to spleen (865)	0	-	-	0	0	-	-	-	-
Injury to kidney (866)	0	-	0	1	0	-	-	-	-
Injury to pelvic organs 867)	0	-	-	0	1	0	1	-	-
Internal injury to unspecified or ill-defined organs (869)	1	-	-	0	0	2	0	1	-
Open wound of ocular adnexa (870)	2	4	3	2	2	2	1	1	-
Open wound of eyeball (871)	3	2	3	2	4	3	2	-	-
Open wound of ear (872)	2	4	5	2	1	1	1	0	1
Other open wound of head (873)	33	124	51	25	15	16	19	45	152
Open wound of neck (874)	0	1	0	1	0	0	-	-	-
Open wound of chest (wall) (875)	0	-	0	1	0	-	-	-	1
Open wound of back (876)	0	0	0	0	0	-	-	-	-
Open wound of buttock (877)	0	-	1	-	0	0	0	-	3
Open wound of genital organs (external), including traumatic amputation (878)	2	5	4	3	2	1	1	2	1
Open wound of other and unspecified sites, except limbs (879)	3	2	3	2	2	2	1	8	12
Open wound of shoulder and upper arm (880)	3	1	2	4	3	3	1	3	3
Open wound of elbow, forearm and wrist (881)	8	2	8	13	6	4	4	30	49
Open wound of hand except finger(s) alone (882)	10	7	7	19	10	8	7	7	15
Open wound of finger(s) (883)	25	21	18	32	27	26	20	21	21
Multiple and unspecified open wounds of upper limb (884)	0	-	0	1	0	0	1	2	1
Traumatic amputation of thumb (complete) (partial) (885)	0	-	-	1	0	-	-	-	-
Traumatic amputation of other finger(s) (complete) (partial) (886)	1	-	1	0	2	2	1	-	-
Traumatic amputation of arm and hand (complete) (partial) (887)	0	-	-	-	-	0	-	0	-
Open wound of hip and thigh (890)	1	1	4	3	1	1	0	1	1
Open wound of knee, leg (except thigh) and ankle (891)	19	5	25	14	8	14	32	87	102

By age-group and sex

Total		0-4		5-15		16-24		25-44		45-64		65-74		75-84		85 and over	
Male	Female	Male	Female	Male	Female	Male	Female	Male	Female	Male	Female	Male	Female	Male	Female	Male	Female
6	3	-	-	2	6	13	7	9	4	5	2	1	2	1	2	-	-
0	1	-	-	1	1	-	-	1	1	-	0	1	1	-	1	6	-
0	0	-	-	0	2	1	-	0	0	-	0	1	1	-	1	-	-
3	2	1	-	2	1	2	1	4	3	4	2	1	4	2	3	-	-
67	63	6	10	16	19	66	50	83	75	101	91	66	83	72	67	42	63
17	14	13	22	14	17	15	10	20	16	23	18	8	6	5	7	-	4
45	55	10	13	71	76	72	66	48	56	28	58	24	46	25	44	48	39
49	37	13	5	47	25	51	30	49	35	56	51	47	50	66	53	53	47
126	89	13	15	94	89	177	112	162	95	135	107	84	67	41	79	-	51
107	114	39	21	120	139	172	123	125	105	83	135	66	138	52	96	30	69
57	72	-	-	4	6	38	55	82	110	94	113	51	61	32	39	30	37
252	235	6	4	58	59	306	324	387	354	308	277	107	139	121	148	196	108
73	74	3	4	41	32	83	62	98	85	85	105	50	91	73	81	59	95
15	12	37	36	38	15	18	22	6	8	6	6	2	7	11	10	24	22
1	0	1	2	1	0	0	0	1	0	0	1	-	-	1	1	-	-
0	0	1	-	-	-	1	-	0	-	0	0	-	-	2	1	-	-
13	10	38	44	27	17	16	9	8	5	3	6	5	5	3	5	6	8
0	0	-	-	0	-	1	1	-	0	0	-	-	-	-	1	-	-
-	0	-	1	-	-	-	-	-	-	-	-	-	-	-	1	-	-
0	0	-	-	-	-	-	1	0	0	0	-	1	-	-	-	-	-
0	0	-	-	1	1	-	0	0	0	0	0	1	1	-	-	-	-
0	0	-	-	-	-	0	-	1	0	-	-	-	-	-	-	-	-
0	0	-	-	1	-	2	0	0	-	-	-	-	-	-	-	-	-
0	0	-	-	-	-	-	0	1	1	0	-	1	-	-	-	-	-
1	0	-	-	-	-	0	-	1	0	2	1	1	-	2	-	-	-
3	1	4	5	4	2	3	-	3	1	3	1	-	1	2	-	-	-
4	2	1	3	4	2	4	1	7	2	3	2	2	2	-	-	-	-
2	2	6	2	5	5	2	2	1	1	0	2	1	1	1	-	-	2
40	26	160	86	71	31	37	14	20	10	17	15	19	19	34	51	155	152
0	0	1	-	-	0	1	0	0	0	0	0	-	-	-	-	-	-
0	0	-	-	0	0	2	-	-	-	0	-	-	-	-	-	-	2
0	0	-	1	1	-	1	-	-	-	0	-	-	-	-	-	-	-
0	0	-	-	1	0	-	-	0	-	1	-	1	-	-	-	6	2
2	2	3	7	5	4	4	2	2	1	0	1	1	1	5	1	6	-
3	3	3	2	4	2	4	1	3	1	1	3	1	0	5	10	-	16
3	2	1	1	3	1	5	3	4	2	3	3	1	1	1	3	-	4
10	6	2	1	10	6	21	6	10	2	4	5	3	5	31	29	65	43
13	6	6	7	9	5	29	8	13	7	10	6	13	1	10	5	12	16
33	17	22	20	24	13	51	14	37	17	33	20	25	15	18	22	36	16
0	1	-	-	0	0	1	1	0	0	0	0	1	1	-	3	6	-
0	-	-	-	-	-	1	-	1	-	-	-	-	-	-	-	-	-
2	1	-	-	0	1	0	-	3	1	4	1	1	1	-	-	-	-
0	-	-	-	-	-	-	-	-	-	0	-	-	-	1	-	-	-
2	1	1	1	4	3	4	1	1	0	1	1	1	-	1	1	-	2
14	25	5	5	32	17	20	8	9	7	8	20	9	51	24	124	24	128

281

Table 25 - *continued*

Disease group	Persons, by age group								
	Total	0-4	5-15	16-24	25-44	45-64	65-74	75-84	85 and over
Open wound of foot except toe(s) alone (892)	5	6	8	6	5	3	5	5	4
Open wound of toe(s) (893)	4	5	3	1	1	7	4	10	7
Multiple and unspecified open wound of lower limb (894)	2	-	2	2	1	2	3	5	10
Traumatic amputation of toe(s) (complete) (partial) (895)	0	-	-	-	0	1	0	-	-
Traumatic amputation of foot (complete) (partial) (896)	0	-	0	-	0	-	0	-	-
Traumatic amputation of leg(s) (complete) (partial) (897)	0	-	-	-	0	0	-	1	-
Injury to blood vessels of head and neck (900)	0	-	0	-	-	-	-	-	-
Injury to blood vessels of abdomen and pelvis (902)	0	-	0	0	0	-	-	0	-
Injury to blood vessels of upper extremity (903)	0	-	-	0	-	0	0	-	-
Injury to blood vessels of lower extremity and unspecified sites (904)	0	-	-	0	0	1	1	0	-
Late effects of musculoskeletal and connective tissue injuries (905)	0	-	0	0	0	1	2	-	1
Late effects of injuries to skin and subcutaneous tissues (906)	0	-	0	0	0	0	1	0	1
Late effects of injuries to the nervous system (907)	1	1	0	1	1	2	2	2	1
Late effects of other and unspecified external causes (909)	1	1	1	2	1	2	1	1	3
Superficial injury of face, neck and scalp except eye (910)	21	73	34	17	11	10	16	34	64
Superficial injury of trunk (911)	15	9	19	16	12	13	19	27	40
Superficial injury of shoulder and upper arm (912)	9	4	11	12	8	6	8	19	30
Superficial injury of elbow, forearm and wrist (913)	2	1	3	2	1	2	3	5	10
Superficial injury of hand(s) except finger(s) alone (914)	18	24	27	21	16	15	12	15	28
Superficial injury of finger(s) (915)	3	5	3	2	2	3	2	3	-
Superficial injury of hip, thigh, leg and ankle (916)	35	17	33	31	24	35	44	102	112
Superficial injury of foot and toe(s) (917)	21	19	34	24	16	18	26	18	25
Superficial injury of eye and adnexa (918)	11	12	11	7	15	12	7	7	-
Superficial injury of other, multiple and unspecified sites (919)	23	33	32	23	19	20	19	31	37
Contusion of face, scalp, and neck except eye(s) (920)	19	66	33	19	10	7	14	30	47
Contusion of eye and adnexa (921)	7	10	12	10	5	4	7	11	19
Contusion of trunk (922)	28	8	18	22	24	30	38	61	151
Contusion of upper limb (923)	29	20	44	37	23	21	30	42	68
Contusion of lower limb and of other and unspecified sites (924)	57	25	62	63	47	50	66	107	166
Crushing injury of face, scalp and neck (925)	0	-	0	0	0	-	-	-	-
Crushing injury of trunk (926)	1	1	1	-	1	0	-	0	-
Crushing injury of upper limb (927)	4	9	5	6	4	5	1	1	-
Crushing injury of lower limb (928)	3	3	2	4	2	3	0	0	-
Crushing injury of multiple and unspecified sites (929)	1	1	0	1	1	1	-	-	-
Foreign body on external eye (930)	12	7	8	13	16	13	10	4	7
Foreign body in ear (931)	4	13	10	1	2	2	2	2	1
Foreign body in nose (932)	1	14	2	-	-	-	-	-	-
Foreign body in pharynx and larynx (933)	1	1	1	1	1	1	1	3	-
Foreign body in trachea, bronchus and lung (934)	0	-	-	-	0	0	-	-	-

By age-group and sex

Total		0-4		5-15		16-24		25-44		45-64		65-74		75-84		85 and over	
Male	Female	Male	Female	Male	Female	Male	Female	Male	Female	Male	Female	Male	Female	Male	Female	Male	Female
6	5	7	5	11	6	7	6	5	5	2	4	7	4	3	6	12	2
4	3	5	5	2	3	1	0	1	1	11	3	6	2	10	10	-	10
2	2	-	-	2	1	2	1	1	0	2	2	2	5	2	6	-	14
0	0	-	-	-	-	-	-	0	-	1	0	-	0	-	-	-	-
0	0	-	-	-	0	-	-	0	-	-	-	-	0	-	-	-	-
0	0	-	-	-	-	-	-	-	-	0	0	0	-	-	-	2	-
0	-	-	-	0	-	-	-	-	-	-	-	-	-	-	-	-	-
0	-	-	-	0	-	0	-	0	-	-	-	-	-	1	-	-	-
-	0	-	-	-	-	-	0	-	-	-	0	-	0	-	-	-	-
0	0	-	-	-	-	-	0	-	0	0	1	1	0	-	1	-	-
0	0	-	-	0	-	1	-	-	0	1	0	1	2	-	-	-	2
0	0	-	-	-	1	0	-	1	0	0	0	1	1	-	1	-	2
2	1	1	1	1	-	2	-	2	0	3	1	2	3	3	1	-	2
1	1	1	-	2	0	1	2	1	1	2	2	2	0	-	2	-	4
20	22	74	71	40	28	17	17	10	11	7	13	9	21	30	36	36	73
15	15	8	10	21	17	16	15	14	10	11	15	13	23	27	27	59	33
9	9	2	6	13	9	13	10	9	6	6	6	5	11	9	25	6	37
2	2	-	1	4	2	2	1	2	1	1	2	3	3	8	3	24	6
22	15	27	22	29	24	26	17	21	10	16	15	15	10	18	12	36	26
3	2	5	6	2	3	2	2	2	2	3	2	2	3	7	1	-	-
26	43	19	16	32	34	35	26	19	30	24	46	21	62	57	129	65	128
20	22	18	20	34	34	25	24	15	17	15	21	31	22	11	22	12	30
13	10	13	11	14	9	9	5	16	14	13	12	10	4	6	8	-	-
19	27	33	33	34	30	19	28	15	24	14	25	14	23	15	41	24	41
19	20	70	62	43	24	21	17	8	11	6	9	4	22	9	42	30	53
7	8	9	11	14	10	9	11	6	5	2	5	2	10	7	14	12	22
26	30	9	8	20	15	24	19	26	23	29	30	26	47	37	76	143	154
30	28	22	17	47	41	38	35	26	20	20	21	26	34	32	49	89	61
49	64	22	27	73	50	69	57	44	51	35	65	39	88	64	133	83	193
0	0	-	-	0	-	0	0	-	0	-	-	-	-	-	-	-	-
1	0	2	-	1	0	-	-	1	1	0	-	-	-	-	1	-	-
7	2	13	6	5	5	9	3	7	1	8	2	1	1	2	1	-	-
4	1	4	3	2	2	6	3	4	1	6	1	-	0	-	1	-	-
1	0	1	-	-	0	1	0	2	0	1	0	-	-	-	-	-	-
19	6	10	4	9	7	23	4	25	7	19	6	15	5	6	3	12	6
4	4	11	15	9	10	1	1	2	2	2	1	2	2	5	-	6	-
1	1	11	18	2	2	-	-	-	-	-	-	-	-	-	-	-	-
1	1	-	2	1	0	1	2	1	2	1	1	1	2	2	3	-	-
0	0	-	-	-	-	-	-	-	0	0	-	-	-	-	-	-	-

Consultations with doctor

Table 25 - *continued*

Disease group	Persons, by age group								
	Total	0-4	5-15	16-24	25-44	45-64	65-74	75-84	85 and over
Foreign body in mouth, oesophagus and stomach (935)	1	4	1	1	1	1	0	-	3
Foreign body in intestine and colon (936)	0	-	0	0	-	-	-	-	-
Foreign body in anus and rectum (937)	0	-	-	-	0	-	-	-	-
Foreign body in digestive system, unspecified (938)	1	3	1	0	0	0	-	-	-
Foreign body in genitourinary tract (939)	2	0	0	3	4	1	-	-	-
Burn confined to eye and adnexa (940)	1	1	1	1	1	1	0	-	-
Burn of face, head and neck (941)	2	5	1	3	2	1	2	0	1
Burn of trunk (942)	3	7	4	1	1	2	9	3	6
Burn of upper limb, except wrist and hand (943)	4	8	1	4	3	4	4	7	6
Burn of wrist(s) and hand(s) (944)	7	18	6	8	7	5	6	7	12
Burn of lower limb(s) (945)	8	15	5	7	6	5	7	24	22
Burns of multiple specified sites (946)	0	-	0	0	0	0	-	0	-
Burn of internal organs (947)	1	-	0	1	1	1	0	-	1
Burns classified according to extent of body surface involved (948)	1	2	0	1	1	0	1	-	-
Burn, unspecified (949)	2	8	1	3	2	2	1	2	7
Injury to other cranial nerve(s) (951)	0	-	-	0	1	0	1	0	-
Spinal cord lesion without evidence of spinal bone injury (952)	0	-	-	-	-	0	1	1	-
Injury to nerve roots and spinal plexus (953)	1	-	0	0	1	1	1	2	-
Injury to other nerve(s) of trunk excluding shoulder and pelvic girdles (954)	0	-	-	0	0	-	-	-	-
Injury to peripheral nerve(s) of shoulder girdle and upper limb (955)	4	-	1	3	6	4	4	1	-
Injury to peripheral nerve(s) of pelvic girdle and lower limb (956)	1	-	-	1	1	2	1	3	-
Injury to other and unspecified nerves (957)	2	9	2	3	2	1	1	1	1
Certain early complications of trauma (958)	4	1	2	4	3	4	5	5	16
Injury, other and unspecified (959)	50	25	52	66	53	44	44	54	90
Poisoning by antibiotics (960)	0	-	-	0	0	0	0	1	-
Poisoning by other anti-infectives (961)	0	-	-	-	-	0	0	0	1
Poisoning by hormones and synthetic substitutes (962)	0	1	-	-	0	-	-	-	-
Poisoning by primarily systemic agents (963)	0	-	-	0	0	-	-	-	-
Poisoning by agents primarily affecting blood constituents (964)	0	0	-	-	-	-	-	-	-
Poisoning by analgesics, antipyretics and antirheumatics (965)	0	0	0	1	0	-	1	-	-
Poisoning by anticonvulsants and anti-Parkinsonism drugs (966)	0	-	-	-	-	0	-	-	-
Poisoning by sedatives and hypnotics (967)	0	-	-	-	-	0	-	-	-
Poisoning by psychotropic agents (969)	0	-	-	1	-	0	-	-	-
Poisoning by agents primarily affecting the cardiovascular system (972)	1	-	-	-	0	0	1	5	9
Poisoning by water, mineral and uric acid metabolism drugs (974)	0	-	-	-	-	-	-	-	1
Poisoning by other and unspecified drugs and medicaments (977)	1	2	0	1	1	0	1	1	-
Poisoning by bacterial vaccines (978)	0	0	0	0	0	-	-	-	-
Poisoning by other vaccines and biological substances (979)	0	1	-	-	0	0	-	-	-
Toxic effect of alcohol (980)	1	-	0	1	1	1	-	-	-
Toxic effect of petroleum products (981)	0	-	-	0	-	-	-	-	-
Toxic effect of solvents other than petroleum-based (982)	0	-	1	1	0	0	-	-	-
Toxic effect of corrosive aromatics, acids and caustic alkalis (983)	0	1	-	-	0	-	-	-	-
Toxic effect of lead and its compounds (including fumes) (984)	0	-	-	0	0	0	-	-	-
Toxic effect of other metals (985)	0	-	0	1	0	-	-	-	-

By age-group and sex

Total		0-4		5-15		16-24		25-44		45-64		65-74		75-84		85 and over	
Male	Female	Male	Female	Male	Female	Male	Female	Male	Female	Male	Female	Male	Female	Male	Female	Male	Female
1	1	5	2	1	1	0	1	0	1	1	0	1	-	-	-	-	4
0	0	-	-	0	0	0	-	-	-	-	-	-	-	-	-	-	-
0	-	-	-	-	-	-	-	0	-	-	-	-	-	-	-	-	-
0	1	4	3	0	1	-	1	0	0	0	0	-	-	-	-	-	-
0	4	1	-	0	1	-	5	-	9	0	3	-	-	-	-	-	-
1	0	-	1	1	1	1	0	1	1	1	0	1	-	-	-	-	-
2	2	9	2	1	2	3	4	2	2	1	1	3	2	-	1	-	2
2	3	7	6	6	2	1	0	1	2	2	2	1	16	2	4	6	6
3	4	7	8	1	1	4	4	3	4	3	5	3	6	1	10	12	4
7	8	16	20	7	4	7	8	7	7	4	7	5	7	6	8	18	10
8	7	16	14	5	5	11	2	5	6	4	7	7	7	42	14	6	28
0	0	-	-	-	0	0	0	0	-	1	-	-	-	-	1	-	-
1	0	-	-	-	0	2	0	1	1	1	1	1	-	-	-	-	2
1	1	2	2	0	0	-	2	1	0	0	0	1	0	-	-	-	-
2	2	8	8	1	1	2	4	1	3	2	1	1	1	2	1	-	10
0	0	-	-	-	-	-	0	1	0	0	1	-	1	-	1	-	-
0	0	-	-	-	-	-	-	-	-	0	0	1	0	2	-	-	-
1	1	-	-	-	0	-	1	1	1	1	2	1	1	-	3	-	-
0	0	-	-	-	-	-	1	0	-	-	-	-	-	-	-	-	-
6	2	-	-	1	1	5	2	10	2	5	3	8	1	3	-	-	-
1	1	-	-	-	-	1	-	1	2	1	2	1	1	3	2	-	-
3	2	13	6	2	2	5	2	2	1	2	1	1	1	1	1	-	2
4	3	1	1	3	2	5	2	4	3	4	4	5	5	7	3	30	12
56	45	24	26	60	42	85	48	65	41	46	42	30	55	32	67	71	97
0	0	-	-	-	-	-	0	-	0	0	0	-	0	-	2	-	-
0	0	-	-	-	-	-	-	-	-	0	0	1	-	-	1	-	2
0	0	1	1	-	-	-	-	0	-	-	-	-	-	-	-	-	-
0	0	-	-	-	-	-	-	1	1	-	-	-	-	-	-	-	-
-	0	-	1	-	-	-	-	-	-	-	-	-	-	-	-	-	-
0	0	-	1	-	0	1	1	0	0	-	-	1	1	-	-	-	-
-	0	-	-	-	-	-	-	-	-	-	0	-	-	-	-	-	-
-	0	-	-	-	-	-	-	-	-	-	0	-	-	-	-	-	-
0	0	-	-	-	-	1	0	-	-	-	1	-	-	-	-	-	-
0	1	-	-	-	-	-	-	0	0	0	0	1	0	2	6	-	12
0	-	-	-	-	-	-	-	-	-	-	-	-	-	-	-	6	-
1	1	2	3	0	-	0	1	1	1	-	0	2	1	1	1	-	-
-	0	-	1	-	1	-	0	-	0	-	-	-	-	-	-	-	-
0	0	1	-	-	-	-	-	0	-	0	0	-	-	-	-	-	-
1	0	-	-	1	0	1	0	1	1	2	-	-	-	-	-	-	-
0	-	-	-	-	-	0	-	-	-	-	-	-	-	-	-	-	-
1	0	-	-	1	0	1	1	0	-	0	-	-	-	-	-	-	-
0	0	1	-	-	-	-	-	0	0	-	-	-	-	-	-	-	-
0	0	-	-	-	0	-	0	-	-	0	-	-	-	-	-	-	-
-	0	-	-	-	0	-	1	-	0	-	-	-	-	-	-	-	-

Table 25 - *continued*

Disease group	Persons, by age group								
	Total	0-4	5-15	16-24	25-44	45-64	65-74	75-84	85 and over
Toxic effect of carbon monoxide (986)	0	0	-	0	0	0	0	-	-
Toxic effect of other gases, fumes or vapours (987)	0	-	0	2	0	0	0	1	1
Toxic effect of noxious substances eaten as food (988)	1	1	1	1	2	1	1	2	3
Toxic effect of other substances, chiefly nonmedicinal as to source (989)	2	2	3	4	2	1	3	3	1
Effects of radiation, unspecified (990)	0	-	-	-	0	1	2	0	-
Effects of reduced temperature (991)	10	4	10	6	6	10	21	22	28
Effects of heat and light (992)	2	3	1	1	2	1	2	2	1
Effects of air pressure (993)	1	-	1	1	1	1	0	-	-
Effects of other external causes (994)	4	9	6	2	3	4	7	7	1
Certain adverse effects not elsewhere classified (995)	320	454	290	315	275	276	310	561	879
Complications peculiar to certain specified procedures (996)	6	1	0	3	3	5	9	34	78
Complications affecting specified body systems, not elsewhere classified (997)	1	-	0	-	0	2	2	0	1
Other complications of procedures, not elsewhere classified (998)	57	21	18	40	72	70	79	83	56
Complications of medical care, not elsewhere classified (999)	1	8	1	1	1	1	1	1	4
Contact with or exposure to communicable diseases (V01)	15	36	28	13	18	5	2	0	3
Carrier or suspected carrier of infectious diseases (V02)	1	1	1	2	2	1	-	0	1
Need for prophylactic vaccination and inoculation against bacterial diseases (V03)	218	225	142	165	217	301	252	178	149
Need for prophylactic vaccination and inoculation against certain viral diseases (V04)	284	138	156	82	109	276	821	1,235	1,525
Need for other prophylactic vaccination and inoculation against single diseases (V05)	4	2	1	6	7	4	1	-	-
Need for prophylactic vaccination and inoculation against combinations of diseases (V06)	276	3,595	130	22	19	10	6	2	1
Need for isolation and other prophylactic measures (V07)	9	3	4	9	12	12	7	1	-
Health supervision of infant or child (V20)	145	2,080	10	1	1	-	0	-	-
Normal pregnancy (V22)	540	1	14	1,231	1,236	5	-	-	-
Supervision of high-risk pregnancy (V23)	5	-	-	12	10	0	-	-	-
Postpartum care and examination (V24)	134	9	2	277	317	1	0	0	-
Contraceptive management (V25)	1,119	4	111	3,836	1,936	92	2	0	1
Procreative management (V26)	12	1	1	33	23	0	-	-	-
Attention to artificial openings (V55)	0	-	-	-	0	0	-	1	1
Housing, household and economic circumstances (V60)	12	8	1	22	14	9	9	22	22
Other family circumstances (V61)	112	19	14	79	149	147	144	179	111
Other psychosocial circumstances (V62)	16	-	3	22	25	19	5	10	28
Other persons seeking consultation without complaint or sickness (V65)	37	33	22	47	42	37	32	33	30
Encounters for administrative purposes (V68)	992	16	16	887	1,377	1,992	273	140	124
General medical examination (V70)	210	46	123	176	172	188	108	988	1,135
Special investigations and examinations (V72)	62	2	6	151	103	43	10	10	4
Special screening examination for viral diseases (V73)	34	1	10	97	63	4	3	-	1
Special screening examination for bacterial and spirochaetal diseases (V74)	1	1	0	2	1	0	0	1	-

By age-group and sex

Total		0-4		5-15		16-24		25-44		45-64		65-74		75-84		85 and over	
Male	Female	Male	Female	Male	Female	Male	Female	Male	Female	Male	Female	Male	Female	Male	Female	Male	Female
0	0	1	-	-	-	-	0	0	0	0	0	-	0	-	-	-	-
1	0	-	-	1	-	2	1	0	0	0	0	-	0	2	-	6	-
1	2	1	1	2	1	1	2	1	3	1	1	1	0	1	2	12	-
2	3	4	1	3	2	2	6	1	3	1	2	2	4	1	3	-	2
0	0	-	-	-	-	-	-	0	-	0	1	1	2	1	-	-	-
5	14	5	3	4	16	1	12	1	11	6	13	22	20	22	23	48	22
1	2	2	4	2	1	1	1	1	3	1	1	2	1	1	2	-	2
1	1	-	-	2	1	1	2	1	1	1	0	1	-	-	-	-	-
3	5	9	9	7	6	1	2	2	3	2	6	4	9	6	8	-	2
255	384	470	436	273	307	253	377	206	344	202	352	249	359	419	646	660	952
9	4	-	1	-	0	4	2	1	5	7	3	17	1	64	16	303	4
1	1	-	-	-	0	-	-	0	1	2	1	2	2	-	1	-	2
49	66	34	8	19	17	25	54	46	99	67	73	94	67	101	73	36	63
1	2	9	7	0	1	0	1	1	2	1	1	-	1	1	1	6	4
14	16	32	41	25	31	11	15	16	20	6	5	2	1	-	1	-	4
1	1	1	1	2	1	1	3	3	2	1	1	-	-	-	1	-	2
194	242	228	221	141	143	141	188	187	248	252	350	228	271	165	186	196	134
227	338	140	137	79	237	63	100	90	128	239	313	794	843	1,225	1,241	1,527	1,525
3	5	1	2	0	1	4	9	7	7	2	6	1	1	-	-	-	-
289	264	3,647	3,541	123	137	17	26	16	23	10	11	3	9	-	3	-	2
8	9	2	4	3	4	6	11	10	13	12	12	9	5	3	-	-	-
148	141	2,040	2,122	10	11	0	1	1	2	-	-	1	-	-	-	-	-
0	1,058	1	2	-	29	-	2,453	0	2,481	0	11	-	-	-	-	-	-
-	9	-	-	-	-	-	24	-	20	-	0	-	-	-	-	-	-
1	262	7	11	-	3	-	553	0	636	0	1	-	0	-	1	-	-
23	2,171	3	4	1	226	10	7,637	63	3,822	8	178	2	2	1	-	-	2
4	19	1	-	-	1	3	63	10	37	0	0	-	-	-	-	-	-
0	0	-	-	-	-	-	-	-	0	-	0	-	-	1	1	6	-
6	17	9	8	2	0	5	39	6	21	6	12	7	11	7	31	36	18
55	168	15	22	9	18	16	143	67	231	71	226	89	188	152	194	166	93
15	17	-	-	4	3	18	25	22	27	20	17	3	7	11	9	42	24
26	46	42	23	17	28	31	62	26	57	24	51	29	36	25	38	36	28
1,145	846	14	19	15	16	868	906	1,465	1,289	2,392	1,585	496	91	205	101	184	104
189	230	52	41	124	121	137	214	154	191	214	162	112	104	994	985	1,105	1,145
2	120	1	3	2	10	1	300	1	205	3	83	-	18	7	12	-	6
8	59	2	1	8	11	17	178	10	116	4	3	3	2	-	-	-	2
1	1	1	2	-	1	3	1	1	1	0	0	1	-	2	-	-	-

Table 25 - *continued*

Disease group	Persons, by age group								
	Total	0-4	5-15	16-24	25-44	45-64	65-74	75-84	85 and over
Special screening examination for other infectious diseases (V75)	1	1	1	2	1	0	0	0	-
Special screening for malignant neoplasms (V76)	238	-	2	295	366	383	72	13	7
Special screening for endocrine, nutritional, metabolic and immunity disorders (V77)	69	2	8	23	62	149	121	84	36
Special screening for disorders of blood and blood-forming organs (V78)	8	1	2	11	10	8	12	14	18
Special screening for mental disorders and developmental handicaps (V79)	8	96	1	2	2	3	2		3
Special screening for neurological, eye and ear diseases (V80)	4	9	2	1	1	5	9	6	9
Special screening for cardiovascular, respiratory and genitourinary diseases (V81)	186	25	31	83	127	329	463	397	218
Special screening for other conditions (V82)	12	19	5	8	11	17	17	11	6

By age-group and sex

Total		0-4		5-15		16-24		25-44		45-64		65-74		75-84		85 and over	
Male	Female	Male	Female	Male	Female	Male	Female	Male	Female	Male	Female	Male	Female	Male	Female	Male	Female
1	1	2	-	2	0	2	3	1	2	0	0	1	-	-	1	-	-
1	466	-	-	-	4	1	587	1	735	0	772	5	126	3	18	-	10
59	79	1	3	8	8	15	31	51	73	131	167	103	136	85	83	53	30
5	12	2	1	2	2	4	18	4	15	7	10	8	15	9	17	18	18
8	9	91	103	2	0	1	2	2	2	3	3	1	2	-	1	6	2
4	4	7	11	3	2	2	0	1	2	4	5	13	6	6	5	12	8
163	208	25	24	33	28	43	122	101	153	321	338	449	474	372	412	244	209
11	13	13	25	6	5	4	12	6	15	19	14	26	10	11	10	12	4

**Table 26   All consultations - rates per 10,000 person years at risk:
home visits and whether consulted doctor or practice
nurse by ICD chapter, category of severity and age**

Disease group	Doctor consultations							
	Ages 0-15		Ages 16-64		Ages 65-74		Ages 75 and over	
	All	Home visits	All	Home visits	All	Home visits	All	Home visits
All diseases and conditions (I-XVIII)	30,833	2,569	32,793	1,427	45,532	6,540	53,902	21,726
Serious	2,147	185	4,204	317	13,666	2,745	18,215	8,325
Intermediate	13,912	1,327	13,360	640	19,020	2,311	20,091	7,503
Minor	14,774	1,056	15,229	470	12,846	1,484	15,596	5,899
All illnesses (I-XVIII)	28,158	2,502	26,915	1,303	43,161	6,382	50,551	20,790
Infectious and parasitic diseases (001-139)	3,588	475	1,684	103	1,150	229	1,223	611
Serious	10	1	11	2	12	4	24	13
Intermediate	2,979	412	1,355	94	914	212	1,033	543
Minor	599	62	318	7	224	12	167	55
II Neoplasms (140-239)	99	5	404	58	1,312	542	1,607	861
Serious	9	1	171	53	1,051	500	1,375	764
Intermediate	90	3	233	5	261	42	232	97
Minor	-	-	-	-	-	-	-	-
III Endocrine, nutritional and metabolic diseases and immunity disorders (240-279)	71	6	680	16	1,885	137	1,578	445
Serious	17	3	345	12	1,331	101	1,306	357
Intermediate	54	3	334	5	554	35	272	88
Minor	-	-	-	-	-	-	-	-
IV Diseases of blood and blood-forming organs (280-289)	80	10	109	3	298	34	618	216
Serious	18	2	8	0	25	2	23	10
Intermediate	62	8	101	3	272	32	595	205
Minor	-	-	-	-	-	-	-	-
V Mental disorders (290-319)	264	9	2,084	91	2,221	400	2,764	1,374
Serious	4	0	381	17	422	110	1,068	662
Intermediate	194	5	1,449	62	1,442	238	1,317	589
Minor	66	4	253	12	357	53	379	123
VI Diseases of the nervous system and sense organs (320-389)	4,700	313	2,059	73	3,434	282	4,058	1,155
Serious	64	8	310	25	889	143	1,427	501
Intermediate	3,294	264	971	39	1,291	99	1,269	332
Minor	1,342	41	778	9	1,254	40	1,362	321
VII Diseases of the circulatory system (390-459)	30	1	1,637	74	8,465	1,043	9,965	3,744
Serious	9	1	497	55	3,485	801	5,738	2,898
Intermediate	12	0	1,126	19	4,936	229	4,130	795
Minor	9	-	14	1	44	14	96	51
VIII Diseases of the respiratory system (460-519)	10,266	1,081	4,752	279	6,695	1,440	6,998	3,519
Serious	1,770	134	900	69	2,508	630	2,491	1,287
Intermediate	2,817	373	1,518	138	2,288	587	2,791	1,583
Minor	5,678	574	2,334	72	1,899	223	1,716	649
IX Diseases of the digestive system (520-579)	631	64	1,446	78	2,726	356	3,175	1,311
Serious	55	14	422	29	865	123	911	380
Intermediate	362	36	494	30	851	108	980	384
Minor	213	15	530	19	1,010	125	1,283	547
X Diseases of the genitourinary system (580-629)	700	40	2,522	77	1,712	201	2,081	796
Serious	11	2	58	9	82	23	108	58
Intermediate	489	30	1,580	57	1,408	167	1,830	694
Minor	199	8	884	11	222	12	144	44
XI Complications of pregnancy, childbirth and the puerperium (630-676)	6	1	281	53	2	0	1	1
Serious	1	0	39	8	-	-	0	0
Intermediate	5	1	235	44	1	0	1	0
Minor	0	-	8	0	1	-	0	0
XII Diseases of the skin and subcutaneous tissue (680-709)	2,855	59	2,061	31	2,377	192	2,647	881
Serious	-	-	-	-	-	-	-	-
Intermediate	2,178	39	1,488	24	1,714	150	1,917	673
Minor	677	20	572	7	664	42	730	208

Nurse consultations

Ages 0-15		Ages 16-64		Ages 65-74		Ages 75 and over		
All	Home visits	All	Home visits	All	Home visits	All	Home visits	
2,471	19	3,338	9	6,294	54	6,099	651	All diseases and conditions (I-XVIII)
179	1	242	1	790	15	561	45	Serious
321	7	733	3	1,964	12	1,514	42	Intermediate
1,970	11	2,363	5	3,540	27	4,024	564	Minor
771	16	1,355	7	3,505	36	2,936	123	All illnesses (I-XVIII)
94	2	41	0	30	1	14	3	Infectious and parasitic diseases (001-139)
0	-	1	-	1	-	2	-	Serious
79	2	35	0	26	1	10	3	Intermediate
14	0	5	0	3	1	2	1	Minor
7	-	25	0	63	2	63	4	II Neoplasms (140-239)
0	-	8	0	43	2	49	4	Serious
6	-	17	0	20	0	15	-	Intermediate
-	-	-	-	-	-	-	-	Minor
5	-	256	0	589	4	279	11	III Endocrine, nutritional and metabolic diseases and immunity disorders (240-279)
0	-	60	0	296	2	218	11	Serious
5	-	196	0	293	1	61	1	Intermediate
-	-	-	-	-	-	-	-	Minor
2	-	32	0	208	0	212	-	IV Diseases of blood and blood-forming organs (280-289)
0	-	1	-	2	-	1	-	Serious
1	-	31	0	206	0	211	-	Intermediate
-	-	-	-	-	-	-	-	Minor
4	-	48	0	40	2	33	6	V Mental disorders (290-319)
0	-	18	0	6	-	11	2	Serious
3	-	29	0	33	2	19	3	Intermediate
1	-	1	0	1	0	3	0	Minor
60	2	139	1	369	4	460	6	VI Diseases of the nervous system and sense organs (320-389)
1	-	7	0	9	1	18	1	Serious
20	2	13	0	33	2	34	1	Intermediate
39	0	118	0	328	1	409	4	Minor
0	-	183	0	1,031	5	653	22	VII Diseases of the circulatory system (390-459)
-	-	22	0	148	4	114	16	Serious
0	-	160	0	882	0	535	5	Intermediate
0	-	1	-	1	-	3	1	Minor
216	7	96	1	184	4	111	13	VIII Diseases of the respiratory system (460-519)
169	1	68	0	156	2	89	4	Serious
10	1	9	0	13	2	12	5	Intermediate
37	5	20	0	15	1	9	4	Minor
7	1	24	0	43	2	27	8	IX Diseases of the digestive system (520-579)
2	-	9	0	23	1	7	3	Serious
4	0	11	0	13	1	11	2	Intermediate
1	0	4	0	7	1	9	3	Minor
8	0	71	0	32	2	43	4	X Diseases of the genitourinary system (580-629)
0	0	1	0	2	0	2	-	Serious
6	0	44	0	25	2	36	4	Intermediate
2	0	25	0	5	0	5	-	Minor
-	-	4	0	-	-	-	-	XI Complications of pregnancy, childbirth and the puerperium (630-676)
-	-	1	0	-	-	-	-	Serious
-	-	3	0	-	-	-	-	Intermediate
-	-	0	-	-	-	-	-	Minor
69	0	111	0	251	-	341	7	XII Diseases of the skin and subcutaneous tissue (680-709)
-	-	-	-	-	-	-	-	Serious
39	0	59	0	126	-	193	5	Intermediate
31	0	52	0	125	-	147	2	Minor

Table 26 - *continued*

Disease group		Doctor consultations							
		Ages 0-15		Ages 16-64		Ages 65-74		Ages 75 and over	
		All	Home visits	All	Home visits	All	Home visits	All	Home visits
XIII	Diseases of the musculoskeletal system and connective tissue (710-739)	485	12	3,203	107	5,842	553	6,553	2,252
	Serious	16	1	948	28	2,836	255	3,403	1,196
	Intermediate	358	8	1,872	68	2,320	224	2,419	821
	Minor	111	3	384	11	687	73	731	235
XIV	Congenital anomalies (740-759)	137	7	49	1	64	5	60	13
	Serious	86	6	26	1	44	5	43	10
	Intermediate	52	1	23	0	20	0	17	3
	Minor	-	-	-	-	-	-	-	-
XV	Certain conditions originating in the perinatal period (760-779)	74	8	1	0	-	-	2	1
	Serious	19	5	0	0	-	-	2	1
	Intermediate	55	4	1	0	-	-	-	-
	Minor	-	-	-	-	-	-	-	-
XVI	Symptoms, signs and ill-defined conditions (780-799)	2,628	327	1,929	165	3,194	645	4,459	2,231
	Serious	0	0	2	1	24	16	59	44
	Intermediate	513	120	185	26	306	97	555	338
	Minor	2,115	207	1,741	138	2,864	532	3,846	1,850
XVII	Injury and poisoning (800-999)	1,546	82	2,014	91	1,784	323	2,761	1,380
	Serious	58	6	86	7	92	33	237	144
	Intermediate	398	21	394	26	442	90	732	358
	Minor	1,090	54	1,534	58	1,250	200	1,791	878
XVIII	Supplementary Classification of factors influencing health status and contact with Health Services (V01-V82)	2,675	67	5,878	124	2,371	158	3,351	937
	Serious	-	-	-	-	-	-	-	-
	Intermediate	-	-	-	-	-	-	-	-
	Minor	2,675	67	5,878	124	2,371	158	3,351	937

Nurse consultations

Ages 0-15		Ages 16-64		Ages 65-74		Ages 75 and over			
All	Home visits	All	Home visits	All	Home visits	All	Home visits		
5	0	68	0	166	3	118	11	XIII	Diseases of the musculoskeletal system and connective tissue (710-739)
0	-	44	0	100	2	37	4		Serious
4	0	19	0	53	1	60	7		Intermediate
1	-	5	0	12	-	21	1		Minor
2	-	3	-	2	-	12	1	XIV	Congenital anomalies (740-759)
1	-	2	-	1	-	10	-		Serious
1	-	1	-	1	-	2	1		Intermediate
-	-	-	-	-	-	-	-		Minor
1	0	0	-			0	-	XV	Certain conditions originating in the perinatal period (760-779)
0	-	-	-	-	-	0	-		Serious
1	0	0	-	-	-	-	-		Intermediate
-	-	-	-	-	-	-	-		Minor
45	2	86	1	155	4	126	17	XVI	Symptoms, signs and ill-defined conditions (780-799)
-	-	-	-	-	-	0	0		Serious
6	0	4	0	7	-	11	2		Intermediate
40	2	82	1	148	4	115	14		Minor
246	1	170	0	344	2	445	9	XVII	Injury and poisoning (800-999)
4	-	3	-	3	-	4	1		Serious
136	0	101	0	234	-	304	3		Intermediate
106	0	67	0	106	2	137	5		Minor
1,699	3	1,983	3	2,789	18	3,163	529	XVIII	Supplementary Classification of factors influencing health status and contact with Health Services (V01-V82)
-	-	-	-	-	-	-	-		Serious
-	-	-	-	-	-	-	-		Intermediate
1,699	3	1,983	3	2,789	18	3,163	529		Minor

All consultations

Table 27   All consultations - rates per 10,000 person years at risk:
home visits and whether consulted doctor or practice nurse
by disease related group and age

Disease group	Doctor consultations							
	Ages 0-15		Ages 16-64		Ages 65-74		Ages 75 and over	
	All	Home visits	All	Home visits	All	Home visits	All	Home visits
All diseases	30,833	2,569	32,793	1,427	45,532	6,540	53,902	21,726
Intestinal infectious diseases (001-009)	1,157	289	344	71	311	141	461	330
Tuberculosis (010-018)	0	-	3	0	6	3	8	4
Zoonotic bacterial diseases (020-027)	1	0	0	-	-	-	-	-
Other bacterial diseases (030-041)	47	6	17	1	18	4	23	12
Poliomyelitis and other non-arthropod-borne viral diseases of central nervous system (045-049)	2	1	2	0	1	1	-	-
Viral diseases accompanied by exanthem (050--57)	539	64	201	11	304	41	310	130
Arthropod-borne viral diseases (060-066)	-	-	-	-	-	-	-	-
Other diseases due to viruses and Chlamydiae (070-079)	945	75	293	11	105	10	86	20
Rickettsioses and other arthropod-borne diseases (080-088)	1	0	1	0	1	-	1	1
Syphilis and other venereal diseases (090-099)	1	0	10	0	6	0	3	1
Other spirochaetal diseases (100-104)	1	-	0	-	1	-	1	-
Mycoses (110-118)	504	17	718	6	372	27	284	91
Helminthiases (120-129)	158	3	19	0	2	-	2	1
Other infectious and parasitic diseases (130-136)	232	20	75	2	23	2	44	22
Late effects of infectious and parasitic diseases (137-139)	0	-	1	-	-	-	1	0
Malignant neoplasm of lip, oral cavity and pharynx (140-149)	-	-	2	1	14	9	14	9
Malignant neoplasm of digestive organs and peritoneum (150-159)	0	-	23	10	212	119	340	236
Malignant neoplasm of respiratory and intrathoracic organs (160-165)	-	-	19	8	139	82	135	91
Malignant neoplasm of bone, connective tissue, skin and breast (170-175)	1	0	45	7	152	32	227	87
Malignant neoplasm of genitourinary organs (179-189)	2	-	32	11	183	70	328	158
Malignant neoplasm of other and unspecified sites (190-199)	1	1	27	11	210	125	204	114
Malignant neoplasm of lymphatic and haematopoietic tissue (200-208)	3	0	8	2	46	20	44	23
Benign neoplasms (210-229)	70	0	194	1	156	5	91	21
Carcinoma in situ (230-234)	-	-	9	3	77	41	78	45
Neoplasms of uncertain behaviour (235-238)	1	0	7	0	20	3	25	11
Neoplasms of unspecified nature (239)	20	3	38	4	103	36	121	67
Disorders of thyroid gland (240-246)	5	0	122	1	343	16	317	83
Diseases of other endocrine glands (250-259)	15	2	237	10	968	80	950	250
Nutritional deficiencies (260-269)	3	0	2	-	12	-	19	5
Other metabolic disorders and immunity disorders (270-279)	48	4	318	5	561	41	293	107
Diseases of blood and blood-forming organs (280-289)	80	10	109	3	298	34	618	216
Organic psychotic conditions (290-294)	1	0	16	3	95	48	683	482
Other psychoses (295-299)	2	0	273	14	328	64	386	181
Neurotic disorders, personality disorders and other nonpsychotic mental disorders (300-316)	260	9	1,789	74	1,796	288	1,694	710
Mental retardation (317-319)	1	-	5	0	2	0	0	0
Inflammatory diseases of the central nervous system (320-326)	3	1	5	1	2	1	3	1
Hereditary and degenerative diseases of the central nervous system (330-337)	6	1	37	3	270	66	448	255
Other disorders of the central nervous system (340-349)	137	11	367	31	228	58	180	87
Disorders of the peripheral nervous system (350-359)	5	0	86	3	135	12	134	32
Disorders of the eye and adnexa (360-379)	1,257	37	578	8	1,381	61	1,837	429
Diseases of the ear and mastoid process (380-389)	3,291	263	987	28	1,418	84	1,455	351
Acute rheumatic fever (390-392)	0	-	0	0	0	-	-	-
Chronic rheumatic heart disease (393-398)	0	-	9	0	31	4	22	5
Hypertensive disease (401-405)	1	-	804	8	4,009	125	2,905	381
Ischaemic heart disease (410-414)	0	-	287	26	1,654	251	1,667	621
Diseases of pulmonary circulation (415-417)	0	-	9	2	50	20	59	32
Other forms of heart disease (420-429)	7	1	94	12	1,151	306	2,952	1,573
Cerebrovascular disease (430-438)	0	-	46	11	445	209	998	655
Diseases of arteries, arterioles and capillaries (440-448)	9	0	61	4	373	43	485	167
Diseases of veins and lymphatics, and other diseases of circulatory system (451-459)	11	0	326	12	753	86	877	310

Nurse consultations

Ages 0-15		Ages 16-64		Ages 65-74		Ages 75 and over		
All	Home visits	All	Home visits	All	Home visits	All	Home visits	
2,471	19	3,338	9	6,294	54	6,099	651	All diseases
7	1	2	0	3	1	2	1	Intestinal infectious diseases (001-009)
-	-	0	-	1	-	-	-	Tuberculosis (010-018
-	-	-	-	-	-	-	-	Zoonotic bacterial diseases (020-027)
0	-	1	-	10	-	1	-	Other bacterial diseases (030-041)
-	-	-	-	-	-	-	-	Poliomyelitis and other non-arthropod-borne viral diseases of central nervous system (045-049)
10	0	3	0	4	0	2	1	Viral diseases accompanied by exanthem (050—057)
-	-	0	-	-	-	-	-	Arthropod-borne viral diseases (060-066)
56	1	21	0	7	-	4	0	Other diseases due to viruses and Chlamydiae (070-079)
-	-	-	-	-	-	-	-	Rickettsioses and other arthropod-borne diseases (080-088)
-	-	0	-	-	-	-	-	Syphilis and other venereal diseases (090-099)
-	-	-	-	-	-	-	-	Other spirochaetal diseases (100-104)
6	-	11	-	4	1	4	0	Mycoses (110-118)
3	-	0	0	-	-	-	-	Helminthiases (120-129)
11	-	2	-	-	-	1	0	Other infectious and parasitic diseases (130-136)
-	-	0	-	-	-	-	-	Late effects of infectious and parasitic diseases (137-139)
-	-	0	-	-	-	-	-	Malignant neoplasm of lip, oral cavity and pharynx (140-149)
-	-	1	0	3	1	2	2	Malignant neoplasm of digestive organs and peritoneum (150-159)
-	-	0	0	-	-	1	-	Malignant neoplasm of respiratory and intrathoracic organs (160-165)
-	-	2	-	17	0	16	0	Malignant neoplasm of bone, connective tissue, skin and breast (170-175)
0	-	3	-	11	1	12	1	Malignant neoplasm of genitourinary organs (179-189)
-	-	1	-	5	0	6	0	Malignant neoplasm of other and unspecified sites (190-199)
-	-	0	-	5	-	7	-	Malignant neoplasm of lymphatic and haematopoietic tissue (200-208)
5	-	15	-	14	-	5	-	Benign neoplasms (210-229)
-	-	0	0	2	-	5	1	Carcinoma in situ (230-234)
0	-	0	-	1	-	1	-	Neoplasms of uncertain behaviour (235-238)
2	-	2	0	6	0	9	-	Neoplasms of unspecified nature (239)
1	-	11	-	30	-	17	0	Disorders of thyroid gland (240-246)
0	-	52	0	267	2	200	10	Diseases of other endocrine glands (250-259)
-	-	2	-	14	-	15	-	Nutritional deficiencies (260-269)
4	-	190	0	278	1	47	1	Other metabolic disorders and immunity disorders (270-279)
2	-	32	0	208	0	212	-	Diseases of blood and blood-forming organs (280-289)
-	-	0	-	1	-	4	2	Organic psychotic conditions (290-294)
0	-	17	0	5	-	6	0	Other psychoses (295-299)
4	-	31	0	34	2	22	4	Neurotic disorders, personality disorders and other nonpsychotic mental disorders (300-316)
-	-	0	-	-	-	-	-	Mental retardation (317-319)
0	-	0	-	1	-	-	-	Inflammatory diseases of the central nervous system (320-326)
-	-	0	0	2	1	3	1	Hereditary and degenerative diseases of the central nervous system (330-337)
1	0	7	0	5	-	3	0	Other disorders of the central nervous system (340-349)
0	-	1	-	0	-	2	-	Disorders of the peripheral nervous system (350-359)
15	0	6	-	15	1	26	1	Disorders of the eye and adnexa (360-379)
44	2	124	0	347	2	426	4	Diseases of the ear and mastoid process (380-389)
-	-	-	-	-	-	-	-	Acute rheumatic fever (390-392)
-	-	3	-	8	-	6	1	Chronic rheumatic heart disease (393-398)
-	-	117	0	650	0	290	2	Hypertensive disease (401-405)
-	-	7	0	34	3	22	4	Ischaemic heart disease (410-414)
-	-	3	-	13	-	13	-	Diseases of pulmonary circulation (415-417)
-	-	4	0	63	0	38	3	Other forms of heart disease (420-429)
-	-	1	-	15	1	21	7	Cerebrovascular disease (430-438)
0	-	2	-	33	1	21	1	Diseases of arteries, arterioles and capillaries (440-448)
0	-	45	0	213	-	243	4	Diseases of veins and lymphatics, and other diseases of circulatory system (451-459)

Table 27 - *continued*

Disease group	Doctor consultations							
	Ages 0-15		Ages 16-64		Ages 65-74		Ages 75 and over	
	All	Home visits	All	Home visits	All	Home visits	All	Home visits
Acute respiratory infections (460-466)	7,613	878	3,039	165	3,485	700	3,950	2,023
Other diseases of upper respiratory tract (470-478)	658	6	537	4	434	12	277	38
Pneumonia and influenza (480-487)	241	67	286	50	306	148	517	375
Chronic obstructive pulmonary disease and allied conditions (490-496)	1,731	128	843	55	2,355	541	2,112	1,010
Pneumoconioses and other lung diseases due to external agents (500-508)	0	-	1	0	8	1	6	3
Other diseases of respiratory system (510-519)	23	2	46	6	108	39	137	71
Diseases of oral cavity, salivary glands and jaws (520-529)	223	13	176	6	178	10	160	44
Diseases of oesophagus, stomach and duodenum (530-537)	74	15	611	27	1,236	127	1,137	375
Appendicitis (540-543)	16	7	14	4	2	1	1	-
Hernia of abdominal cavity (550-553)	37	4	79	2	292	26	336	107
Noninfective enteritis and colitis (555-558)	27	8	77	5	86	13	80	44
Other diseases of intestines and peritoneum (560-569)	246	17	414	21	760	129	1,235	603
Other diseases of digestive system (570-579)	8	1	77	13	172	50	226	139
Nephritis, nephrotic syndrome and nephrosis (580-589)	4	1	14	1	47	15	72	41
Other diseases of urinary system (590-599)	288	26	600	43	974	151	1,392	593
Diseases of male genital organs (600-608)	197	10	112	3	225	18	179	44
Disorders of breast (610-611)	35	1	181	2	64	3	37	9
Inflammatory disease of female pelvic organs (614-616)	51	1	204	9	62	2	68	22
Other disorders of female genital tract (617-629)	125	2	1,411	18	340	13	334	88
Pregnancy with abortive outcome(630-639)	1	0	54	8	-	-	-	-
Complications mainly related to pregnancy (640-648)	1	1	117	28	-	-	0	0
Normal delivery, and other indications for care in pregnancy, labour and delivery (650-659)	1	0	49	6	-	-	-	-
Complications occurring mainly in the course of labour and delivery (660-669)	2	0	21	4	-	-	-	-
Complications of the puerperium (670-676)	1	-	39	6	2	0	1	1
Infections of skin and subcutaneous tissue (680-686)	584	17	410	16	493	84	693	331
Other inflammatory conditions of skin and subcutaneous tissue (690-698)	1,668	27	922	7	1,199	47	1,118	281
Other diseases of skin and subcutaneous tissue (700-709)	604	15	729	8	684	60	836	269
Arthropathies and related disorders (710-719)	166	4	991	21	2,823	262	3,549	1,264
Dorsopathies (720-724)	90	3	1,301	69	1,414	169	1,321	516
Rheumatism, excluding the back (725-729)	147	4	842	15	1,419	89	1,429	358
Osteopathies, chondropathies and acquired musculoskeletal deformities (730-739)	82	1	70	2	185	31	254	115
Congenital anomalies (740-759)	137	7	49	1	64	5	60	13
Certain conditions originating in the perinatal period (760-779)	74	8	1	0	-	-	2	1
Symptoms, signs and ill-defined conditions (780-789)	2,403	259	1,761	154	2,931	601	4,027	1,976
Nonspecific abnormal findings (790-796)	214	67	145	9	196	18	144	43
Ill-defined and unknown causes of morbidity and mortality (797-799)	12	1	22	2	66	26	288	212
Fracture of skull (800-804)	7	0	12	1	5	1	6	3
Fracture of spine and trunk (805-809)	2	0	28	2	36	13	86	49
Fracture of upper limb (810-819)	62	2	64	1	75	13	107	48
Fracture of lower limb (820-829)	23	1	63	4	74	27	187	120
Dislocation (830-839)	12	1	20	1	18	5	22	13
Sprains and strains of joints and adjacent muscles (840-848)	342	8	956	33	603	78	552	234
Intracranial injury, excluding those with skull fracture (850-854)	60	7	17	2	10	2	20	12
Internal injury of chest, abdomen and pelvis (860-869)	1	0	2	0	2	1	2	1
Open wound of head, neck and trunk (870-879)	94	5	29	1	25	3	82	48
Open wound of upper limb (880-887)	34	1	51	1	33	3	68	22
Open wound of lower limb (890-897)	33	0	22	1	46	7	112	40
Injury to blood vessels (900-904)	0	-	1	-	1	-	1	0
Late effects of injuries, poisonings, toxic effects and other external causes (905-909)	2	0	3	0	6	3	4	2

Nurse consultations

Ages 0-15		Ages 16-64		Ages 65-74		Ages 75 and over		
All	Home visits	All	Home visits	All	Home visits	All	Home visits	
40	6	17	1	21	2	19	8	Acute respiratory infections (460-466)
6	0	9	-	4	0	1	-	Other diseases of upper respiratory tract (470-478)
1	0	2	0	2	0	2	1	Pneumonia and influenza (480-487)
168	0	67	0	155	2	89	4	Chronic obstructive pulmonary disease and allied conditions (490-496)
-	-	-	-	0	-	-	-	Pneumoconioses and other lung diseases due to external agents (500-508)
-	-	1	0	2	-	0	0	Other diseases of respiratory system (510-519)
2	-	2	0	2	-	2	-	Diseases of oral cavity, salivary glands and jaws (520-529)
0	-	4	0	8	2	5	1	Diseases of oesophagus, stomach and duodenum (530-537)
1	-	1	-	-	-	0	0	Appendicitis (540-543)
1	0	1	-	9	0	3	0	Hernia of abdominal cavity (550-553)
1	0	5	0	4	-	1	0	Noninfective enteritis and colitis (555-558)
1	0	8	0	8	0	12	4	Other diseases of intestines and peritoneum (560-569)
0	-	2	-	12	-	5	1	Other diseases of digestive system (570-579)
-	-	1	0	1	0	2	-	Nephritis, nephrotic syndrome and nephrosis (580-589)
3	0	7	0	15	2	18	2	Other diseases of urinary system (590-599)
2	0	2	-	3	0	6	0	Diseases of male genital organs (600-608)
0	-	4	-	2	-	0	-	Disorders of breast (610-611)
1	-	6	-	1	-	2	1	Inflammatory disease of female pelvic organs (614-616)
3	-	50	0	10	-	16	-	Other disorders of female genital tract (617-629)
-	-	1	0	-	-	-	-	Pregnancy with abortive outcome(630-639)
-	-	1	0	-	-	-	-	Complications mainly related to pregnancy (640-648)
-	-	0	0	-	-	-	-	Normal delivery, and other indications for care in pregnancy, labour and delivery (650-659)
-	-	0	0	-	-	-	-	Complications occurring mainly in the course of labour and delivery (660-669)
-	-	1	0	-	-	-	-	Complications of the puerperium (670-676)
20	0	40	0	57	-	67	3	Infections of skin and subcutaneous tissue (680-686)
18	-	12	0	18	-	18	3	Other inflammatory conditions of skin and subcutaneous tissue (690-698)
31	0	59	0	175	-	225	1	Other diseases of skin and subcutaneous tissue (700-709)
2	0	46	0	103	2	43	5	Arthropathies and related disorders (710-719)
1	-	9	0	11	1	10	3	Dorsopathies (720-724)
1	-	11	0	42	-	64	3	Rheumatism, excluding the back (725-729)
0	-	2	-	9	-	2	-	Osteopathies, chondropathies and acquired musculoskeletal deformities (730-739)
2	-	3	-	2	-	12	1	Congenital anomalies (740-759)
1	0	0	-	-	-	0	-	Certain conditions originating in the perinatal period (760-779)
43	2	56	1	95	4	87	13	Symptoms, signs and ill-defined conditions (780-789)
2	0	28	0	57	-	30	1	Nonspecific abnormal findings (790-796)
1	-	2	-	4	-	9	3	Ill-defined and unknown causes of morbidity and mortality (797-799)
-	-	0	-	1	-	-	-	Fracture of skull (800-804)
-	-	0	-	-	-	1	1	Fracture of spine and trunk (805-809)
3	-	1	-	2	-	4	-	Fracture of upper limb (810-819)
1	-	2	-	1	-	3	1	Fracture of lower limb (820-829)
1	-	1	-	-	-	1	-	Dislocation (830-839)
14	0	10	0	11	1	8	1	Sprains and strains of joints and adjacent muscles (840-848)
3	-	1	-	-	-	1	-	Intracranial injury, excluding those with skull fracture (850-854)
0	-	-	-	-	-	-	-	Internal injury of chest, abdomen and pelvis (860-869)
43	0	11	-	10	-	15	-	Open wound of head, neck and trunk (870-879)
29	-	36	-	49	-	51	-	Open wound of upper limb (880-887)
27	0	19	-	127	-	192	2	Open wound of lower limb (890-897)
-	-	0	-	-	-	-	-	Injury to blood vessels (900-904)
0	-	0	-	-	-	0	-	Late effects of injuries, poisonings, toxic effects and other external causes (905-909)

Table 27 - *continued*

Disease group	Doctor consultations							
	Ages 0-15		Ages 16-64		Ages 65-74		Ages 75 and over	
	All	Home visits	All	Home visits	All	Home visits	All	Home visits
Superficial injury (910-919)	204	8	133	3	156	21	280	122
Contusion with intact skin surface (920-924)	156	6	118	4	155	29	297	168
Crushing injury (925-929)	10	0	9	0	1	-	2	-
Effects of foreign body entering through orifice (930-939)	29	2	22	0	13	0	9	0
Burns (940-949)	33	2	24	1	30	2	47	17
Injury to nerves and spinal cord (950-957)	5	1	9	0	8	0	6	3
Certain traumatic complications and unspecified injuries (958-959)	45	2	56	2	49	8	69	34
Poisoning by drugs, medicaments and biological substances (960-979)	2	0	2	0	3	1	8	6
Toxic effects of substances chiefly nonmedicinal as to source (980-989)	5	1	6	1	4	1	5	2
Other and unspecified effects of external causes (990-995)	362	31	296	18	341	71	664	354
Complications of surgical and medical care not elsewhere classified (996-999)	22	4	71	13	90	31	124	82
Persons with potential health hazards related to communicable diseases (V01-V07)	1,631	24	441	5	1,089	76	1,476	459
Persons encountering health services in circumstances related to reproduction and development (V20-V28)	785	37	2,770	88	3	0	1	-
Persons encountering health services for specific procedures and aftercare (V50-V59)	-	-	0	-	-	-	1	0
Persons encountering health services in other circumstances (V60-V68)	63	3	1,694	29	463	57	368	114
Persons without reported diagnosis encountered during examination and investigation of individuals and populations (V70-V82)	195	3	974	2	817	25	1,505	364

Nurse consultations

Ages 0-15		Ages 16-64		Ages 65-74		Ages 75 and over		
All	Home visits	All	Home visits	All	Home visits	All	Home visits	
42	0	24	0	42	-	86	-	Superficial injury (910-919) -
14	0	6	0	7	-	8	0	Contusion with intact skin surface (920-924)
3	-	2	-	1	-	0	-	Crushing injury (925-929)
3	-	3	-	3	-	1	-	Effects of foreign body entering through orifice (930-939)
21	-	15	0	19	-	19	0	Burns (940-949)
0	-	0	-	-	-	1	-	Injury to nerves and spinal cord (950-957)
8	-	5	-	8	0	5	1	Certain traumatic complications and unspecified injuries (958-959)
0	-	0	-	0	-	0	-	Poisoning by drugs, medicaments and biological substances (960-979)
0	-	0	-	1	-	0	-	Toxic effects of substances chiefly nonmedicinal as to source (980-989)
29	0	23	0	40	1	42	3	Other and unspecified effects of external causes (990-995)
3	-	11	0	23	-	9	-	Complications of surgical and medical care not elsewhere classified (996-999)
1,577	3	892	1	1,866	14	1,565	84	Persons with potential health hazards related to communicable diseases (V01-V07)
10	0	135	0	1	-	-	-	Persons encountering health services in circumstances related to reproduction and development (V20-V28)
-	-	-	-	-	-	-	-	Persons encountering health services for specific procedures and aftercare (V50-V59)
5	-	25	0	14	0	11	3	Persons encountering health services in other circumstances (V60-V68)
108	-	931	1	908	3	1,587	442	Persons without reported diagnosis encountered during examination and investigation of individuals and populations (V70-V82)

Table 28 Age standardised patient consulting ratios (SPCR) (study population = 100) with approximate 95 per cent upper and lower confidence limits: comparison by age, sex, and broad geographical region

	Disease group		Ages 0-15						Ages 16-64						Ages 65 and over					
			North		Midlands and Wales		South		North		Midlands and Wales		South		North		Midlands and Wales		South	
			M	F	M	F	M	F	M	F	M	F	M	F	M	F	M	F	M	F
	All diseases and conditions (I-XVIII)	SPCR	98	97	102	103	100	100	102	99	101	101	97	100	100	100	101	100	100	100
		Lower cl	96	96	100	101	99	98	101	98	100	100	96	99	98	98	98	98	97	98
		Upper cl	99	99	104	104	102	102	103	100	102	102	98	101	102	101	103	102	102	102
	Serious	SPCR	97	91	105	108	98	100	106	102	101	100	94	98	100	100	104	102	97	98
		Lower cl	92	86	100	103	94	95	104	99	98	98	92	97	97	98	100	99	94	96
		Upper cl	101	96	109	113	102	105	109	104	103	102	96	100	103	102	107	104	99	101
	Intermediate	SPCR	96	96	102	103	102	101	101	99	102	101	97	100	98	98	100	101	102	100
		Lower cl	94	94	100	101	100	99	99	97	101	100	96	99	95	96	98	99	99	98
		Upper cl	98	98	104	105	104	103	102	100	104	102	98	101	100	100	103	104	104	103
	Minor	SPCR	97	96	105	106	98	98	102	98	102	102	96	100	98	98	102	101	100	101
		Lower cl	95	94	103	104	97	96	101	97	101	101	95	99	95	96	99	99	98	99
		Upper cl	99	98	107	107	100	100	103	99	104	103	97	101	101	100	104	103	103	103
	All illnesses (I-XVII)	SPCR	98	98	102	102	99	99	102	99	101	101	97	100	100	100	101	101	99	99
		Lower cl	97	97	100	101	98	97	101	98	100	100	96	99	98	98	99	99	97	98
		Upper cl	100	100	104	104	101	101	103	100	103	102	98	101	102	102	104	103	101	101
I	Infectious and parasitic diseases (001-139)	SPCR	101	99	102	103	97	98	102	94	100	103	99	102	99	101	95	102	106	97
		Lower cl	97	96	99	99	94	95	98	92	97	100	96	100	91	95	87	96	98	92
		Upper cl	104	102	106	106	100	101	105	97	103	105	102	104	106	107	103	107	114	103
II	Neoplasms (140-239)	SPCR	88	91	87	90	122	117	94	88	94	99	110	111	95	92	99	98	105	109
		Lower cl	71	74	70	74	103	99	88	83	87	94	103	106	87	85	90	90	97	101
		Upper cl	106	108	104	106	141	135	101	92	101	104	117	116	104	100	108	106	114	118
III	Endocrine, nutritional and metabolic diseases and immunity disorders (240-279)	SPCR	121	99	93	98	89	103	110	104	101	98	91	98	91	91	104	108	105	101
		Lower cl	95	76	71	77	68	82	104	100	96	94	86	95	84	86	96	102	98	95
		Upper cl	147	121	116	119	109	124	115	108	106	102	95	102	98	97	111	114	112	107
IV	Diseases of blood and blood-forming organs (280-289)	SPCR	73	74	97	114	126	110	102	97	116	105	84	98	112	105	103	102	86	93
		Lower cl	54	56	76	92	104	89	83	89	95	97	68	91	96	95	88	92	73	84
		Upper cl	91	92	117	135	148	130	122	105	137	113	101	106	127	115	119	112	100	102
V	Mental disorders (290-319)	SPCR	93	78	102	109	103	111	99	100	103	102	99	98	96	96	102	102	102	102
		Lower cl	83	67	92	97	93	100	95	97	99	99	95	96	89	91	94	97	94	98
		Upper cl	104	88	113	120	113	123	103	103	107	105	102	101	104	100	110	107	109	107
VI	Diseases of the nervous system and sense organs (320-389)	SPCR	93	93	101	103	104	103	99	96	101	102	100	102	96	95	106	100	99	105
		Lower cl	90	90	98	100	102	100	96	94	99	99	97	100	92	92	101	96	95	101
		Upper cl	96	96	105	107	107	106	101	98	104	104	102	104	100	99	110	104	103	108
VII	Diseases of the circulatory system (390-459)	SPCR	94	120	96	78	109	103	104	101	104	101	93	98	97	98	102	98	101	103
		Lower cl	62	84	65	50	77	72	101	98	101	98	90	95	93	95	98	95	98	100
		Upper cl	126	156	127	106	141	134	108	105	108	105	96	101	100	101	105	101	105	106
VIII	Diseases of the respiratory system (460-519)	SPCR	100	99	103	104	97	97	101	100	103	102	96	98	106	107	100	101	94	93
		Lower cl	98	96	101	102	95	95	99	99	101	100	95	97	102	104	96	97	91	90
		Upper cl	103	101	105	107	99	99	103	102	105	103	98	100	110	110	104	104	98	96
IX	Diseases of the digestive system (520-579)	SPCR	107	104	108	105	88	92	104	99	99	99	97	101	97	97	101	102	101	101
		Lower cl	99	96	100	97	82	86	101	96	96	97	94	99	92	92	96	98	96	97
		Upper cl	114	112	115	112	94	99	108	102	103	102	100	104	103	101	107	107	107	105
X	Diseases of the genitourinary system (580-629)	SPCR	88	89	109	109	101	101	100	99	104	105	96	96	93	95	105	106	102	99
		Lower cl	81	83	101	102	94	94	95	97	99	103	91	94	86	90	97	101	95	94
		Upper cl	96	96	117	116	108	107	106	101	110	107	101	98	100	100	113	111	109	104
XI	Complications of pregnancy, childbirth and the puerperium (630-679)	SPCR	-	*84*	-	*111*	-	*103*	-	*91*	-	*104*	-	*103*	-	*49*	-	*209*	-	*49*
		Lower cl	-	*40*	-	*63*	-	*58*	-	*86*	-	*99*	-	*99*	-	*0*	-	*64*	-	*0*
		Upper cl	-	*128*	-	*160*	-	*148*	-	*96*	-	*109*	-	*108*	-	*117*	-	*353*	-	*117*

Table 28 - *continued*

Disease group			Ages 0-15						Ages 16-64						Ages 65 and over					
			North		Midlands and Wales		South		North		Midlands and Wales		South		North		Midlands and Wales		South	
			M	F	M	F	M	F	M	F	M	F	M	F	M	F	M	F	M	F
XII	Diseases of the skin and subcutaneous tissue (680-709)	SPCR	95	96	102	102	102	102	98	97	103	101	99	101	95	92	98	100	106	108
		Lower cl	91	93	98	98	99	98	96	95	100	99	96	99	90	88	93	95	101	104
		Upper cl	99	100	106	105	106	105	101	100	105	104	101	103	100	96	104	104	112	113
XIII	Diseases of the musculoskeletal system and connective tissue (710-739)	SPCR	91	85	109	117	99	97	103	99	104	105	93	96	99	99	105	103	97	99
		Lower cl	84	78	101	108	91	90	101	97	102	103	91	94	95	96	100	100	93	96
		Upper cl	99	93	117	125	107	105	106	101	107	107	96	98	103	102	109	106	101	102
XIV	Congenital anomalies (740-759)	SPCR	97	82	103	106	100	110	99	85	109	111	92	103	56	55	172	168	77	80
		Lower cl	83	66	90	88	87	93	83	72	93	97	78	90	31	38	128	137	49	59
		Upper cl	111	98	117	124	112	126	116	98	126	126	107	115	81	72	217	199	105	101
XV	Certain conditions originating in the perinatal period (760-779)	SPCR	85	89	103	97	108	111	-	83	154	124	133	93	103	-	211	231	-	74
		Lower cl	65	69	82	77	89	91	-	29	0	61	0	42	0	-	0	0	-	0
		Upper cl	105	109	125	118	128	131	-	136	455	187	393	143	305	-	503	492	-	218
XVI	Symptoms, signs and ill-defined conditions (780-799)	SPCR	100	97	120	119	82	85	104	101	115	116	84	85	101	101	115	112	86	87
		Lower cl	96	94	116	115	79	82	101	99	112	114	81	83	96	97	109	109	82	84
		Upper cl	104	101	124	123	85	88	107	104	118	118	86	87	105	104	120	116	91	91
XVII	Injury and poisoning (800-999)	SPCR	88	89	112	113	99	97	103	95	102	103	96	101	94	93	104	105	102	102
		Lower cl	84	85	108	108	96	93	100	93	100	101	94	99	88	89	98	100	97	98
		Upper cl	91	94	117	118	103	102	105	98	105	105	98	103	100	97	110	109	108	106
XVIII	Supplementary classification of factors influencing health status and contact with health services (VO1-V82)	SPCR	86	83	105	109	107	106	104	95	103	104	94	101	90	91	102	97	108	112
		Lower cl	83	80	102	106	104	103	102	94	101	102	92	100	87	88	98	95	104	109
		Upper cl	89	86	108	112	110	109	106	96	105	105	96	102	94	93	105	100	111	114

Table 29 Age standardised patient consulting ratios (SPCR) for people aged 16-64 (study population=100) with approximate 95 per cent upper and lower confidence limits: comparison by sex, tenure, urban/rural, and ethnic group

Disease group			Tenure								Urban / rural			
			Owner occupier		Council house		Other rented		Communal		Urban		Rural	
			M	F	M	F	M	F	M	F	M	F	M	F
	All diseases and conditions (I-XVIII)	SPCR	98	99	105	103	108	105	103	103	100	100	97	99
		Lower cl	97	98	104	101	106	103	97	98	100	99	95	97
		Upper cl	99	99	107	104	111	107	109	108	101	101	99	101
	Serious	SPCR	89	91	142	134	122	117	120	117	102	101	90	92
		Lower cl	88	89	137	130	117	112	104	103	100	100	86	89
		Upper cl	91	92	146	137	127	121	135	131	103	103	93	95
	Intermediate	SPCR	96	97	112	112	109	106	99	96	101	100	96	96
		Lower cl	95	96	110	110	106	104	92	90	100	100	93	94
		Upper cl	97	97	115	113	112	108	107	102	102	101	98	98
	Minor	SPCR	97	98	108	104	111	106	101	99	101	100	94	97
		Lower cl	96	98	106	103	108	104	94	93	100	100	92	95
		Upper cl	98	99	110	106	114	108	108	104	102	101	96	99
	All illnesses (I-XVII)	SPCR	97	98	108	106	108	105	102	103	101	100	96	98
		Lower cl	97	97	106	104	106	103	96	98	100	100	94	96
		Upper cl	98	99	110	107	110	107	108	108	101	101	98	99
I	Infectious and parasitic diseases (001-139)	SPCR	97	95	106	115	112	110	99	96	100	100	98	99
		Lower cl	95	93	102	111	106	105	85	86	98	99	92	95
		Upper cl	99	97	111	118	118	114	114	106	102	102	103	103
II	Neoplasms (140-239)	SPCR	101	102	94	88	108	111	*73*	*52*	100	100	101	101
		Lower cl	96	98	84	81	93	100	*37*	*28*	96	97	90	92
		Upper cl	105	105	105	95	122	122	*109*	*75*	105	103	113	109
III	Endocrine, nutritional and metabolic diseases and immunity disorders (240-279)	SPCR	93	88	124	145	125	119	93	112	100	102	97	85
		Lower cl	90	86	115	138	113	110	57	82	97	100	89	79
		Upper cl	96	91	133	153	137	128	130	142	104	105	105	91
IV	Diseases of blood and blood-forming organs (280-289)	SPCR	91	94	133	130	120	101	*165*	*95*	101	102	93	81
		Lower cl	78	88	99	117	76	86	*3*	*51*	89	97	64	69
		Upper cl	103	99	166	143	164	116	*326*	*139*	114	107	123	93
V	Mental disorders (290-319)	SPCR	80	86	163	154	155	124	183	84	105	103	70	80
		Lower cl	78	84	155	149	145	118	155	70	102	101	65	76
		Upper cl	82	87	171	159	164	129	212	99	107	105	76	84
VI	Diseases of the nervous system and sense organs (320-389)	SPCR	98	97	108	112	106	101	112	90	100	101	98	95
		Lower cl	96	96	103	108	101	97	96	78	99	99	94	91
		Upper cl	99	99	112	115	112	106	128	102	102	102	103	99
VII	Diseases of the circulatory system (390-459)	SPCR	95	94	125	129	108	104	71	86	102	101	90	93
		Lower cl	92	91	120	124	100	97	49	64	100	99	84	87
		Upper cl	97	96	131	134	115	111	94	109	104	103	95	98
VIII	Diseases of the respiratory system (460-519)	SPCR	96	95	113	117	109	104	103	106	101	101	95	93
		Lower cl	95	94	109	114	105	101	93	98	100	100	92	91
		Upper cl	98	97	116	119	113	107	113	114	102	102	98	96
IX	Diseases of the digestive system (520-579)	SPCR	90	92	141	133	115	106	105	78	102	102	87	87
		Lower cl	88	90	135	129	108	101	86	64	100	100	82	83
		Upper cl	92	94	147	138	122	112	125	93	104	104	92	91
X	Diseases of the genitourinary system (580-629)	SPCR	97	95	116	119	100	105	102	92	101	101	98	92
		Lower cl	93	94	107	116	89	101	71	83	97	100	89	89
		Upper cl	100	96	125	122	110	108	132	101	104	102	106	95
XI	Complications of pregnancy, childbirth and the puerperium (630-679)	SPCR	-	97	-	117	-	99	-	39	-	99	-	105
		Lower cl	-	94	-	110	-	91	-	25	-	96	-	96
		Upper cl	-	101	-	124	-	106	-	53	-	102	-	114
XII	Diseases of the skin and subcutaneous tissue (680-709)	SPCR	98	95	105	116	110	106	88	97	101	101	94	92
		Lower cl	96	94	101	113	105	102	76	86	99	100	89	88
		Upper cl	100	97	109	120	115	110	100	108	103	103	98	95

White M	White F	Black Afro-caribbean M	F	Indian M	F	Pakistani/ Bangladeshi M	F	Other M	F		Disease group	
100	100	99	102	102	97	103	100	96	99	SPCR	All diseases and conditions	
99	99	90	95	94	90	93	90	90	93	Lower cl	(I-XVIII)	
101	101	108	109	110	104	114	110	102	104	Upper cl		
100	100	114	111	118	120	142	157	93	89	SPCR	Serious	
98	99	94	94	100	102	117	128	80	77	Lower cl		
101	101	134	127	136	138	167	187	106	100	Upper cl		
100	100	96	108	99	99	105	105	93	93	SPCR	Intermediate	
99	99	85	100	89	91	92	93	86	87	Lower cl		
101	101	107	117	109	108	118	118	100	99	Upper cl		
100	100	103	104	112	97	120	105	97	100	SPCR	Minor	
99	99	92	96	102	90	107	94	90	94	Lower cl		
101	101	113	111	122	105	134	116	104	105	Upper cl		
100	100	99	106	100	100	102	103	97	98	SPCR	All illnesses (I-XVII)	
99	99	90	98	92	92	92	92	90	93	Lower cl		
101	101	108	113	108	107	113	113	103	104	Upper cl		
100	100	110	106	101	91	126	96	93	89	SPCR	Infectious and parasitic	I
98	99	85	90	79	75	94	74	77	78	Lower cl	diseases (001-139)	
102	102	135	121	123	106	157	117	109	100	Upper cl		
101	101	*48*	*67*	*72*	*57*	*108*	*40*	*75*	102	SPCR	Neoplasms (140-239)	II
97	98	*10*	*36*	*30*	*28*	*41*	*5*	*40*	72	Lower cl		
105	104	*86*	*99*	*115*	*85*	*174*	*75*	*109*	131	Upper cl		
99	100	111	141	158	120	208	166	91	77	SPCR	Endocrine, nutritional and	III
96	97	66	103	111	85	139	105	62	55	Lower cl	metabolic diseases and	
102	102	155	179	204	155	277	228	121	99	Upper cl	immunity disorders (240-279)	
99	97	*124*	209	*152*	332	*81*	262	*144*	127	SPCR	Diseases of blood and blood-	IV
88	92	*0*	127	*0*	228	*0*	130	*3*	78	Lower cl	forming organs (280-289)	
111	101	*296*	291	*324*	436	*239*	395	*285*	176	Upper cl		
100	100	89	96	68	68	95	74	101	88	SPCR	Mental disorders (290-319)	V
98	99	61	77	46	52	61	49	80	74	Lower cl		
103	102	117	115	90	84	129	98	122	102	Upper cl		
100	100	87	100	108	110	114	129	103	88	SPCR	Diseases of the nervous system	VI
98	99	67	83	88	93	88	102	87	76	Lower cl	and sense organs (320-389)	
102	101	107	116	128	127	141	156	118	99	Upper cl		
100	100	117	141	125	113	119	*72*	104	99	SPCR	Diseases of the circulatory	VII
98	98	86	110	97	85	84	*38*	81	78	Lower cl	system (390-459)	
102	102	148	172	154	141	154	*106*	126	119	Upper cl		
99	100	114	97	124	104	142	115	107	101	SPCR	Diseases of the respiratory	VIII
98	99	98	86	108	92	121	98	96	93	Lower cl	system (460-519)	
101	101	130	108	139	116	162	133	118	110	Upper cl		
99	100	125	100	116	114	184	239	93	93	SPCR	Diseases of the digestive system	IX
97	98	95	79	91	92	142	192	75	78	Lower cl	(520-579)	
101	101	154	121	142	137	225	285	111	108	Upper cl		
100	100	108	106	90	82	154	107	93	88	SPCR	Diseases of the genitourinary	X
97	99	64	93	53	70	92	88	64	79	Lower cl	system (580-629)	
103	101	151	120	126	94	216	126	123	97	Upper cl		
-	100	-	95	-	80	-	137	-	95	SPCR	Complications of pregnancy,	XI
-	97	-	65	-	49	-	83	-	72	Lower cl	childbirth and the puerperium	
-	103	-	126	-	111	-	191	-	118	Upper cl	(630-679)	
100	100	93	109	120	115	161	136	103	107	SPCR	Diseases of the skin and	XII
98	98	73	93	99	98	131	110	88	95	Lower cl	subcutaneous tissue (680-709)	
101	101	113	126	141	133	191	162	117	120	Upper cl		

Table 29 - *continued*

| Disease group | | | Tenure | | | | | | | | Urban / rural | | | |
| | | | Owner occupier | | Council house | | Other rented | | Communal | | Urban | | Rural | |
			M	F	M	F	M	F	M	F	M	F	M	F
XIII	Diseases of the musculoskeletal	SPCR	94	93	129	131	108	108	72	82	101	102	91	89
	system and connective tissue	Lower cl	92	91	125	127	103	104	60	70	100	100	88	86
	(710-739)	Upper cl	95	94	133	134	113	113	84	94	103	103	95	92
XIV	Congenital anomalies (740-759)	SPCR	90	91	150	118	99	133	*113*	*138*	105	104	70	76
		Lower cl	80	82	120	97	68	103	*23*	*52*	94	95	48	56
		Upper cl	101	100	181	140	130	162	*204*	*223*	116	113	92	96
XV	Certain conditions originating in	SPCR	*68*	*84*	*337*	*182*	-	*87*	-	-	*117*	109	-	*27*
	the perinatal period (760-779)	Lower cl	*0*	*46*	*0*	*74*	-	*2*	-	-	*0*	71	-	*0*
		Upper cl	*201*	*122*	*998*	*289*	-	*171*	-	-	*279*	146	-	*79*
XVI	Symptoms, signs and ill-defined	SPCR	91	91	134	136	113	111	102	95	103	102	81	84
	conditions (780-799)	Lower cl	90	89	129	132	107	106	86	84	101	101	77	80
		Upper cl	93	92	140	139	119	115	118	106	105	104	85	87
XVII	Injury and poisoning (800-999)	SPCR	95	93	117	126	111	109	94	105	101	101	93	94
		Lower cl	93	91	113	122	106	104	83	92	99	99	89	90
		Upper cl	97	95	121	129	116	113	106	118	103	102	97	98
XVIII	Supplementary classification of	SPCR	95	98	114	103	121	109	112	89	101	100	93	97
	factors influencing health status	Lower cl	93	97	111	102	116	107	100	83	100	100	90	95
	and contact with health services	Upper cl	96	99	118	105	125	112	124	95	102	101	96	99
	(VO1-V82)														

Ethnic group										Disease group		
White		Black Afro-caribbean		Indian		Pakistani/ Bangladeshi		Other				
M	F	M	F	M	F	M	F	M	F			
100	99	95	118	104	150	129	166	94	94	SPCR	Diseases of the musculoskeletal	XIII
99	98	77	100	86	131	105	136	80	82	Lower cl	system and connective tissue	
101	101	113	135	121	170	154	196	107	106	Upper cl	(710-739)	
101	100	*122*	*102*	*135*	*133*	-	*52*	*20*	*60*	SPCR	Congenital anomalies (740-759)	XIV
91	92	*0*	*2*	*3*	*16*	-	*0*	*0*	*1*	Lower cl		
111	108	*261*	*201*	*266*	*250*	-	*155*	*60*	*119*	Upper cl		
103	100	-	-	-	-	-	*741*	-	-	SPCR	Certain conditions originating in	XV
0	66	-	-	-	-	-	*0*	-	-	Lower cl	the perinatal period (760-779)	
246	135	-	-	-	-	-	*2,193*	-	-	Upper cl		
99	99	143	144	140	131	168	188	109	122	SPCR	Symptoms, signs and ill-defined	XVI
97	98	115	125	115	112	133	157	92	108	Lower cl	conditions (780-799)	
101	100	171	163	164	150	203	219	126	135	Upper cl		
100	100	103	112	93	86	83	108	78	80	SPCR	Injury and poisoning (800-999)	XVII
99	99	84	94	76	70	63	83	66	68	Lower cl		
102	102	122	130	109	103	103	134	89	92	Upper cl		
100	100	97	109	140	92	143	95	97	95	SPCR	Supplementary classification of	XVIII
98	99	81	100	123	83	121	83	86	89	Lower cl	factors influencing health status	
101	101	112	118	157	101	165	107	108	102	Upper cl	and contact with health services (VO1-V82)	

Table 30 Age standardised patient consulting ratios (SPCR) for people aged 16-64 (study population=100) with approximate
95 per cent upper and lower confidence limits:
comparison by sex, marital status, cohabiting status and social class (as defined by occupation)

Disease group			Marital status						Cohabiting status					
			Single		Married		Widowed/divorced		Single		Married/cohabiting		Sep/wid/div not cohabiting	
			M	F	M	F	M	F	M	F	M	F	M	F
	All diseases and conditions (I-XVIII)	SPCR	99	99	100	100	112	105	97	97	100	100	112	105
		Lower cl	97	97	99	99	109	103	96	95	100	100	109	103
		Upper cl	100	100	101	101	115	107	98	98	101	101	115	107
	Serious	SPCR	106	99	96	97	129	118	104	97	96	98	131	118
		Lower cl	103	96	94	96	122	114	101	94	95	96	125	114
		Upper cl	109	101	97	99	135	122	108	100	98	99	138	122
	Intermediate	SPCR	99	97	99	100	119	111	96	95	100	100	119	110
		Lower cl	97	96	98	99	115	108	95	93	99	99	115	108
		Upper cl	100	98	100	100	123	113	98	96	101	101	123	113
	Minor	SPCR	98	98	100	100	114	107	96	95	101	101	114	107
		Lower cl	96	97	99	99	110	105	94	94	100	100	110	105
		Upper cl	99	99	101	101	117	109	97	97	102	101	117	109
	All illnesses (I-XVII)	SPCR	99	98	99	100	114	107	97	97	100	100	114	107
		Lower cl	98	97	99	99	111	105	96	96	99	99	111	105
		Upper cl	100	100	100	100	117	109	99	98	101	101	117	109
I	Infectious and parasitic diseases (001-139)	SPCR	99	98	98	98	129	121	96	96	100	99	130	121
		Lower cl	96	96	96	96	119	116	93	93	98	97	120	116
		Upper cl	102	100	101	100	139	126	99	98	102	101	141	126
II	Neoplasms (140-239)	SPCR	98	103	100	97	107	111	91	103	102	99	98	105
		Lower cl	90	96	95	94	89	102	83	95	98	95	81	96
		Upper cl	107	110	105	101	124	120	100	110	107	102	115	114
III	Endocrine, nutritional and metabolic diseases and immunity disorders (240-279)	SPCR	110	103	97	98	112	108	111	103	98	98	105	107
		Lower cl	101	97	94	95	100	101	102	96	95	95	93	100
		Upper cl	118	110	100	101	124	115	119	110	101	101	117	114
IV	Diseases of blood and blood-forming organs (280-289)	SPCR	101	88	97	104	135	98	110	86	94	104	143	99
		Lower cl	75	79	84	99	85	84	80	76	82	98	90	85
		Upper cl	128	97	109	110	186	112	139	96	107	109	196	113
V	Mental disorders (290-319)	SPCR	122	102	83	91	190	151	122	99	84	91	218	158
		Lower cl	117	99	81	89	177	145	117	95	82	89	204	152
		Upper cl	126	105	86	93	203	157	127	103	87	93	233	164
VI	Diseases of the nervous system and sense organs (320-389)	SPCR	100	98	100	99	105	109	99	97	100	99	105	108
		Lower cl	97	95	98	98	98	105	95	94	98	98	98	104
		Upper cl	103	100	102	101	112	113	102	100	102	101	113	113
VII	Diseases of the circulatory system (390-459)	SPCR	106	92	98	100	115	106	104	90	98	100	118	106
		Lower cl	100	87	95	98	107	100	98	84	96	98	109	101
		Upper cl	112	97	100	103	123	111	110	95	100	102	126	111
VIII	Diseases of the respiratory system (460-519)	SPCR	97	98	100	98	115	118	96	98	101	98	114	118
		Lower cl	96	97	99	97	109	114	94	96	100	97	108	115
		Upper cl	99	100	102	99	120	121	98	100	103	99	120	122
IX	Diseases of the digestive system (520-579)	SPCR	99	96	98	98	129	119	94	92	100	99	129	119
		Lower cl	95	92	95	96	120	113	90	88	97	97	119	113
		Upper cl	103	99	100	101	138	124	98	95	102	101	138	124
X	Diseases of the genitourinary system (580-629)	SPCR	94	91	101	102	113	113	91	87	103	102	103	111
		Lower cl	88	89	97	100	98	109	84	85	99	101	89	108
		Upper cl	100	93	105	103	127	116	97	89	107	104	118	115
XI	Complications of pregnancy, childbirth and the puerperium (630-679)	SPCR	-	63	-	131	-	89	-	43	-	134	-	70
		Lower cl	-	60	-	127	-	77	-	39	-	129	-	60
		Upper cl	-	67	-	136	-	100	-	46	-	138	-	80
XII	Diseases of the skin and subcutaneous tissue (680-709)	SPCR	100	101	98	98	122	111	99	102	99	97	123	115
		Lower cl	98	99	96	96	114	107	96	99	97	95	114	110
		Upper cl	103	103	100	99	130	116	101	104	101	99	131	119

* Social class of married/cohabiting women is based on their partner's occupation.

Social class										Disease group		
I & II		IIIN		IIIM		IV & V		Other				
M	F	M	F	M	F	M	F	M	F			
98	99	100	100	101	101	103	102	97	97	SPCR	All diseases and conditions	
96	98	97	98	100	100	101	100	95	95	Lower cl	(I-XVIII)	
99	100	102	101	102	102	104	103	100	99	Upper cl		
81	90	92	92	106	114	120	115	117	105	SPCR	Serious	
79	87	88	90	104	109	117	112	110	101	Lower cl		
83	92	96	94	109	119	124	118	124	109	Upper cl		
94	97	99	99	103	105	106	106	96	95	SPCR	Intermediate	
93	95	96	98	102	102	104	104	93	93	Lower cl		
95	98	101	100	105	107	108	107	99	97	Upper cl		
97	100	101	100	101	103	103	102	97	95	SPCR	Minor	
96	99	99	99	100	100	101	101	94	93	Lower cl		
98	101	104	101	103	105	105	103	100	96	Upper cl		
96	99	99	99	102	102	104	103	97	96	SPCR	All illnesses (I-XVII)	
95	97	97	98	101	100	103	102	94	95	Lower cl		
97	100	102	101	103	105	106	105	99	98	Upper cl		
103	101	104	98	99	104	99	105	93	93	SPCR	Infectious and parasitic	I
99	98	98	96	95	99	95	102	87	90	Lower cl	diseases (001-139)	
107	104	110	100	102	109	103	108	99	97	Upper cl		
115	109	102	104	92	96	84	91	112	89	SPCR	Neoplasms (140-239)	II
108	103	89	99	85	85	75	85	92	80	Lower cl		
123	115	115	109	99	107	92	97	133	98	Upper cl		
97	83	104	94	98	117	108	118	92	107	SPCR	Endocrine, nutritional and	III
92	78	94	90	93	107	101	113	74	99	Lower cl	metabolic diseases and	
102	87	114	98	103	126	116	123	111	115	Upper cl	immunity disorders (240-279)	
89	84	104	99	102	113	111	116	*111*	96	SPCR	Diseases of blood and blood-	IV
71	76	67	91	82	95	85	106	*51*	82	Lower cl	forming organs (280-289)	
108	92	141	107	121	131	137	127	*172*	110	Upper cl		
78	83	101	92	99	109	128	122	144	110	SPCR	Mental disorders (290-319)	V
74	80	94	90	95	103	122	119	132	105	Lower cl		
81	86	108	95	103	115	133	126	156	115	Upper cl		
98	95	99	99	99	102	103	104	109	103	SPCR	Diseases of the nervous system	VI
95	93	94	97	96	97	100	101	102	99	Lower cl	and sense organs (320-389)	
101	98	104	102	101	107	107	106	116	107	Upper cl		
90	87	101	95	103	110	111	115	110	103	SPCR	Diseases of the circulatory	VII
86	83	94	92	100	103	106	111	96	96	Lower cl	system (390-459)	
93	90	108	98	107	118	116	119	125	109	Upper cl		
99	96	102	97	99	105	102	109	98	97	SPCR	Diseases of the respiratory	VIII
97	94	99	96	97	101	100	107	94	94	Lower cl	system (460-519)	
101	98	106	99	101	108	105	111	102	99	Upper cl		
87	86	93	98	107	108	115	115	90	100	SPCR	Diseases of the digestive system	IX
84	83	87	95	103	102	110	111	82	95	Lower cl	(520-579)	
91	89	99	101	111	115	120	119	99	105	Upper cl		
96	95	102	99	99	106	108	108	100	93	SPCR	Diseases of the genitourinary	X
90	93	91	97	94	102	100	106	86	90	Lower cl	system (580-629)	
101	97	112	101	105	110	115	110	114	96	Upper cl		
-	107	-	97	-	112	-	103	-	83	SPCR	Complications of pregnancy,	XI
-	101	-	92	-	101	-	96	-	76	Lower cl	childbirth and the puerperium	
-	113	-	102	-	124	-	109	-	91	Upper cl	(630-679)	
100	91	101	100	99	103	98	106	106	104	SPCR	Diseases of the skin and	XII
97	88	96	98	96	98	95	103	101	100	Lower cl	subcutaneous tissue (680-709)	
103	93	106	103	102	108	102	109	111	107	Upper cl		

Table 30 - *continued*

Disease group			Marital status						Cohabiting status					
			Single		Married		Widowed/ divorced		Single		Married/ cohabiting		Sep/wid/div not cohabiting	
			M	F	M	F	M	F	M	F	M	F	M	F
XIII	Diseases of the musculoskeletal system and connective tissue (710-739)	SPCR	93	95	101	98	120	116	89	93	102	99	117	115
		Lower cl	90	92	99	97	114	112	86	90	100	97	111	111
		Upper cl	96	98	102	100	126	120	92	96	103	100	124	118
XIV	Congenital anomalies (740-759)	SPCR	110	105	96	97	*89*	108	115	107	94	94	99	121
		Lower cl	92	89	84	87	*50*	82	95	89	83	85	57	94
		Upper cl	128	121	108	106	*128*	133	134	125	106	104	142	148
XV	Certain conditions originating in the perinatal period (760-779)	SPCR	-	77	*161*	119	-	*94*	-	*63*	*141*	117	-	*131*
		Lower cl	-	*32*	*0*	68	-	*0*	-	*16*	*0*	70	-	*0*
		Upper cl	-	*123*	*385*	170	-	*224*	-	*109*	*337*	164	-	*278*
XVI	Symptoms, signs and ill-defined conditions (780-799)	SPCR	101	97	97	98	129	120	99	94	99	99	127	120
		Lower cl	98	95	95	96	120	115	95	91	96	97	119	116
		Upper cl	104	100	99	100	137	124	102	96	101	101	136	125
XVII	Injury and poisoning (800-999)	SPCR	97	101	100	97	124	119	96	99	101	98	121	118
		Lower cl	95	98	98	95	117	114	93	96	99	96	113	113
		Upper cl	100	103	102	98	132	124	98	102	103	99	128	122
XVIII	Supplementary classification of factors influencing health status and contact with health services (VO1-V82)	SPCR	99	97	99	100	118	110	96	92	100	102	121	109
		Lower cl	97	96	97	99	113	108	94	91	98	101	115	107
		Upper cl	102	98	100	101	123	113	99	94	101	103	126	112

Social class										Disease group		
I & II		IIIN		IIIM		IV & V		Other				
M	F	M	F	M	F	M	F	M	F			
80	89	93	94	113	114	118	118	87	93	SPCR	Diseases of the musculoskeletal	XIII
78	87	88	92	111	109	114	115	81	89	Lower cl	system and connective tissue	
82	92	97	96	116	119	121	121	94	97	Upper cl	(710-739)	
99	95	97	93	81	73	112	112	162	121	SPCR	Congenital anomalies (740-759)	XIV
82	79	67	80	66	47	89	94	117	97	Lower cl		
116	111	126	106	96	98	135	130	208	146	Upper cl		
146	*127*	-	*82*	*149*	*196*	-	*96*	-	*48*	SPCR	Certain conditions originating in	XV
0	*48*	-	*31*	*0*	*24*	-	*25*	-	*0*	Lower cl	the perinatal period (760-779)	
431	*205*	-	*133*	*441*	*369*	-	*168*	-	*116*	Upper cl		
89	88	100	99	104	105	114	117	93	93	SPCR	Symptoms, signs and ill-defined	XVI
86	86	95	96	101	100	110	114	87	89	Lower cl	conditions (780-799)	
92	91	106	101	107	109	118	120	100	97	Upper cl		
80	92	92	95	114	113	119	116	82	92	SPCR	Injury and poisoning (800-999)	XVII
78	89	88	93	111	107	116	112	78	88	Lower cl		
82	95	96	98	117	118	123	119	87	96	Upper cl		
92	102	99	101	103	105	107	102	109	88	SPCR	Supplementary classification of	XVIII
90	100	95	99	101	103	104	100	104	86	Lower cl	factors influencing health status	
94	104	103	102	105	108	110	103	115	90	Upper cl	and contact with health services (VO1-V82)	

Table 31 Age standardised patient consulting ratios (SPCR) for people aged 16 and over (study population = 100) with approximate 95 per cent upper and lower confidence limits: comparison by age, sex, and smoking status

Disease group			Aged 16-64				Aged 65 and over			
			Smoked last week		Did not smoke		Smoked last week		Did not smoke	
			M	F	M	F	M	F	M	F
	All diseases and conditions (I-XVIII)	SPCR	102	102	99	99	96	98	101	100
		Lower cl	101	101	98	98	93	95	100	99
		Upper cl	103	104	100	100	99	101	103	101
	Serious	SPCR	109	116	95	94	96	102	101	100
		Lower cl	107	113	94	92	92	97	99	98
		Upper cl	112	118	97	95	100	106	103	101
	Intermediate	SPCR	105	107	98	97	94	99	102	100
		Lower cl	103	105	97	96	91	96	100	99
		Upper cl	106	108	99	98	97	103	104	101
	Minor	SPCR	101	103	99	99	93	96	102	101
		Lower cl	100	102	98	98	90	93	100	99
		Upper cl	103	104	100	99	96	100	104	102
	All illnesses (I-XVII)	SPCR	103	104	99	98	96	99	101	100
		Lower cl	101	103	98	98	93	96	100	99
		Upper cl	104	105	99	99	99	102	103	101
I	Infectious and parasitic diseases SPCR (001-139)	100	100	106	100	98	86	96	104	100
		Lower cl	97	103	98	96	77	87	99	97
		Upper cl	104	108	102	99	95	105	110	104
II	Neoplasms (140-239)	SPCR	97	97	102	101	96	97	101	101
		Lower cl	90	92	97	97	85	84	95	95
		Upper cl	104	103	107	105	107	110	107	106
III	Endocrine, nutritional and metabolic diseases and immunity disorders (240-279)	SPCR	87	100	107	100	74	88	108	102
		Lower cl	82	95	103	97	67	80	103	98
		Upper cl	92	104	111	103	82	96	113	106
IV	Diseases of blood and blood-forming organs (280-289)	SPCR	94	81	102	108	88	94	104	101
		Lower cl	75	73	88	102	70	77	93	95
		Upper cl	113	88	116	114	106	111	114	107
V	Mental disorders (290-319)	SPCR	139	139	80	84	116	121	95	97
		Lower cl	134	136	78	82	105	113	90	94
		Upper cl	143	142	83	86	126	130	100	100
VI	Diseases of the nervous system and sense organs (320-389)	SPCR	100	105	100	98	93	95	102	101
		Lower cl	98	102	98	97	88	89	99	99
		Upper cl	103	107	102	100	98	100	105	103
VII	Diseases of the circulatory system (390-459)	SPCR	93	95	103	102	86	87	104	102
		Lower cl	90	92	101	100	81	82	102	100
		Upper cl	97	99	106	104	90	91	107	104
VIII	Diseases of the respiratory system (460-519)	SPCR	98	109	101	96	100	117	100	97
		Lower cl	96	107	100	95	95	112	97	95
		Upper cl	100	111	102	97	105	123	103	99
IX	Diseases of the digestive system (520-579)	SPCR	115	116	92	93	93	99	102	100
		Lower cl	112	113	90	92	87	92	98	97
		Upper cl	119	120	94	95	100	106	105	103
X	Diseases of the genitourinary system (580-629)	SPCR	99	111	101	95	93	83	102	103
		Lower cl	93	109	97	94	84	76	97	99
		Upper cl	104	113	104	97	102	90	107	106
XI	Complications of pregnancy, childbirth and the puerperium (630-679)	SPCR	-	103	-	99	-	*156*	-	*89*
		Lower cl	-	98	-	95	-	*0*	-	*31*
		Upper cl	-	109	-	102	-	*333*	-	*148*
XII	Diseases of the skin and subcutaneous tissue (680-709)	SPCR	101	107	100	97	92	100	103	100
		Lower cl	98	105	98	96	85	92	99	97
		Upper cl	104	110	102	99	98	107	106	103

Table 31 - *continued*

Disease group			Aged 16-64				Aged 65 and over			
			Smoked last week		Did not smoke		Smoked last week		Did not smoke	
			M	F	M	F	M	F	M	F
XIII	Diseases of the musculoskeletal system and connective tissue (710-739)	SPCR	110	114	95	94	93	96	102	101
		Lower cl	107	112	93	93	88	91	99	99
		Upper cl	112	117	97	96	98	100	105	103
XIV	Congenital anomalies (740-759)	SPCR	80	93	111	103	93	92	103	101
		Lower cl	65	78	98	94	55	55	80	85
		Upper cl	95	107	123	113	130	128	125	116
XV	Certain conditions originating in the perinatal period (760-779)	SPCR	-	*125*	*155*	89	-	-	*126*	*108*
		Lower cl	-	*57*	*0*	51	-	-	*0*	*2*
		Upper cl	-	*193*	*371*	128	-	-	*301*	*214*
XVI	Symptoms, signs and ill-defined conditions (780-799)	SPCR	107	116	97	94	95	100	101	100
		Lower cl	103	113	94	92	89	94	98	98
		Upper cl	110	118	99	95	101	106	105	102
XVII	Injury and poisoning (800-999)	SPCR	109	114	95	94	91	97	103	100
		Lower cl	106	111	94	93	84	91	99	98
		Upper cl	112	117	97	96	98	104	107	103
XVIII	Supplementary classification of factors influencing health status and contact with health services (VO1-V82)	SPCR	103	104	99	98	87	90	104	102
		Lower cl	101	103	97	98	84	86	102	100
		Upper cl	105	105	100	99	91	94	106	103

Table 32 Age standardised patient consulting ratios (SPCR) for people aged 16-64 (study population = 100) with approximate 95 per cent upper and lower confidence limits: comparison by sex, living alone, sole adult with children, children in household

Disease group			All adults				Sole adults			
			Living alone		Living accompanied		Sole adult without children		Sole adult with children	
			M	F	M	F	M	F	M	F
	All diseases and conditions (I-XVIII)	SPCR	109	103	99	100	100	99	101	102
		Lower cl	106	100	99	99	97	96	90	99
		Upper cl	112	105	100	100	102	101	111	105
	Serious	SPCR	129	114	98	99	100	97	92	107
		Lower cl	124	109	96	98	96	93	72	100
		Upper cl	135	119	99	100	105	101	111	114
	Intermediate	SPCR	113	104	99	100	100	97	103	105
		Lower cl	109	101	98	99	97	94	90	102
		Upper cl	116	106	100	100	103	99	116	109
	Minor	SPCR	111	104	99	100	100	98	100	103
		Lower cl	108	101	98	99	97	96	88	100
		Upper cl	114	106	100	100	103	100	112	106
	All illnesses (I-XVII)	SPCR	110	103	99	100	100	98	103	103
		Lower cl	107	101	99	99	97	96	92	100
		Upper cl	113	106	100	100	102	100	114	106
I	Infectious and parasitic diseases (001-139)	SPCR	120	110	99	99	97	94	145	107
		Lower cl	112	104	97	98	91	89	111	101
		Upper cl	128	116	101	101	104	99	178	113
II	Neoplasms (140-239)	SPCR	111	119	99	99	102	102	*66*	96
		Lower cl	94	106	95	96	87	91	*13*	81
		Upper cl	127	132	103	102	117	113	*118*	111
III	Endocrine, nutritional and metabolic diseases and immunity disorders (240-279)	SPCR	121	109	98	99	101	99	*68*	102
		Lower cl	109	100	95	97	91	91	*28*	88
		Upper cl	133	118	101	102	112	107	*108*	116
IV	Diseases of blood and blood-forming organs (280-289)	SPCR	129	95	98	100	92	94	*248*	110
		Lower cl	82	77	86	96	59	76	*5*	86
		Upper cl	177	113	109	105	126	111	*490*	135
V	Mental disorders (290-319)	SPCR	198	148	93	97	100	96	101	107
		Lower cl	186	141	91	95	94	91	76	100
		Upper cl	210	156	95	98	106	101	126	114
VI	Diseases of the nervous system and sense organs (320-389)	SPCR	107	104	99	100	100	96	103	108
		Lower cl	101	99	98	98	94	91	77	101
		Upper cl	113	109	101	101	106	101	129	115
VII	Diseases of the circulatory system (390-459)	SPCR	117	101	99	100	99	98	115	109
		Lower cl	109	95	97	98	93	92	76	95
		Upper cl	125	108	101	102	106	104	154	122
VIII	Diseases of the respiratory system (460-519)	SPCR	110	106	99	100	99	96	111	107
		Lower cl	105	102	98	99	95	92	91	102
		Upper cl	114	110	101	101	104	99	130	112
IX	Diseases of the digestive system (520-579)	SPCR	122	105	98	100	100	94	95	112
		Lower cl	113	99	96	98	93	88	66	103
		Upper cl	130	112	100	101	107	100	124	120
X	Diseases of the genitourinary system (580-629)	SPCR	106	97	100	100	99	90	*124*	113
		Lower cl	93	92	96	99	87	86	*65*	108
		Upper cl	118	101	103	101	111	94	*183*	119
XI	Complications of pregnancy, childbirth and the puerperium (630-679)	SPCR	-	43	-	103	-	60	-	133
		Lower cl	-	35	-	100	-	48	-	117
		Upper cl	-	52	-	106	-	72	-	149
XII	Diseases of the skin and subcutaneous tissue (680-709)	SPCR	121	109	99	99	100	97	99	105
		Lower cl	114	104	97	98	94	92	74	99
		Upper cl	128	115	100	101	106	102	123	111

Children in household								Disease group		
None		Under 5s only		5-15s only		Under 5s and 5-15s				
M	F	M	F	M	F	M	F			
100	100	105	104	98	98	103	101	SPCR	All diseases and conditions	
99	99	102	102	96	97	100	99	Lower cl	(I-XVIII)	
101	101	107	106	99	100	106	103	Upper cl		
102	100	95	104	94	98	101	100	SPCR	Serious	
100	99	90	99	91	95	95	95	Lower cl		
104	102	101	108	97	101	107	105	Upper cl		
100	99	105	107	98	99	104	103	SPCR	Intermediate	
99	98	102	105	96	98	101	101	Lower cl		
101	99	108	109	100	101	108	106	Upper cl		
100	100	105	106	97	97	105	101	SPCR	Minor	
99	99	102	105	95	96	102	99	Lower cl		
101	100	108	108	99	98	108	103	Upper cl		
100	99	105	104	98	99	103	101	SPCR	All illnesses (I-XVII)	
99	99	102	102	97	98	100	99	Lower cl		
100	100	107	105	100	101	106	103	Upper cl		
99	97	108	112	97	97	102	109	SPCR	Infectious and parasitic	I
97	95	102	108	93	94	95	105	Lower cl	diseases (001-139)	
102	98	114	116	101	99	109	114	Upper cl		
101	102	107	97	101	100	81	90	SPCR	Neoplasms (140-239)	II
95	98	92	88	92	93	66	79	Lower cl		
106	106	122	107	111	106	96	100	Upper cl		
104	99	89	98	87	102	99	104	SPCR	Endocrine, nutritional and	III
101	96	77	89	81	96	85	94	Lower cl	metabolic diseases and	
108	102	101	107	94	108	112	115	Upper cl	immunity disorders (240-279)	
102	90	*59*	132	114	106	*62*	113	SPCR	Diseases of blood and blood-	IV
89	84	*20*	116	84	97	*19*	96	Lower cl	forming organs (280-289)	
115	96	*98*	148	144	116	*105*	131	Upper cl		
108	98	83	107	84	100	92	104	SPCR	Mental disorders (290-319)	V
105	96	76	102	80	96	83	98	Lower cl		
111	100	90	112	89	103	100	110	Upper cl		
99	98	109	109	98	100	105	106	SPCR	Diseases of the nervous system	VI
97	96	103	104	94	97	99	101	Lower cl	and sense organs (320-389)	
101	99	115	113	102	103	112	111	Upper cl		
102	99	81	121	94	95	99	106	SPCR	Diseases of the circulatory	VII
100	97	72	113	89	90	88	97	Lower cl	system (390-459)	
105	101	90	130	100	100	109	115	Upper cl		
97	98	116	110	97	98	114	107	SPCR	Diseases of the respiratory	VIII
96	97	112	107	95	96	110	104	Lower cl	system (460-519)	
98	99	120	113	100	100	119	111	Upper cl		
98	98	108	102	100	102	105	103	SPCR	Diseases of the digestive system	IX
96	96	101	97	96	99	97	97	Lower cl	(520-579)	
101	101	115	107	105	106	113	109	Upper cl		
99	97	97	108	103	102	103	107	SPCR	Diseases of the genitourinary	X
95	95	87	105	96	100	90	104	Lower cl	system (580-629)	
103	98	108	111	111	104	116	111	Upper cl		
-	74	-	196	-	57	-	98	SPCR	Complications of pregnancy,	XI
-	70	-	187	-	52	-	91	Lower cl	childbirth and the puerperium	
-	78	-	205	-	62	-	106	Upper cl	(630-679)	
100	99	100	100	99	100	101	108	SPCR	Diseases of the skin and	XII
98	97	95	96	95	97	94	103	Lower cl	subcutaneous tissue (680-709)	
102	101	105	104	102	103	107	112	Upper cl		

Table 32 - *continued*

Disease group			All adults				Sole adults			
			Living alone		Living accompanied		Sole adult without children		Sole adult with children	
			M	F	M	F	M	F	M	F
XIII	Diseases of the musculoskeletal system and connective tissue (710-739)	SPCR	108	109	99	99	100	97	95	108
		Lower cl	103	105	98	98	95	93	73	101
		Upper cl	114	114	101	101	105	101	118	115
XIV	Congenital anomalies (740-759)	SPCR	119	139	99	97	106	98	-	103
		Lower cl	78	102	89	89	70	72	-	65
		Upper cl	159	175	108	105	142	125	-	141
XV	Certain conditions originating in the perinatal period (760-779)	SPCR	-	*173*	*108*	96	-	*98*	-	*102*
		Lower cl	-	*0*	*0*	62	-	*0*	-	*0*
		Upper cl	-	*369*	*258*	130	-	*209*	-	*217*
XVI	Symptoms, signs and ill-defined conditions (780-799)	SPCR	125	107	98	100	100	92	109	113
		Lower cl	118	102	96	98	94	87	82	107
		Upper cl	133	112	100	101	106	97	136	120
XVII	Injury and poisoning (800-999)	SPCR	109	108	99	99	100	95	96	108
		Lower cl	103	102	98	98	95	90	74	101
		Upper cl	114	114	101	101	106	100	118	115
XVIII	Supplementary classification of factors influencing health status and contact with health services (VO1-V82)	SPCR	120	105	99	100	100	98	91	103
		Lower cl	115	101	97	99	96	95	74	99
		Upper cl	125	108	100	100	105	101	108	107

\multicolumn{8}{l}{Children in household}								Disease group	
None		Under 5s only		5-15s only		Under 5s and 5-15s			
M	F	M	F	M	F	M	F		
99	99	100	95	103	103	106	104	SPCR	Diseases of the musculoskeletal XIII
97	98	94	91	100	100	100	99	Lower cl	system and connective tissue
100	101	105	99	106	105	112	109	Upper cl	(710-739)
105	102	78	88	101	96	74	111	SPCR	Congenital anomalies (740-759) XIV
93	92	50	64	80	79	43	80	Lower cl	
118	113	106	111	122	113	106	142	Upper cl	
-	*115*	-	*109*	*195*	*63*	*648*	*79*	SPCR	Certain conditions originating in XV
-	*64*	-	*28*	*0*	*1*	*0*	*0*	Lower cl	the perinatal period (760-779)
-	*165*	-	*190*	*577*	*125*	*1918*	*168*	Upper cl	
99	96	104	108	98	103	110	108	SPCR	Symptoms, signs and ill-defined XVI
97	95	98	104	94	100	103	103	Lower cl	conditions (780-799)
101	98	110	112	102	106	117	113	Upper cl	
99	101	100	93	101	101	109	100	SPCR	Injury and poisoning (800-999) XVII
97	99	95	89	98	98	104	95	Lower cl	
101	103	104	97	104	104	115	105	Upper cl	
102	100	100	114	91	92	103	100	SPCR	Supplementary classification of XVIII
101	99	96	112	89	90	98	97	Lower cl	factors influencing health status
104	101	104	116	94	93	107	102	Upper cl	and contact with health services (VO1-V82)

Table 33 Age standardised patient consulting ratios (SPCR) for people aged 16-64 (study population = 100) with approximate 95 per cent upper and lower confidence limits: comparison by sex, economic position last week and one year ago

Disease group			Economic position last week									
			Working full time		Working part time		Waiting/seeking work		Long-term sick		Home/family	
			M	F	M	F	M	F	M	F	M	F
	All diseases and conditions (I-XVIII)	SPCR	98	100	101	99	104	106	129	110	115	101
		Lower cl	97	99	96	98	102	103	126	106	103	100
		Upper cl	98	101	106	100	107	109	133	114	126	102
	Serious	SPCR	83	89	93	91	125	126	252	244	133	107
		Lower cl	82	87	84	88	120	117	244	233	109	104
		Upper cl	85	91	102	93	131	134	261	256	157	110
	Intermediate	SPCR	96	98	103	99	109	111	141	125	119	104
		Lower cl	95	97	96	97	106	107	137	120	104	102
		Upper cl	97	99	109	100	112	115	146	130	133	105
	Minor	SPCR	97	100	100	99	104	105	141	114	129	102
		Lower cl	96	99	94	97	101	102	137	109	115	100
		Upper cl	98	101	106	100	106	109	145	118	143	103
	All illnesses (I-XVII)	SPCR	97	99	100	99	105	107	133	117	115	101
		Lower cl	97	98	95	98	103	104	130	113	103	100
		Upper cl	98	100	106	100	108	110	137	121	127	102
I	Infectious and parasitic diseases (001-139)	SPCR	98	98	113	99	104	109	127	130	107	104
		Lower cl	96	96	97	97	98	102	117	119	75	102
		Upper cl	100	100	128	102	110	117	138	141	138	107
II	Neoplasms (140-239)	SPCR	94	103	82	92	94	104	177	151	*96*	96
		Lower cl	89	98	56	86	80	86	154	128	*33*	90
		Upper cl	98	108	109	98	108	122	199	174	*159*	102
III	Endocrine, nutritional and metabolic diseases and immunity disorders (240-279)	SPCR	89	88	103	93	112	148	183	171	122	111
		Lower cl	86	84	82	88	100	129	168	153	72	106
		Upper cl	93	92	123	97	124	167	198	189	172	117
IV	Diseases of blood and blood-forming organs (280-289)	SPCR	85	79	*117*	102	104	105	222	159	*161*	132
		Lower cl	73	72	*41*	93	62	78	162	122	*0*	121
		Upper cl	98	86	*193*	111	146	131	282	197	*383*	143
V	Mental disorders (290-319)	SPCR	74	85	136	89	185	151	337	264	186	114
		Lower cl	71	82	117	86	175	140	319	248	139	111
		Upper cl	76	87	156	92	196	162	356	280	234	118
VI	Diseases of the nervous system and sense organs (320-389)	SPCR	95	95	105	100	105	107	160	159	117	103
		Lower cl	93	93	93	97	100	99	151	149	90	100
		Upper cl	96	97	117	103	111	114	169	170	145	106
VII	Diseases of the circulatory system (390-459)	SPCR	87	86	94	93	98	112	194	168	121	113
		Lower cl	85	83	81	89	91	98	184	154	87	109
		Upper cl	89	89	106	97	106	126	204	182	155	118
VIII	Diseases of the respiratory system (460-519)	SPCR	97	100	93	100	103	101	144	128	118	100
		Lower cl	96	98	85	98	99	96	138	121	98	98
		Upper cl	98	101	101	102	107	106	151	135	139	102
IX	Diseases of the digestive system (520-579)	SPCR	92	93	102	95	128	125	188	181	92	109
		Lower cl	89	90	87	91	120	114	176	167	63	105
		Upper cl	94	96	116	98	135	135	200	196	122	113
X	Diseases of the genitourinary system (580-629)	SPCR	95	95	100	101	103	118	180	115	*105*	108
		Lower cl	91	94	76	99	92	111	162	108	*54*	106
		Upper cl	98	97	123	103	114	124	199	123	*157*	110
XI	Complications of pregnancy, childbirth and the puerperium (630-679)	SPCR	-	74	-	91	-	107	-	51	-	174
		Lower cl	-	71	-	85	-	93	-	33	-	166
		Upper cl	-	78	-	97	-	122	-	69	-	182
XII	Diseases of the skin and subcutaneous tissue (680-709)	SPCR	96	96	118	96	105	112	139	141	119	105
		Lower cl	94	94	105	94	99	105	130	131	91	102
		Upper cl	98	98	131	99	110	120	148	152	148	108

Working full time		Working part time		Waiting/seeking work		Long-term sick		Home/family		Disease group		
M	F	M	F	M	F	M	F	M	F			
98	101	102	99	102	103	127	109	111	100	SPCR	All diseases and conditions	
98	100	96	98	99	98	124	105	99	99	Lower cl	(I-XVIII)	
99	101	108	100	105	107	131	114	123	101	Upper cl		
87	92	96	91	127	126	244	237	131	105	SPCR	Serious	
86	90	86	89	120	115	236	225	105	102	Lower cl		
88	94	105	94	134	137	253	248	157	108	Upper cl		
98	99	100	99	106	109	138	123	111	102	SPCR	Intermediate	
97	98	93	98	103	103	134	118	96	101	Lower cl		
99	100	107	101	110	114	143	128	126	104	Upper cl		
98	101	103	99	102	102	138	112	120	100	SPCR	Minor	
97	100	96	98	98	97	134	108	105	99	Lower cl		
99	102	110	100	105	107	143	117	135	101	Upper cl		
98	100	101	100	104	105	131	116	111	100	SPCR	All illnesses (I-XVII)	
97	99	96	98	101	100	127	111	99	99	Lower cl		
99	101	107	101	107	110	135	120	124	102	Upper cl		
99	99	111	99	102	111	123	128	111	102	SPCR	Infectious and parasitic	I
97	97	94	96	94	101	112	117	76	99	Lower cl	diseases (001-139)	
101	101	128	102	110	121	134	140	146	105	Upper cl		
96	105	91	93	86	86	154	142	*75*	96	SPCR	Neoplasms (140-239)	II
92	100	60	87	69	64	132	119	*15*	89	Lower cl		
101	110	123	99	104	109	176	165	*135*	102	Upper cl		
91	92	98	91	117	153	182	162	*104*	113	SPCR	Endocrine, nutritional and	III
88	88	76	87	102	127	166	144	*55*	108	Lower cl	metabolic diseases and	
94	96	120	96	132	178	198	180	*154*	119	Upper cl	immunity disorders (240-279)	
90	85	*63*	106	*93*	111	225	157	*184*	121	SPCR	Diseases of blood and blood-	IV
78	79	*1*	97	*43*	74	162	118	*0*	110	Lower cl	forming organs (280-289)	
103	92	*125*	116	*144*	148	288	195	*439*	132	Upper cl		
81	89	150	89	187	155	329	256	186	115	SPCR	Mental disorders (290-319)	V
79	86	127	86	173	140	310	240	135	112	Lower cl		
83	91	173	92	201	171	348	273	238	119	Upper cl		
96	96	103	99	98	101	163	160	107	104	SPCR	Diseases of the nervous system	VI
94	94	90	96	91	91	153	149	79	101	Lower cl	and sense organs (320-389)	
98	98	117	101	105	111	172	171	135	106	Upper cl		
89	89	95	96	99	115	189	163	108	110	SPCR	Diseases of the circulatory	VII
87	86	81	92	90	97	179	149	74	106	Lower cl	system (390-459)	
92	92	108	100	109	133	199	177	142	114	Upper cl		
97	99	98	99	104	106	144	127	122	101	SPCR	Diseases of the respiratory	VIII
96	97	88	97	99	99	137	120	99	99	Lower cl	system (460-519)	
99	100	108	101	109	113	151	135	145	104	Upper cl		
94	96	113	95	131	129	183	180	100	106	SPCR	Diseases of the digestive system	IX
91	94	96	92	121	115	171	166	67	102	Lower cl	(520-579)	
96	99	130	99	141	144	195	195	133	110	Upper cl		
96	97	95	102	100	117	180	115	*108*	106	SPCR	Diseases of the genitourinary	X
92	95	70	100	86	109	160	107	*52*	104	Lower cl	system (580-629)	
99	99	120	104	115	126	199	122	*165*	109	Upper cl		
-	94	-	98	-	95	-	44	-	139	SPCR	Complications of pregnancy,	XI
-	90	-	91	-	76	-	26	-	132	Lower cl	childbirth and the puerperium	
-	98	-	105	-	114	-	61	-	146	Upper cl	(630-679)	
97	96	110	97	100	116	138	145	114	105	SPCR	Diseases of the skin and	XII
95	94	96	94	93	106	129	133	84	102	Lower cl	subcutaneous tissue (680-709)	
99	98	124	100	107	127	148	156	145	108	Upper cl		

SPCRs

Table 33 - *continued*

Disease group			Economic position last week									
			Working full time		Working part time		Waiting/seeking work		Long-term sick		Home/family	
			M	F	M	F	M	F	M	F	M	F
XIII	Diseases of the musculoskeletal	SPCR	93	96	88	98	116	116	181	184	120	97
	system and connective tissue	Lower cl	91	94	79	96	110	108	173	174	96	95
	(710-739)	Upper cl	95	98	98	101	121	124	189	194	143	100
XIV	Congenital anomalies (740-759)	SPCR	88	78	*130*	99	116	121	251	303	*59*	110
		Lower cl	77	67	*50*	83	81	71	182	213	*0*	92
		Upper cl	98	90	*211*	115	151	170	320	392	*174*	129
XV	Certain conditions originating in	SPCR	*118*	*75*	-	*45*	-	*219*	-	*176*	-	*196*
	the perinatal period (760-779)	Lower cl	*0*	*31*	-	*0*	-	*0*	-	*0*	-	*100*
		Upper cl	*281*	*119*	-	*97*	-	*468*	-	*520*	-	*292*
XVI	Symptoms, signs and ill-defined	SPCR	93	94	99	95	125	126	176	169	129	112
	conditions (780-799)	Lower cl	91	91	86	93	118	118	166	158	97	109
		Upper cl	95	96	111	98	132	134	187	180	160	115
XVII	Injury and poisoning (800-999)	SPCR	99	102	97	100	107	113	131	137	162	97
		Lower cl	98	100	86	97	102	105	123	126	132	94
		Upper cl	101	104	107	102	112	121	140	148	192	100
XVIII	Supplementary classification of	SPCR	92	101	92	97	102	106	197	126	159	103
	factors influencing health status	Lower cl	91	100	84	95	98	101	190	120	136	102
	and contact with health services	Upper cl	93	102	100	98	106	110	204	131	182	105
	(VO1-V82)											

| Economic position 1 year ago | | | | | | | | | | Disease group | |
| Working full time | | Working part time | | Waiting/seeking work | | Long-term sick | | Home/family | | | |
M	F	M	F	M	F	M	F	M	F		
96	98	92	99	110	120	174	179	115	96	SPCR	Diseases of the musculoskeletal XIII
94	96	81	97	103	109	166	169	90	94	Lower cl	system and connective tissue
97	100	103	101	116	131	182	189	140	99	Upper cl	(710-739)
92	83	*100*	102	102	*149*	273	305	*140*	103	SPCR	Congenital anomalies (740-759) XIV
81	71	*20*	85	60	*74*	197	212	*0*	85	Lower cl	
102	95	*179*	118	145	*224*	349	397	*334*	121	Upper cl	
112	*126*	-	32	-	*132*	-	-	-	144	SPCR	Certain conditions originating in XV
0	*71*	-	0	-	*0*	-	-	-	59	Lower cl	the perinatal period (760-779)
268	*182*	-	77	-	*391*	-	-	-	229	Upper cl	
95	95	106	97	126	119	174	167	133	110	SPCR	Symptoms, signs and ill-defined XVI
93	93	91	95	118	108	163	156	99	107	Lower cl	conditions (780-799)
97	97	121	100	135	130	184	178	168	113	Upper cl	
100	102	102	100	106	121	121	132	140	96	SPCR	Injury and poisoning (800-999) XVII
99	100	90	97	99	109	113	121	109	93	Lower cl	
102	104	115	103	112	132	130	143	170	99	Upper cl	
94	104	95	97	99	101	189	121	128	99	SPCR	Supplementary classification of XVIII
93	102	86	96	93	95	182	115	106	98	Lower cl	factors influencing health status
96	105	104	99	104	106	196	127	151	101	Upper cl	and contact with health services
											(VO1-V82)

Table 34 Age standardised patient consulting ratios (SPCR) for people aged 16-64 (study population = 100) with approximate 95 per cent upper and lower confidence limits: comparison by sex and occupation.

Disease group			1(a) M	1(a) F	1(b) M	1(b) F	2(a) M	2(a) F	2(b) M	2(b) F	2(c) M	2(c) F	2(d) M	2(d) F
	All diseases and conditions (I-XVIII)	SPCR	99	102	97	101	96	102	57	87	100	99	97	98
		Lower cl	97	99	95	98	93	93	52	79	96	96	93	93
		Upper cl	102	105	100	104	99	110	63	95	104	101	100	102
	Serious	SPCR	79	85	97	99	78	85	46	63	74	78	76	90
		Lower cl	75	79	91	93	72	67	36	47	67	73	70	81
		Upper cl	83	91	103	105	84	103	56	78	81	83	83	99
	Intermediate	SPCR	96	99	95	100	89	91	48	65	96	94	91	96
		Lower cl	93	96	92	96	85	82	42	57	91	91	86	91
		Upper cl	99	102	99	103	93	101	55	73	101	97	96	102
	Minor	SPCR	99	103	95	100	96	101	52	86	102	99	97	98
		Lower cl	96	100	92	97	92	92	45	78	97	97	92	93
		Upper cl	102	106	98	103	100	110	58	95	106	102	101	102
	All illnesses (I-XVII)	SPCR	98	101	96	100	94	97	49	74	99	98	95	96
		Lower cl	96	98	93	97	91	88	44	66	94	95	91	92
		Upper cl	100	104	99	103	97	105	55	81	103	100	99	101
I	Infectious and parasitic diseases (001-139)	SPCR	99	107	100	96	107	99	45	61	116	109	114	97
		Lower cl	93	100	91	90	97	81	30	46	103	102	102	87
		Upper cl	106	114	108	103	117	118	60	76	129	115	126	107
II	Neoplasms (140-239)	SPCR	107	117	98	101	126	126	*92*	110	120	119	125	120
		Lower cl	93	101	80	86	104	76	*48*	63	94	105	98	94
		Upper cl	120	133	115	115	149	177	*135*	157	147	133	152	145
III	Endocrine, nutritional and metabolic diseases and immunity disorders (240-279)	SPCR	101	89	123	98	79	*51*	66	*48*	76	65	94	88
		Lower cl	92	77	109	87	66	*23*	39	*22*	62	56	78	71
		Upper cl	110	101	137	110	92	*79*	92	*75*	91	73	111	106
IV	Diseases of blood and blood-forming organs (280-289)	SPCR	75	72	*80*	69	*115*	*23*	*40*	*36*	*84*	86	*115*	72
		Lower cl	45	53	*38*	50	*57*	*0*	*0*	*0*	*26*	67	*44*	42
		Upper cl	106	91	*122*	87	*173*	*55*	*120*	*77*	*142*	104	*186*	102
V	Mental disorders (290-319)	SPCR	67	77	88	91	71	62	*31*	39	94	66	89	91
		Lower cl	61	71	79	84	61	44	*17*	24	81	60	77	79
		Upper cl	73	84	97	99	80	80	*45*	53	107	72	102	103
VI	Diseases of the nervous system and sense organs (320-389)	SPCR	102	98	88	96	95	89	32	66	113	98	99	99
		Lower cl	96	91	81	90	87	71	22	50	102	92	90	88
		Upper cl	107	104	94	102	102	107	42	82	123	104	109	109
VII	Diseases of the circulatory system (390-459)	SPCR	96	78	99	99	81	61	52	58	87	78	87	89
		Lower cl	90	70	91	90	72	36	36	34	76	71	76	75
		Upper cl	102	87	107	108	90	87	68	81	97	85	98	104
VIII	Diseases of the respiratory system (460-519)	SPCR	99	94	97	97	100	89	43	59	109	100	101	98
		Lower cl	95	90	92	92	94	76	34	48	101	95	94	90
		Upper cl	103	99	102	101	106	101	52	70	117	104	108	105
IX	Diseases of the digestive system (520-579)	SPCR	90	91	94	94	84	73	33	46	75	75	76	87
		Lower cl	84	83	86	86	75	52	21	29	65	69	66	75
		Upper cl	95	99	103	102	93	94	46	63	85	82	86	100
X	Diseases of the genitourinary system (580-629)	SPCR	106	98	94	103	86	76	*40*	57	107	85	76	92
		Lower cl	95	93	80	97	71	63	*17*	45	87	81	59	84
		Upper cl	116	103	107	108	100	90	*63*	69	127	90	92	100
XI	Complications of pregnancy, childbirth and the puerperium (630-679)	SPCR	-	101	-	108	-	108	-	109	-	118	-	114
		Lower cl	-	87	-	93	-	73	-	69	-	101	-	91
		Upper cl	-	115	-	123	-	144	-	149	-	136	-	138
XII	Diseases of the skin and subcutaneous tissue (680-709)	SPCR	102	94	95	96	101	78	51	45	104	93	100	89
		Lower cl	96	87	88	89	93	61	37	31	93	87	90	79
		Upper cl	108	101	102	103	109	95	64	58	114	99	110	99

* See appendix C for description of each group.

3(a)		3(b)		3(c)		4(a)		4(b)				
M	F	M	F	M	F	M	F	M	F			
95	102	105	98	102	101	100	100	107	100	SPCR	All diseases and conditions	
91	95	96	96	98	98	97	99	88	98	Lower cl	(I-XVIII)	
99	108	114	101	105	105	102	101	126	102	Upper cl		
85	82	114	93	84	96	98	91	117	86	SPCR	Serious	
77	69	95	87	78	88	92	88	78	82	Lower cl		
94	95	133	98	91	103	103	94	155	89	Upper cl		
93	97	102	95	99	96	101	99	109	98	SPCR	Intermediate	
88	89	92	92	95	92	98	97	85	96	Lower cl		
98	104	113	98	103	100	105	100	133	100	Upper cl		
95	101	108	97	101	100	100	100	90	100	SPCR	Minor	
90	94	98	94	97	96	97	99	70	98	Lower cl		
100	108	119	100	105	104	103	102	111	102	Upper cl		
94	98	103	97	100	99	100	100	110	99	SPCR	All illnesses (I-XVII)	
90	91	94	94	97	96	97	98	90	97	Lower cl		
99	104	112	100	104	103	103	101	129	101	Upper cl		
103	103	102	95	104	99	104	95	*114*	99	SPCR	Infectious and parasitic	I
91	89	78	89	94	91	96	92	*58*	94	Lower cl	diseases (001-139)	
115	118	126	101	115	107	111	98	*171*	103	Upper cl		
139	100	*112*	96	120	114	96	103	*124*	116	SPCR	Neoplasms (140-239)	II
107	67	*55*	82	96	94	80	95	*2*	106	Lower cl		
170	134	*168*	109	144	133	112	111	*246*	127	Upper cl		
93	77	140	78	89	75	104	96	*109*	85	SPCR	Endocrine, nutritional and	III
73	52	93	68	74	62	91	89	*28*	77	Lower cl	metabolic diseases and	
113	102	187	88	104	88	116	102	*190*	92	Upper cl	immunity disorders (240-279)	
138	*105*	*121*	99	*108*	104	*74*	99	206	98	SPCR	Diseases of blood and blood-	IV
48	*54*	*0*	77	*47*	76	*35*	87	0	83	Lower cl	forming organs (280-289)	
228	*157*	*288*	120	*169*	132	*113*	110	610	113	Upper cl		
71	73	117	81	90	93	112	89	*68*	89	SPCR	Mental disorders (290-319)	V
59	58	86	75	79	84	103	85	*18*	84	Lower cl		
83	88	148	88	101	102	122	93	*118*	94	Upper cl		
99	90	93	93	110	93	103	100	138	101	SPCR	Diseases of the nervous system	VI
89	76	73	87	101	85	96	96	87	97	Lower cl	and sense organs (320-389)	
109	104	112	99	119	100	109	103	190	105	Upper cl		
85	82	109	90	92	86	106	94	*119*	88	SPCR	Diseases of the circulatory	VII
72	61	81	81	82	75	97	89	*64*	82	Lower cl	system (390-459)	
98	104	138	99	102	97	114	99	*173*	94	Upper cl		
97	89	115	91	104	99	100	98	92	96	SPCR	Diseases of the respiratory	VIII
89	79	99	87	98	93	96	96	61	93	Lower cl	system (460-519)	
104	99	131	96	110	104	105	100	123	99	Upper cl		
97	66	123	74	95	101	96	99	*131*	93	SPCR	Diseases of the digestive system	IX
85	51	95	67	85	90	88	95	*71*	88	Lower cl	(520-579)	
110	81	151	81	105	111	103	103	*192*	98	Upper cl		
87	92	*70*	96	95	95	108	96	*116*	98	SPCR	Diseases of the genitourinary	X
68	81	*36*	91	78	89	95	93	*23*	95	Lower cl	system (580-629)	
107	103	*105*	101	111	101	121	98	*210*	102	Upper cl		
-	107	-	111	-	84	-	97	-	90	SPCR	Complications of pregnancy,	XI
-	77	-	97	-	69	-	90	-	81	Lower cl	childbirth and the puerperium	
-	137	-	124	-	99	-	104	-	99	Upper cl	(630-679)	
89	90	106	82	113	90	102	100	*93*	100	SPCR	Diseases of the skin and	XII
79	76	84	76	103	82	96	96	*50*	96	Lower cl	subcutaneous tissue (680-709)	
98	104	127	87	122	98	108	103	*136*	105	Upper cl		

Table 34 - *continued*

Disease group			Occupation (Sub-major Groups)											
			5(a)		5(b)		5(c)		6(a)		6(b)		7(a)	
			M	F	M	F	M	F	M	F	M	F	M	F
	All diseases and conditions (I-XVIII)	SPCR	99	103	100	98	101	100	103	104	107	102	100	102
		Lower cl	96	85	97	87	99	97	98	95	102	101	95	95
		Upper cl	101	121	102	109	103	103	107	114	111	104	104	108
	Serious	SPCR	110	98	94	99	106	113	99	106	124	112	86	93
		Lower cl	104	57	90	74	102	106	91	85	114	108	78	79
		Upper cl	116	140	99	124	111	120	108	128	134	116	95	106
	Intermediate	SPCR	100	101	102	102	104	103	103	100	110	106	98	98
		Lower cl	96	79	99	88	101	99	97	89	104	104	92	91
		Upper cl	103	122	105	115	106	106	108	111	116	108	103	105
	Minor	SPCR	97	104	99	99	100	101	106	105	108	103	100	102
		Lower cl	94	84	96	87	98	98	101	95	103	101	95	95
		Upper cl	101	123	101	111	102	104	111	115	113	105	106	109
	All illnesses (I-XVII)	SPCR	100	99	100	99	102	101	103	103	108	104	99	101
		Lower cl	97	80	98	87	100	98	98	94	103	102	94	94
		Upper cl	103	118	103	111	104	104	107	113	112	106	104	108
I	Infectious and parasitic diseases (001-139)	SPCR	93	144	97	96	97	102	101	115	115	109	115	99
		Lower cl	85	96	90	71	91	95	89	93	103	105	101	85
		Upper cl	101	191	103	121	102	109	113	137	128	113	129	113
II	Neoplasms (140-239)	SPCR	95	*26*	95	*48*	85	91	99	*109*	111	97	98	120
		Lower cl	78	*0*	81	*6*	74	76	73	*57*	82	88	70	83
		Upper cl	112	*76*	109	*90*	97	105	125	*161*	140	105	126	157
III	Endocrine, nutritional and metabolic diseases and immunity disorders (240-279)	SPCR	84	*18*	91	133	90	120	105	*50*	133	118	104	99
		Lower cl	72	*0*	81	76	81	107	85	*20*	109	110	83	71
		Upper cl	96	*53*	101	190	98	133	124	*80*	156	126	124	127
IV	Diseases of blood and blood-forming organs (280-289)	SPCR	*75*	*170*	*67*	*108*	122	126	*82*	*113*	*127*	100	*77*	*111*
		Lower cl	*33*	*0*	*35*	*13*	84	100	*16*	*35*	*44*	87	*10*	*58*
		Upper cl	*118*	*362*	*99*	*203*	160	153	*148*	*191*	*211*	114	*145*	*164*
V	Mental disorders (290-319)	SPCR	97	*114*	89	103	102	114	99	97	141	115	94	87
		Lower cl	88	*60*	81	71	96	106	85	71	124	110	79	71
		Upper cl	107	*169*	96	135	109	123	113	122	159	120	109	104
VI	Diseases of the nervous system and sense organs (320-389)	SPCR	96	*65*	100	91	99	99	93	99	96	105	100	85
		Lower cl	89	*31*	95	66	94	93	83	77	86	101	89	72
		Upper cl	103	*99*	106	116	104	106	103	120	106	109	111	99
VII	Diseases of the circulatory system (390-459)	SPCR	95	*84*	99	155	104	107	104	127	118	111	90	67
		Lower cl	87	*22*	92	106	98	98	90	88	103	105	77	48
		Upper cl	104	*146*	106	204	111	117	117	165	133	117	103	86
VIII	Diseases of the respiratory system (460-519)	SPCR	92	92	99	96	96	101	108	102	111	108	98	101
		Lower cl	87	64	95	78	93	97	100	87	103	105	89	91
		Upper cl	97	120	103	114	99	106	115	117	119	111	106	112
IX	Diseases of the digestive system (520-579)	SPCR	107	*104*	97	102	104	118	100	92	131	107	96	91
		Lower cl	98	*49*	90	69	98	108	88	66	117	102	83	74
		Upper cl	116	*158*	104	136	110	127	113	118	146	113	110	109
X	Diseases of the genitourinary system (580-629)	SPCR	92	97	96	100	97	104	114	93	109	112	122	108
		Lower cl	79	65	85	79	88	99	92	77	87	109	98	96
		Upper cl	106	130	107	121	107	110	135	109	131	115	147	119
XI	Complications of pregnancy, childbirth and the puerperium (630-679)	SPCR	-	*134*	-	*100*	-	122	-	107	-	104	-	104
		Lower cl	-	*41*	-	*47*	-	106	-	65	-	95	-	74
		Upper cl	-	*226*	-	*152*	-	139	-	148	-	112	-	133
XII	Diseases of the skin and subcutaneous tissue (680-709)	SPCR	89	*69*	101	89	100	101	99	93	104	104	101	94
		Lower cl	82	*35*	95	65	95	94	88	73	94	100	89	80
		Upper cl	95	*103*	106	113	104	108	109	113	114	108	112	108

* See appendix C for description of each group.

7(b) M	7(b) F	8(a) M	8(a) F	8(b) M	8(b) F	9(a) M	9(a) F	9(b) M	9(b) F		Disease group	
99	100	102	102	103	102	99	96	104	102	SPCR	All diseases and conditions	
94	98	100	99	101	92	91	88	102	100	Lower cl	(I-XVIII)	
104	102	105	104	106	112	108	104	107	104	Upper cl		
94	101	112	124	114	122	112	102	131	115	SPCR	Serious	
84	97	107	118	109	98	95	85	126	111	Lower cl		
105	106	117	130	120	145	129	119	137	119	Upper cl		
100	101	106	107	105	112	98	92	108	107	SPCR	Intermediate	
94	99	103	104	101	100	88	83	105	105	Lower cl		
106	104	109	110	108	125	108	102	111	109	Upper cl		
101	101	102	103	106	98	101	93	105	102	SPCR	Minor	
95	98	99	101	103	88	92	85	102	100	Lower cl		
106	103	105	106	110	109	111	102	108	104	Upper cl		
100	100	104	104	103	106	99	95	106	104	SPCR	All illnesses (I-XVII)	
94	98	101	101	100	96	90	87	104	101	Lower cl		
105	102	106	106	106	117	107	104	109	106	Upper cl		
100	100	104	104	97	96	89	95	95	105	SPCR	Infectious and parasitic	I
87	95	97	98	90	75	68	76	88	100	Lower cl	diseases (001-139)	
113	104	111	110	105	118	110	114	102	110	Upper cl		
64	91	90	87	96	95	77	87	84	90	SPCR	Neoplasms (140-239)	II
38	81	76	75	81	45	34	47	70	81	Lower cl		
90	101	104	100	112	144	121	128	99	99	Upper cl		
105	103	102	122	119	175	152	103	112	117	SPCR	Endocrine, nutritional and	III
79	95	91	111	107	120	107	69	100	109	Lower cl	metabolic diseases and	
132	112	113	134	131	230	196	137	124	125	Upper cl	immunity disorders (240-279)	
155	108	115	130	121	169	45	115	129	114	SPCR	Diseases of blood and blood-	IV
40	92	73	107	75	69	0	44	82	98	Lower cl	forming organs (280-289)	
269	124	157	154	167	269	133	186	176	130	Upper cl		
103	105	104	126	107	151	71	83	154	126	SPCR	Mental disorders (290-319)	V
85	100	95	118	98	118	48	62	143	121	Lower cl		
120	111	112	133	116	184	94	103	164	132	Upper cl		
94	100	103	103	101	121	77	79	107	103	SPCR	Diseases of the nervous system	VI
82	96	97	97	95	97	60	62	100	99	Lower cl	and sense organs (320-389)	
106	105	108	109	107	146	94	95	113	108	Upper cl		
91	108	109	124	106	115	115	116	113	113	SPCR	Diseases of the circulatory	VII
74	101	102	115	98	79	90	88	105	107	Lower cl	system (390-459)	
108	115	117	133	113	151	141	144	121	119	Upper cl		
107	99	102	111	103	97	81	85	106	110	SPCR	Diseases of the respiratory	VIII
99	96	98	106	98	82	68	73	102	107	Lower cl	system (460-519)	
116	102	107	115	108	113	93	98	111	114	Upper cl		
96	105	113	125	114	93	86	109	123	115	SPCR	Diseases of the digestive system	IX
81	99	106	117	106	66	64	84	115	109	Lower cl	(520-579)	
111	111	121	133	122	120	108	133	131	120	Upper cl		
83	109	114	107	108	103	82	82	105	107	SPCR	Diseases of the genitourinary	X
61	105	102	102	95	85	47	68	92	103	Lower cl	system (580-629)	
105	112	126	112	121	121	116	96	117	110	Upper cl		
-	105	-	118	-	124	-	72	-	91	SPCR	Complications of pregnancy,	XI
-	95	-	104	-	73	-	35	-	80	Lower cl	childbirth and the puerperium	
-	114	-	132	-	175	-	108	-	102	Upper cl	(630-679)	
101	102	99	109	101	108	97	112	98	109	SPCR	Diseases of the skin and	XII
89	98	93	102	95	84	78	92	92	105	Lower cl	subcutaneous tissue (680-709)	
112	107	105	115	108	131	115	132	104	114	Upper cl		

Table 34 - *continued*

Disease group			Occupation (Sub-major Groups)*												
			1(a)		1(b)		2(a)		2(b)		2(c)		2(d)	
			M	F	M	F	M	F	M	F	M	F	M	F
XIII	Diseases of the musculoskeletal system and connective tissue (710-739)	SPCR	85	88	90	99	74	87	34	55	73	79	70	84
		Lower cl	81	82	84	93	69	70	25	41	66	74	63	75
		Upper cl	89	93	95	104	80	105	42	69	80	84	77	93
XIV	Congenital anomalies (740-759)	SPCR	84	113	95	93	*75*	-	-	*39*	*158*	97	*109*	*53*
		Lower cl	55	69	55	55	*34*	-	-	*0*	*85*	61	*50*	*7*
		Upper cl	113	156	136	132	*116*	-	-	*115*	*232*	133	*168*	*99*
XV	Certain conditions originating in the perinatal period (760-779)	SPCR	-	*219*	*890*	-	-	-	-	-	-	90	-	*186*
		Lower cl	-	*0*	*0*	-	-	-	-	-	-	0	-	*0*
		Upper cl	-	*467*	*2,635*	-	-	-	-	-	-	268	-	*551*
XVI	Symptoms, signs and ill-defined conditions (780-799)	SPCR	91	95	89	93	88	73	40	48	90	82	86	87
		Lower cl	86	88	82	87	80	57	27	35	80	77	77	78
		Upper cl	97	101	96	99	96	89	52	62	100	88	96	97
XVII	Injury and poisoning (800-999)	SPCR	84	92	86	102	78	84	21	46	78	79	71	93
		Lower cl	80	85	80	95	71	65	14	32	70	73	64	83
		Upper cl	89	99	92	109	84	102	29	61	87	85	79	104
XVIII	Supplementary classification of factors influencing health status and contact with health services (VO1-V82)	SPCR	91	105	92	100	90	105	68	105	96	98	87	100
		Lower cl	87	101	87	96	84	94	57	93	89	94	80	94
		Upper cl	94	109	97	104	95	115	79	116	103	102	93	106

* See appendix C for description of each group.

3(a) M	3(a) F	3(b) M	3(b) F	3(c) M	3(c) F	4(a) M	4(a) F	4(b) M	4(b) F		Disease group	
91	88	105	89	78	86	96	94	83	85	SPCR	Diseases of the musculoskeletal	XIII
82	74	87	84	72	79	91	91	49	82	Lower cl	system and connective tissue	
100	101	124	95	84	93	102	97	117	89	Upper cl	(710-739)	
126	43	79	135	121	88	96	74	357	109	SPCR	Congenital anomalies (740-759)	XIV
57	0	0	91	65	42	59	56	0	81	Lower cl		
194	102	188	180	176	135	134	91	853	137	Upper cl		
-	-	-	248	-	-	-	122	-	132	SPCR	Certain conditions originating in	XV
-	-	-	5	-	-	-	32	-	3	Lower cl	the perinatal period (760-779)	
-	-	-	492	-	-	-	212	-	261	Upper cl		
80	87	113	78	97	90	106	94	117	93	SPCR	Symptoms, signs and ill-defined	XVI
70	73	89	73	88	83	99	91	66	89	Lower cl	conditions (780-799)	
90	100	137	84	106	98	113	97	168	97	Upper cl		
73	104	95	85	86	95	92	94	89	92	SPCR	Injury and poisoning (800-999)	XVII
66	88	77	79	79	87	87	91	51	88	Lower cl		
81	119	112	92	94	104	97	97	127	97	Upper cl		
93	109	112	101	96	101	100	102	91	99	SPCR	Supplementary classification of	XVIII
85	101	96	97	90	96	95	100	61	97	Lower cl	factors influencing health status	
100	118	128	104	102	105	104	104	120	102	Upper cl	and contact with health services (VO1-V82)	

Table 34 - *continued*

Disease group			Occupation (Sub-major Groups)*											
			5(a)		5(b)		5(c)		6(a)		6(b)		7(a)	
			M	F	M	F	M	F	M	F	M	F	M	F
XIII	Diseases of the musculoskeletal system and connective tissue (710-739)	SPCR	112	102	107	93	116	116	113	111	118	113	89	102
		Lower cl	106	60	102	69	112	109	103	90	108	109	80	88
		Upper cl	119	143	112	117	121	123	122	133	128	117	98	116
XIV	Congenital anomalies (740-759)	SPCR	62	173	85	-	87	69	86	179	69	104	104	127
		Lower cl	30	0	54	-	60	35	30	4	18	80	36	25
		Upper cl	94	511	116	-	113	103	143	355	120	128	172	229
XV	Certain conditions originating in the perinatal period (760-779)	SPCR	-	-	-	-	-	157	-	-	-	166	-	-
		Lower cl	-	-	-	-	-	0	-	-	-	43	-	-
		Upper cl	-	-	-	-	-	374	-	-	-	289	-	-
XVI	Symptoms, signs and ill-defined conditions (780-799)	SPCR	102	104	93	94	108	107	96	113	125	115	92	104
		Lower cl	94	63	87	69	103	100	85	91	112	110	80	89
		Upper cl	109	146	99	119	114	113	107	136	137	119	104	118
XVII	Injury and poisoning (800-999)	SPCR	113	127	106	90	116	113	116	137	112	113	86	101
		Lower cl	106	77	101	63	111	106	106	110	102	109	76	86
		Upper cl	119	177	111	116	120	121	126	163	121	118	95	117
XVIII	Supplementary classification of factors influencing health status and contact with health services (VO1-V82)	SPCR	100	112	96	96	100	105	113	107	114	104	92	104
		Lower cl	94	88	91	82	97	101	105	95	106	102	84	96
		Upper cl	105	135	100	111	104	109	121	119	122	106	100	113

* See appendix C for description of each group.

7(b)		8(a)		8(b)		9(a)		9(b)			Disease group
M	F	M	F	M	F	M	F	M	F		
96	105	116	124	114	114	103	99	123	122	SPCR	Diseases of the musculoskeletal XIII
86	101	110	118	109	92	86	82	117	118	Lower cl	system and connective tissue
107	109	121	130	120	137	120	117	128	126	Upper cl	(710-739)
105	99	127	124	84	*49*	-	-	112	111	SPCR	Congenital anomalies (740-759) XIV
32	72	88	85	50	*0*	-	-	74	83	Lower cl	
178	126	166	164	118	*146*	-	-	150	139	Upper cl	
-	-	-	*117*	*759*	-	-	-	-	*43*	SPCR	Certain conditions originating in XV
-	-	-	*0*	*0*	-	-	-	-	*0*	Lower cl	the perinatal period (760-779)
-	-	-	*280*	*2,247*	-	-	-	-	*128*	Upper cl	
104	112	108	115	111	115	104	75	118	121	SPCR	Symptoms, signs and ill-defined XVI
91	108	101	109	104	92	83	59	111	116	Lower cl	conditions (780-799)
117	117	114	122	118	139	126	91	125	126	Upper cl	
101	104	118	119	120	131	126	113	126	115	SPCR	Injury and poisoning (800-999) XVII
91	99	112	112	114	104	107	92	120	110	Lower cl	
111	109	123	126	126	159	146	135	132	120	Upper cl	
101	100	100	105	119	101	105	91	114	100	SPCR	Supplementary classification of XVIII
92	97	96	102	114	88	91	81	109	97	Lower cl	factors influencing health status
110	102	104	109	124	113	120	101	118	102	Upper cl	and contact with health services
											(VO1-V82)

Table 35 Age standardised patient consulting ratios (SPCR) for married/cohabiting women aged 16-64 (study population = 100) with approximate 95 per cent upper and lower confidence limits: comparison by economic position of partner last week and one year ago

Disease group			Economic position of partner last week					Economic position of partner 1 year ago				
			Working full time	Working part time	Waiting/ seeking work	Long-term sick	Home/ family	Working full time	Working part time	Waiting/ seeking work	Long-term sick	Home/ family
	All diseases and conditions (I-XVIII)	SPCR	100	97	102	103	106	100	99	101	103	107
		Lower cl	99	92	99	99	94	99	93	97	99	94
		Upper cl	100	102	105	107	119	101	105	105	107	120
	Serious	SPCR	96	92	119	135	157	97	87	124	136	163
		Lower cl	95	82	112	127	124	95	77	115	127	127
		Upper cl	98	101	126	143	190	99	98	134	144	198
	Intermediate	SPCR	99	97	107	111	114	99	98	107	112	111
		Lower cl	98	91	104	107	98	98	91	103	107	95
		Upper cl	100	103	110	116	130	100	105	112	117	128
	Minor	SPCR	100	99	102	106	108	100	99	101	106	107
		Lower cl	99	93	99	101	94	99	92	97	101	92
		Upper cl	100	105	105	110	122	101	106	105	110	121
	All illnesses (I-XVII)	SPCR	99	97	103	106	107	100	97	103	106	106
		Lower cl	99	92	100	102	93	99	91	99	102	92
		Upper cl	100	103	106	110	120	100	104	107	111	120
I	Infectious and parasitic diseases (001-139)	SPCR	99	108	109	115	127	99	121	111	114	115
		Lower cl	97	93	102	104	94	97	104	102	102	82
		Upper cl	100	122	115	126	160	101	139	120	125	148
II	Neoplasms (140-239)	SPCR	101	108	79	91	*115*	101	104	75	99	*116*
		Lower cl	97	80	66	74	*47*	97	74	58	80	*44*
		Upper cl	105	136	91	108	*183*	105	135	92	118	*188*
III	Endocrine, nutritional and metabolic diseases and immunity disorders (240-279)	SPCR	95	99	123	144	*99*	96	89	120	144	*120*
		Lower cl	91	80	110	129	*49*	93	70	102	127	*61*
		Upper cl	98	118	136	160	*150*	99	109	138	160	*179*
IV	Diseases of blood and blood-forming organs (280-289)	SPCR	99	117	107	122	*167*	99	121	104	124	*159*
		Lower cl	93	71	85	90	*43*	93	70	75	90	*32*
		Upper cl	105	163	128	155	*291*	105	173	133	158	*286*
V	Mental disorders (290-319)	SPCR	94	102	140	150	197	96	102	151	144	176
		Lower cl	92	86	131	137	148	94	85	138	131	127
		Upper cl	96	117	149	163	247	98	119	164	157	225
VI	Diseases of the nervous system and sense organs (320-389)	SPCR	99	98	105	112	137	99	99	103	113	143
		Lower cl	97	86	98	103	104	97	86	94	104	107
		Upper cl	101	110	111	120	170	101	113	111	122	179
VII	Diseases of the circulatory system (390-459)	SPCR	97	91	113	119	113	97	92	112	122	116
		Lower cl	94	77	103	108	71	95	78	98	112	70
		Upper cl	99	104	123	129	155	100	107	126	133	161
VIII	Diseases of the respiratory system (460-519)	SPCR	98	97	108	125	115	99	97	109	128	122
		Lower cl	97	88	104	118	93	97	87	102	120	98
		Upper cl	100	106	113	132	137	100	107	115	135	146
IX	Diseases of the digestive system (520-579)	SPCR	96	97	124	130	132	97	99	129	130	140
		Lower cl	94	83	116	118	91	95	83	117	117	96
		Upper cl	99	112	133	141	173	99	115	141	142	185
X	Diseases of the genitourinary system (580-629)	SPCR	99	100	112	104	116	99	101	114	103	109
		Lower cl	98	90	107	97	92	98	90	107	96	85
		Upper cl	100	110	118	112	140	101	113	121	111	133
XI	Complications of pregnancy, childbirth and the puerperium (630-679)	SPCR	99	89	115	78	*106*	100	*73*	113	81	*87*
		Lower cl	95	59	104	52	*48*	96	*41*	97	52	*33*
		Upper cl	102	119	126	104	*163*	103	*105*	128	110	*142*
XII	Diseases of the skin and subcutaneous tissue (680-709)	SPCR	98	101	113	119	105	99	90	116	119	114
		Lower cl	96	88	106	109	75	97	77	107	108	80
		Upper cl	100	114	120	129	136	101	104	125	129	147

Table 35 - *continued*

Disease group			Economic position of partner last week					Economic position of partner 1 year ago				
			Working full time	Working part time	Waiting/ seeking work	Long-term sick	Home/ family	Working full time	Working part time	Waiting/ seeking work	Long-term sick	Home/ family
XIII	Diseases of the musculoskeletal system and connective tissue (710-739)	SPCR	98	95	117	128	122	98	90	125	127	125
		Lower cl	96	85	111	120	94	97	79	116	119	94
		Upper cl	99	105	123	135	150	100	101	134	135	155
XIV	Congenital anomalies (740-759)	SPCR	98	*117*	121	*94*	*82*	97	*143*	*152*	*97*	-
		Lower cl	87	*36*	77	*45*	*0*	86	*44*	*86*	*44*	-
		Upper cl	109	*197*	165	*144*	*243*	108	*241*	*219*	*150*	-
XV	Certain conditions originating in the perinatal period (760-779)	SPCR	*96*	-	*123*	-	*1,135*	100	-	78	-	*1,189*
		Lower cl	*53*	-	*0*	-	*0*	57	-	0	-	*0*
		Upper cl	*139*	-	*262*	-	*3,359*	142	-	231	-	*3,521*
XVI	Symptoms, signs and ill-defined conditions (780-799)	SPCR	97	86	128	134	126	97	90	133	138	128
		Lower cl	95	74	121	124	94	96	78	124	128	95
		Upper cl	98	97	135	143	158	99	103	143	148	162
XVII	Injury and poisoning (800-999)	SPCR	99	92	111	117	156	99	84	117	116	132
		Lower cl	97	79	104	107	117	97	70	107	106	95
		Upper cl	101	104	118	127	194	101	97	126	126	169
XVIII	Supplementary classification of factors influencing health status and contact with health services (VO1-V82)	SPCR	100	98	99	100	115	100	97	96	99	113
		Lower cl	99	90	96	95	97	99	89	92	94	95
		Upper cl	101	105	103	106	132	101	105	101	105	132

Table 36   Age standardised patient consulting ratios (SPCR) for married/cohabiting women aged 16-64
(study population = 100) with approximate 95 per cent upper and lower confidence limits:
comparison by own social class (as defined by occupation)

Disease group			Own social class				
			I & II	IIIN	IIIM	IV & V	Other
	All diseases and conditions (I-XVIII)	SPCR	100	100	101	101	98
		Lower cl	99	99	98	99	95
		Upper cl	102	101	103	102	100
	Serious	SPCR	91	93	115	113	106
		Lower cl	88	90	109	110	101
		Upper cl	94	95	121	116	112
	Intermediate	SPCR	97	98	104	105	99
		Lower cl	95	97	101	103	96
		Upper cl	99	100	107	107	102
	Minor	SPCR	100	100	102	101	97
		Lower cl	99	98	99	99	94
		Upper cl	102	101	105	102	100
	All illnesses (I-XVII)	SPCR	99	99	102	103	98
		Lower cl	97	98	99	101	95
		Upper cl	100	100	105	104	101
I	Infectious and parasitic diseases (001-139)	SPCR	101	97	104	102	99
		Lower cl	97	95	98	99	93
		Upper cl	104	100	111	106	105
II	Neoplasms (140-239)	SPCR	108	103	96	92	87
		Lower cl	101	97	83	85	75
		Upper cl	115	109	109	99	99
III	Endocrine, nutritional and metabolic diseases and immunity disorders (240-279)	SPCR	83	94	114	116	117
		Lower cl	78	89	103	110	106
		Upper cl	88	98	125	122	128
IV	Diseases of blood and blood-forming organs (280-289)	SPCR	82	100	112	115	106
		Lower cl	72	91	91	103	86
		Upper cl	91	109	133	127	127
V	Mental disorders (290-319)	SPCR	83	92	111	122	117
		Lower cl	79	89	103	117	109
		Upper cl	86	95	118	126	125
VI	Diseases of the nervous system and sense organs (320-389)	SPCR	97	99	102	103	104
		Lower cl	94	96	96	100	99
		Upper cl	100	102	108	106	110
VII	Diseases of the circulatory system (390-459)	SPCR	87	95	109	115	107
		Lower cl	82	91	101	110	99
		Upper cl	91	99	118	119	114
VIII	Diseases of the respiratory system (460-519)	SPCR	96	97	104	108	100
		Lower cl	94	95	99	105	96
		Upper cl	98	99	108	110	104
IX	Diseases of the digestive system (520-579)	SPCR	85	97	104	114	114
		Lower cl	82	94	97	110	107
		Upper cl	89	100	112	119	122
X	Diseases of the genitourinary system (580-629)	SPCR	95	99	107	105	99
		Lower cl	93	97	102	103	95
		Upper cl	98	101	112	108	104
XI	Complications of pregnancy, childbirth and the puerperium (630-679)	SPCR	112	94	105	88	121
		Lower cl	105	89	94	81	108
		Upper cl	118	99	117	94	134
XII	Diseases of the skin and subcutaneous tissue (680-709)	SPCR	93	99	104	106	107
		Lower cl	89	97	98	102	100
		Upper cl	96	102	111	109	113

Table 36 - *continued*

Disease group			Own social class				
			I & II	IIIN	IIIM	IV & V	Other
XIII	Diseases of the musculoskeletal system and connective tissue (710-739)	SPCR	90	95	113	117	94
		Lower cl	87	92	108	114	88
		Upper cl	92	97	119	120	99
XIV	Congenital anomalies (740-759)	SPCR	104	94	75	105	118
		Lower cl	84	78	43	84	78
		Upper cl	124	111	107	125	157
XV	Certain conditions originating in the perinatal period (760-779)	SPCR	*123*	*89*	*106*	*110*	*51*
		Lower cl	*32*	*27*	*0*	*22*	*0*
		Upper cl	*214*	*150*	*253*	*198*	*151*
XVI	Symptoms, signs and ill-defined conditions (780-799)	SPCR	87	99	103	115	101
		Lower cl	84	96	97	111	95
		Upper cl	90	102	109	118	107
XVII	Injury and poisoning (800-999)	SPCR	92	95	114	114	94
		Lower cl	88	92	107	110	88
		Upper cl	95	98	120	118	100
XVIII	Supplementary classification of factors influencing health status and contact with health services (VO1-V82)	SPCR	102	99	104	99	95
		Lower cl	100	98	100	97	91
		Upper cl	104	101	107	101	98

Table 37   Age standardised patient consulting ratios (SPCR) for children aged 0-15
(study population=100) with approximate 95 per cent upper and lower confidence limits:
comparison by sex, tenure, urban/rural, and ethnic group.

Disease group			Tenure								Urban / rural			
			Owner occupier		Council house		Other rented		Communal		Urban		Rural	
			M	F	M	F	M	F	M	F	M	F	M	F
	All diseases and conditions (I-XVIII)	SPCR	99	98	101	103	104	105	107	113	100	100	101	99
		Lower cl	98	97	99	101	101	101	95	95	99	99	98	96
		Upper cl	100	100	103	105	108	108	120	131	101	101	104	102
	Serious	SPCR	95	95	115	115	102	104	92	*97*	100	100	95	96
		Lower cl	92	91	109	109	93	93	64	*48*	98	97	87	87
		Upper cl	98	98	120	122	111	114	121	*146*	103	104	102	106
	Intermediate	SPCR	99	98	102	106	102	103	96	97	100	100	102	99
		Lower cl	98	96	100	104	97	99	82	76	98	99	98	96
		Upper cl	100	99	105	109	106	107	111	117	101	101	105	103
	Minor	SPCR	99	98	103	104	103	105	118	123	101	100	96	98
		Lower cl	97	96	100	102	99	102	103	102	99	99	93	94
		Upper cl	100	99	105	107	107	109	133	145	102	102	99	101
	All illnesses (I-XVII)	SPCR	99	98	102	104	103	105	95	106	100	100	100	99
		Lower cl	98	97	100	102	99	102	83	88	99	99	97	96
		Upper cl	100	99	104	106	106	109	106	124	101	101	103	102
I	Infectious and parasitic diseases (001-139)	SPCR	96	93	113	119	98	108	84	81	101	101	96	95
		Lower cl	94	90	109	115	92	102	61	50	99	99	91	89
		Upper cl	98	95	117	123	104	115	107	111	103	103	101	100
II	Neoplasms (140-239)	SPCR	113	106	75	89	*66*	89	-	-	99	100	100	103
		Lower cl	99	93	55	68	*35*	55	-	-	88	89	68	72
		Upper cl	127	118	95	109	*98*	122	-	-	111	111	131	134
III	Endocrine, nutritional and metabolic diseases and immunity disorders (240-279)	SPCR	98	87	97	121	120	146	*180*	*187*	100	97	98	100
		Lower cl	82	73	69	91	69	93	*0*	*0*	85	84	58	62
		Upper cl	114	102	125	151	171	199	*383*	*447*	114	111	138	139
IV	Diseases of blood and blood-forming organs (280-289)	SPCR	102	98	96	118	101	*72*	-	-	104	102	82	94
		Lower cl	87	84	71	91	59	*38*	-	-	91	89	49	59
		Upper cl	116	112	121	145	144	*106*	-	-	117	115	114	128
V	Mental disorders (290-319)	SPCR	89	86	126	134	123	129	*93*	*105*	103	104	85	75
		Lower cl	82	78	111	117	99	103	*24*	*2*	96	96	68	57
		Upper cl	96	93	141	150	147	156	*162*	*207*	109	111	102	92
VI	Diseases of the nervous system and sense organs (320-389)	SPCR	104	102	91	96	92	98	117	105	99	99	105	106
		Lower cl	102	100	87	92	86	92	90	71	98	97	100	101
		Upper cl	106	104	95	99	98	104	145	140	101	101	110	112
VII	Diseases of the circulatory system (390-459)	SPCR	103	100	*89*	111	*110*	80	*91*	-	91	105	*159*	*58*
		Lower cl	79	77	*50*	69	*38*	21	*0*	-	72	84	*87*	*15*
		Upper cl	126	122	*128*	154	*182*	139	*269*	-	111	126	*230*	*101*
VIII	Diseases of the respiratory system (460-519)	SPCR	98	97	107	109	99	102	72	106	101	101	92	96
		Lower cl	96	95	105	106	95	98	58	81	100	99	88	92
		Upper cl	100	98	110	112	104	107	86	130	103	102	96	100
IX	Diseases of the digestive system (520-579)	SPCR	95	93	119	122	87	101	*84*	*64*	100	101	98	96
		Lower cl	91	88	110	112	75	87	*32*	*1*	96	97	86	83
		Upper cl	100	98	128	132	100	115	*136*	*127*	105	106	111	109
X	Diseases of the genitourinary system (580-629)	SPCR	99	93	103	123	101	102	*48*	*60*	101	102	93	89
		Lower cl	94	88	94	113	86	89	*6*	*16*	96	97	80	78
		Upper cl	105	97	112	132	116	116	*90*	*105*	106	106	105	100
XI	Complications of pregnancy, childbirth and the puerperium (630-679)	SPCR	-	70	-	*165*	-	*186*	-	-	-	113	-	-
		Lower cl	-	41	-	*84*	-	*48*	-	-	-	80	-	-
		Upper cl	-	100	-	*246*	-	*324*	-	-	-	146	-	-
XII	Diseases of the skin and subcutaneous tissue (680-709)	SPCR	97	96	108	111	103	102	112	102	101	101	93	95
		Lower cl	94	93	103	107	95	95	84	66	99	98	87	89
		Upper cl	99	98	113	116	110	110	140	138	103	103	99	101

White		Black Afro-Caribbean		Indian		Pakistani/Bangladeshi		Other		Disease group		
M	F	M	F	M	F	M	F	M	F			
100	100	100	101	105	102	107	109	97	97	SPCR	All diseases and conditions	
99	99	88	90	93	90	95	97	91	90	Lower cl	(I-XVIII)	
101	101	112	113	117	114	120	121	104	103	Upper cl		
100	100	133	141	127	88	73	76	108	111	SPCR	Serious	
97	97	99	100	94	55	47	46	91	90	Lower cl		
102	103	168	181	160	121	99	107	125	133	Upper cl		
100	100	95	92	100	89	97	101	96	95	SPCR	Intermediate	
99	99	81	79	86	75	83	87	88	87	Lower cl		
101	101	108	105	114	102	111	115	104	103	Upper cl		
100	100	105	106	120	108	122	125	103	101	SPCR	Minor	
98	99	92	93	106	95	106	110	95	93	Lower cl		
101	101	119	119	135	122	137	140	110	109	Upper cl		
100	100	100	100	104	103	109	111	96	95	SPCR	All illnesses (I-XVII)	
99	99	88	88	92	90	96	99	89	88	Lower cl		
101	101	112	111	116	115	121	124	102	102	Upper cl		
100	100	99	83	95	77	118	131	100	92	SPCR	Infectious and parasitic	I
98	98	77	65	73	59	94	107	88	80	Lower cl	diseases (001-139)	
102	102	120	102	116	96	142	155	112	104	Upper cl		
103	102	41	68	-	-	-	35	80	75	SPCR	Neoplasms (140-239)	II
91	92	0	0	-	-	-	0	16	15	Lower cl		
114	113	121	162	-	-	-	103	143	134	Upper cl		
96	100	130	107	124	57	339	57	182	138	SPCR	Endocrine, nutritional and	III
82	87	0	0	0	0	42	0	63	36	Lower cl	metabolic diseases and	
109	113	310	256	297	170	636	169	301	241	Upper cl	immunity disorders (240-279)	
98	98	53	273	210	201	330	94	81	100	SPCR	Diseases of blood and blood-	IV
86	86	0	54	4	4	66	0	10	20	Lower cl	forming organs (280-289)	
111	110	157	491	416	398	594	224	151	180	Upper cl		
101	101	94	29	91	47	56	62	83	102	SPCR	Mental disorders (290-319)	V
95	94	24	0	24	0	1	1	47	56	Lower cl		
107	108	164	70	158	101	111	123	120	148	Upper cl		
101	101	69	70	97	76	87	82	86	80	SPCR	Diseases of the nervous system	VI
99	99	52	54	76	58	67	63	76	70	Lower cl	and sense organs (320-389)	
103	103	87	86	118	94	107	100	97	91	Upper cl		
98	99	-	-	117	372	-	122	253	86	SPCR	Diseases of the circulatory	VII
78	80	-	-	0	0	-	0	50	0	Lower cl	system (390-459)	
117	118	-	-	346	792	-	361	455	205	Upper cl		
99	100	111	109	129	118	126	127	106	100	SPCR	Diseases of the respiratory	VIII
98	98	95	93	111	101	108	110	97	91	Lower cl	system (460-519)	
101	101	128	124	146	136	144	145	115	109	Upper cl		
100	100	101	68	98	127	226	183	76	86	SPCR	Diseases of the digestive system	IX
96	95	53	30	50	71	152	116	54	60	Lower cl	(520-579)	
104	104	149	107	145	182	300	249	99	113	Upper cl		
100	101	124	85	63	102	51	47	116	68	SPCR	Diseases of the genitourinary	X
96	97	67	45	22	56	13	16	85	46	Lower cl	system (580-629)	
105	105	181	126	105	147	88	78	146	90	Upper cl		
-	100	-	-	-	296	-	-	-	104	SPCR	Complications of pregnancy,	XI
-	70	-	-	-	0	-	-	-	0	Lower cl	childbirth and the puerperium	
-	130	-	-	-	875	-	-	-	307	Upper cl	(630-679)	
100	99	114	98	104	97	123	155	91	107	SPCR	Diseases of the skin and	XII
98	97	87	75	79	73	94	124	77	93	Lower cl	subcutaneous tissue (680-709)	
102	102	141	121	129	121	151	185	104	122	Upper cl		

Table 37 - *continued*

Disease group			Tenure								Urban / rural			
			Owner occupier		Council house		Other rented		Communal		Urban		Rural	
			M	F	M	F	M	F	M	F	M	F	M	F
XIII	Diseases of the musculoskeletal system and connective tissue (710-739)	SPCR	98	94	107	118	101	103	92	134	100	101	99	91
		Lower cl	93	89	96	107	83	86	53	66	95	96	85	78
		Upper cl	104	100	117	129	118	120	130	201	105	106	112	105
XIV	Congenital anomalies (740-759)	SPCR	99	102	105	94	89	98	114	219	100	104	105	65
		Lower cl	90	90	89	73	64	66	0	0	91	93	81	40
		Upper cl	109	115	122	114	114	130	243	523	108	115	129	90
XV	Certain conditions originating in the perinatal period (760-779)	SPCR	88	89	134	108	99	147	-	936	100	100	104	109
		Lower cl	74	74	105	82	60	102	-	0	87	87	65	69
		Upper cl	102	103	164	134	137	192	-	2,234	113	113	142	148
XVI	Symptoms, signs and ill-defined conditions (780-799)	SPCR	95	92	114	119	105	111	64	67	101	102	88	83
		Lower cl	92	90	109	114	97	103	41	35	99	100	82	78
		Upper cl	98	95	119	124	112	118	87	99	104	105	94	89
XVII	Injury and poisoning (800-999)	SPCR	95	94	111	111	116	120	105	67	100	99	105	109
		Lower cl	92	91	105	105	107	110	80	34	97	96	98	100
		Upper cl	98	97	116	116	125	130	130	99	102	102	113	117
XVIII	Supplementary classification of factors influencing health status and contact with health services (VO1-V82)	SPCR	98	98	96	99	113	110	291	222	100	101	101	99
		Lower cl	96	96	92	96	106	103	240	173	98	99	95	93
		Upper cl	101	100	100	103	120	116	341	272	102	102	106	104

Ethnic group										Disease group		
White		Black Afro-Caribbean		Indian		Pakistani/ Bangladeshi		Other				
M	F	M	F	M	F	M	F	M	F			
100	100	99	74	142	75	93	89	78	107	SPCR	Diseases of the musculoskeletal	XIII
95	96	45	28	83	29	40	39	50	74	Lower cl	system and connective tissue	
105	105	152	119	202	122	145	140	106	141	Upper cl	(710-739)	
101	99	154	163	69	37	70	111	65	134	SPCR	Congenital anomalies (740-759)	XIV
93	89	40	20	0	0	0	0	25	55	Lower cl		
109	109	269	306	148	109	150	236	105	213	Upper cl		
103	102	108	46	-	-	118	113	15	69	SPCR	Certain conditions originating in	XV
90	89	0	0	-	-	0	0	0	1	Lower cl	the perinatal period (760-779)	
115	114	258	135	-	-	282	270	45	136	Upper cl		
99	99	114	122	170	119	149	168	117	115	SPCR	Symptoms, signs and ill-defined	XVI
96	97	87	96	137	92	118	136	102	99	Lower cl	conditions (780-799)	
101	101	141	148	204	147	181	200	133	130	Upper cl		
100	101	112	81	96	109	116	64	89	90	SPCR	Injury and poisoning (800-999)	XVII
98	98	83	55	70	77	85	40	74	73	Lower cl		
103	103	141	108	122	141	146	88	104	107	Upper cl		
100	100	119	105	127	107	108	86	103	104	SPCR	Supplementary classification of	XVIII
98	98	95	85	102	85	85	67	91	92	Lower cl	factors influencing health status	
101	102	143	125	153	129	132	106	115	116	Upper cl	and contact with health services (VO1-V82)	

Table 38   Age standardised patient consulting ratios (SPCR) for children aged 0-15
(study population=100) with approximate 95 per cent upper and lower confidence limits:
comparison by sex, household structure and social class of parent (as defined by occupation)

Disease group			Living with sole adult M	F	Not living with sole adult M	F	I & II M	F	IIIN M	F	IIIM M	F	IV & V M	F	Other M	F
	All diseases and conditions	SPCR	100	103	100	100	99	98	100	101	100	101	101	101	103	104
	(I-XVIII)	Lower cl	97	100	99	99	97	96	97	98	98	99	99	99	98	99
		Upper cl	103	106	101	101	101	99	103	104	102	102	103	104	107	109
	Serious	SPCR	110	112	99	98	92	92	98	105	106	104	106	107	95	85
		Lower cl	102	103	96	95	88	87	91	96	101	98	100	100	84	73
		Upper cl	118	122	101	102	97	97	106	114	111	110	112	114	106	98
	Intermediate	SPCR	101	105	100	99	98	96	100	102	102	101	101	103	98	103
		Lower cl	97	101	99	98	96	94	96	98	99	99	99	100	93	98
		Upper cl	105	108	101	101	100	98	103	106	104	103	104	106	104	109
	Minor	SPCR	99	103	100	100	97	97	100	101	101	101	102	103	105	106
		Lower cl	96	99	99	98	95	95	97	97	99	98	100	100	100	100
		Upper cl	103	106	101	101	99	99	103	104	103	103	105	105	110	111
	All illnesses (I-XVII)	SPCR	101	104	100	99	99	97	100	101	101	101	102	102	100	103
		Lower cl	98	101	99	98	97	95	97	98	99	99	99	100	95	98
		Upper cl	104	107	101	101	100	99	103	105	102	103	104	105	105	108
I	Infectious and parasitic diseases (001-139)	SPCR	107	112	99	98	92	88	99	99	104	104	108	112	102	111
		Lower cl	102	106	97	97	89	85	94	94	100	100	103	108	94	103
		Upper cl	113	117	101	100	95	91	105	105	107	107	112	116	111	120
II	Neoplasms (140-239)	SPCR	87	98	102	100	130	111	102	125	91	81	75	94	*48*	*112*
		Lower cl	57	69	90	89	109	92	70	91	72	65	54	72	*15*	*63*
		Upper cl	116	128	113	111	151	129	135	158	109	98	97	116	*81*	*161*
III	Endocrine, nutritional and metabolic diseases and immunity disorders (240-279)	SPCR	110	122	99	97	89	87	93	82	120	102	91	125	*104*	*114*
		Lower cl	68	81	84	84	67	66	54	48	93	79	62	93	*43*	*52*
		Upper cl	153	164	113	110	111	107	132	116	146	126	121	158	*166*	*177*
IV	Diseases of blood and blood-forming organs (280-289)	SPCR	96	80	101	103	79	81	81	*60*	135	123	102	122	*63*	*97*
		Lower cl	61	50	88	90	60	62	48	*33*	109	99	75	92	*19*	*44*
		Upper cl	131	111	113	115	97	99	113	*87*	160	147	130	151	*107*	*150*
V	Mental disorders (290-319)	SPCR	138	121	95	97	82	82	99	101	107	102	119	119	107	130
		Lower cl	116	99	89	90	72	72	81	81	96	90	104	103	78	95
		Upper cl	159	143	102	104	92	93	117	121	118	114	134	136	135	164
VI	Diseases of the nervous system and sense organs (320-389)	SPCR	91	95	101	101	103	102	101	101	100	101	96	93	91	99
		Lower cl	86	90	99	99	100	99	95	96	97	98	92	90	83	91
		Upper cl	96	100	103	103	107	106	106	106	103	105	100	97	99	106
VII	Diseases of the circulatory system (390-459)	SPCR	*76*	*111*	103	98	117	104	*68*	*98*	106	116	*90*	*70*	*57*	*97*
		Lower cl	*26*	*53*	82	79	81	71	*21*	*42*	71	79	*48*	*35*	*0*	*12*
		Upper cl	*126*	*170*	124	118	153	138	*116*	*153*	142	152	*131*	*106*	*121*	*182*
VIII	Diseases of the respiratory system (460-519)	SPCR	100	106	100	99	96	94	101	101	102	101	104	107	96	102
		Lower cl	96	102	99	98	93	92	97	97	100	99	101	104	90	96
		Upper cl	104	110	101	101	98	96	105	105	105	104	107	110	102	108
IX	Diseases of the digestive system (520-579)	SPCR	96	111	100	99	90	89	97	103	106	104	112	115	90	83
		Lower cl	84	98	96	94	83	82	85	90	99	96	102	105	73	66
		Upper cl	108	125	105	103	96	96	108	115	114	111	122	126	107	100
X	Diseases of the genitourinary system (580-629)	SPCR	109	116	99	98	94	86	95	107	106	103	105	115	96	99
		Lower cl	96	103	94	94	87	80	82	95	98	95	95	106	76	81
		Upper cl	123	128	103	102	102	93	107	119	114	110	115	125	115	117
XI	Complications of pregnancy, childbirth and the puerperium (630-679)	SPCR	-	*176*	-	90	-	*53*	-	*78*	-	*124*	-	*135*	-	*184*
		Lower cl	-	*61*	-	61	-	*16*	-	*2*	-	*65*	-	*59*	-	*4*
		Upper cl	-	*291*	-	120	-	*89*	-	*155*	-	*183*	-	*212*	-	*365*
XII	Diseases of the skin and subcutaneous tissue (680-709)	SPCR	106	103	99	100	94	94	98	102	103	101	104	107	109	103
		Lower cl	99	96	97	97	90	90	92	96	100	97	99	102	99	93
		Upper cl	112	109	102	102	98	97	104	108	107	105	108	112	119	112

Table 38 - *continued*

Disease group			Household composition													
			Living with sole adult		Not living with sole adult		Social class of parent									
							I & II		IIIN		IIIM		IV & V		Other	
			M	F	M	F	M	F	M	F	M	F	M	F	M	F
XIII	Diseases of the musculoskeletal system and connective tissue (710-739)	SPCR	105	110	99	99	100	88	95	109	100	100	101	110	107	122
		Lower cl	91	95	94	94	92	80	81	95	92	92	90	99	85	98
		Upper cl	120	124	104	104	108	95	109	124	109	109	112	122	128	145
XIV	Congenital anomalies (740-759)	SPCR	97	111	100	99	89	94	98	126	108	104	109	94	94	*74*
		Lower cl	74	80	92	88	76	77	75	92	93	86	90	72	60	*35*
		Upper cl	120	143	109	109	102	112	121	159	123	123	127	116	128	*112*
XV	Certain conditions originating in the perinatal period (760-779)	SPCR	93	96	101	101	69	81	82	87	113	106	138	123	*111*	*122*
		Lower cl	57	60	88	88	51	62	49	54	90	84	106	93	*53*	*64*
		Upper cl	129	132	114	113	87	100	114	120	137	129	171	153	*169*	*180*
XVI	Symptoms, signs and ill-defined conditions (780-799)	SPCR	107	112	99	98	93	89	104	105	100	102	113	112	91	109
		Lower cl	101	105	97	96	89	85	97	98	96	98	107	106	82	99
		Upper cl	114	119	101	101	97	92	110	111	104	105	118	117	100	119
XVII	Injury and poisoning (800-999)	SPCR	109	108	99	99	92	94	99	98	104	102	107	106	103	102
		Lower cl	101	100	96	96	88	90	92	90	100	98	101	100	92	90
		Upper cl	116	116	101	102	96	99	106	106	109	107	112	112	114	115
XVIII	Supplementary classification of factors influencing health status and contact with health services (VO1-V82)	SPCR	91	97	101	100	101	99	98	98	99	99	95	100	121	115
		Lower cl	86	92	99	98	98	96	93	93	96	96	91	96	111	106
		Upper cl	97	103	103	102	105	102	104	103	102	103	99	104	130	123

Table 39 Age standardised patient consulting ratios (SPCR) for children aged 0-15 (study population = 100) with approximate 95 per cent upper and lower confidence limits: comparison by sex and economic position of parent last week and one year ago

Disease group			Economic position of parent last week									
			Working full time		Working part time		Waiting/seeking work		Long-term sick		Home/family	
			M	F	M	F	M	F	M	F	M	F
	All diseases and conditions (I-XVIII)	SPCR	100	99	99	101	100	102	102	103	102	104
		Lower cl	99	98	94	95	97	98	94	95	98	100
		Upper cl	101	100	104	106	104	105	110	110	105	107
	Serious	SPCR	98	97	107	110	103	102	105	126	113	114
		Lower cl	95	94	93	93	94	92	85	101	103	102
		Upper cl	101	101	121	126	112	112	125	151	122	125
	Intermediate	SPCR	100	99	101	103	100	102	106	107	103	105
		Lower cl	98	98	95	96	96	98	96	97	99	100
		Upper cl	101	100	108	109	104	106	116	116	107	109
	Minor	SPCR	100	99	98	102	100	103	101	106	102	104
		Lower cl	98	98	92	96	96	99	93	97	98	100
		Upper cl	101	100	104	108	104	106	110	114	106	108
	All illnesses (I-XVII)	SPCR	100	99	100	101	101	102	104	105	102	105
		Lower cl	98	98	95	96	98	99	96	97	99	101
		Upper cl	101	100	106	107	105	106	112	113	106	108
I	Infectious and parasitic diseases (001-139)	SPCR	97	95	95	104	112	115	109	122	113	118
		Lower cl	95	93	85	94	106	109	93	106	106	111
		Upper cl	99	97	105	114	119	122	124	138	119	124
II	Neoplasms (140-239)	SPCR	106	105	*109*	*80*	82	73	*62*	*79*	*78*	98
		Lower cl	93	93	*52*	*35*	49	44	*1*	*16*	*43*	61
		Upper cl	119	117	*166*	*125*	116	102	*123*	*142*	*114*	135
III	Endocrine, nutritional and metabolic diseases and immunity disorders (240-279)	SPCR	100	92	*96*	*134*	92	111	*84*	*175*	*95*	116
		Lower cl	85	78	*25*	*58*	48	65	*0*	*54*	*48*	67
		Upper cl	116	106	*168*	*210*	136	156	*178*	*297*	*141*	166
IV	Diseases of blood and blood-forming organs (280-289)	SPCR	107	101	*86*	*87*	60	135	*116*	*84*	*93*	*68*
		Lower cl	93	87	*26*	*30*	29	90	*14*	*2*	*52*	*33*
		Upper cl	122	114	*145*	*143*	91	180	*218*	*166*	*134*	*102*
V	Mental disorders (290-319)	SPCR	91	89	146	161	119	131	161	*120*	137	121
		Lower cl	84	82	107	117	96	105	101	*67*	112	95
		Upper cl	97	96	186	204	142	156	221	*173*	163	148
VI	Diseases of the nervous system and sense organs (320-389)	SPCR	102	102	90	96	89	93	96	102	94	92
		Lower cl	100	100	81	87	84	87	82	88	88	87
		Upper cl	104	104	99	105	95	98	110	116	99	98
VII	Diseases of the circulatory system (390-459)	SPCR	102	97	*101*	*115*	*91*	*95*	*148*	*89*	*65*	*152*
		Lower cl	80	76	*2*	*14*	*28*	*33*	*0*	*0*	*8*	*66*
		Upper cl	125	119	*200*	*216*	*154*	*157*	*317*	*212*	*122*	*238*
VIII	Diseases of the respiratory system (460-519)	SPCR	99	98	102	103	103	104	112	108	105	109
		Lower cl	97	97	95	95	98	99	101	98	100	104
		Upper cl	101	100	109	110	107	109	123	119	110	114
IX	Diseases of the digestive system (520-579)	SPCR	98	95	109	119	101	105	153	143	105	123
		Lower cl	94	91	86	95	87	91	112	103	91	107
		Upper cl	103	100	133	144	114	119	194	182	120	139
X	Diseases of the genitourinary system (580-629)	SPCR	99	95	93	125	102	105	91	164	111	116
		Lower cl	94	90	70	103	88	91	57	128	95	101
		Upper cl	104	99	116	147	117	118	125	199	127	132
XI	Complications of pregnancy, childbirth and the puerperium (630-679)	SPCR	-	93	-	*229*	-	*128*	-	-	-	120
		Lower cl	-	61	-	*5*	-	*16*	-	-	-	2
		Upper cl	-	126	-	*454*	-	*240*	-	-	-	237
XII	Diseases of the skin and subcutaneous tissue (680-709)	SPCR	98	98	107	105	107	107	104	105	110	106
		Lower cl	95	96	95	93	100	99	87	89	102	99
		Upper cl	100	100	119	116	114	114	121	121	117	114

Economic position of parent 1 year ago												Disease group	
Working full time		Working part time		Waiting/seeking work		Long-term sick		Home/family					
M	F	M	F	M	F	M	F	M	F			
100	99	100	103	98	102	102	100	100	102	SPCR	All diseases and conditions	
99	98	95	97	94	97	94	92	97	98	Lower cl	(I-XVIII)	
101	101	106	108	103	106	110	108	104	106	Upper cl		
98	97	108	121	104	107	107	131	110	108	SPCR	Serious	
96	94	94	103	92	94	86	103	100	96	Lower cl		
101	100	123	139	115	121	128	158	120	119	Upper cl		
100	99	101	105	98	100	106	105	101	103	SPCR	Intermediate	
99	98	94	98	93	95	96	95	97	99	Lower cl		
101	101	107	111	103	106	116	115	106	108	Upper cl		
100	99	100	103	99	102	101	104	99	102	SPCR	Minor	
99	98	94	97	94	97	92	94	95	98	Lower cl		
101	101	106	109	104	107	111	113	104	106	Upper cl		
100	99	100	103	100	102	104	103	101	103	SPCR	All illnesses (I-XVII)	
99	98	95	97	95	98	95	94	97	99	Lower cl		
101	100	106	109	104	107	112	111	105	107	Upper cl		
98	97	100	108	116	111	111	123	109	117	SPCR	Infectious and parasitic	I
96	95	90	97	107	102	94	106	102	110	Lower cl	diseases (001-139)	
100	99	110	118	124	119	127	139	116	124	Upper cl		
103	101	112	96	102	77	86	89	71	103	SPCR	Neoplasms (140-239)	II
91	90	53	46	53	38	11	18	36	64	Lower cl		
116	113	171	147	150	117	162	161	105	142	Upper cl		
104	93	99	117	74	133	62	199	77	112	SPCR	Endocrine, nutritional and	III
89	80	26	44	23	68	0	61	33	62	Lower cl	metabolic diseases and	
120	107	172	189	126	198	148	337	120	163	Upper cl	immunity disorders (240-279)	
104	100	33	110	88	151	104	71	110	62	SPCR	Diseases of blood and blood-	IV
90	87	0	45	38	88	2	0	64	28	Lower cl	forming organs (280-289)	
118	114	71	175	137	214	206	151	156	96	Upper cl		
93	91	151	171	110	124	167	123	130	125	SPCR	Mental disorders (290-319)	V
86	84	110	125	82	91	103	66	104	98	Lower cl		
99	98	191	216	138	157	231	180	155	153	Upper cl		
102	102	95	97	86	90	94	102	90	92	SPCR	Diseases of the nervous system	VI
100	100	85	87	78	82	79	87	85	86	Lower cl	and sense organs (320-389)	
104	104	104	106	93	97	108	117	96	98	Upper cl		
104	98	78	167	76	108	220	101	70	107	SPCR	Diseases of the circulatory	VII
82	77	0	43	2	22	4	0	9	33	Lower cl	system (390-459)	
126	119	166	291	151	194	436	241	131	181	Upper cl		
100	99	101	106	102	104	110	106	103	105	SPCR	Diseases of the respiratory	VIII
98	97	94	99	96	98	98	95	98	100	Lower cl	system (460-519)	
101	100	109	114	108	110	121	118	108	110	Upper cl		
99	97	102	120	106	96	138	156	103	117	SPCR	Diseases of the digestive system	IX
95	93	79	95	87	78	97	112	88	101	Lower cl	(520-579)	
104	102	126	146	124	114	179	200	118	133	Upper cl		
99	96	94	108	103	104	98	147	115	124	SPCR	Diseases of the genitourinary	X
94	92	70	87	83	86	61	111	98	108	Lower cl	system (580-629)	
104	101	117	128	122	121	135	183	131	140	Upper cl		
-	97	-	240	-	88	-	-	-	96	SPCR	Complications of pregnancy,	XI
-	65	-	5	-	0	-	-	-	0	Lower cl	childbirth and the puerperium	
-	128	-	476	-	210	-	-	-	205	Upper cl	(630-679)	
99	99	104	105	101	107	106	105	103	104	SPCR	Diseases of the skin and	XII
97	96	92	94	91	98	87	87	95	97	Lower cl	subcutaneous tissue (680-709)	
102	101	116	117	110	117	124	122	111	112	Upper cl		

Table 39 - *continued*

Disease group			Working full time		Working part time		Waiting/seeking work		Long-term sick		Home/family	
			M	F	M	F	M	F	M	F	M	F
XIII	Diseases of the musculoskeletal system and connective tissue (710-739)	SPCR	97	97	112	96	101	102	148	123	120	120
		Lower cl	92	92	87	74	85	86	109	89	100	100
		Upper cl	102	103	136	118	118	119	186	157	140	140
XIV	Congenital anomalies (740-759)	SPCR	103	99	*83*	*148*	97	83	*45*	*88*	87	105
		Lower cl	94	88	*42*	*80*	72	53	*1*	*11*	63	70
		Upper cl	113	111	*123*	*216*	122	114	*89*	*165*	112	140
XV	Certain conditions originating in the perinatal period (760-779)	SPCR	97	98	*63*	*30*	133	96	*73*	*67*	104	129
		Lower cl	83	84	*1*	*0*	87	57	*0*	*0*	65	85
		Upper cl	110	112	*125*	*71*	178	134	*174*	*161*	143	172
XVI	Symptoms, signs and ill-defined conditions (780-799)	SPCR	97	96	105	105	110	115	112	127	109	118
		Lower cl	95	93	93	93	102	108	94	108	102	110
		Upper cl	100	98	117	117	117	123	130	145	117	126
XVII	Injury and poisoning (800-999)	SPCR	97	97	100	107	108	109	112	127	119	111
		Lower cl	94	94	88	93	99	100	94	105	109	101
		Upper cl	99	100	113	120	116	118	131	148	128	121
XVIII	Supplementary classification of factors influencing health status and contact with health services (VO1-V82)	SPCR	101	100	88	98	95	99	79	85	99	98
		Lower cl	98	98	78	88	89	93	65	72	93	92
		Upper cl	103	102	98	108	101	105	93	98	105	104

| Working full time | | Working part time | | Waiting/seeking work | | Long-term sick | | Home/family | | | Disease group | |
M	F	M	F	M	F	M	F	M	F			
97	98	116	111	99	94	143	128	119	113	SPCR	Diseases of the musculoskeletal	XIII
92	92	91	87	78	74	103	91	99	93	Lower cl	system and connective tissue	
102	103	141	135	120	114	184	165	140	133	Upper cl	(710-739)	
103	101	95	96	103	72	50	100	76	110	SPCR	Congenital anomalies (740-759)	XIV
94	90	51	39	68	34	1	12	52	73	Lower cl		
111	113	139	153	137	110	99	188	99	146	Upper cl		
102	104	64	65	94	97	120	78	77	62	SPCR	Certain conditions originating in	XV
88	90	1	1	43	44	0	0	41	31	Lower cl	the perinatal period (760-779)	
116	118	126	130	145	149	257	185	112	93	Upper cl		
98	97	109	109	117	118	119	127	105	116	SPCR	Symptoms, signs and ill-defined	XVI
95	94	97	96	107	108	99	107	97	107	Lower cl	conditions (780-799)	
100	99	122	121	127	128	139	147	113	124	Upper cl		
98	98	101	105	104	109	112	118	119	111	SPCR	Injury and poisoning (800-999)	XVII
95	95	88	91	94	97	92	96	110	101	Lower cl		
100	101	113	119	115	121	131	140	129	121	Upper cl		
101	101	96	103	90	96	80	85	88	89	SPCR	Supplementary classification of	XVIII
99	99	85	93	83	88	65	71	82	83	Lower cl	factors influencing health status	
103	103	106	114	98	104	95	99	95	94	Upper cl	and contact with health services (VO1-V82)	

Economic position of parent 1 year ago

Table 40 Age standardised patient consulting ratios (SPCR) for people aged 65 and over (study population=100) with approximate 95 per cent upper and lower confidence limits: comparison by sex, tenure, urban/rural, and ethnic group.

Disease group			Tenure								Urban / rural			
			Owner occupier		Council house		Other rented		Communal		Urban		Rural	
			M	F	M	F	M	F	M	F	M	F	M	F
	All diseases and conditions (I-XVIII)	SPCR	99	99	100	100	101	101	110	108	100	100	100	99
		Lower cl	98	97	97	98	97	97	102	103	99	99	96	95
		Upper cl	101	100	103	102	106	105	118	112	101	101	104	102
	Serious	SPCR	95	94	108	108	106	102	117	114	100	101	96	94
		Lower cl	93	92	104	105	100	97	106	108	98	99	91	89
		Upper cl	98	96	112	111	113	107	127	119	102	102	101	98
	Intermediate	SPCR	99	98	101	103	101	101	109	101	100	100	99	98
		Lower cl	97	97	98	100	95	96	99	96	98	99	94	94
		Upper cl	101	100	105	105	107	105	118	106	102	102	104	102
	Minor	SPCR	100	99	98	99	104	103	111	108	100	100	100	98
		Lower cl	98	97	95	96	99	99	102	104	98	99	96	94
		Upper cl	102	101	101	101	110	107	120	113	102	102	104	101
	All illnesses (I-XVII)	SPCR	99	98	101	101	101	101	109	106	100	100	99	98
		Lower cl	97	97	98	99	96	97	101	102	99	99	95	95
		Upper cl	101	100	104	104	106	105	117	111	102	101	103	101
I	Infectious and parasitic diseases (001-139)	SPCR	96	95	105	103	99	104	140	120	100	100	99	101
		Lower cl	91	91	95	96	83	93	109	106	95	97	86	90
		Upper cl	102	100	115	110	115	116	171	135	105	104	112	111
II	Neoplasms (140-239)	SPCR	100	101	99	98	99	102	117	97	103	100	85	101
		Lower cl	93	95	88	89	80	86	85	79	97	95	71	86
		Upper cl	107	108	110	107	117	118	148	114	109	105	99	116
III	Endocrine, nutritional and metabolic diseases and immunity disorders (240-279)	SPCR	100	92	99	117	111	98	87	101	99	101	100	90
		Lower cl	94	88	90	110	95	87	63	86	95	98	88	80
		Upper cl	105	96	107	125	127	110	111	116	104	105	112	99
IV	Diseases of blood and blood-forming organs (280-289)	SPCR	95	93	107	103	104	120	133	109	100	100	102	103
		Lower cl	84	86	88	91	72	99	82	89	90	93	76	85
		Upper cl	106	101	126	115	135	142	184	129	109	106	127	122
V	Mental disorders (290-319)	SPCR	89	87	107	110	104	100	236	161	101	101	92	93
		Lower cl	84	83	97	104	88	90	199	148	96	98	79	85
		Upper cl	95	90	117	116	121	109	273	174	106	104	104	102
VI	Diseases of the nervous system and sense organs (320-389)	SPCR	99	99	99	97	105	112	111	107	100	101	96	94
		Lower cl	96	96	93	92	96	104	96	99	98	98	89	87
		Upper cl	102	102	104	101	114	119	126	115	103	103	103	100
VII	Diseases of the circulatory system (390-459)	SPCR	99	99	103	106	103	101	89	88	100	100	101	103
		Lower cl	96	96	98	102	95	95	78	82	98	98	95	97
		Upper cl	102	101	107	109	110	107	100	94	102	102	107	108
VIII	Diseases of the respiratory system (460-519)	SPCR	93	91	114	114	102	97	131	121	101	102	95	87
		Lower cl	90	89	109	110	94	91	117	113	98	100	89	82
		Upper cl	96	94	119	118	110	104	146	129	103	104	102	93
IX	Diseases of the digestive system (520-579)	SPCR	96	95	107	109	107	102	116	106	99	99	103	108
		Lower cl	92	91	101	104	96	93	98	96	96	96	94	100
		Upper cl	99	98	114	114	118	110	134	115	103	102	112	116
X	Diseases of the genitourinary system (580-629)	SPCR	96	97	98	98	101	98	174	135	101	100	98	102
		Lower cl	91	93	89	93	86	88	143	122	96	97	85	93
		Upper cl	102	101	107	104	117	107	204	147	105	103	110	111
XI	Complications of pregnancy, childbirth and the puerperium (630-679)	SPCR	-	-	-	-	-	-	-	-	-	-	-	-
		Lower cl	-	-	-	-	-	-	-	-	-	-	-	-
		Upper cl	-	-	-	-	-	-	-	-	-	-	-	-
XII	Diseases of the skin and subcutaneous tissue (680-709)	SPCR	98	98	104	100	94	101	124	116	100	100	93	103
		Lower cl	94	94	97	95	83	92	103	106	97	97	84	95
		Upper cl	102	101	111	105	105	109	145	126	104	102	102	111

White		Black Afro-Caribbean		Indian		Pakistani/ Bangladeshi		Other			Disease group	
M	F	M	F	M	F	M	F	M	F			
100	100	103	101	104	86	68	85	93	88	SPCR	All diseases and conditions	
99	99	71	70	76	65	33	26	72	70	Lower cl	(I-XVIII)	
101	101	136	132	131	107	104	144	113	107	Upper cl		
100	100	114	75	109	91	80	119	82	85	SPCR	Serious	
98	99	67	38	71	61	28	24	55	61	Lower cl		
102	102	161	112	147	121	133	215	108	109	Upper cl		
100	100	116	102	105	93	63	85	101	87	SPCR	Intermediate	
98	99	75	65	72	67	22	17	75	66	Lower cl		
102	101	157	138	138	118	104	154	127	109	Upper cl		
100	100	118	103	110	91	85	94	103	100	SPCR	Minor	
98	99	78	67	78	66	39	24	78	78	Lower cl		
101	101	159	138	143	116	131	164	129	122	Upper cl		
100	100	100	103	99	90	67	89	94	88	SPCR	All illnesses (I-XVII)	
99	99	67	71	72	68	30	27	72	69	Lower cl		
101	101	133	135	127	112	103	150	115	106	Upper cl		
100	100	123	100	109	67	112	105	85	117	SPCR	Infectious and parasitic	I
95	97	2	2	13	8	0	0	17	51	Lower cl	diseases (001-139)	
105	103	243	197	205	126	268	310	154	183	Upper cl		
100	100	94	100	31	-	-	210	41	78	SPCR	Neoplasms (140-239)	II
95	95	0	0	0	-	-	0	0	2	Lower cl		
106	105	224	238	93	-	-	621	97	154	Upper cl		
99	100	252	197	168	188	143	100	157	39	SPCR	Endocrine, nutritional and	III
95	96	96	60	58	93	0	0	72	1	Lower cl	metabolic diseases and	
104	103	408	333	278	283	305	297	243	77	Upper cl	immunity disorders (240-279)	
100	100	142	78	91	184	-	-	-	178	SPCR	Diseases of blood and blood-	IV
91	94	0	0	0	4	-	-	-	35	Lower cl	forming organs (280-289)	
109	106	421	230	270	364	-	-	-	320	Upper cl		
100	100	200	122	46	86	118	-	44	61	SPCR	Mental disorders (290-319)	V
96	97	40	32	0	30	0	-	0	21	Lower cl		
105	103	360	213	109	143	282	-	94	100	Upper cl		
100	100	51	105	57	114	148	160	106	99	SPCR	Diseases of the nervous system	VI
98	98	6	43	17	66	46	3	62	62	Lower cl	and sense organs (320-389)	
103	102	97	166	96	162	251	316	149	137	Upper cl		
100	100	109	115	120	93	25	57	99	66	SPCR	Diseases of the circulatory	VII
98	98	56	60	73	57	0	0	65	40	Lower cl	system (390-459)	
102	102	162	170	167	129	60	137	134	91	Upper cl		
100	100	101	89	114	108	71	125	91	105	SPCR	Diseases of the respiratory	VIII
98	98	46	39	65	67	9	3	56	71	Lower cl	system (460-519)	
102	102	156	140	163	149	133	248	127	139	Upper cl		
100	100	182	43	73	102	164	121	108	89	SPCR	Diseases of the digestive system	IX
97	97	79	0	19	47	33	0	55	45	Lower cl	(520-579)	
103	103	285	91	127	157	295	288	161	132	Upper cl		
100	100	192	72	65	58	-	-	97	113	SPCR	Diseases of the genitourinary	X
96	97	38	1	0	12	-	-	25	58	Lower cl	system (580-629)	
104	103	346	143	138	105	-	-	169	168	Upper cl		
-	-	-	-	-	-	-	-	-	-	SPCR	Complications of pregnancy,	XI
-	-	-	-	-	-	-	-	-	-	Lower cl	childbirth and the puerperium	
-	-	-	-	-	-	-	-	-	-	Upper cl	(630-679)	
100	100	63	116	124	86	117	61	146	85	SPCR	Diseases of the skin and	XII
97	97	1	36	51	35	2	0	82	42	Lower cl	subcutaneous tissue (680-709)	
103	103	126	196	198	137	232	181	210	127	Upper cl		

Table 40 - *continued*

Disease group			Tenure								Urban / rural			
			Owner occupier		Council house		Other rented		Communal		Urban		Rural	
			M	F	M	F	M	F	M	F	M	F	M	F
XIII	Diseases of the musculoskeletal system and connective tissue (710-739)	SPCR	99	97	106	108	101	107	78	83	101	101	97	90
		Lower cl	96	95	101	104	92	100	65	77	98	99	90	85
		Upper cl	102	100	111	111	110	113	91	89	103	103	104	95
XIV	Congenital anomalies (740-759)	SPCR	104	118	101	81	*97*	*84*	-	*48*	102	110	*100*	*29*
		Lower cl	80	97	61	56	*30*	*42*	-	*10*	81	94	*46*	*6*
		Upper cl	129	138	140	105	*165*	*127*	-	*87*	123	126	*154*	*53*
XV	Certain conditions originating in the perinatal period (760-779)	SPCR	*83*	*146*	*200*	-	-	*226*	-	-	*116*	*115*	-	-
		Lower cl	*0*	*0*	*0*	-	-	*0*	-	-	*0*	*2*	-	-
		Upper cl	*245*	*310*	*591*	-	-	*670*	-	-	*277*	*228*	-	-
XVI	Symptoms, signs and ill-defined conditions (780-799)	SPCR	92	92	111	109	119	109	126	113	102	102	87	86
		Lower cl	89	90	105	104	108	102	109	105	99	99	79	80
		Upper cl	95	95	117	113	129	117	143	121	105	104	94	92
XVII	Injury and poisoning (800-999)	SPCR	97	96	104	106	99	105	133	103	100	100	102	100
		Lower cl	93	93	97	101	86	96	111	94	96	97	91	93
		Upper cl	101	99	111	111	111	113	155	111	104	103	112	108
XVIII	Supplementary classification of factors influencing health status and contact with health services (VO1-V82)	SPCR	102	102	89	91	109	104	115	115	100	100	103	104
		Lower cl	100	100	85	88	102	99	104	108	98	98	98	99
		Upper cl	105	104	93	93	117	109	127	121	102	101	109	109

White		Black Afro-Caribbean		Indian		Pakistani/Bangladeshi		Other			Disease group
M	F	M	F	M	F	M	F	M	F		
100	100	107	105	129	117	99	147	79	74	SPCR	Diseases of the musculoskeletal XIII
97	98	46	52	72	76	20	18	43	46	Lower cl	system and connective tissue
103	102	167	158	185	158	179	276	114	102	Upper cl	(710-739)
100	100	-	436	-	-	-	-	238	-	SPCR	Congenital anomalies (740-759) XIV
81	86	-	0	-	-	-	-	0	-	Lower cl	
119	114	-	1291	-	-	-	-	706	-	Upper cl	
100	101	-	-	-	-	-	-	-	-	SPCR	Certain conditions originating in XV
0	2	-	-	-	-	-	-	-	-	Lower cl	the perinatal period (760-779)
240	199	-	-	-	-	-	-	-	-	Upper cl	
100	100	156	146	105	125	138	166	96	129	SPCR	Symptoms, signs and ill-defined XVI
97	98	68	72	46	74	28	3	50	86	Lower cl	conditions (780-799)
103	102	244	220	164	176	248	330	141	172	Upper cl	
100	100	140	130	54	80	36	111	80	81	SPCR	Injury and poisoning (800-999) XVII
97	98	36	50	1	33	0	0	28	41	Lower cl	
104	103	244	211	107	128	106	265	132	121	Upper cl	
100	100	128	99	129	79	87	46	90	102	SPCR	Supplementary classification of XVIII
98	98	73	53	84	49	27	0	60	73	Lower cl	factors influencing health status
102	102	183	145	174	110	147	110	121	131	Upper cl	and contact with health services (VO1-V82)

Table 41 Age standardised patient consulting ratios (SPCR) for people aged 65 and over (study population=100) with approximate 95 per cent upper and lower confidence limits: comparison by sex, marital status, cohabiting status and social class (as defined by occupation)*

Disease group			Marital status						Cohabiting status					
			Single		Married		Widowed/ divorced		Single		Married/ cohabiting		Sep/wid/div not cohabiting	
			M	F	M	F	M	F	M	F	M	F	M	F
	All diseases and conditions (I-XVIII)	SPCR	96	97	100	100	100	101	95	97	100	100	100	101
		Lower cl	90	93	99	98	97	99	89	93	99	98	97	99
		Upper cl	101	101	102	102	103	102	101	101	102	102	103	102
	Serious	SPCR	95	90	100	98	102	103	94	90	100	98	102	103
		Lower cl	88	85	98	95	98	101	87	85	98	95	98	101
		Upper cl	103	95	102	100	106	105	102	95	102	100	106	105
	Intermediate	SPCR	94	92	100	99	101	102	93	92	100	99	101	102
		Lower cl	87	88	98	97	97	100	86	88	98	97	97	100
		Upper cl	100	96	102	101	105	103	99	97	102	101	105	103
	Minor	SPCR	91	93	101	101	98	100	90	93	101	101	98	100
		Lower cl	85	89	99	99	95	99	84	89	99	99	95	99
		Upper cl	97	98	103	103	102	102	97	98	103	103	101	102
	All illnesses (I-XVII)	SPCR	96	96	100	99	101	101	95	96	100	99	101	101
		Lower cl	90	92	99	98	98	100	89	92	99	98	97	100
		Upper cl	101	100	102	101	104	103	101	100	102	101	104	103
I	Infectious and parasitic diseases (001-139)	SPCR	85	86	99	98	107	103	87	87	99	98	107	104
		Lower cl	68	75	94	93	97	99	68	75	94	92	96	99
		Upper cl	103	98	104	103	118	108	105	98	104	103	117	108
II	Neoplasms (140-239)	SPCR	78	89	105	103	90	99	77	89	104	104	91	99
		Lower cl	58	73	98	96	79	92	56	72	98	96	80	92
		Upper cl	98	106	111	111	101	106	97	106	111	112	102	105
III	Endocrine, nutritional and metabolic diseases and immunity disorders (240-279)	SPCR	117	87	99	104	98	98	115	87	99	104	98	99
		Lower cl	98	75	94	99	88	94	95	75	95	98	88	94
		Upper cl	136	99	104	109	107	103	134	99	104	109	108	104
IV	Diseases of blood and blood-forming organs (280-289)	SPCR	136	112	95	96	108	101	135	112	95	97	108	100
		Lower cl	92	90	84	86	89	93	90	90	84	87	89	92
		Upper cl	180	134	105	106	127	108	179	134	105	107	128	108
V	Mental disorders (290-319)	SPCR	117	95	91	91	124	107	116	95	91	91	124	107
		Lower cl	97	85	86	87	113	103	95	85	86	86	113	103
		Upper cl	138	105	96	96	135	111	137	105	96	95	135	111
VI	Diseases of the nervous system and sense organs (320-389)	SPCR	92	93	102	98	96	102	89	94	102	99	95	102
		Lower cl	82	86	99	95	90	99	79	86	99	95	90	99
		Upper cl	102	101	105	102	101	105	99	101	105	102	101	105
VII	Diseases of the circulatory system (390-459)	SPCR	89	90	100	100	101	101	89	90	101	100	101	101
		Lower cl	81	84	98	97	96	99	81	84	98	97	96	99
		Upper cl	98	96	103	103	106	104	98	96	103	103	106	104
VIII	Diseases of the respiratory system (460-519)	SPCR	82	80	100	97	104	105	81	80	100	96	103	106
		Lower cl	73	74	98	94	99	103	72	74	98	93	98	103
		Upper cl	90	86	103	100	109	108	89	86	103	99	108	108
IX	Diseases of the digestive system (520-579)	SPCR	91	86	101	104	100	99	90	86	101	104	99	99
		Lower cl	78	77	97	100	93	96	77	77	97	100	92	96
		Upper cl	103	94	104	108	107	103	103	94	105	108	106	103
X	Diseases of the genitourinary system (580-629)	SPCR	99	71	101	105	97	100	99	70	100	106	99	100
		Lower cl	81	62	95	101	88	96	80	61	95	101	90	96
		Upper cl	118	80	106	110	107	104	118	79	105	110	109	104
XI	Complications of pregnancy, childbirth and the puerperium (630-679)	SPCR	-	-	-	-	-	-	-	-	-	-	-	-
		Lower cl	-	-	-	-	-	-	-	-	-	-	-	-
		Upper cl	-	-	-	-	-	-	-	-	-	-	-	-
XII	Diseases of the skin and subcutaneous tissue (680-709)	SPCR	98	96	100	98	100	102	95	96	100	99	101	101
		Lower cl	84	87	96	94	93	98	82	86	96	95	93	98
		Upper cl	111	105	104	102	107	105	109	105	104	103	108	105

* Social class of married/cohabiting women is based on their partners's occupation.

Social class*										Disease group		
I & II		IIIN		IIIM		IV & V		Other				
M	F	M	F	M	F	M	F	M	F			
100	100	100	100	101	100	98	100	105	99	SPCR	All diseases and conditions	
98	97	96	98	98	98	95	98	98	96	Lower cl	(I-XVIII)	
103	102	104	103	103	102	100	103	113	102	Upper cl		
94	95	97	99	105	102	99	105	102	98	SPCR	Serious	
91	92	92	96	102	98	96	102	93	94	Lower cl		
98	98	103	103	108	105	103	108	112	102	Upper cl		
103	100	99	100	101	101	96	102	98	95	SPCR	Intermediate	
99	97	94	97	98	98	93	99	90	92	Lower cl		
106	103	104	103	104	104	100	104	107	98	Upper cl		
102	102	101	100	100	100	96	100	104	98	SPCR	Minor	
99	99	96	97	98	97	93	97	95	95	Lower cl		
105	104	106	103	103	103	100	102	112	101	Upper cl		
100	99	100	101	101	100	98	101	104	98	SPCR	All illnesses (I-XVII)	
97	97	95	98	99	98	95	99	97	96	Lower cl		
102	101	104	103	104	103	100	103	112	101	Upper cl		
108	98	80	99	103	100	96	102	88	101	SPCR	Infectious and parasitic	I
99	90	67	90	95	93	87	95	64	92	Lower cl	diseases (001-139)	
117	105	93	107	111	108	106	109	111	109	Upper cl		
105	115	106	97	104	93	84	97	111	96	SPCR	Neoplasms (140-239)	II
95	103	89	86	94	83	73	88	81	84	Lower cl		
115	126	123	109	113	104	94	107	141	108	Upper cl		
107	90	99	92	104	110	93	108	51	95	SPCR	Endocrine, nutritional and	III
99	83	85	84	97	102	84	101	34	86	Lower cl	metabolic diseases and	
115	97	112	100	111	118	101	116	68	104	Upper cl	immunity disorders (240-279)	
94	92	114	99	97	111	113	108	60	88	SPCR	Diseases of blood and blood-	IV
77	79	85	85	82	97	93	95	25	75	Lower cl	forming organs (280-289)	
110	105	144	113	112	126	133	120	95	101	Upper cl		
99	89	104	101	102	99	92	105	125	106	SPCR	Mental disorders (290-319)	V
91	83	89	94	94	92	83	99	98	99	Lower cl		
108	95	118	108	110	105	101	111	153	113	Upper cl		
106	103	103	106	100	100	93	97	88	94	SPCR	Diseases of the nervous system	VI
101	98	95	101	96	95	88	93	75	89	Lower cl	and sense organs (320-389)	
111	108	111	112	105	105	98	101	101	99	Upper cl		
100	96	99	102	105	105	95	103	85	92	SPCR	Diseases of the circulatory	VII
96	92	93	98	101	100	91	100	74	88	Lower cl	system (390-459)	
104	100	106	106	108	109	100	107	96	96	Upper cl		
92	93	95	94	104	99	104	111	113	99	SPCR	Diseases of the respiratory	VIII
88	89	88	90	100	95	99	107	100	94	Lower cl	system (460-519)	
96	97	102	99	108	103	109	115	126	104	Upper cl		
99	102	97	98	104	100	96	103	98	95	SPCR	Diseases of the digestive system	IX
94	97	87	92	99	95	89	98	82	88	Lower cl	(520-579)	
105	108	106	104	110	106	102	108	115	101	Upper cl		
102	105	101	94	97	97	101	99	111	106	SPCR	Diseases of the genitourinary	X
94	98	87	88	89	90	91	93	86	99	Lower cl	system (580-629)	
110	111	115	101	104	103	110	105	135	114	Upper cl		
-	-	-	-	-	-	-	-	-	-	SPCR	Complications of pregnancy,	XI
-	-	-	-	-	-	-	-	-	-	Lower cl	childbirth and the puerperium	
-	-	-	-	-	-	-	-	-	-	Upper cl	(630-679)	
111	102	101	99	94	97	93	101	110	100	SPCR	Diseases of the skin and	XII
105	96	91	93	89	92	86	96	91	93	Lower cl	subcutaneous tissue (680-709)	
118	108	111	105	100	103	100	106	129	106	Upper cl		

* Social class of married/cohabiting women is based on their partners's occupation.

SPCRs

Table 41 - *continued*

Disease group			Marital status						Cohabiting status					
			Single		Married		Widowed/divorced		Single		Married/cohabiting		Sep/wid/div not cohabiting	
			M	F	M	F	M	F	M	F	M	F	M	F
XIII	Diseases of the musculoskeletal system and connective tissue (710-739)	SPCR	87	84	101	98	100	104	86	84	101	98	99	104
		Lower cl	78	78	98	95	95	101	76	78	98	95	94	101
		Upper cl	97	90	104	101	106	106	96	90	104	101	105	106
XIV	Congenital anomalies (740-759)	SPCR	*146*	*126*	91	94	120	101	*154*	*128*	92	92	116	102
		Lower cl	*51*	*68*	70	72	72	81	*53*	*69*	71	70	69	83
		Upper cl	*242*	*184*	112	116	169	121	*255*	*187*	113	113	163	122
XV	Certain conditions originating in the perinatal period (760-779)	SPCR	-	-	*76*	*259*	*173*	*70*	-	-	*76*	*263*	*173*	*70*
		Lower cl	-	-	*0*	*0*	*0*	*0*	-	-	*0*	*0*	*0*	*0*
		Upper cl	-	-	*226*	*619*	*513*	*167*	-	-	*225*	*627*	*513*	*167*
XVI	Symptoms, signs and ill-defined conditions (780-799)	SPCR	98	95	99	96	105	103	98	95	99	96	105	104
		Lower cl	87	88	95	92	98	101	86	88	95	92	98	101
		Upper cl	110	103	102	99	111	106	110	103	102	99	111	106
XVII	Injury and poisoning (800-999)	SPCR	103	90	98	95	107	105	105	91	98	95	106	105
		Lower cl	88	82	94	91	99	101	89	82	94	91	98	101
		Upper cl	118	99	102	99	114	108	120	99	102	99	113	108
XVIII	Supplementary classification of factors influencing health status and contact with health services (VO1-V82)	SPCR	89	91	102	106	95	97	88	91	102	106	95	97
		Lower cl	81	85	100	103	91	95	80	85	100	103	91	95
		Upper cl	96	96	105	109	99	99	96	96	105	108	99	100

Social class*											Disease group
I & II		IIIN		IIIM		IV & V		Other			
M	F	M	F	M	F	M	F	M	F		
97	99	94	100	106	100	98	106	93	91	SPCR	Diseases of the musculoskeletal XIII
93	95	86	96	102	96	93	102	80	87	Lower cl	system and connective tissue
102	103	101	105	110	104	103	110	106	96	Upper cl	(710-739)
81	105	*122*	126	92	108	110	85	*208*	78	SPCR	Congenital anomalies (740-759) XIV
49	73	*56*	88	61	75	68	59	*54*	46	Lower cl	
114	136	*188*	164	123	141	152	111	*361*	110	Upper cl	
-	-	-	289	*145*	*325*	*223*	-	-	-	SPCR	Certain conditions originating in XV
-	-	-	*0*	*0*	*0*	*0*	-	-	-	Lower cl	the perinatal period (760-779)
-	-	-	*689*	*430*	*774*	*659*	-	-	-	Upper cl	
96	96	98	97	102	99	104	109	94	97	SPCR	Symptoms, signs and ill-defined XVI
90	91	89	92	98	94	98	104	80	91	Lower cl	conditions (780-799)
101	100	107	102	107	104	110	113	109	102	Upper cl	
102	100	90	101	104	92	92	106	118	99	SPCR	Injury and poisoning (800-999) XVII
96	95	80	95	98	87	85	101	97	93	Lower cl	
109	106	101	107	110	97	99	111	138	105	Upper cl	
106	106	100	100	98	102	94	93	106	102	SPCR	Supplementary classification of XVIII
103	102	94	96	94	98	91	90	95	98	Lower cl	factors influencing health status
110	109	106	104	101	105	98	96	116	106	Upper cl	and contact with health services
											(VO1-V82)

* Social class of married/cohabiting women is based on their partners's occupation.

Table 42 Age standardised patient consulting ratios (SPCR) for people aged 65 and over (study population = 100) with approximate 95 per cent upper and lower confidence limits: comparison by sex, living alone, sole adult with children, children in household

Disease group			All adults				Sole adults			
			Living alone		Living accompanied		Sole adult without children		Sole adult with children	
			M	F	M	F	M	F	M	F
	All diseases and conditions (I-XVIII)	SPCR	99	100	100	100	100	100	107	98
		Lower cl	95	98	99	99	97	98	46	64
		Upper cl	102	101	102	102	103	102	167	133
	Serious	SPCR	98	100	100	100	100	100	92	131
		Lower cl	94	98	98	98	96	98	18	78
		Upper cl	102	102	102	102	104	102	166	185
	Intermediate	SPCR	99	101	100	99	100	100	115	100
		Lower cl	96	99	98	98	96	98	40	60
		Upper cl	103	103	102	101	104	102	190	140
	Minor	SPCR	97	99	101	100	100	100	93	108
		Lower cl	93	97	99	99	96	98	29	67
		Upper cl	101	101	102	102	104	102	157	148
	All illnesses (I-XVII)	SPCR	99	100	100	100	100	100	103	99
		Lower cl	96	98	99	98	97	98	42	64
		Upper cl	102	102	102	101	103	102	164	134
I	Infectious and parasitic diseases (001-139)	SPCR	100	99	100	101	100	100	-	132
		Lower cl	89	93	95	96	89	94	-	3
		Upper cl	111	104	105	105	112	105	-	261
II	Neoplasms (140-239)	SPCR	90	96	102	103	100	100	153	203
		Lower cl	78	88	96	96	86	92	0	0
		Upper cl	102	104	108	109	113	108	452	432
III	Endocrine, nutritional and metabolic diseases and immunity disorders (240-279)	SPCR	97	95	101	103	100	100	-	93
		Lower cl	86	89	96	99	89	94	-	0
		Upper cl	107	100	105	108	111	106	-	198
IV	Diseases of blood and blood-forming organs (280-289)	SPCR	97	101	101	99	100	100	-	135
		Lower cl	77	92	91	91	79	91	-	0
		Upper cl	118	110	111	107	122	109	-	322
V	Mental disorders (290-319)	SPCR	112	102	97	99	99	100	256	103
		Lower cl	100	97	92	95	89	95	0	13
		Upper cl	123	106	102	102	110	104	546	194
VI	Diseases of the nervous system and sense organs (320-389)	SPCR	92	102	102	98	100	100	104	92
		Lower cl	86	99	99	96	94	97	0	28
		Upper cl	98	106	105	101	106	103	221	155
VII	Diseases of the circulatory system (390-459)	SPCR	98	101	100	99	100	100	135	106
		Lower cl	93	99	98	97	95	97	27	48
		Upper cl	103	104	103	101	105	103	243	163
VIII	Diseases of the respiratory system (460-519)	SPCR	97	100	101	100	100	100	51	127
		Lower cl	91	97	98	98	95	97	0	60
		Upper cl	102	103	103	103	106	103	121	193
IX	Diseases of the digestive system (520-579)	SPCR	98	97	100	102	100	100	49	109
		Lower cl	91	93	97	99	93	96	0	22
		Upper cl	106	101	104	105	108	104	144	197
X	Diseases of the genitourinary system (580-629)	SPCR	88	93	103	105	100	100	106	51
		Lower cl	78	88	98	101	89	95	0	0
		Upper cl	97	97	108	108	111	105	314	122
XI	Complications of pregnancy, childbirth and the puerperium (630-679)	SPCR	-	-	-	-	-	-	-	-
		Lower cl	-	-	-	-	-	-	-	-
		Upper cl	-	-	-	-	-	-	-	-
XII	Diseases of the skin and subcutaneous tissue (680-709)	SPCR	98	101	100	99	100	100	108	71
		Lower cl	90	97	97	96	92	96	0	1
		Upper cl	106	105	104	103	108	104	257	141

None		Under 5s only		5-15s only		Under 5s and 5-15s		Disease group		
M	F	M	F	M	F	M	F			
100	100	98	99	95	97	101	103	SPCR	All diseases and conditions	
99	99	76	78	83	86	75	82	Lower cl	(I-XVIII)	
101	101	121	120	108	107	127	124	Upper cl		
100	100	114	123	97	112	117	117	SPCR	Serious	
98	98	81	90	80	96	80	87	Lower cl		
102	101	147	155	114	127	154	148	Upper cl		
100	100	105	103	94	99	101	104	SPCR	Intermediate	
98	99	77	78	79	87	70	80	Lower cl		
102	101	133	128	109	111	131	129	Upper cl		
100	100	86	105	92	96	102	101	SPCR	Minor	
99	99	62	80	78	85	73	78	Lower cl		
102	101	111	129	106	108	132	124	Upper cl		
100	100	101	98	94	97	105	107	SPCR	All illnesses (I-XVII)	
99	99	77	76	81	87	78	85	Lower cl		
101	101	124	119	107	108	132	128	Upper cl		
100	100	79	92	101	123	122	128	SPCR	Infectious and parasitic	I
95	96	10	28	57	85	24	55	Lower cl	diseases (001-139)	
105	103	148	156	146	160	220	200	Upper cl		
101	100	92	186	58	84	54	152	SPCR	Neoplasms (140-239)	II
95	95	2	57	18	40	0	39	Lower cl		
106	105	183	314	97	127	129	264	Upper cl		
100	100	66	107	100	125	107	114	SPCR	Endocrine, nutritional and	III
96	96	8	41	59	88	21	46	Lower cl	metabolic diseases and	
104	103	123	174	141	163	193	181	Upper cl	immunity disorders (240-279)	
100	100	67	117	125	93	74	166	SPCR	Diseases of blood and blood-	IV
91	94	0	0	25	35	0	20	Lower cl	forming organs (280-289)	
109	106	199	250	225	151	218	311	Upper cl		
100	100	82	57	110	113	116	128	SPCR	Mental disorders (290-319)	V
95	97	10	15	63	83	23	67	Lower cl		
105	103	154	100	156	143	210	188	Upper cl		
100	100	93	98	96	97	95	78	SPCR	Diseases of the nervous system	VI
97	98	50	57	72	77	47	43	Lower cl	and sense organs (320-389)	
103	102	136	139	121	118	142	113	Upper cl		
100	100	103	96	96	102	117	126	SPCR	Diseases of the circulatory	VII
98	98	66	62	75	84	73	88	Lower cl	system (390-459)	
102	102	140	130	116	120	161	163	Upper cl		
100	100	106	147	117	108	116	109	SPCR	Diseases of the respiratory	VIII
97	98	66	103	93	89	70	72	Lower cl	system (460-519)	
102	102	145	191	140	128	163	145	Upper cl		
100	100	114	74	96	89	130	117	SPCR	Diseases of the digestive system	IX
97	98	56	30	67	65	62	64	Lower cl	(520-579)	
103	103	172	118	126	113	199	169	Upper cl		
100	100	140	75	89	67	55	108	SPCR	Diseases of the genitourinary	X
96	97	49	26	48	44	0	52	Lower cl	system (580-629)	
105	103	232	124	130	91	116	165	Upper cl		
-	-	-	-	-	-	-	-	SPCR	Complications of pregnancy,	XI
-	-	-	-	-	-	-	-	Lower cl	childbirth and the puerperium	
-	-	-	-	-	-	-	-	Upper cl	(630-679)	
100	100	121	114	84	120	93	125	SPCR	Diseases of the skin and	XII
97	97	60	60	55	92	32	70	Lower cl	subcutaneous tissue (680-709)	
103	102	183	168	113	148	154	180	Upper cl		

Table 42 - *continued*

Disease group			All adults				Sole adults			
			Living alone		Living accompanied		Sole adult without children		Sole adult with children	
			M	F	M	F	M	F	M	F
XIII	Diseases of the musculoskeletal system and connective tissue (710-739)	SPCR	102	106	100	96	100	100	120	127
		Lower cl	96	103	97	94	94	97	2	63
		Upper cl	109	109	102	98	106	103	237	191
XIV	Congenital anomalies (740-759)	SPCR	143	105	92	97	100	100	-	-
		Lower cl	86	82	72	79	60	78	-	-
		Upper cl	200	128	112	115	140	122	-	-
XV	Certain conditions originating in the perinatal period (760-779)	SPCR	223	48	64	155	100	100	-	-
		Lower cl	0	0	0	0	0	0	-	-
		Upper cl	660	144	191	330	296	297	-	-
XVI	Symptoms, signs and ill-defined conditions (780-799)	SPCR	101	101	100	99	100	100	74	117
		Lower cl	94	98	97	96	93	97	0	44
		Upper cl	108	105	103	102	107	103	177	189
XVII	Injury and poisoning (800-999)	SPCR	101	105	100	97	100	100	181	88
		Lower cl	93	101	96	94	91	96	0	18
		Upper cl	110	109	104	100	108	104	386	159
XVIII	Supplementary classification of factors influencing health status and contact with health services (VO1-V82)	SPCR	94	96	101	103	100	100	93	104
		Lower cl	90	94	99	100	95	97	11	51
		Upper cl	99	99	103	105	105	103	174	156

Children in household								Disease group	
None		Under 5s only		5-15s only		Under 5s and 5-15s			
M	F	M	F	M	F	M	F		
100	100	132	114	94	105	130	108	SPCR	Diseases of the musculoskeletal XIII
97	98	84	76	70	87	76	73	Lower cl	system and connective tissue
102	102	180	152	117	124	184	144	Upper cl	(710-739)
100	97	-	200	171	203	-	557	SPCR	Congenital anomalies (740-759) XIV
80	83	-	0	0	4	-	0	Lower cl	
119	111	-	591	407	402	-	1,187	Upper cl	
101	101	-	-	-	-	-	-	SPCR	Certain conditions originating in XV
0	2	-	-	-	-	-	-	Lower cl	the perinatal period (760-779)
242	201	-	-	-	-	-	-	Upper cl	
100	100	102	112	102	99	98	135	SPCR	Symptoms, signs and ill-defined XVI
97	98	52	67	74	78	45	88	Lower cl	conditions (780-799)
103	102	152	156	130	120	151	182	Upper cl	
100	100	89	87	123	109	192	129	SPCR	Injury and poisoning (800-999) XVII
96	97	31	41	84	83	98	76	Lower cl	
103	102	148	132	162	134	287	181	Upper cl	
100	100	69	88	87	103	92	71	SPCR	Supplementary classification of XVIII
98	98	41	59	70	87	56	46	Lower cl	factors influencing health status
102	102	97	118	105	119	127	97	Upper cl	and contact with health services
									(VO1-V82)

Appendices

Appendix A Socio-economic interview record

MSGP4   SOCIO-ECONOMIC INTERVIEW RECORD

NAME .... ID No. ....

Date of birth .... Sex ....

TO BE COMPLETED FOR ALL PERSONS

TO BE COMPLETED FOR PERSONS AGED 16 AND OVER
(For those living in communal establishments, QUESTIONS 6, 7 and 8 **DO NOT** apply)

1 SOURCE OF INFORMATION

   1. Patient   2. Proxy   3. Total refusal

2 MARITAL STATUS   R

   1. Single not cohabiting   6. Divorced not cohabiting

   2. Single cohabiting   7. Divorced cohabiting

   3. Married   8. Widowed not cohabiting

   4. Separated not cohabiting   9. Widowed cohabiting

   5. Separated cohabiting   NK

3 TENURE OF HOUSEHOLD   R
Owner occupier:

   1. Buying   2. Owns outright

Renting:

   3. With job   7. Private furnished

   4. Council   8. Private unfurnished

   5. New Town   9. Communal

   6. Housing Assn   NK

4 ETHNIC GROUP   R

   1. White   6. Bangladeshi

   2. Black-Caribbean   7. Chinese

   3. Black-African   8. Sri Lankan

   4. Indian   9. Other

   5. Pakistani   NK

5 COUNTRY OF BIRTH....................................... R

                          Code [ ][ ]

6 SOLE ADULT IN HOUSEHOLD   R

   1. Yes   2. No   NK

7 CHILDREN UNDER 5 IN HOUSEHOLD   R

   1 Yes   2. No   NK

8 CHILDREN AGED 5-15 IN HOUSEHOLD   R

   1. Yes   2. No   NK

9 HAS PATIENT SMOKED AT ALL IN LAST WEEK   R

   1. Yes   2. No   NK

10 ECONOMIC POSITION LAST WEEK   R

   1. Working full-time   6. Student

   2. Working part-time   7. Permanently sick

   3. Training scheme   8. Retired

   4. Waiting to start work   9. Home / family care

   5. Seeking work   NK

11 ECONOMIC POSITION ONE YEAR AGO   R

   1. Working full-time   6. Student

   2. Working part-time   7. Permanently sick

   3. Training scheme   8. Retired

   4. Waiting to start work   9. Home / family care

   5. Seeking work   NK

12 OCCUPATION   R

                          Code [ ][ ][ ]

Industry information

13 EMPLOYMENT STATUS   R

   1. Employee NEC   4. Foreman / supervisor

   2. Self employed-employing   5. Manager

   3. Self employed-alone   6. Non worker

TO BE COMPLETED FOR PERSONS UNDER 16 LIVING IN PRIVATE HOUSEHOLDS
(For those living in communal establishments, these questions **DO NOT** apply)

14 LIVING WITH SOLE ADULT   R

   1. Yes   2. No   NK

15 ECONOMIC POSITION OF PARENT LAST WEEK   R

   1. Working full-time   6. Student

   2. Working part-time   7. Permanently sick

   3. Training scheme   8. Retired

   4. Waiting to start work   9. Home / family care

   5. Seeking work   NK

16 ECONOMIC POSITION OF PARENT ONE YEAR AGO   R

   1. Working full-time   6. Student

   2. Working part-time   7. Permanently sick

   3. Training scheme   8. Retired

   4. Waiting to start work   9. Home / family care

   5. Seeking work   NK

17 OCCUPATION OF PARENT   R

Code

Industry information

18 EMPLOYMENT STATUS OF PARENT   R

   1. Employee NEC   4. Foreman / supervisor

   2. Self employed-employing   5. Manager

   3. Self employed-alone   6. Non worker

TO BE COMPLETED FOR WOMEN WHO ARE MARRIED OR COHABITING

19 ECONOMIC POSITION OF PARTNER LAST WEEK   R

   1. Working full-time   6. Student

   2. Working part-time   7. Permanently sick

   3. Training scheme   8. Retired

   4. Waiting to start work   9. Home / family care

   5. Seeking work   NK

20 ECONOMIC POSITION OF PARTNER ONE YEAR AGO   R

   1. Working full-time   6. Student

   2. Working part-time   7. Permanently sick

   3. Training scheme   8. Retired

   4. Waiting to start work   9. Home / family care

   5. Seeking work   NK

21 OCCUPATION OF PARTNER   R

Code

Industry information

22 EMPLOYMENT STATUS OF PARTNER   R

   1. Employee NEC   4. Foreman / supervisor

   2. Self employed-employing   5. Manager

   3. Self employed-alone   6. Non worker

Additional information

TB1/1 1/91

Appendix B Glossary

Age: as at 1 March 1992, the mid-study date; derived from date of birth.

Age standardised ratio: the ratio between the observed and expected numbers of occurrences in a subgroup of the population, where the expected number is the number which would be expected if those in that subgroup were to experience the same morbidity in each (five-year) age group as the study population as a whole.

All diseases and conditions: includes any diagnosis in ICD Chapters I-XVII or in the ICD Supplementary Classification.

All illnesses: includes any diagnosis in ICD Chapters I-XVII.

Broad geographical region: North: Northern, Yorkshire, Mersey, North Western
(by regional health authorities) Midlands and Wales: Trent, East Anglia, West Midlands, Wales
  South: North West Thames, North East Thames, South East Thames, South West Thames, Wessex, Oxford, South Western.

Category of severity: assigned by OPCS to each diagnostic code, irrespective of the condition of an individual patient or the doctor's opinion.

> *Serious:* Invariably or frequently serious or possibly life threatening, *or*
> Invariably or frequently requiring major surgery or intensive care, *or*
> With a high probability of serious complications or significant disability.
>
> *intermediate:* Other than serious or minor.
>
> *Minor:* Illnesses commonly treated without recourse to medical advice, *or*
> Minor self-limiting illnesses which require no specific treatment, *or*
> Reasons for contact in the ICD9 supplementary classification.

Cohabiting status: single not cohabiting; married/cohabiting; separated/widowed/divorced not cohabiting.

Consultation: each diagnosis or reason for contact recorded during a contact; for each contact one or more consultations were recorded.

Consultation type: recorded for each illness or reason recorded by the doctor or practice nurse.

> *First*: first consultation ever in his life by a patient with any general practitioner or practice nurse for that illness or reason.
>
> *New*: first consultation for a new occurrence of an illness or reason for which the patient has previously consulted any general practitioner or practice nurse.
>
> *Ongoing*: any consultation for continuing illness following a first or new consultation.

Contact: a face-to-face meeting between a GP or practice nurse and a person registered as an NHS patient with a practice participating in the study; telephone or written contacts and contacts with other members of the practice team were excluded. Contacts with a practice nurse which followed contacts with a doctor during the same visit were also excluded.

Doctor: principal, assistant, trainee or locum general practitioners.

Economic position: working full-time (more than 30 hours per week/on government employment or training scheme); working part-time (one to 30 hours per week); unemployed (looking for a job/waiting to start a job already accepted); permanently sick and unable to work; looking after home/family; other(at school or other full-time education/retired from paid work).

Episode: a single or sequence of consultations covering the duration of a continuing illness or reason for consulting, derived at OPCS from the consultation types reported by grouping the consultations for that illness or reason chronologically.

Episode type: derived by OPCS from the earliest consultation type recorded for that episode of illness or reason.

First: first ever episode of an illness or reason for consulting a GP or practice nurse.
New: new episode of illness for which the patient has previously consulted a GP or practice nurse.
Ongoing: an episode for which the patient had consulted a GP or practice nurse before the start of the study year.

Ethnic group: White; Afro-Caribbean; Indian; Pakistani/Bangladeshi; other.

Household composition:
children whether living with sole adult:
adults whether sole adult in household:
sole adult with or without children aged 0-5, 5-15 or both, living alone.

ICD9: Ninth revision of the International Statistical Classification of diseases, injuries and causes of death.

Incidence rates: first and new episode rates (the sum of first and new episodes reported during the study year).

Marital status: single; married; widowed/divorced.

Nurse: practice employed nurse; nurses employed by other agencies such as a health authority were excluded.

Parent (guardian): in priority order if living in the same house, child's father, stepfather, mother's cohabitee, mother (if sole adult in household), head of household.

Patient: a person who was registered as an NHS patient for part or all of the year with a practice participating in the study; temporary or private patients were excluded.

Patient consulting rates: rates of patients who consulted at least once during the year at a defined level of diagnostic detail (eg for any illness, or for a respiratory illness, or for acute bronchitis).

Person years at risk: the sum of the number of days each patient in a particular category, such as men aged 16-24 years living in council housing, was registered with a study practice during the year, divided by the number of days (366) in the year.

Place of contact: surgery; patient's home; elsewhere. If not stated, allocated to surgery.

Prevalence (period prevalence): the number of patients who consulted at least once during the study year for a condition or group of conditions.

Prevalence rates: patient consulting rates (period prevalence rates) at each level of detail of diagnostic coding.

Prevention health care codes: the ICD Supplementary Classification codes V01-V07, V20, V22-V26, V70, V72-V82.

Rates: rates for persons are per 10,000 person years at risk. This applies to each sex, age and socio-economic group, e.g. the number of male patients aged 0-4 years in Social Class IIIN who consulted for every 10,000 males- aged 0-4 years in Social Class IIIN years at risk.

Read Clinical Classification: developed for use in general practice and managed by the NHS Centre for Coding and Classification; the diagnostic part only was used corresponding to ICD9 Chapters I-XVII and selected codes in the ICD Supplementary Classification (V codes).

Referrals: referral by a GP to a medically or dentally qualified practitioner; to inpatients, outpatients, accident and emergency departments, for private (non-NHS) consultation, domiciliary consultation or some other.

Supplementary Classification: ICD supplementary classification of factors influencing health status and contact with health services (V codes). This classification is sometimes referred to as ICD Chapter XVIII in this volume.

Tenure of housing: owner occupied (with or without a loan/mortgage); council housing (local authority, new-town corporation or housing action trust); other rented (with job, housing association, private landlord); communal establishment.

Urban/rural place of residence: derived from patient's postcode reported by practice, by linking it to the enumeration district and assigning the urban or rural indicator designated to each enumeration district by the Department of the Environment.

Appendix C Standard Occupational Classification: the definition of sub-major groups

Major group	Sub-major group
1 Managers and administrators	a) Corporate managers and administrators b) Managers/proprietors in agriculture and services
2 Professional occupations	a) Science and engineering professionals b) Health professionals c) Teaching professionals d) Other professional occupations
3 Associate professional and technical occupations	a) Science and engineering associate professionals b) Health associate professionals c) Other associate professional occupations
4 Clerical and secretarial occupations	a) Clerical occupations b) Secretarial occupations
5 Craft and related occupations	a) Skilled construction trades b) Skilled engineering trades c) Other skilled trades
6 Personal and protective service occupations	a) Protective service occupations b) Personal service occupations
7 Sales occupations	a) Buyers, brokers and sales reps. b) Other sales occupations
8 Plant and machine operatives	a) Industrial plant and machine operators, assemblers b) Drivers and mobile machine operators
9 Other occupations	a) Other occupations in agriculture, forestry and fishing b) Other elementary occupations

Appendix D Table index

	Table number	Page number	Age groups — All	0-15	16 and over	16-64	65 and over	All diseases and conditions (ICD chapters I-XVIII)	Category of severity within all diseases and conditions	All illnesses (ICD chapters I-XVII)	ICD chapters	Category of severity within ICD chapter	Disease related groups (ICD subheadings)	ICD 3 digits	Sex	Total population	Broad geographical region	Urban/rural residence	Tenure of housing	Marital status
Population	1		x												x	x	x			
	2		x												x				x	
	3		x												x			x		
	4		x												x					
	5		x												x					x
	6				x										x					
	7		x												x					
	8				x										x					
	9				x										x					
	10				x										x					
	11				x										x					
	12					x									x					
	13				x										x					
	14				x										x					
	15				x										x					
	16			x											x					
	17			x											x					
	18			x											x					
Patient consulting rates	19		x					x	x	x	x	x			x					
	20		x										x		x					
	21		x											x	x					
Incidence rates	22		x											x	x					
Consultation rates	23		x					x	x	x	x	x			x					
	24		x										x		x					
	25		x											x	x					
	26		x					x	x	x	x	x			x					
	27		x										x		x					
Standardised patient consulting ratios	28		x					x	x	x	x				x		x			
	29				x			x	x	x	x				x			x	x	
	30				x			x	x	x	x				x					x
	31				x			x	x	x	x				x					
	32				x			x	x	x	x				x					
	33				x			x	x	x	x				x					
	34				x			x	x	x	x				x					
	35				x			x	x	x	x				x					
	36				x			x	x	x	x				x					
	37			x				x	x	x	x				x			x	x	
	38			x				x	x	x	x				x					
	39			x				x	x	x	x				x					
	40						x	x	x	x	x				x			x	x	
	41						x	x	x	x	x				x					x
	42						x	x	x	x	x				x					

* Partner's social class for married/cohabiting women

362

Category	Table number	Page number	With practice nurse	With doctor	Home visits	All consultations	Parent's economic position	Parents' social class	Women's partners economic position	Women's own social class	Smoking status	Ethnic group	Economic position	Occupation	Social class*	Household composition	Cohabiting status
							Socio-economic Characteristics – continued										
Population	1																
	2																
	3																
	4												x				
	5																
	6																x
	7														x		
	8											x					
	9															x	
	10												x				
	11												x				
	12													x			
	13							x									
	14							x									
	15									x							
	16															x	
	17						x										
	18						x										
Patient consulting rates	19																
	20																
	21																
Incidence rates	22																
Consultation rates	23			x													
	24			x													
	25			x													
	26		x	x	x	x											
	27		x	x	x	x											
Standardised patient consulting ratios	28																
	29											x					
	30														x		x
	31									x							
	32															x	
	33											x					
	34										x						
	35							x									
	36									x							
	37											x					
	38							x								x	
	39						x										
	40											x					
	41														x		x
	42														x		

Appendix E Standard tables available on disk

All tables published in the volume and additional tables are available on disk. Tables will include:

Population tables with age groups 0-4, 5-15, 16-24, 25-44, 45-64, 65-74, 75-84, 85 and over, by sex, broad geographical region, urban or rural place of residence, housing tenure, marital status, cohabiting status, household composition, social class (as defined by occupation), occupation, economic position, ethnic group and smoking status, as person years at risk.

Population tables with age groups 0-4, 5-14, 15-24, 25-44, 45-64, 65-74, 75-84, 85 and over, by sex and broad geographical region, as person years at risk.

Patients consulting tables with age groups 0-4, 5-15, 16-24, 25-44, 45-64, 65-74, 75-84, 85 and over, by ICD chapter and category of severity, ICD subheadings (disease related groups), first 3 ICD digits and 4 ICD digits, by sex, as rates per 10,000 person years at risk.

Patients consulting tables with age groups 0-4, 5-14, 15-24, 25-44, 45-64, 65-74, 75-84, 85 and over, by ICD chapter and category of severity, ICD subheadings (disease related groups) and first 3 ICD digits and 4 ICD digits, by sex, as rates per 10,000 person years at risk.

Patients consulting tables with age groups 0-4, 5-14, 15-24, 25-44, 45-64, 65-74, 75-84, 85 and over, by all diseases and conditions, and ICD chapter, by sex and selected socio-economic characteristics, as rates per 10,000 persons.

Age standardised patient consulting ratios with 95% confidence limits, with age groups 0-15, 16-64, 65 and over, by category of severity, ICD chapter and ICD subheadings (disease related groups), by sex, broad geographical region, urban or rural place of residence, housing tenure, marital status, cohabiting status, household composition, economic position, occupation, social class, ethnic group and smoking status.

Episode tables with age groups 0-4, 5-15, 16-24, 25-44, 45-64, 65-74, 75-84, 85 and over for all episodes, first episodes and new episodes by first 3 ICD digits, by sex, as rates per 10,000 person years at risk.

Age standardised first and new episode ratios with 95% confidence limits, with age groups 0-15, 16-64, 65 and over by first 3 ICD digits, sex, broad geographical region, urban or rural place of residence, housing tenure, marital status, cohabiting status, household composition, social class, occupation, economic position, ethnic group and smoking status.

New and first episodes by month, by first 3 ICD digits, as rates per 10,000 person years at risk.

Consultation with doctor tables with age groups 0-4, 5-15, 16-24, 25-44, 45-64, 65-74, 75-84, 85 and over, by ICD chapter and category of severity, ICD subheadings (disease related groups) and first 3 ICD digits, by sex, as rates per 10,000 person years at risk.

Consultation tables with age groups 0-15, 16-64, 65-74, 75 and over, for all consultations, home visits and whether seen by a doctor or practice nurse, by ICD chapter and severity of condition, ICD subheadings (disease related groups) and first 3 ICD digits.

Age standardised ratios with 95% confidence limits contacts with doctor, contacts with practice nurse, all consultations with doctor, all ICD chapters I-XVII consultations, all preventive health care consultations, all referrals and patients referred, by sex, broad geographical region, urban or rural place of residence, housing tenure, marital status, cohabiting status, household composition, social class, occupation, economic position, ethnic group and smoking status.

Contacts with doctor by week, with age groups 0-4, 5-15, 16-24, 25-44, 45-64, 65-74, 75-84, 85 and over, by sex as rates per 10,000 person years at risk.

Tables comparable with 1981-82 Study (MSGP3)

Patients consulting with age groups 0-4, 5-14, 15-24, 25-44, 45-64, 65-75, 75 and over, by ICD chapter and category of severity (SIT), by sex, as rates per 10,000 person years at risk.

Patients consulting with age groups 0-4, 5-14, 15-24, 25-44, 45-64, 65-74, 75 and over, by college diagnostic code by sex, as rates per 10,000 person years at risk.

Age standardised patient consulting ratios with 95% confidence limits by tenure (all ages), marital status, economic position and social class (16 and over), household composition and social class of parent (0-15), and whether living alone (16-24, 65 and over).

Consultations with doctor with age groups 0-4, 5-14, 15-24, 25-44, 45-64, 65-74, 75 and over by ICD chapter and category of severity (SIT) by sex, as rates per 10,000 person years at risk.

For further information and an order form please contact

John Charlton
Health Statistics Division
OPCS
10 Kingsway
London WC2B 6JP

Telephone 071 396 2219

Appendix F Standard datasets of individual records available on disk

Seven standard datasets of individual records are available from MSGP4. These cover selected data aggregated to ICD chapter level, plus half a dozen or so individual disease groups. Each file takes up 11 to 15 MBytes of disk space when expanded onto a PC hard disc. Other datasets, tailored to the user's specific requirements, can be made available upon request. The contents of the standard datasets are summarised below.

SDIR1   Children aged 0-15

Urban/rural indicator, days in study, 5-year age group, sex, tenure, lives with sole adult, ethnic group, social class (as defined by occupation) of guardian, economic position of guardian last week, economic position of guardian last year,
number of consultations for:
    any reason, serious illness, intermediate illness, minor reasons, ICD chapters, ICD E codes, ICD V codes, preventive health care, total with GP, total with practice nurse,
number of referrals for:
    ICD chapters, ICD V codes
number of home visits:
    by doctor, by practice nurse
number of consultations for specified diagnoses:
    ICD 140-208, 250, 300-316, 493, 530-537,
distance between patient's home and practice (km)

SDIR2   Males aged 16-39

Urban/rural indicator, days in study, 5-year age group, sex, tenure, marital status, cohabiting status, lives with other adult, dependent children in household, ethnic group, smoked last week, social class (as defined by occupation), economic position last week, economic position last year,
number of consultations for:
    any reason, serious illness, intermediate illness, minor reasons, ICD chapters, ICD E codes, ICD V codes, preventive health care, total with GP, total with practice nurse,
number of referrals for:
    ICD chapters, ICD V codes
number of home visits:
    by doctor, by practice nurse
number of consultations for specified diagnoses:
    ICD 140-208, 250, 300-316, 401-405, 410-414, 430-438, 493, 530-537,
distance between patient's home and practice (km)

SDIR3   Females aged 16-39

as for SDIR2

SDIR4   Males aged 40-64

as for SDIR2

SDIR5   Females aged 40-64

as for SDIR2

SDIR6   Persons aged 65 and over

Urban/rural indicator, days in study, 5-year age group, sex, tenure, marital status, cohabiting status, lives with other adult, dependent children in household, ethnic group, smoked last week, social class (as defined by occupation), economic position last week, economic position last year,
number of consultations for:
    any reason, serious illness, intermediate illness, minor reasons, ICD chapters, ICD E codes, ICD V codes, preventive health care, total with GP, total with practice nurse,
number of referrals for:
    ICD chapters, ICD V codes
number of home visits:
    by doctor, by practice nurse
number of consultations for specified diagnoses:
    ICD 140-208, 250, 300-316, 401-405, 410-414, 430-438, 493, 530-537,
distance between patient's home and practice (km)

SDIR7   Married/cohabiting women

Urban/rural indicator, days in study, 5-year age group, sex, tenure, marital status, cohabiting status, lives with other adult, dependent children in household, ethnic group, smoked last week, social class (own), social class of partner, economic position last week (own), economic position last year (own), economic position last week (partner), economic position last year (partner),
number of consultations for:
    any reason, serious illness, intermediate illness, minor reasons, ICD chapters, ICD E codes, ICD V codes, preventive health care, total with GP, total with practice nurse,
number of referrals for:
    ICD chapters, ICD V codes
number of home visits:
    by doctor, by practice nurse
number of consultations for specified diagnoses:
    ICD 140-208, 250, 300-316, 401-405, 410-414, 430-438, 493, 530-537,
distance between patient's home and practice (km)

For further information and an order form please contact
    John Charlton
    Health Statistics Division
    OPCS
    10 Kingsway
    London WC2B 6JP

    Telephone 071 396 2219

References

1. GRO. *Morbidity statistics from general practice, 1955-56 (vols I-III)*. Studies on Medical and Population Subjects No 14, HMSO (London 1958).

2. RCGP, OPCS and DHSS. *Morbidity statistics from general practice: second national study, 1970-71*. Studies on Medical and Population Subjects No 26, HMSO (London 1974).

3. RCGP, OPCS and DHSS. *Morbidity statistics from general practice, 1971-72: second national study*. Studies on Medical and Population Subjects No 36, HMSO (London 1979).

4. RCGP, OPCS and DHSS. *Morbidity statistics from general practice, 1970-71: socio-economic analysis*. Studies on Medical and Population Subjects no 46, HMSO (London 1982).

5. RCGP, OPCS and DHSS. *Morbidity statistics from general practice: third national study, 1981-82*. Series MB5 No 1, HMSO (London 1986).

6. RCGP, OPCS and DH. *Morbidity statistics from general practice. Third morbidity study: socio-economic analysis 1981-82*. Series MB5 No 2, HMSO (London 1990).

7. OPCS. *General Household Survey, 1992*. Series GHS No 23, HMSO (London 1994).

8. Chisholm J. The Read clinical classification. *Br Med J* 1990;300:1092.

9. OPCS. *Standard Occupational Classification (Vols 1 and 2)*. HMSO (London 1990).

10. OPCS. *Health Survey for England, 1992*. HMSO (London 1994).

11. Crombie DL, Cross KW, Fleming DM. The problem of diagnostic variability in general practice. *J Epidemiol Community Health* 1992;46:447-54.

12. OPCS. *Cancer statistics - registrations 1988*. Series MB1 No 21, HMSO (London 1994).

13. Hofman A, Rocca WA, Brayne C et al. The prevalence of dementia in Europe: a collaborative study of 1980-1990 findings. *Int J Epidemiol* 1991;20:736-48.

14. Francis B, Green M, Payne C (eds). *GLIM 4. The statistical system for generalised linear interactive modelling*. Clarendon Press (Oxford 1993).

15. Connor MJ, Gillings D. An empiric study of ecological inference. *Am J Public Health* 1984;74:555-9.

16. Haskey J. The ethnic minority populations resident in private households — estimates by county and metropolitan district of England and Wales. *Population Trends* 1991;63:22-35.

17. National Center for Health Statistics. *Synthetic state estimates of disability*. PHS Publication No 1759. 1968 Washington DC.

18. Skinner C. *The use of synthetic estimation techniques to produce small area estimates*. New methodology series No NM18, OPCS (1993).

19. Marsh C, Teague A. Samples of anonymised records from the 1991 census. *Population Trends* 1992,69:17-26.